RED BOOK®
ATLAS
OF PEDIATRIC INFECTIOUS DISEASES

2ND EDITION

Editor

Carol J. Baker, MD, FAAP

American Academy of Pediatrics

141 Northwest Point Blvd

Elk Grove Village, IL 60007-1019

American Academy of Pediatrics Department of Marketing and Publications Staff

Maureen DeRosa, MPA, Director, Department of Marketing and Publications
Mark Grimes, Director, Division of Product Development
Martha Cook, MS, Sr Product Development Editor
Carrie Peters, Editorial Assistant
Sandi King, MS, Director, Division of Publishing and Production Services
Theresa Wiener, Manager, Publications Production and Manufacturing
Kate Larson, Manager, Editorial Services
Peg Mulcahy, Manager Graphic Design and Production
Linda Smessaert, Manger, Clinical and Professional Publications Marketing

Library of Congress Control Number LOC 2012941376
ISBN: 978-1-58110-753-1
eISBN: 978-1-58110-795-1
MA0651

The recommendations in this publication do not indicate an exclusive course of treatment or serve as a standard of medical care. Variations, taking into account individual circumstances, may be appropriate.

The publishers have made every effort to trace the copyright holders for borrowed material. If they have inadvertently overlooked any, they will be pleased to make the necessary arrangements at first opportunity.

1 2 3 4 5 6 7 8 9 10

Table of Contents

Introduction

The American Academy of Pediatrics (AAP) *Red Book® Atlas of Pediatric Infectious Diseases,* 2nd Edition, is a summary of key disease information from the AAP *Red Book®: 2012 Report of the Committee on Infectious Diseases.* It is intended to be a study guide for students, residents, and practitioners.

Visual representations of common and atypical clinical manifestations of infectious diseases provide diagnostic information not found in the print version of the *Red Book.* The juxtaposition of these visuals with a summary of the clinical features, epidemiology, diagnostic methods, and treatment information serves as a training tool and quick reference. The *Red Book Atlas* is not intended to provide detailed treatment and management information but rather a big-picture approach that can be refined by consulting reference texts or infectious disease specialists. Complete disease and treatment information from the AAP can be found on *Red Book® Online* (www.aapredbook.org), the electronic version of the *Red Book.*

This *Red Book Atlas* could not have been completed without the superb assistance of Martha Cook at the AAP and of those physicians who photographed disease manifestations in their patients and shared these with the AAP. Some diseases rarely are seen today because of improved preventive strategies, especially immunization programs. While photographs can't replace hands-on experience, they have helped me to consider the likelihood of a correct diagnosis, and I hope this will be so for the reader. I also want to thank those individuals at the Centers for Disease Control and Prevention who generously have provided many photographs of the etiologic agents, vectors, and life cycles of parasites and protozoa relevant to these largely domestic infections.

The study of pediatric infectious diseases has been a challenging and changing professional life that has brought me great joy. To gather information with my ears and eyes (the history and physical examination), place this into the context of relevant epidemiology and incubation, and then select appropriate diagnostic studies is still exciting. Putting these many pieces together to arrive at the correct diagnosis is akin to solving a crime. On many occasions, just seeing *the* clue (eg, a characteristic rash, an asymmetry, a swelling) will solve the medical puzzle, lead to recovery with the proper management, and bring satisfaction almost nothing can replace. It is my hope that the readers of the second edition of the *Red Book Atlas* might find a similar enthusiasm for the field.

Carol J. Baker, MD, FAAP
Editor

1

Actinomycosis

Clinical Manifestations

Actinomycosis results from pathogen introduction following a breakdown in mucocutaneous protective barriers. Spread within the host is by direct invasion of adjacent tissues, typically forming sinus tracts that cross tissue planes.

There are 3 common anatomic sites of infection. **Cervicofacial** is most common, often occurring after tooth extraction, oral surgery, other oral/facial trauma, or even from carious teeth. Localized pain and induration can progress to cervical abscess and "woody hard" nodular lesions ("lumpy jaw"), which can develop draining sinus tracts, usually at the angle of the jaw or in the submandibular region. Infection also may contribute to chronic tonsillar airway obstruction. **Thoracic** disease can be an extension of cervicofacial infection but most commonly it is secondary to aspiration of oropharyngeal secretions. It rarely occurs after esophageal disruption during or nonpenetrating trauma. Presentations include pneumonia, which can be complicated by lung abscesses, empyema and, rarely, pleurodermal sinuses. Focal or multifocal mediastinal and pulmonary masses may be mistaken for tumors. **Abdominal** actinomycosis usually is attributable to penetrating trauma or intestinal perforation. The appendix and cecum are the most common sites; symptoms are similar to appendicitis. Slowly developing masses can simulate abdominal or retroperitoneal neoplasms. Intraabdominal abscesses and peritoneal-dermal draining sinuses occur with chronic infection often forming draining sinus tracts with purulent discharge. **Other sites** of infection include liver, pelvis (which, in some cases, has been linked to use of intrauterine devices), heart, testicles, and brain (typically associated with a primary pulmonary focus). Noninvasive primary cutaneous actinomycosis has occurred.

Etiology

Actinomyces israelii is the most common species causing human disease but at least 5 other *Actinomyces* species are human pathogens. All are slow-growing, microaerophilic or facultative anaerobic, gram-positive, filamentous branching bacilli. *Actinomyces* species frequently are copathogens in tissues harboring multiple other anaerobic and/or aerobic species. *Actinobacillus actinomycetemcomitans* is a frequent copathogen, and its isolation may predict the presence of actinomycosis.

Epidemiology

Actinomyces species occur worldwide, being components of endogenous oral gastrointestinal tract and vaginal flora. *Actinomyces* species are opportunistic pathogens (reported in patients with HIV and chronic granulomatous disease), with disease usually following penetrating and nonpenetrating trauma. Infection is uncommon in infants and children, with 80% of cases occurring in adults. The male-to-female ratio in children is 1.5:1. Overt, microbiologically confirmed, monomicrobial disease caused by *Actinomyces* species is rare.

Incubation Period

Varies from several days to several years.

Diagnostic Tests

Microscopic demonstration of beaded, branched, non-acid fast, gram-positive bacilli in purulent material or tissue specimens suggests the diagnosis. Yellow "sulfur granules" visualized microscopically or macroscopically in drainage or loculations of purulent material also suggest the diagnosis. A Gram stain of "sulfur granules" discloses a dense aggregate of bacterial filaments mixed with inflammatory debris. Immunofluorescent stains for *Actinomyces* species and 16s rRNA sequencing and polymerase chain reaction assay are available for tissue specimens. Only normally sterile site specimens should be submitted for culture, and specimens must be obtained, transported, and cultured anaerobically on special media for greatest diagnostic sensitivity.

Treatment

Initial therapy should include intravenous penicillin G or ampicillin for 4 to 6 weeks, followed by high doses of oral penicillin typically for a total of 4 to 12 months. Amoxicillin, erythromycin, clindamycin, doxycycline, and tetracycline are alternative antimicrobial choices. Surgical drainage or debridement often is a necessary adjunct to medical management and may allow for a shorter duration of antimicrobial treatment.

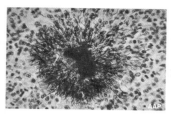

Image 1.1
Tissue showing filamentous branching rods of *Actinomyces israelii* (Brown and Brenn stain). *Actinomyces* have fastidious growth requirements. Staining of a crushed sulfur granule reveals branching bacilli.

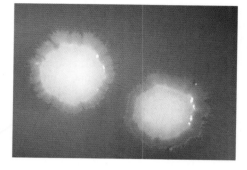

Image 1.2
A brain heart infusion agar plate culture of *Actinomyces* sp, magnification x573, at 10 days of incubation. Courtesy of Centers for Disease Control and Prevention/Dr George.

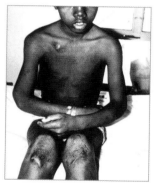

Image 1.3
A 10-year-old boy with chronic pulmonary, abdominal, and lower extremity abscesses with chronic draining sinus tracts from which *Actinomyces israelii* was isolated. Prolonged antimicrobial treatment and surgical drainage were required for resolution of this infectious process.

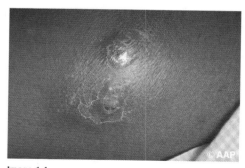

Image 1.4
Actinomycotic abscesses of the thigh of the child in Image 1.3. *Actinomyces* infections are often polymicrobial. *Actinobacillus actinomycetemcomitans,* one of the HACEK group of organisms, may accompany *Actinomyces israelii* and may cause endocarditis.

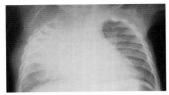

Image 1.5
An 8-month-old infant with pulmonary actinomycosis, an uncommon infection in infancy that may follow aspiration. As in this infant, most cases of actinomycosis are caused by *Actinomyces israelii*.

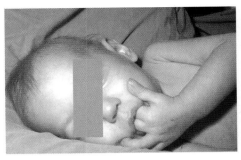

Image 1.6
Clubbing of the thumb and fingers of the 8-month-old boy in Image 1.5 with chronic pulmonary actinomycosis. Blood cultures were repeatedly negative without clinical signs of endocarditis. Courtesy of Edgar O. Ledbetter, MD, FAAP.

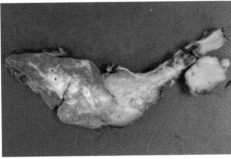

Image 1.7
The resected right lower lobe, diaphragm, and portion of the liver in a 3-year-old previously healthy girl with an unknown source for her pulmonary actinomycosis. Courtesy of Carol J. Baker, MD.

2

Adenovirus Infections

Clinical Manifestations

Adenovirus infections of the upper respiratory tract are common and, although often subclinical, can result in symptoms of the common cold, pharyngitis, tonsillitis, otitis media, and pharyngoconjunctival fever. Life-threatening disseminated infection, severe pneumonia, hepatitis, meningitis, and encephalitis occur occasionally, especially among young infants and immunocompromised hosts. Adenoviruses occasionally cause a pertussis-like syndrome, croup, bronchiolitis, exudative tonsillitis, hemorrhagic cystitis, and gastroenteritis. Ocular adenovirus infections can present as a follicular conjunctivitis or as epidemic keratoconjunctivitis. In epidemic keratoconjunctivitis, there is an autoimmune infiltration of the cornea in addition to the follicular conjunctivitis. In both cases, ophthalmologic illness frequently presents acutely in one eye followed by involvement of the other eye. In epidemic keratoconjunctivitis, corneal inflammation produces symptoms including light sensitivity and vision loss.

Etiology

Adenoviruses are double-stranded, nonenveloped DNA viruses; at least 51 distinct serotypes divided into 6 species (A through F) cause human infections. Some adenovirus types are associated primarily with respiratory tract disease, and others are associated primarily with gastroenteritis (types 40 and 41). Adenovirus type 14 is emerging as a type that can cause severe and sometimes fatal respiratory tract illness in patients of all ages, including healthy young adults, such as military recruits.

Epidemiology

Infection in infants and children can occur at any age. Adenoviruses causing respiratory tract infections usually are transmitted by respiratory tract secretions through person-to-person contact, airborne droplets, and fomites, the latter because adenoviruses are stable in the environment. The conjunctiva can provide a portal of entry. Community outbreaks of adenovirus-associated pharyngoconjunctival fever have been attributed to water exposure from contaminated swimming pools and fomites, such as shared towels. Health care–associated transmission of adenoviral respiratory tract, conjunctival, and gastrointestinal tract infections can occur in hospitals, residential institutions, and nursing homes from exposures between infected health care personnel, patients, or contaminated equipment. Adenovirus infections in transplant recipients can occur from donor tissues. Epidemic keratoconjunctivitis commonly occurs by direct contact, has been associated with equipment used during eye examinations, and is caused principally by types 8 and 19. Enteric strains of adenoviruses are transmitted by the fecal-oral route. Adenoviruses causing respiratory and enteric infections circulate throughout the year. Enteric disease primarily affects children younger than 4 years. Adenovirus infections are most communicable during the first few days of an acute illness, but persistent and intermittent shedding for longer periods, even months, is common. Asymptomatic infections are common. Reinfection can occur.

Incubation Period

Respiratory tract infection, 2 to 14 days; gastroenteritis, 3 to 10 days.

Diagnostic Tests

The preferred methods for diagnosis of adenovirus infection include cell culture, antigen detection, and DNA detection. Adenoviruses associated with respiratory tract disease can be isolated from pharyngeal and eye secretions and feces by inoculation of specimens into susceptible cell cultures. A pharyngeal or ocular isolate suggests recent infection, but a fecal isolate indicates either recent infection or prolonged carriage. Rapid detection of adenovirus antigens is possible in a variety of body fluids by commercial immunoassay techniques. These rapid assays can be useful for diagnosis of respiratory tract infections, ocular disease, and diarrheal disease. Enteric adenovirus types 40 and 41 usually cannot be isolated in standard cell cultures. Adenoviruses also can be identified by electron microscopic examination of respiratory tract or stool specimens, but this modality lacks sensitivity. Polymerase chain reaction assays for adenovirus DNA rapidly are replacing other detection methods because of improved sensitivity and increasing commercial availability. Adenovirus typing is available from some reference and research laboratories.

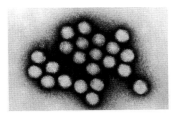

Image 2.1
Transmission electron micrograph of adenovirus. Adenoviruses have a characteristic icosahedral structure. Courtesy of Centers for Disease Control and Prevention/Dr William Gary, Jr.

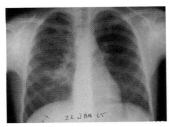

Image 2.3
Adenoviral pneumonia in an 8-year-old girl with diffuse pulmonary infiltrate bilaterally. Most adenoviral infections in the normal host are self-limited and require no specific treatment. Lobar consolidation is unusual.

Treatment

Treatment of adenovirus infection is supportive. Randomized clinical trials evaluating specific antiviral therapy have not been performed. However, the successful use of intravenous cidofovir has been reported in immunocompromised patients with severe adenoviral disease.

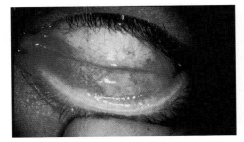

Image 2.2
Acute follicular adenovirus conjunctivitis. Adenoviruses are resistant to alcohol, detergents, and chlorhexidine and may contaminate ophthalmologic solutions and equipment. Instruments can be disinfected by steam autoclaving or immersion in 1% sodium hypochlorite for 10 minutes.

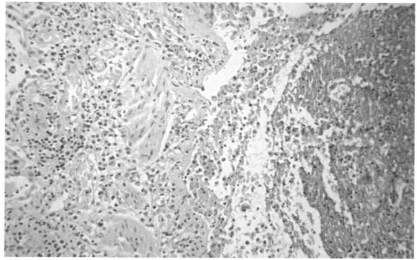

Image 2.4
Histopathology of the lung with bronchiolar occlusion in an immunocompromised child who died with adenoviral pneumonia. Note interstitial mononuclear cell infiltration and hyaline membranes. Adenoviruses types 3 and 7 can cause necrotizing bronchitis and bronchiolitis. Courtesy of Edgar O. Ledbetter, MD, FAAP.

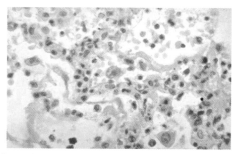

Image 2.5
Pulmonary histopathology of the immuno-compromised child in Image 2.4 showing multiple adenovirus intranuclear inclusion cells. Courtesy of Edgar O. Ledbetter, MD, FAAP.

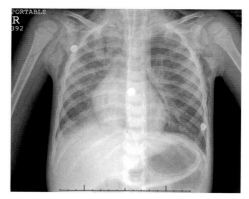

Image 2.6
A previously healthy 3-year-old boy who presented with respiratory failure requiring intensive care for adenovirus type 7 pneumonia. He eventually recovered with mild impairment in pulmonary function studies. Note the pneuo-mediastinum. Courtesy of Carol J. Baker, MD.

3

Amebiasis

Clinical Manifestations

Clinical syndromes associated with *Entamoeba histolytica* infection include noninvasive intestinal tract infection, intestinal amebiasis (amebic colitis), ameboma, and liver abscess. Disease is more severe in young children, the elderly, malnourished people, and pregnant women. Patients with noninvasive intestinal tract infection can be asymptomatic or can have nonspecific intestinal tract complaints. Patients with intestinal amebiasis generally have a gradual onset of symptoms over 1 to 3 weeks. The mildest form of intestinal tract disease is nondysenteric colitis. However, amebic dysentery is the most common manifestation of amebiasis and generally includes diarrhea with either gross or microscopic blood in the stool, lower abdominal pain, and tenesmus. Weight loss is common, but fever occurs in only about 8% to 38% of patients. Symptoms can be chronic and mimic those of inflammatory bowel disease. Progressive involvement of the colon can produce toxic megacolon, fulminant colitis, ulceration of the colon and perianal area and, rarely, perforation. Colonic progression can occur at multiple sites and carries a high fatality rate. Progression can occur in patients inappropriately treated with corticosteroids or antimotility drugs. An ameboma may occur as an annular lesion of the colon and may present as a palpable mass on physical examination. Amebomas can occur in any area of the colon but are more common in the cecum. Amebomas may be mistaken for colonic carcinoma. Amebomas usually resolve with antiamebic therapy and do not require surgery.

In a small proportion of patients, extraintestinal disease can occur. The liver is the most common extraintestinal site, and infection can spread from there to the pleural space, lungs, and pericardium. Liver abscess can be acute, with fever, abdominal pain, tachypnea, liver tenderness, and hepatomegaly, or may be chronic, with weight loss, vague abdominal symptoms, and irritability. Rupture of a liver abscess into the abdomen or chest may lead to death. Evidence of recent intestinal tract infection usually is absent. Infection also can spread from the colon to the genitourinary tract and the skin. The organism rarely spreads hematogenously to the brain and other areas of the body.

Etiology

The genus *Entamoeba* includes 6 species that live in the human intestine. Three of these species are identical morphologically: *E histolytica, Entamoeba dispar,* and *Entamoeba moshkovskii.* The pathogenic *E histolytica* and the nonpathogenic *E dispar* and *E moshkovskii* are excreted as cysts or trophozoites in stools of infected people.

Epidemiology

E histolytica can be found worldwide but is more prevalent in people of lower socioeconomic status who live in resource-limited countries, where the prevalence of amebic infection may be as high as 50% in some communities. Groups at increased risk of infection in industrialized countries include immigrants from or long-term visitors to areas with endemic infection, institutionalized people, and men who have sex with men. *E histolytica* is transmitted via amebic cysts by the fecal-oral route. Ingested cysts, which are unaffected by gastric acid, undergo excystation in the alkaline small intestine and produce trophozoites that infect the colon. Cysts that develop subsequently are the source of transmission, especially from asymptomatic cyst excreters. Infected patients excrete cysts intermittently, sometimes for years if untreated. Transmission has been associated with contaminated food or water. Fecal-oral transmission also can occur in the setting of anal sexual practices or direct rectal inoculation through colonic irrigation devices.

Incubation Period

Variable, ranging from a few days to months or years but commonly 2 to 4 weeks.

Diagnostic Tests

A presumptive diagnosis of intestinal tract infection depends on identifying trophozoites or cysts in stool specimens. Examination of serial specimens may be necessary. Specimens of stool can be examined microscopically by wet mount within 30 minutes of collection or may be fixed in formalin or polyvinyl alcohol (available in kits) for concentration, permanent staining, and subsequent microscopic examination. Biopsy specimens and endoscopy scrapings (not swabs) can be examined using similar methods. Polymerase chain reaction, isoenzyme analysis, and monoclonal antibody-based antigen detection assays can differentiate *E histolytica* from *E dispar* and *E moshkovskii*.

Commercially available enzyme immunoassay (EIA) kits for serum can diagnose amebiasis. The EIA detects antibody specific for *E histolytica* in approximately 95% of patients with extraintestinal amebiasis, 70% of patients with active intestinal tract infection, and 10% of asymptomatic people who are passing cysts of *E histolytica*. Positive serologic tests persist even after adequate therapy.

Ultrasonography, computed tomography, and magnetic resonance imaging can identify liver abscesses and other extraintestinal sites of infection. Aspirates from a liver abscess usually show neither trophozoites nor leukocytes.

Treatment

Treatment involves elimination of the tissue-invading trophozoites as well as organisms in the intestinal lumen. *E dispar* and *E mosh-*

kovskii infections are considered to be nonpathogenic and do not require treatment. Corticosteroids and antimotility drugs administered to people with amebiasis can worsen symptoms and the disease process. The following regimens are recommended:

- Asymptomatic cyst excreters (intraluminal infections): treat with a luminal amebicide, such as iodoquinol, paromomycin, or diloxanide. Metronidazole is not effective.

- Patients with intestinal tract symptoms or extraintestinal disease (including liver abscess): treat with metronidazole or tinidazole, followed by a therapeutic course of a luminal amebicide (iodoquinol or paromomycin). An alternate treatment for liver abscess is chloroquine administered concomitantly with metronidazole or tinidazole, followed by a therapeutic course of a luminal amebicide.

Percutaneous or surgical aspiration of large liver abscesses occasionally can be required when response to medical therapy is unsatisfactory. In most cases of liver abscess, though, drainage is not required.

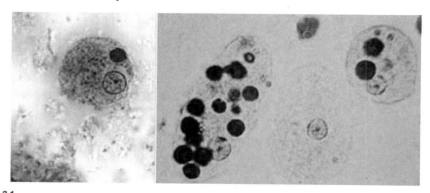

Image 3.1
Trophozoites of *Entamoeba histolytica* with ingested erythrocytes. Trichrome stain. The ingested erythrocytes appear as dark inclusions. Erythrophagocytosis is the only characteristic that can be used to differentiate morphologically *E histolytica* from the nonpathogenic *E dispar*. In these specimens, the parasite nuclei have the typical small, centrally located karyosome and thin, uniform peripheral chromatin. Courtesy of Centers for Disease Control and Prevention.

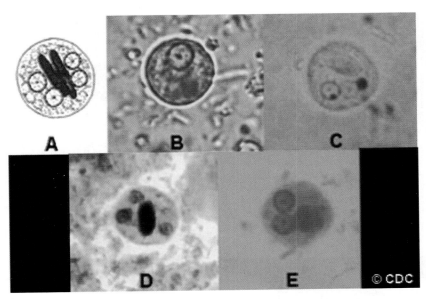

Image 3.2
Cysts of *Entamoeba histolytica* and *Entamoeba dispar.* Line drawing (A), wet mounts (B; iodine C), and permanent preparations stained with trichrome (D, E). The cysts are usually spherical and often have a halo (B, C). Mature cysts have 4 nuclei. The cyst in B appears uninucleate, while in C, D, and E, 2 to 3 nuclei are visible in the focal plane (the fourth nucleus is coming into focus in D). The nuclei have characteristically centrally located karyosomes and fine, uniformly distributed peripheral chromatin. The cysts in C, D, and E contain chromatoid bodies, with the one in D being particularly well demonstrated, with typically blunted ends. *E histolytica* cysts usually measure 12 to 15 μm. Courtesy of Centers for Disease Control and Prevention.

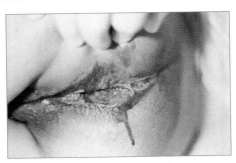

Image 3.3
This amebiasis patient presented with tissue destruction and granulation of the anoperineal region due to an *Entamoeba histolytica* infection. Courtesy of Centers for Disease Control and Prevention.

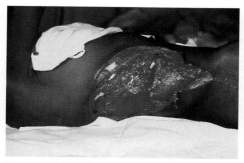

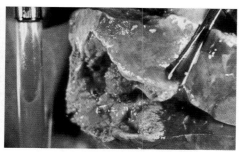

Image 3.4

This patient presented with a case of invasive extraintestinal amebiasis affecting the cutaneous region of the right flank. Courtesy of Centers for Disease Control and Prevention/Kerrison Juniper, MD, and George Healy, PhD, DPDx.

Image 3.5

Gross pathology of amebic (*Entamoeba histolytica*) abscess of liver. Tube of "chocolate-like" pus from abscess. Amebic liver abscesses are usually singular, large, and in the right lobe of the liver. Bacterial hepatic abscesses are more likely to be multiple. Courtesy of Centers for Disease Control and Prevention/Dr Mae Melvin; Dr E. West.

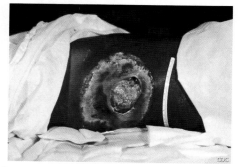

Image 3.6

This patient presented with a case of invasive extraintestinal amebiasis affecting the cutaneous region of the right flank causing severe tissue necrosis. Here we see the site of tissue destruction, pre-debridement. Courtesy of Centers for Disease Control and Prevention/ Kerrison Juniper, MD, and George Healy, PhD, DPDx.

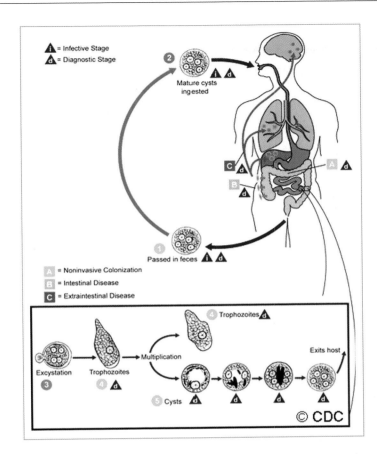

Image 3.7

Cysts are passed in feces (1). Infection by *Entamoeba histolytica* occurs by ingestion of mature cysts (2) in fecally contaminated food, water, or hands. Excystation (3) occurs in the small intestine and trophozoites (4) are released, which migrate to the large intestine. The trophozoites multiply by binary fission and produce cysts (5), which are passed in the feces (1). Because of the protection conferred by their walls, the cysts can survive days to weeks in the external environment and are responsible for transmission. (Trophozoites can also be passed in diarrheal stools, but are rapidly destroyed once outside the body, and if ingested would not survive exposure to the gastric environment.) In many cases, the trophozoites remain confined to the intestinal lumen (A: noninvasive infection) of individuals who are asymptomatic carriers, passing cysts in their stool. In some patients the trophozoites invade the intestinal mucosa (B: intestinal disease) or, through the bloodstream, extraintestinal sites such as the liver, brain, and lungs (C: extraintestinal disease), with resultant pathologic manifestations. The invasive and noninvasive forms represent 2 separate species, respectively *E histolytica* and *E dispar*; however, not all persons infected with *E histolytica* will have invasive disease. These 2 species are morphologically indistinguishable. Transmission can also occur through fecal exposure during sexual contact (in which case not only cysts, but also trophozoites, could prove infective). Courtesy of Centers for Disease Control and Prevention.

4

Amebic Meningoence- phalitis and Keratitis

(*Naegleria fowleri, Acanthamoeba* species, and *Balamuthia mandrillaris*)

Clinical Manifestations

Naegleria fowleri causes a rapidly progressive, almost always fatal, primary amebic meningo- encephalitis. Early symptoms include fever, headache, vomiting, and sometimes distur- bances of smell and taste, then progresses rap- idly to signs of meningoencephalitis including nuchal rigidity, lethargy, confusion, personal- ity changes, and altered level of consciousness. Seizures are common, and death generally occurs within a week of onset of symptoms. No distinct clinical features differentiate this disease from fulminant bacterial meningitis or other causes of meningoencephalitis.

Granulomatous amebic encephalitis (GAE) caused by *Acanthamoeba* species and *Balamu- thia mandrillaris* has a more insidious onset and progression of manifestations occurring weeks to months after exposure. Signs and symptoms include personality changes, sei- zures, headaches, nuchal rigidity, ataxia, cra- nial nerve palsies, hemiparesis, and other focal deficits. Fever often is low grade and intermit- tent. Chronic granulomatous skin lesions (pus- tules, nodules, ulcers) may be present without central nervous system (CNS) involvement, particularly in patients with acquired immu- nodeficiency syndrome, and lesions on the midface may present for months before CNS involvement in immunocompetent hosts.

The most common symptoms of amebic kera- titis, usually attributable to *Acanthamoeba* species, are pain (often out of proportion to clinical signs), photophobia, tearing, and foreign body sensation. Characteristic signs include radial keratoneuritis and stromal ring infiltrate. *Acanthamoeba* keratitis generally follows an indolent course and initially can resemble herpes simplex or bacterial keratitis; delay in diagnosis is associated with poor outcome.

Etiology

Naegleria fowleri, Acanthamoeba species, and *Balamuthia mandrillaris* are free-living ame- bae that exist as motile, infectious trophozoites and environmentally hardy cysts.

Epidemiology

N fowleri is found in warm freshwater and moist soil. Most infections have been associ- ated with swimming in warm freshwater, such as ponds, lakes, and hot springs, but other sources have included tap water from geother- mal sources and contaminated and poorly chlorinated swimming pools. Disease has been reported worldwide but is uncommon. In the United States, infection occurs primarily in the summer and usually affects children and young adults. The trophozoites of the parasite invade the brain directly from the nose along the olfactory nerves via the cribriform plate. In infections with *N fowleri,* trophozoites but not cysts can be visualized in sections of brain or in cerebrospinal fluid (CSF).

Acanthamoeba species are distributed world- wide and are found in soil; dust; cooling towers of electric and nuclear power plants; heating, ventilating, and air-conditioning units; fresh and brackish water; whirlpool baths; and physiotherapy pools. The environmental niche of *B mandrillaris* is not delineated clearly, although it has been isolated from soil. CNS infection attributable to *Acanthamoeba* occurs primarily in debilitated and immunocompro- mised people. However, some patients infected with *B mandrillaris* have had no demonstrable underlying disease or disability. CNS infection by both amebae probably occurs by inhalation or direct contact with contaminated soil or water. The primary foci of these infections most likely are skin or respiratory tract, fol- lowed by hematogenous spread to the brain. *Acanthamoeba* keratitis occurs primarily in people who wear contact lenses, although it also has been associated with corneal trauma. Poor contact lens hygiene or disinfection prac- tices as well as swimming with contact lenses are risk factors.

Incubation Period

Incubation period for *N fowleri* is typically 3 to 7 days. *Acanthamoeba* and *Balamuthia* GAE incubation periods are unknown but are thought to range from several weeks to months for CNS disease and within a few weeks for *Acanthamoeba* keratitis.

Diagnostic Tests

In *N fowleri* infection, computed tomography scans of the head without contrast are unremarkable or show only cerebral edema; contrast meningeal enhancement of the basilar cisterns and sulci may be found. However, these changes are nonspecific. CSF pressure usually is elevated (300 to >600 mm H_2O), and CSF can have polymorphonuclear pleocytosis, increased protein concentration, and a normal to very low glucose concentration. *N fowleri* infection can be documented by microscopic demonstration of the motile trophozoites on a wet mount of centrifuged CSF. Smears of CSF should be stained with Giemsa, trichrome, or Wright stains to identify the trophozoites, if present; Gram stain is not useful.

In infection with *Acanthamoeba* species and *B mandrillaris*, trophozoites and cysts can be visualized in sections of brain, lungs, and skin; in cases of *Acanthamoeba* keratitis, they also can be visualized in corneal scrapings and by confocal microscopy in vivo in the cornea. In GAE infections, CSF indices typically reveal a lymphocytic pleocytosis and an increased protein concentration, with normal or low glucose concentrations. Computed tomography and magnetic resonance imaging scans of the head reveal single or multiple space-occupying, ring-enhancing lesions that can mimic brain abscesses, tumors, cerebrovascular accidents, or other diseases. *N fowleri* and *Acanthamoeba* species, but not *Balamuthia* species, can be cultured on special media; *B mandrillaris* can be grown using mammalian cell culture. Like *N fowleri*, immunofluorescence and PCR assays can be performed on clinical specimens to identify *Acanthamoeba* species and *Balamuthia* species; these tests are available through the Centers for Disease Control and Prevention.

Treatment

Although an effective treatment regimen for primary amebic meningoencephalitis due to *N fowleri* has not been identified, amphotericin B is the drug of choice. However, treatment usually is unsuccessful, with only a few cases of complete recovery documented. Two survivors recovered after treatment with amphotericin B in combination with an azole drug. Early diagnosis and institution of high-dose drug therapy is thought to be important for optimizing outcome. Effective treatment for infections caused by *Acanthamoeba* species and *B mandrillaris* has not been established. Several patients with *Acanthamoeba* GAE and *Acanthamoeba* cutaneous infections without CNS involvement have been treated successfully with a multidrug regimen consisting of various combinations of pentamidine, sulfadiazine, flucytosine, either fluconazole or itraconazole, trimethoprim-sulfamethoxazole, and topical application of chlorhexidine gluconate and ketoconazole for skin lesions. Patients with keratitis should be evaluated by an ophthalmologist. Early diagnosis and therapy are important for a good outcome.

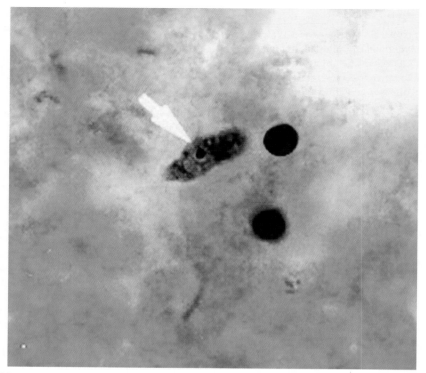

Image 4.1
Naegleria fowleri trophozoite in spinal fluid. Trichrome stain. Note the typically large karyosome and the monopodial locomotion. Courtesy of Centers for Disease Control and Prevention.

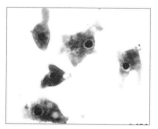

Image 4.2
Naegleria fowleri trophozoites cultured from cerebrospinal fluid. These cells have characteristically large nuclei, with a large, dark-staining karyosome. The amebae are very active and extend and retract pseudopods (trichrome stain). From a patient who died of primary amebic meningoencephalitis in Virginia. Courtesy of Centers for Disease Control and Prevention.

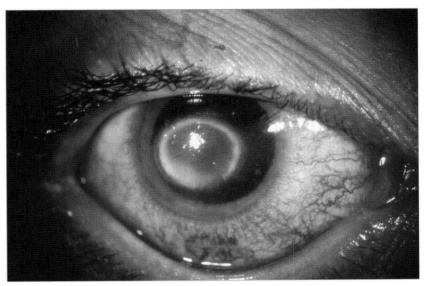

Image 4.3
Acanthamoeba keratitis. Courtesy of Susan Lehman, MD, FAAP.

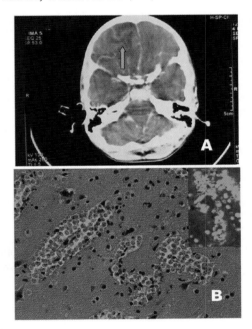

Image 4.4
(A) Computed tomographic scan: note the right fronto-basal collection (arrow) with a midline shift right to left. (B) Brain histology: 3 large clusters of amebic vegetative forms are seen (hematoxylin-eosin stain, x250). Inset: positive indirect immunofluorescent analysis on tissue section with anti-*Naegleria fowleri* serum. Courtesy of Cogo PE, Scagli M, Giatti S, et al. Fatal *Naegleria fowleri* meningoencephalitis, Italy. *Emerg Infect Dis.* 2004;10(10):1835–1837.

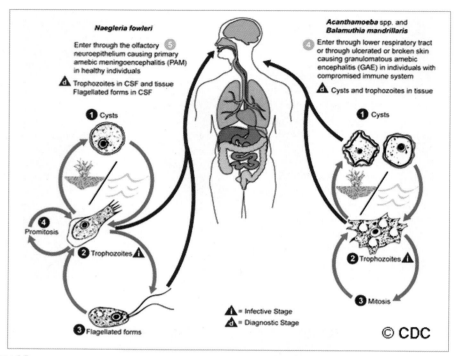

Image 4.5

Free-living amebae belonging to the genera *Acanthamoeba, Balamuthia,* and *Naegleria* are important causes of disease in humans and animals. *Fowleri* produces an acute, and usually lethal, central nervous system disease called primary amebic meningoencephalitis. *N fowleri* has 3 stages: cysts (1), trophozoites (2), and flagellated forms (3), in its life cycle. The trophozoites replicate by promitosis (nuclear membrane remains intact) (4). *N fowleri* is found in freshwater, soil, thermal discharges of power plants, heated swimming pools, hydrotherapy and medicinal pools, aquariums, and sewage. Trophozoites can turn into temporary flagellated forms, which usually revert back to the trophozoite stage. Trophozoites infect humans or animals by entering the olfactory neuroepithelium (5) and reaching the brain. *N fowleri* trophozoites are found in cerebrospinal fluid (CSF) and tissue, while flagellated forms are found in CSF. *Acanthamoeba* spp and *B mandrillaris* are opportunistic free-living amebae capable of causing granulomatous amebic encephalitis in individuals with compromised immune systems. *Acanthamoeba* spp have been found in soil; fresh, brackish, and sea water; sewage; swimming pools; contact lens equipment; medicinal pools; dental treatment units; dialysis machines; heating, ventilating, and air-conditioning systems; mammalian cell cultures; vegetables; human nostrils and throats; and human and animal brain, skin, and lung tissues. *B mandrillaris,* however, has not been isolated from the environment but has been isolated from autopsy specimens of infected humans and animals. Unlike *N fowleri, Acanthamoeba* and *Balamuthia* have only 2 stages: cysts (1) and trophozoites (2), in their life cycle. No flagellated stage exists as part of the life cycle. The trophozoites replicate by mitosis (nuclear membrane does not remain intact) (3). The trophozoites are the infective forms and are believed to gain entry into the body through the lower respiratory tract or ulcerated or broken skin and invade the central nervous system by hematogenous dissemination (4). *Acanthamoeba* spp and *B mandrillaris* cysts and trophozoites are found in tissue. Courtesy of Centers for Disease Control and Prevention.

5

Anthrax

Clinical Manifestations

Depending on the route of infection, anthrax can occur in 3 forms: cutaneous, inhalational, and gastrointestinal. **Cutaneous** anthrax begins as a pruritic papule or vesicle that enlarges and ulcerates in 1 to 2 days, with subsequent formation of a central black eschar. The lesion itself characteristically is painless, with surrounding edema, hyperemia, and painful regional lymphadenopathy. Patients may have associated fever, lymphangitis, and extensive edema. **Inhalational** anthrax is a frequently lethal form of the disease and is a medical emergency. A nonspecific prodrome of fever, sweats, nonproductive cough, chest pain, headache, myalgia, malaise, and nausea and vomiting may occur initially, but illness progresses to the fulminant phase 2 to 5 days later. In some cases, the illness is biphasic with a period of improvement between prodromal symptoms and overwhelming illness. Fulminant manifestations include hypotension, dyspnea, hypoxia, cyanosis, and shock occurring as a result of hemorrhagic mediastinal lymphadenitis, hemorrhagic pneumonia, and hemorrhagic pleural effusions, bacteremia, and toxemia. In addition, the liver and central nervous system (CNS) may be involved. A widened mediastinum is the classic finding on imaging of the chest. Chest radiography also may show pleural effusions and/or infiltrates, each of which may be hemorrhagic in nature. **Gastrointestinal tract** disease can present as 2 clinical syndromes—intestinal or oropharyngeal. Patients with the intestinal form have symptoms of nausea, anorexia, vomiting, and fever progressing to severe abdominal pain, massive ascites, hematemesis, bloody diarrhea, and submucosal intestinal hemorrhage. Oropharyngeal anthrax also may have dysphagia with posterior oropharyngeal necrotic ulcers, which may be associated with marked, often unilateral neck swelling, regional adenopathy, fever, and sepsis. Hemorrhagic meningitis can result from hematogenous spread of the organism after acquiring any form of disease and may develop without any other apparent clinical presentation. The case-fatality rate for patients with appropriately treated cutaneous anthrax usually is less than 1%, but for inhalation or gastrointestinal tract disease, mortality often exceeds 50% and approaches 100% for meningitis in the absence of antimicrobial therapy.

Etiology

Bacillus anthracis is an aerobic, gram-positive, encapsulated, spore-forming, nonhemolytic, nonmotile rod. *B anthracis* has 3 major virulence factors: an antiphagocytic capsule and 2 exotoxins, called lethal and edema toxins. The toxins are responsible for the significant morbidity and clinical manifestations of hemorrhage, edema, and necrosis.

Epidemiology

Anthrax is a zoonotic disease most commonly affecting domestic and wild herbivores that occurs in many rural regions of the world. *B anthracis* spores can remain viable in the soil for decades, representing a potential source of infection for livestock or wildlife through ingestion. In susceptible hosts, the spores germinate to become viable bacteria. Natural infection of humans occurs through contact with infected animals or contaminated animal products, including carcasses, hides, hair, wool, meat, and bone meal. Outbreaks of gastrointestinal tract anthrax have occurred after ingestion of undercooked or raw meat from infected animals. Historically, most (~95%) cases of anthrax in the United States were cutaneous infections among animal handlers or mill workers. Discharge from cutaneous lesions potentially is infectious, but person-to-person transmission rarely has been reported.

The incidence of naturally occurring human anthrax decreased in the United States from an estimated 130 cases annually in the early 1900s to 0 to 2 cases per year by the end of the first decade of the 21st century. Recent cases of inhalation, cutaneous, and gastrointestinal tract anthrax have occurred in drum makers working with animal hides contaminated with *B anthracis* spores or people exposed to drumming events where spore-contaminated drums were used.

B anthracis is one of the most likely agents to be used as a biological weapon because (1) its spores are highly stabile; (2) spores can infect via the respiratory route; and (3) the resulting inhalational anthrax has a high mortality rate. In 1979, an accidental release of *B anthracis* spores from a military microbiology facility in the former Soviet Union resulted in at least 69 deaths. In 2001, 22 cases of anthrax (11 inhalational, 11 cutaneous) were identified in the United States after intentional contamination of the mail; 5 (45%) of the inhalational anthrax cases were fatal. In addition to aerosolization, there is a theoretical health risk associated with *B anthracis* spores being introduced into food products or water supplies. Use of *B anthracis* in a biological attack would require immediate response and mobilization of public health resources. Anthrax meets the definition of a nationally and immediately notifiable condition as specified by the US Council of State and Territorial Epidemiologists; therefore, every suspected case should be reported immediately to the local or state health department.

Incubation Period

Typically 1 week or less for cutaneous or gastrointestinal tract anthrax: for inhalational 1 to 43 days in humans.

Diagnostic Tests

Depending on the clinical presentation, Gram stain, culture, and PCR for anthrax should be performed on pleural fluid, cerebrospinal fluid, and tissue biopsy specimens or on swabs of vesicular fluid or eschar material from cutaneous or oropharyngeal lesions, rectal swabs, or stool. These tests should be obtained before initiating antimicrobial therapy because previous treatment with antimicrobial agents makes isolation by culture unlikely. Definitive identification of suspect *B anthracis* isolates can be performed through the Laboratory Response Network in each state. Additional diagnostic tests for anthrax can be accessed through state health departments, including tissue immunohistochemistry, an enzyme immunoassay that measures immunoglobulin G antibodies against *B anthracis* protective antigen in paired sera, or a MALDI-TOF mass spectrometry assay measuring lethal factor activity in serum

samples. The commercially available Quick-ELISA Anthrax-PA Kit can be used as a screening test.

Treatment

A high index of suspicion and rapid administration of appropriate antimicrobial therapy to people suspected of being infected, along with access to critical care support, are essential for effective treatment of anthrax. No controlled trials in humans have been performed to validate current treatment recommendations for anthrax. Case reports suggest that naturally occurring cutaneous disease can be treated effectively with a variety of antimicrobial agents, including penicillins and tetracyclines for 7 to 10 days. For bioterrorism-associated cutaneous disease in adults or children, ciprofloxacin or doxycycline (for children 8 years of age or older) is recommended for initial treatment until antimicrobial susceptibility data are available. Because of the risk of spore dormancy in mediastinal lymph nodes, the antimicrobial regimen should be continued for a total of 60 days to provide postexposure prophylaxis, in conjunction with administration of vaccine. A multidrug approach is recommended if there also are signs of systemic disease, extensive edema, or lesions of the head and neck.

Ciprofloxacin (intravenously) is recommended as the primary antimicrobial agent as part of an initial multidrug regimen for treating inhalational anthrax, anthrax meningitis, cutaneous anthrax with systemic signs or extensive edema, and gastrointestinal tract/oropharyngeal anthrax until results of antimicrobial susceptibility testing are known. Meningitis treatment requires agents with known CNS penetration; meningeal involvement should be suspected in cases of inhalational anthrax or other systemic anthrax infections. The addition of 1 or 2 other agents with adequate CNS penetration is recommended for use in conjunction with ciprofloxacin; the list of additional antimicrobial agents to consider includes clindamycin, rifampin, penicillin, ampicillin, vancomycin, meropenem, chloramphenicol, and clarithromycin. Because of intrinsic resistance, cephalosporins and trimethoprim-sulfamethoxazole should not be used. Treatment should continue for at least 60 days, but a switch from intravenous to oral therapy may occur when clinically appropriate. For severe anthrax, anthrax-specific hyperimmune globulin 5% should be considered in consultation with the Centers for Disease Control and Prevention (CDC) under the CDC-sponsored investigational new drug use protocol. In addition, aggressive pleural fluid drainage is recommended if effusions exist and is recommended for treatment of all patients with inhalational anthrax.

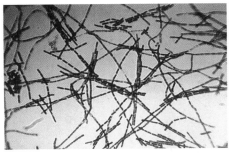

Image 5.1
A photomicrograph of *Bacillus anthracis* bacteria using Gram stain technique. Courtesy of Centers for Disease Control and Prevention.

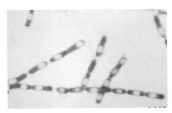

Image 5.2
Sporulation of *Bacillus anthracis,* a gram-positive, nonmotile, encapsulated bacillus.

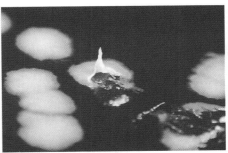

Image 5.3
Bacillus anthracis tenacity positive on sheep blood agar. *B anthracis* colony characteristics: Consistency sticky (tenacious). When teased with loop, colony will stand up like beaten egg white. Courtesy of Centers for Disease Control and Prevention/Larry Stauffer, Oregon State Public Health Laboratory.

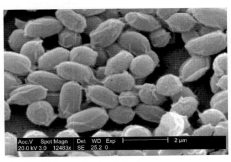

Image 5.4
An electron micrograph of spores from the Sterne strain of *Bacillus anthracis* bacteria. These spores can live for many years, enabling the bacteria to survive in a dormant state. Courtesy of Centers for Disease Control and Prevention/ Janice Haney Carr.

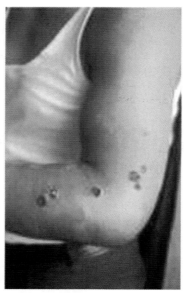

Image 5.5
Cutaneous anthrax. Notice edema and typical lesions. Courtesy of Centers for Disease Control and Prevention.

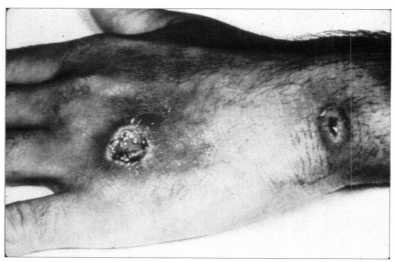

Image 5.6
Cutaneous anthrax on the hand. Courtesy of Gary Overturf, MD.

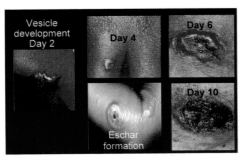

Image 5.7
Cutaneous anthrax. Vesicle development occurs from day 2 through day 10 of progression. Courtesy of Centers for Disease Control and Prevention.

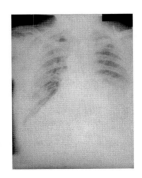

Image 5.8
Posteroanterior chest radiograph taken on the fourth day of illness, which shows a large pleural effusion and marked widening of the mediastinal shadow. Courtesy of Centers for Disease Control and Prevention.

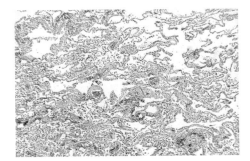

Image 5.9
Photomicrograph of lung tissue demonstrating hemorrhagic pneumonia in a case of fatal human inhalation anthrax (magnification x50). Courtesy of Centers for Disease Control and Prevention/Dr LaForce.

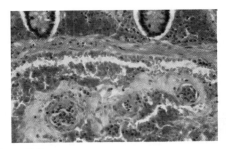

Image 5.10
This micrograph reveals submucosal hemorrhage in the small intestine in a case of fatal human anthrax (hematoxylin-eosin stain, magnification x240). The first symptoms of gastrointestinal (GI) anthrax are nausea, loss of appetite, bloody diarrhea, and fever, followed by severe stomach pain. One-fourth to more than half of GI anthrax cases lead to death. Note the associated arteriolar degeneration. Courtesy of Centers for Disease Control and Prevention/Dr Marshal Fox.

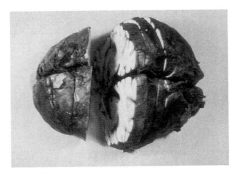

Image 5.11
Gross pathology of fixed, cut brain showing hemorrhagic meningitis secondary to inhalational anthrax. Courtesy of Centers for Disease Control and Prevention.

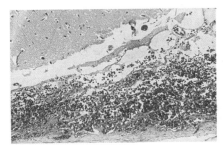

Image 5.12
Photomicrograph of meninges demonstrating hemorrhagic meningitis due to fatal inhalational anthrax (magnification x125). Courtesy of Centers for Disease Control and Prevention/Dr LaForce.

6

Arboviruses

(Also see Dengue, p 130, and West Nile
Virus, p 620.)

(Including California Serogroup, Chikungunya,
Colorado Tick Fever, Eastern Equine Enceph-
alitis, Japanese Encephalitis, Powassan, St
Louis Encephalitis, Tickborne Encephalitis,
Venezuelan Equine Encephalitis, Western
Equine Encephalitis, and Yellow Fever Viruses)

Clinical Manifestations

More than 150 arthropodborne viruses (arboviruses) are known to cause human disease.
Although most infections are subclinical,
symptomatic illness usually manifests as 1 of
3 primary clinical syndromes: systemic febrile
illness, neuroinvasive disease, or hemorrhagic
fever (Table 6.1).

- *Systemic febrile illness.* Most arboviruses
  are capable of causing a systemic febrile illness that often includes headache, arthralgia, myalgia, and rash. Some viruses also
  can cause more characteristic clinical
  manifestations, including severe joint pain
  (eg, chikungunya) or jaundice (yellow fever).
  With some arboviruses, fatigue, malaise,
  and weakness can linger for weeks following
  the initial infection.

- *Neuroinvasive disease.* Many arboviruses
  cause neuroinvasive diseases, including
  aseptic meningitis, encephalitis, or acute
  flaccid paralysis. Illness usually presents
  with a prodrome similar to the systemic
  febrile illness followed by neurologic symptoms and signs. The manifestations vary
  by virus and clinical syndrome but can
  include vomiting, stiff neck, mental status

Table 6.1
Clinical Manifestations for Select Domestic and International Arboviral Diseases

Virus	Systemic Febrile Illness	Neuroinvasive Disease[a]	Hemorrhagic Fever
Domestic			
Colorado tick fever	Yes	Rare	No
Dengue	Yes	Rare	Yes
Eastern equine encephali-tis	Yes	Yes	No
California serogroup[b]	Yes	Yes	No
Powassan	Yes	Yes	No
St Louis encephalitis	Yes	Yes	No
Western equine encephali-tis	Yes	Yes	No
West Nile	Yes	Yes	No
International			
Chikungunya	Yes[c]	Rare	No
Japanese encephalitis	Yes	Yes	No
Tickborne encephalitis	Yes	Yes	No
Venezuelan equine encephalitis	Yes	Yes	No
Yellow fever	Yes	No	Yes

[a] Aseptic meningitis, encephalitis, or acute flaccid paralysis.
[b] In this group, most human cases are caused by La Crosse virus. Other known or suspected human pathogens in the group include California encephalitis, Jamestown Canyon, snowshoe hare, and trivittatus viruses.
[c] Most often characterized by sudden onset of high fever and severe joint pain.

changes, seizures, or focal neurologic deficits. The severity and long-term outcome of the illness vary by etiologic agent and the underlying characteristics of the host, such as age, immune status, and preexisting medical condition.

- *Hemorrhagic fever.* Hemorrhagic fevers can be caused by dengue or yellow fever viruses. After several days of nonspecific febrile illness, the patient may develop overt signs of hemorrhage (eg, petechiae, ecchymoses, bleeding from nose and gums, hematemesis, and melena) and septic shock (eg, decreased peripheral circulation, azotemia, tachycardia, and hypotension). Hemorrhagic fever caused by dengue and yellow fever viruses can be confused with hemorrhagic fevers transmitted by rodents (eg, Argentine hemorrhagic fever, Bolivian hemorrhagic fever, and Lassa fever) or those caused by Ebola or Marburg viruses. For information on other infections causing hemorrhagic manifestations, see pages 186–189.

Etiology

Arboviruses are RNA viruses that are transmitted to humans primarily through bites of infected arthropods (mosquitoes, ticks, sandflies, and biting midges). The viral families responsible for most arboviral infections in humans are Flaviviridae (genus *Flavivirus*), Togaviridae (genus *Alphavirus*), and Bunyaviridae (genus *Bunyavirus*). Reoviridae (genus *Coltivirus*) also is responsible for a smaller number of human arboviral infections (eg, Colorado tick fever) (Table 6.2).

Epidemiology

Most arboviruses maintain cycles of transmission between birds or small mammals and arthropod vectors. Humans and domestic animals usually are infected incidentally as "dead-end" hosts (Table 6.2). Important exceptions are dengue, yellow fever, and chikungunya viruses, which can be spread from person to arthropod to person (anthroponotic transmission). For other arboviruses, humans usually do not develop a sustained or high enough level of viremia to infect arthropod vectors. Direct person-to-person spread of arboviruses can occur through blood transfusion, organ transplantation, intrauterine transmission, and possibly human milk. Percutaneous and aerosol transmission of arboviruses can occur in the laboratory setting.

In the northern United States, arboviral infections occur during summer and autumn, when mosquitoes and ticks are most active. In the southern United States, cases occur throughout the year because of warmer temperatures, which are conducive to year-round arthropod activity. The number of domestic or imported arboviral disease cases reported in the United States varies greatly by specific etiology and year (Table 6.2).

Overall, the risk of severe clinical disease for most arboviral infections in the United States is higher among adults than among children. One notable exception is La Crosse virus infections, for which children are at highest risk of severe neurologic disease and possible long-term sequelae. Eastern equine encephalitis virus causes a low incidence of disease but high case-fatality rate (40%) across all age groups.

Incubation Period

Typically ranges between 2 and 15 days. Longer incubation periods can occur in immunocompromised people and for tickborne viruses.

Diagnostic Tests

Arboviral infections are confirmed most frequently by measurement of virus-specific antibody in serum or cerebrospinal fluid (CSF). Acute-phase serum specimens should be tested for virus-specific immunoglobulin (Ig) M using an enzyme immunoassay (EIA) or microsphere immunoassay (MIA). With clinical and epidemiologic correlation, a positive IgM test has good diagnostic predictive value, but cross-reaction with related arboviruses from the same family can occur. For most arboviral infections, IgM is detectable 3 to 8 days after onset of illness and persists for 30 to 90 days. A positive IgM test result occasionally may reflect a past infection. Serum collected within 10 days of illness onset may not have detectable IgM, and the test should be repeated on a convalescent sample. IgG antibody generally is detectable shortly after IgM and persists for years. A plaque-reduction neutralization test (PRNT) can be performed to

Table 6.2

Genus, Geographic Location, Vectors, and Average Number of Annual Cases
for Selected Domestic and International Arboviral Diseases

Virus	Genus	United States	Non-United States	Vectors	Number of US Cases/Year (Range)[a]
			Geographic Location		
Domestic					
Colorado tick fever	*Coltivirus*	West	Canada	Ticks	8 (2–12)
Dengue	*Flavivirus*	Puerto Rico, Florida, Texas, and Hawaii	Worldwide in tropical areas	Mosquitoes	45 (20–71)[b]
Eastern equine encephalitis	*Alphavirus*	Eastern and gulf states	Canada, Central and South America	Mosquitoes	8 (3–21)
California serogroup	*Bunyavirus*	Widespread, most prevalent in midwest and east	Canada	Mosquitoes	93 (46–167)
Powassan	*Flavivirus*	Northeast and north central	Canada, Russia	Ticks	2 (0–7)
St Louis encephalitis	*Flavivirus*	Widespread	Canada, Caribbean, Mexico, Central and South America	Mosquitoes	21 (2–79)
Western equine encephalitis	*Alphavirus*	Central and west	Central and South America	Mosquitoes	<1
West Nile	*Flavivirus*	Widespread	Canada, Europe, Africa, Asia	Mosquitoes	1215 (19–2946)[c]
International					
Chikungunya	*Alphavirus*	Imported only	Asia, Africa	Mosquitoes	27 (12–42)[d]
Japanese encephalitis	*Flavivirus*	Imported only	Asia	Mosquitoes	<1
Tickborne encephalitis	*Flavivirus*	Imported only	Europe, northern Asia	Ticks	<1
Venezuelan equine encephalitis	*Alphavirus*	Imported only	Mexico, Central and South America	Mosquitoes	<1
Yellow fever	*Flavivirus*	Imported only	South America, Africa	Mosquitoes	<1

[a] Average annual number of domestic and/or imported cases from 2000 to 2009 unless otherwise noted.
[b] Domestic and imported cases from 1997–2006; excludes indigenous transmission in Puerto Rico.
[c] Neuroinvasive disease only.
[d] Cases imported to the United States from 2006 to 2009 only.

measure virus-specific neutralizing antibodies. A fourfold or greater increase in virus-specific neutralizing antibodies between acute- and convalescent-phase serum specimens collected 2 to 3 weeks apart may be used to confirm recent infection or discriminate between cross-reacting antibodies in primary arboviral infections. For some arboviral infections (eg, Colorado tick fever), the immune response may be delayed, with IgM antibodies not appearing until 2 to 3 weeks after onset of illness and neutralizing antibodies taking up to a month to develop. Immunization history, date of symptom onset, and information regarding other arboviruses known to circulate in the geographic area that may cross-react in serologic assays should be considered when interpreting results.

Viral culture and nucleic acid amplification tests (NAATs) for RNA can be performed on acute-phase serum, CSF, or tissue specimens.

Arboviruses that are more likely to be detected using culture or NAATs early in the illness include chikungunya, dengue, and yellow fever viruses. Immunohistochemical staining (IHC) can detect specific viral antigen in fixed tissue.

Antibody testing for common domestic arboviral diseases is performed in most state public health laboratories and many commercial laboratories. Confirmatory PRNTs, viral culture, NAATs, IHC, and testing for less common domestic and international arboviruses are performed only at the Centers for Disease Control and Prevention.

Treatment

The primary treatment for all arboviral disease is supportive. Although various therapies have been evaluated for several arboviral diseases, none have shown specific benefit.

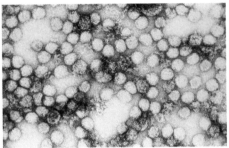

Image 6.1
An electron micrograph of yellow fever virus virions. Virions are spheroidal, uniform in shape, and 40 to 60 nm in diameter. The name "yellow fever" is due to the ensuing jaundice that affects some patients. The vector is the *Aedes aegypti* or *Haemagogus* spp mosquito.

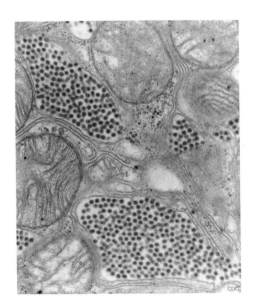

Image 6.2
This colorized transmission electron micrograph depicts a salivary gland that had been extracted from a mosquito that was infected by the eastern equine encephalitis virus, which has been colorized red (magnification x83,900). Courtesy of Centers for Disease Control and Prevention/Dr Fred Murphy; Sylvia Whitfield.

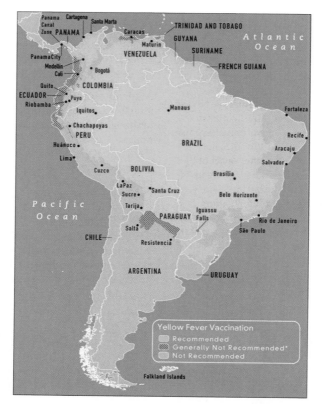

Image 6.3
Yellow fever vaccine recommendations in the Americas, 2010. Courtesy of Centers for Disease Control and Prevention.

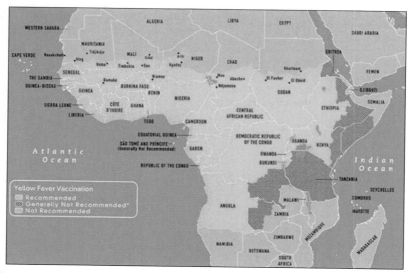

Image 6.4
Yellow fever vaccine recommendations in Africa, 2010. Courtesy of Centers for Disease Control and Prevention.

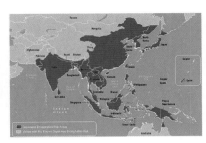

Image 6.5
Geographic distribution of Japanese encephalitis.
Courtesy of Centers for Disease Control and Prevention.

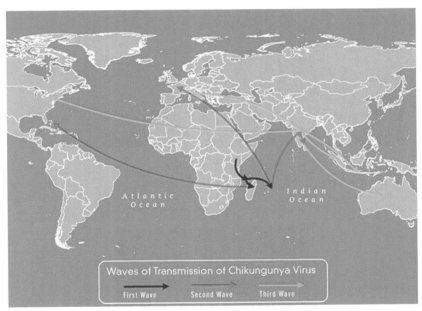

Image 6.6
Global spread of chikungya virus during 2005–2009. Courtesy of *Morbidity and Mortality Weekly Report.*

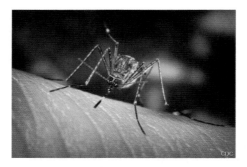

Image 6.7
A close-up anterior view of a *Culex tarsalis* mosquito as it was about to begin feeding. The epidemiologic importance of *C tarsalis* lies in its ability to spread western equine encephalitis, St Louis encephalitis, and California encephalitis, and is currently the main vector of West Nile virus in the western United States. Courtesy of Centers for Disease Control and Prevention/James Gathany.

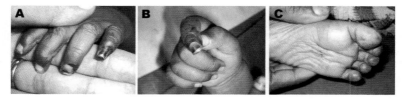

Image 6.8
Digital gangrene in an 8-month-old girl during week 3 of hospitalization. She was admitted to the hospital with fever, multiple seizures, and a widespread rash; chikungunya virus was detected in her plasma. (A) Little finger of the left hand; (B) index finger of the right hand; and (C) 4 toes on the right foot. Courtesy of Centers for Disease Control and Prevention/*Emerging Infectious Diseases*.

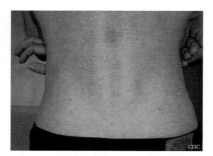

Image 6.9
Cutaneous eruption of chikungunya infection, a generalized exanthema comprising non-coalescent lesions occurs during the first week of the disease as seen in this patient with erythematous maculopapular lesions with islands of normal skin. Courtesy of Hochedez P, Jaureguiberry S, Debruyne M, et al. Chikungunya infection in travelers. *Emerg Infect Dis.* 2006;12(10):1565–1567.

7

Arcanobacterium haemolyticum Infections

Clinical Manifestations

Acute pharyngitis attributable to *Arcanobacterium haemolyticum* often is indistinguishable from that caused by group A streptococci. Fever, pharyngeal exudate, lymphadenopathy, rash, and pruritus are common, but palatal petechiae and strawberry tongue are absent. In almost half of all reported cases, a maculopapular or scarlatiniform exanthem is present, beginning on the extensor surfaces of the distal extremities, spreading centripetally to the chest and back, and sparing the face, palms, and soles. Rash is associated primarily with cases presenting with pharyngitis and typically develops 1 to 4 days after onset of sore throat, although cases have been reported with rash preceding pharyngitis. Respiratory tract infections that mimic diphtheria, including membranous pharyngitis, sinusitis, and pneumonia, and skin and soft tissue infections, including chronic ulceration, cellulitis, paronychia, and wound infection, have been attributed to *A haemolyticum*. Invasive infections, including septicemia, peritonsillar abscess, Lemierre syndrome, brain abscess, orbital cellulitis, meningitis, endocarditis, pyogenic arthritis, osteomyelitis, urinary tract infection, pneumonia, spontaneous bacterial peritonitis, and pyothorax have been reported. No nonsuppurative sequelae have been reported.

Etiology

A haemolyticum is a catalase-negative, weakly acid-fast, facultative, hemolytic, anaerobic, gram-positive, slender, sometimes club-shaped bacillus formerly classified as *Corynebacterium haemolyticum*.

Epidemiology

Humans are the primary reservoir of *A haemolyticum,* and spread is person to person, presumably via droplet respiratory tract secretions. Severe disease occurs almost exclusively among immunocompromised people. Pharyngitis occurs primarily in adolescents and young adults. Although long-term pharyngeal carriage with *A haemolyticum* has been described after an episode of acute pharyngitis, isolation of the bacterium from the nasopharynx of asymptomatic people is rare. An estimated 0.5% to 3% of acute pharyngitis is attributable to *A haemolyticum*.

Incubation Period

Unknown.

Diagnostic Tests

A haemolyticum grows on blood-enriched agar, but colonies are small, have a narrow band of hemolysis, and may not be visible for 48 to 72 hours. Detection is enhanced by culture on rabbit or human blood agar rather than on more commonly used sheep blood agar because of larger colony size and wider zones of hemolysis. Growth also is enhanced by addition of 5% carbon dioxide. Routine throat cultures are inoculated onto sheep blood agar, and *A haemolyticum* may be missed if laboratory personnel are not trained to look for the organism. Pits characteristically form under the colonies on blood agar plates. Two biotypes of *A haemolyticum* have been identified: a rough biotype predominates in respiratory tract infections and a smooth biotype is most commonly associated with skin and soft-tissue infections.

Treatment

Erythromycin is the drug of choice for treating tonsillopharyngitis attributable to *A haemolyticum*. *A haemolyticum* is also susceptible in vitro to azithromycin, clindamycin, cefuroxime, vancomycin, and tetracycline. Failures in treatment of pharyngitis with penicillin have been reported, perhaps because of this intracellular residing pathogen. In the rare case of disseminated infection, susceptibility tests should be performed. In disseminated infection, parenteral penicillin plus an aminoglycoside may be used initially as empirical treatment.

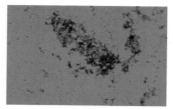

Image 7.1
Arcanobacterium haemolyticum (Gram stain).
A haemolyticum appears strongly gram-positive
in young cultures but becomes more gram-
variable after 24 hours of incubation as in
this photograph. Copyright Noni MacDonald,
MD, FAAP.

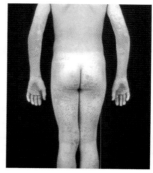

Image 7.2
Arcanobacterium haemolyticum was isolated on
pharyngeal culture from this 12-year-old boy with
an erythematous rash that was followed by mild
desquamation. Copyright Williams/Karofsky.

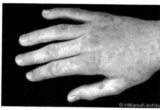

Image 7.3
Arcanobacterium haemolyticum–associated
rash on dorsal surface of hand in the 12-year-old
boy in images 7.2, 7.4, and 7.5. Copyright
Williams/Karofsky.

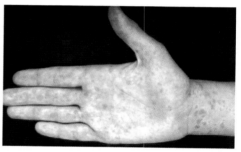

Image 7.4
Note that the palms are affected in this patient,
though they are often spared. Copyright
Williams/Karofsky.

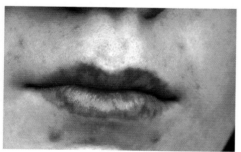

Image 7.5
Although not present in this patient with facial
skin lesions associated with *Arcanobacterium
haemolyticum* pharyngitis, a pharyngeal
membrane similar to that of diphtheria may
occur with *A haemolyticum* pharyngeal
infection. Copyright Williams/Karofsky.

8

Ascaris lumbricoides Infections

Clinical Manifestations

Most infections with *Ascaris lumbricoides* are asymptomatic, although moderate to heavy infections can lead to malnutrition and non-specific gastrointestinal tract symptoms. During the larval migratory phase, an acute transient pneumonitis (Löffler syndrome) associated with fever and marked eosinophilia can occur. Acute intestinal obstruction has been associated with heavy infestations. Children are prone to this complication because of the small diameter of the intestinal lumen and their propensity to acquire large worm burdens. Worm migration can cause peritonitis secondary to intestinal wall perforation and common bile duct obstruction resulting in biliary colic, cholangitis, or pancreatitis. Adult worms can be stimulated to migrate by stressful conditions (eg, fever, illness, or anesthesia) and by some anthelmintic drugs. *A lumbricoides* has been found in the appendiceal lumen in patients with acute appendicitis.

Etiology

A lumbricoides is the most prevalent of all human intestinal nematodes (roundworms), with more than 1 billion people infected worldwide.

Epidemiology

Adult worms live in the lumen of the small intestine. Female worms produce approximately 200,000 eggs per day, which are excreted in stool and must incubate in soil for 2 to 3 weeks for an embryo to become infectious. Following ingestion of embryonated eggs, usually from contaminated soil, larvae hatch in the small intestine, penetrate the mucosa, and are transported passively by portal blood to the liver and lungs. After migrating into the airways, larvae ascend through the tracheobronchial tree to the pharynx, are swallowed, and mature into adults in the small intestine. Infection with *A lumbricoides* is most common in resource-limited countries, including rural and urban communities characterized by poor sanitation. Adult worms can live for 12 to 18 months, resulting in daily fecal excretion of large numbers of ova. Female worms are longer than male worms and can measure 40 cm in length and 6 mm in diameter.

Incubation Period

Approximately 8 weeks (interval between ingestion of eggs and development of egg-laying adults).

Diagnostic Tests

Ova routinely are detected by examination of a fresh stool specimen using light microscopy. Infected people also may pass adult worms from the rectum, from the nose after migration through the nares, and from the mouth, usually in vomitus. Adult worms may be detected by computed tomographic scan of the abdomen or by ultrasonographic examination of the biliary tree.

Treatment

Albendazole (taken with food in a single dose), mebendazole for 3 days, or ivermectin (taken on an empty stomach in a single dose) are recommended for treatment of ascariasis. The safety of ivermectin in children weighing less than 15 kg and in pregnant women has not been established. In 1-year-old children, the World Health Organization recommends reducing the albendazole dose to half of that given to older children and adults. Reexamination of stool specimens 2 weeks after therapy to determine whether the worms have been eliminated is helpful for assessing effectiveness of therapy.

Conservative management of small bowel obstruction, including nasogastric suction and intravenous fluids, may result in resolution of major symptoms before administration of anthelmintic therapy. Surgical intervention occasionally is necessary to relieve intestinal or biliary tract obstruction or for volvulus or peritonitis secondary to perforation. Endoscopic retrograde cholangiopancreatography has been used successfully for extraction of worms from the biliary tree.

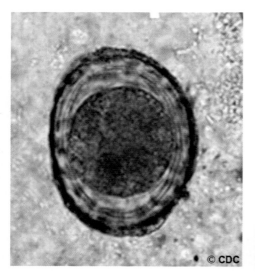

Image 8.1
A fertilized ascaris egg, still at the unicellular stage, which is the usual stage when the eggs are passed in the stool (complete development of the larva requires 18 days under favorable conditions). Courtesy of Centers for Disease Control and Prevention.

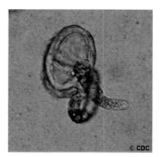

Image 8.2
Larva hatching from an ascaris egg. This occurs in the small intestine. Courtesy of Centers for Disease Control and Prevention.

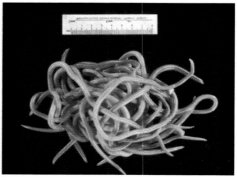

Image 8.4
A mass of large round worms *(A lumbricoides)* from a human infestation.

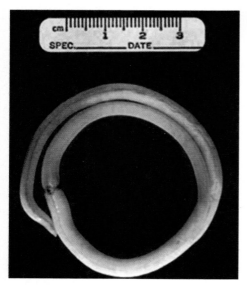

Image 8.3
An adult ascaris. Diagnostic characteristics: tapered ends; length 15 to 35 cm (the females tend to be larger). This worm is a female, as evidenced by the size and genital girdle (the dark circular groove at bottom area of image). Courtesy of Centers for Disease Control and Prevention.

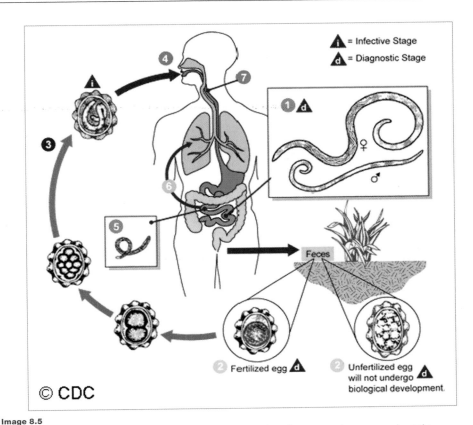

© CDC

Image 8.5

Adult worms (1) live in the lumen of the small intestine. A female may produce approximately 200,000 eggs per day, which are passed with the feces (2). Unfertilized eggs may be ingested but are not infective. Fertile eggs embryonate and become infective after 18 days to several weeks (3), depending on the environmental conditions (optimum: moist, warm, shaded soil). After infective eggs are swallowed (4), the larvae hatch (5), invade the intestinal mucosa, and are carried via the portal, then systemic circulation to the lungs (6). The larvae mature further in the lungs (10–14 days), penetrate the alveolar walls, ascend the bronchial tree to the throat, and are swallowed (7). On reaching the small intestine, they develop into adult worms (8). Between 2 and 3 months are required from ingestion of the infective eggs to oviposition by the adult female. Adult worms can live 1 to 2 years. Courtesy of Centers for Disease Control and Prevention.

9

Aspergillosis

Clinical Manifestations

Aspergillosis manifests as invasive, noninvasive, chronic, or allergic disease depending on the immune status of the host. **Invasive aspergillosis** occurs almost exclusively in immunocompromised patients with prolonged neutropenia (eg, cytotoxic chemotherapy), graft-versus-host disease, or impaired phagocyte function (eg, chronic granulomatous disease, immunosuppressive therapy, corticosteroids). Children at highest risk include children with new-onset or a relapse of hematologic malignancy and allogeneic hematopoietic stem cell transplant recipients. Invasive infection usually involves pulmonary, sinus, cerebral, or cutaneous sites. Rarely, endocarditis, osteomyelitis, meningitis, infection of the eye or orbit, and esophagitis occur. The hallmark of invasive aspergillosis is angioinvasion with resulting thrombosis, dissemination to other organs and, occasionally, erosion of the blood vessel wall with catastrophic hemorrhage. However, aspergillosis in patients with chronic granulomatous disease rarely displays angioinvasion. **Aspergillomas and otomycosis** are 2 syndromes of nonallergic colonization by *Aspergillus* species in immunocompetent children. Aspergillomas ("fungal balls") grow in preexisting pulmonary cavities or bronchogenic cysts without invading pulmonary tissue; almost all patients have underlying lung disease, such as cystic fibrosis or tuberculosis. Patients with otomycosis have chronic otitis media with colonization of the external auditory canal by a fungal mat that produces a dark discharge. **Allergic bronchopulmonary aspergillosis** is a hypersensitivity lung disease that manifests as episodic wheezing, expectoration of brown mucus plugs, low-grade fever, eosinophilia, and transient pulmonary infiltrates. This form of aspergillosis occurs most commonly in immunocompetent children with asthma or cystic fibrosis and can be a trigger for asthmatic flares. **Allergic sinusitis** is a far less common allergic response to colonization by *Aspergillus* species than is allergic bronchopulmonary aspergillosis. Allergic sinusitis occurs in children with nasal polyps or previous episodes of sinusitis or children who have undergone sinus surgery. Allergic sinusitis is characterized by symptoms of chronic sinusitis with dark plugs of nasal discharge.

Etiology

Aspergillus species are ubiquitous molds that grow on decaying vegetation and in soil. *Aspergillus fumigatus* is the most common cause of invasive aspergillosis, with *Aspergillus flavus* being the next most common. Several other species, including *Aspergillus terreus, Aspergillus nidulans,* and *Aspergillus niger,* also cause invasive human infections.

Epidemiology

The principal route of transmission is inhalation of conidia (spores) originating from multiple environmental sources (plants, vegetables, dust from construction or demolition), soil, and water supplies (eg, shower heads). Incidence of disease in transplant recipients is highest during periods of neutropenia or during treatment for graft-versus-host disease. Health care–associated outbreaks of invasive pulmonary aspergillosis in susceptible hosts have occurred in which the probable source of the fungus was a nearby construction site or faulty ventilation system. Transmission by direct inoculation of skin abrasions or wounds is less likely. Person-to-person spread does not occur.

Incubation Period

Unknown.

Diagnostic Tests

Dichotomously branched and septate hyphae, identified by microscopic examination of 10% potassium hydroxide wet preparations or of Gomori methenamine silver nitrate stain of tissue or bronchoalveolar lavage specimens, are suggestive of the diagnosis. Isolation of *Aspergillus* species is required for definitive diagnosis. The organism usually is not recoverable from blood (except *A terreus*) but is isolated readily from lung, sinus, and skin biopsy specimens when cultured on fungal media. *Aspergillus* species can be a laboratory contaminant, but when evaluating results from ill, immunocompromised patients, recovery of this organism frequently indicates infection.

Biopsy of a lesion usually is required to confirm the diagnosis, and care should be taken to distinguish aspergillosis from zygomycosis, which appears similar by diagnostic imaging studies. An enzyme immunosorbent assay serologic test for detection of galactomannan, a molecule found in the cell wall of *Aspergillus* species, is available commercially and has been found to be useful in children and adults. Monitoring of serum antigen concentrations twice weekly in periods of highest risk (eg, neutropenia and active graft-versus-host disease) may be useful for early detection of invasive aspergillosis in at-risk patients. False-positive test results have been reported and can be related to consumption of food products containing galactomannan (eg, rice and pasta) or from cross-reactivity with antimicrobial agents derived from fungi (eg, penicillins). A negative galactomannan test result does not exclude diagnosis of invasive aspergillosis. False-negative galactomannan test results consistently occur in patients with chronic granulomatous disease, so the test should not be used in these patients. Unlike adults, children frequently do not manifest cavitation or the air crescent or halo signs on chest radiography, and lack of these characteristic signs does not exclude the diagnosis of invasive aspergillosis. In allergic aspergillosis, diagnosis is suggested by a typical clinical syndrome with elevated total concentrations of immunoglobulin (Ig) E (≥1,000 ng/mL) and *Aspergillus*-specific serum IgE, eosinophilia, and a positive result from a skin test for *Aspergillus* antigens. In children with cystic fibrosis, the diagnosis is more difficult, because wheezing and eosinophilia not associated with allergic bronchopulmonary aspergillosis often are present.

Treatment

Voriconazole is the drug of choice for invasive aspergillosis, except in neonates, for whom amphotericin B deoxycholate in high doses is recommended. Voriconazole has been shown to be superior to amphotericin B in a large, randomized trial in adults. Therapy is continued for at least 12 weeks, but treatment duration should be individualized. Monitoring of serum galactomannan serum concentrations twice weekly may be useful to assess response to therapy concomitant with clinical and radiologic evaluation. Voriconazole is metabolized in a linear fashion in children, so the recommended adult dosing is too low for children.

Caspofungin has been studied in pediatric patients older than 3 months as salvage therapy for invasive aspergillosis. Itraconazole alone is an alternative for mild to moderate cases of aspergillosis, although extensive drug interactions and poor absorption (capsular form) limit the utility of itraconazole. Lipid formulations of amphotericin B can be considered, but *A terreus* is resistant to all amphotericin B products. The efficacy and safety of combination antifungal therapy for invasive aspergillosis in children have not been evaluated adequately. Immune reconstitution can occur during treatment in some patients. Decreasing immunosuppression, if possible, specifically decreasing corticosteroid dose, is important to disease control.

Surgical excision of a localized invasive lesion (eg, cutaneous eschars, a single pulmonary lesion, sinus debris, accessible cerebral lesions) usually is warranted. In pulmonary disease, surgery is indicated only when a mass is impinging on a great vessel. Allergic bronchopulmonary aspergillosis is treated with corticosteroids, and adjunctive antifungal therapy is recommended. Allergic sinus aspergillosis also is treated with corticosteroids, and surgery has been reported to be beneficial in many cases. Antifungal therapy has not been found to be useful.

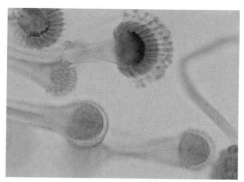

Image 9.1
Aspergillus fumigatus. Copyright Tufts University.

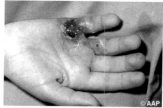

Image 9.2
Aspergilloma of the hand in a 7-year-old boy with chronic granulomatous disease.

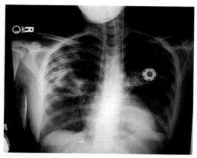

Image 9.4
Aspergillus pneumonia, bilateral, in a 16-year-old boy with acute myelogenous leukemia. Note pulmonary cavitation in the right lung field and perihilar and retrocardiac densities in the left lung field. Copyright Michael Rajnik, MD, FAAP.

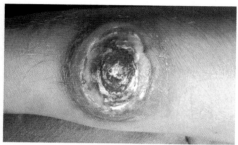

Image 9.3
Aspergilloma at intravenous line site in a 9-year-old boy with acute lymphoblastic leukemia.

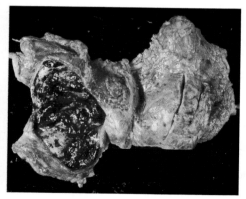

Image 9.5
Pulmonary aspergillosis in a patient with acute lymphatic leukemia. Courtesy of Dimitris P. Agamanolis, MD.

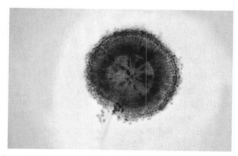

Image 9.6
Conidial head of an *Aspergillus niger* fungal organism showing a double row of sterigmata. Conidial heads of *Aspergillus niger* are large, globose, and dark brown, and contain the fungal spores, facilitating propagation of the organism. This is one of the most common species associated with invasive pulmonary aspergillosis. Courtesy of Centers for Disease Control and Prevention/Lucille K. Georg, MD.

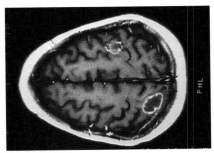

Image 9.7
Aspergillomas in a 10-year-old with Hodgkins lymphoma. Copyright Benjamin Estrada, MD.

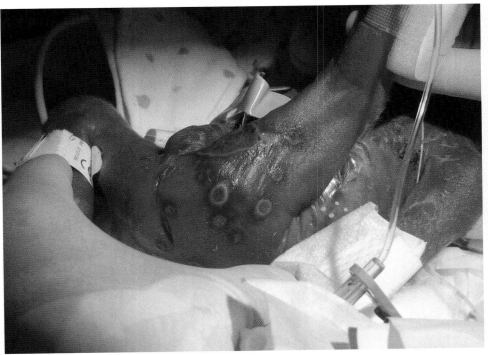

Image 9.8
Cutaneous aspergilosis in a 23-week gestation preterm infant. Copyright David Kaufman, MD.

10

Astrovirus Infections

Clinical Manifestations

Illness is characterized by diarrhea of short duration accompanied by vomiting, fever and, occasionally, abdominal pain and mild dehydration. Infection in an immunocompetent host is self-limited, lasting a median of 5 to 6 days. Asymptomatic infections are common.

Etiology

Astroviruses are nonenveloped, singlestranded RNA viruses with a characteristic starlike appearance when visualized by electron microscopy. Eight human antigenic types originally were described, and several novel species have been identified since 2008.

Epidemiology

Human astroviruses have a worldwide distribution. Multiple antigenic types cocirculate in the same region. Astroviruses have been detected in as many as 10% to 34% of sporadic cases of nonbacterial gastroenteritis among young children but uncommonly cause severe childhood gastroenteritis requiring hospitalization. Astrovirus infections occur predominantly in children younger than 4 years; these infections peak during the late winter and spring in the United States. Transmission is person to person via the fecal-oral route. Outbreaks tend to occur in closed populations of young and elderly persons. Excretion lasts a median of 5 days after illness onset, but asymptomatic excretion can last for several weeks.

Incubation Period

1 to 4 days.

Diagnostic Tests

Commercial tests for diagnosis are not available in the United States. Some reference laboratories test fecal specimens by electron microscopy for detection of viral particles, enzyme immunoassay for detection of viral antigen, and reverse transcriptase PCR assay for detection of viral RNA in stool.

Treatment

No antiviral therapy is available. Oral or parenteral fluids and electrolytes are given to prevent and correct dehydration.

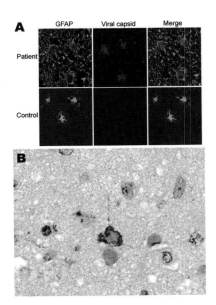

Image 10.1

Astrovirus encephalitis in a boy with X-linked agammaglobulinemia. Encephalitis is a major cause of death worldwide. Although more than 100 pathogens have been identified as causative agents, the pathogen is not determined for up to 75% of cases. This diagnostic failure impedes effective treatment and underscores the need for better tools and new approaches for detecting novel pathogens or determining new manifestations of known pathogens. Although astroviruses are commonly associated with gastroenteritis, they have not been associated with central nervous system disease. Using unbiased pyrosequencing, astrovirus was determined to be the causative agent for encephalitis in a 15-year-old boy with agammaglobulinemia. Courtesy of Quan PL, Wagner TA, Briese T, et al. Astrovirus encephalitis in boy with X-linked agammaglobulinemia. *Emerg Infect Dis.* 2010;16(6): 918–925.

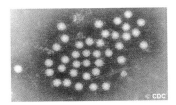

Image 10.2

Electron micrograph of astrovirus obtained from stool of a child with gastroenteritis. Note the characteristic starlike appearance. Courtesy of Centers for Disease Control and Prevention.

11

Babesiosis

Clinical Manifestations

Babesia infection often is asymptomatic or associated with mild, nonspecific symptoms. The infection also can be severe and life-threatening, particularly in people who are asplenic, immunocompromised, or elderly. Babesiosis, like malaria, is characterized by the presence of fever and hemolytic anemia; however, some infected people who are immunocompromised or at the extremes of age (eg, preterm infants) are afebrile. Patients can have a prodromal illness, with gradual onset of malaise, anorexia, and fatigue, followed by fever and other influenza-like symptoms (eg, chills, sweats, myalgia, arthralgia, headache, anorexia, nausea, vomiting). Less common manifestations include hyperesthesia, sore throat, abdominal pain, conjunctival injection, photophobia, weight loss, and nonproductive cough. Clinical signs generally are minimal, (eg, fever and tachycardia), although hypotension, respiratory distress, mild hepatosplenomegaly, jaundice, and dark urine may be noted. Thrombocytopenia is common; disseminated intravascular coagulation can be a complication of severe babesiosis. If untreated, illness can last for several weeks or months. Asymptomatic people can have persistent low-level parasitemia for more than 1 year. The possibility of concurrent *Borrelia burgdorferi* or *Anaplasma* infection should be considered.

Etiology

Babesia species are intraerythrocytic protozoa. The etiologic agents of babesiosis in the United States include *Babesia microti,* which has caused most of the reported cases, and several other genetically and antigenically distinct organisms, such as *Babesia duncani* (formerly the WA1-type parasite).

Epidemiology

Babesiosis predominantly is a tickborne zoonosis. Transmission of *Babesia* species also can occur through blood transfusion and congenital/perinatal routes. In the United States, the primary reservoir host for *B microti* is the white-footed mouse (*Peromyscus leucopus*), and the primary vector is the tick *Ixodes scapularis,* which also can transmit *B burgdorferi* and *Anaplasma phagocytophilum,* the causative agents of Lyme disease and human granulocytic anaplasmosis, respectively. Humans become infected through tick bites, which typically are not noticed. The white-tailed deer *(Odocoileus virginianus)* is an important host for tick blood meals but is not a reservoir host of *B microti*. An increase in the deer population in some geographic areas, including some suburban areas, is thought to be a major factor in the spread of *I scapularis* and the increase in numbers of reported babesiosis cases. The reported vectorborne cases of *B microti* infection have been acquired in the Northeast (Connecticut, Massachusetts, New Jersey, New York, and Rhode Island) and in the upper Midwest (Wisconsin and Minnesota). Occasional human cases of babesiosis caused by other species have been described in the United States; tick vectors and reservoir hosts for these agents typically have not yet been identified. Most vectorborne cases of babesiosis occur during late spring, summer, or autumn.

Incubation Period

1 week to several months.

Diagnostic Tests

The provisional diagnosis is made by microscopic identification of the organism on Giemsa- or Wright-stained thick or thin blood smears. If seen, the tetrad (Maltese-cross) form is pathognomonic. *B microti* and other *Babesia* species can be difficult to distinguish from *Plasmodium falciparum;* examination of blood smears by a reference laboratory should be considered for confirmation of the diagnosis. Serologic and molecular testing is performed at the Centers for Disease Control and Prevention and are important adjunctive tests.

Treatment

Clindamycin plus oral quinine or atovaquone plus azithromycin had comparable efficacy among adult patients who did not have life-threatening babesiosis. Therapy with atovaquone plus azithromycin is associated with fewer adverse effects, but clindamycin and quinine remain the combination for severely ill patients. In addition, exchange blood transfusions should be considered for patients who are critically ill (eg, hemodynamically unstable), especially but not exclusively for patients with parasitemia concentrations 10% or greater.

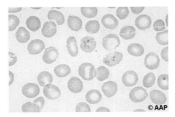

Image 11.1
Babesia microti in a peripheral blood smear. Note the typical intraerythrocytic location of the organisms. Babesiosis is often asymptomatic or associated with mild symptoms. The infection can be life-threatening in people who are asplenic or immunocompromised.

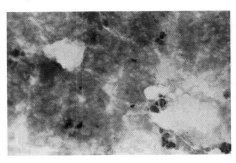

Image 11.2
A Giemsa stain of a blood film from an infected human used to identify the parasite *Babesia microti*. Babesiosis is caused by hemo-protozoan parasites of the genus *Babesia*. While more than 100 species have been reported, *B microti* and *B divergens* have been identified in most human cases. Courtesy of Centers for Disease Control and Prevention/Dr George Healy.

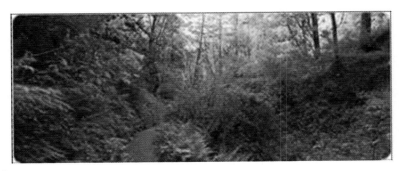

Image 11.3
Babesiosis is caused by parasites that infect red blood cells and are spread by certain ticks. In the United States, tickborne transmission is most common in parts of the Northeast and upper Midwest and it usually peaks during the warm months. Although many people who are infected with *Babesia* do not have symptoms, effective treatment is available if symptoms develop. Babesiosis is preventable if simple steps are taken to reduce exposure to ticks. Courtesy of Centers for Disease Control and Prevention.

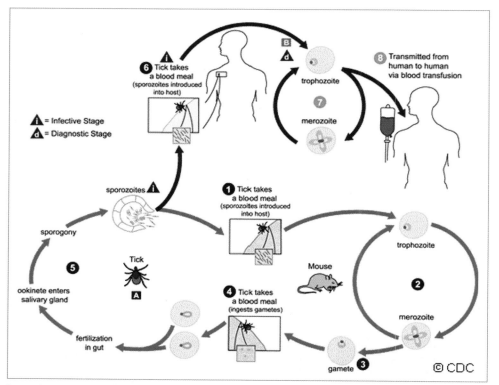

Image 11.4

The *Babesia microti* life cycle involves 2 hosts, which include a rodent, primarily the white-footed mouse *(Peromyscus leucopus)*. During a blood meal, a *Babesia*-infected tick introduces sporozoites into the mouse host (1). Sporozoites enter erythrocytes and undergo asexual reproduction (budding) (2). In the blood, some parasites differentiate into male and female gametes, although these cannot be distinguished at the light microscope level (3). The definitive host is a tick, in this case the deer tick *(Ixodes dammini [I scapularis])*. Once ingested by an appropriate tick (4), gametes unite and undergo a sporogonic cycle resulting in sporozoites (5). Transovarial transmission (also known as vertical, or hereditary, transmission) has been documented for "large" *Babesia* spp but not for the "small" *Babesia,* such as *B microti* (A).

During a blood meal, a *Babesia*-infected tick introduces sporozoites into the human host (6). Sporozoites enter erythrocytes (B) and undergo asexual replication (budding) (7). Multiplication of the blood stage parasites is responsible for the clinical manifestations of the disease. There is little, if any, subsequent transmission that occurs from ticks feeding on infected persons. However, human-to-human transmission is well recognized to occur through blood transfusions (8). Deer are the hosts on which the adult ticks feed and are indirectly part of the *Babesia* cycle, as they influence the tick population. When deer populations increase, the tick population also increases. Courtesy of Centers for Disease Control and Prevention.

12

Bacillus cereus Infections

Clinical Manifestations

Two clinical syndromes are associated with *Bacillus cereus* foodborne illness. The first is the emetic syndrome, which has a short incubation period and is characterized by nausea, vomiting, abdominal cramps and, in approximately 30% of patients, diarrhea. The second is the diarrhea syndrome, which has a slightly longer incubation period and is characterized predominantly by moderate to severe abdominal cramps and watery diarrhea, with vomiting in approximately 25% of patients. Both syndromes are mild, usually are not associated with fever, and abate within 24 hours.

B cereus also can cause local skin and wound infections (some can be severe, resembling gas gangrene), periodontitis, ocular infections, and invasive disease, including bacteremia, central line–associated bloodstream infection, endocarditis, osteomyelitis, pneumonia, brain abscess, and meningitis. Ocular involvement includes panophthalmitis, endophthalmitis, and keratitis.

Etiology

B cereus is an aerobic and facultatively anaerobic, spore-forming, gram-positive bacillus. The emetic syndrome is caused by a preformed heat-stable enterotoxin. The emetic toxin is cytotoxic, can cause rhabdomyolysis, and has been associated with fulminant liver failure. The diarrhea syndrome is caused by in vivo production of 1 or 2 heat-labile enterotoxins.

Epidemiology

B cereus is ubiquitous in the environment. It commonly is present in small numbers in raw, dried, and processed foods. It is a common cause of foodborne illness in the United States, but is rarely diagnosed because clinical laboratories do not test for it. Spores of *B cereus* are heat resistant and can survive pasteurization, brief cooking, or boiling. Vegetative forms can grow and produce enterotoxins over a wide range of temperatures, from 25°C to 42°C (77°F–108°F). The emetic syndrome occurs after eating food containing preformed toxin, most commonly fried rice. Disease can result from eating food contaminated with *B cereus* spores. Spore-associated disease most commonly is caused by contaminated meat or vegetables and manifests as the diarrhea syndrome. Foodborne illness caused by *B cereus* is not transmissible from person-to-person.

Risk factors for invasive disease attributable to *B cereus* include history of injection drug use, presence of indwelling intravascular catheters or implanted devices, neutropenia or immunosuppression, and preterm birth. *B cereus* endophthalmitis has occurred after penetrating ocular trauma and injection drug use. *Bacillus*-contaminated 70% alcohol pads can lead to outbreaks if not labeled as sterile.

Incubation Period

Emetic syndrome 0.5 to 6 hours; diarrhea syndrome 6 to 24 hours.

Diagnostic Tests

For foodborne illness, isolation of *B cereus* in a concentration of 10^5 colony-forming units/gram or greater of epidemiologically incriminated food establishes the diagnosis. Because stool specimens from some well people may contain *B cereus,* presence of the organism in feces or vomitus of ill people does not provide definitive evidence of infection. Food can be tested for the diarrhea syndrome toxins using commercially available tests. Phage typing, DNA hybridization, plasmid analysis, enzyme electrophoresis, and multilocus sequence typing have been used as epidemiologic tools in outbreaks of foodborne illness.

In patients with risk factors for invasive disease, isolation of *B cereus* from wounds, blood, or other usually sterile body fluids is diagnostic.

Treatment

People with *B cereus* food poisoning require only supportive treatment. Oral rehydration or, occasionally, intravenous fluid and electrolyte replacement for patients with severe dehydration is indicated. Antimicrobial agents are not indicated.

In patients with invasive disease, vancomycin is the drug of choice. Prompt removal of any potentially infected foreign bodies, such as central lines or implants, is essential. *B cereus* is susceptible to alternative drugs, including clindamycin, meropenem, imipenem, and ciprofloxacin. *B cereus* is resistant to beta-lactam antimicrobial agents.

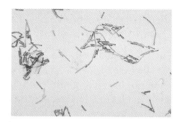

Image 12.1
Bacillus cereus subsp *mycoides* (Gram stain). *B cereus* is a known cause of toxin-induced food poisoning. These organisms may appear gram-variable as shown here. Courtesy of Centers for Disease Control and Prevention/ Dr William A. Clark.

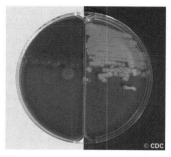

Image 12.2
Blood agar and bicarbonate agar plate cultures of *Bacillus cereus*. Negative encapsulation test. Rough colonies of *B cereus* on both blood and bicarbonate agars. Courtesy of Centers for Disease Control and Prevention/Dr James Feeley.

13

Bacterial Vaginosis

Clinical Manifestations

Bacterial vaginosis (BV), a polymicrobial clinical syndrome diagnosed primarily in sexually active postpubertal females, is characterized by changes in the vaginal flora. Classic signs, when present, include a thin white or grey, homogenous, adherent vaginal discharge with a fishy odor often noted to increase after intercourse. Although 84% of females with BV have no symptoms, the remainder have vaginal discharge that rarely can be accompanied by abdominal pain, pruritus, or dysuria. In pregnant women, BV has been associated with chorioamnionitis, preterm delivery, and postpartum endometritis.

Vaginitis and vulvitis in prepubertal girls rarely, if ever, are manifestations of BV. Causes of vaginitis in prepubertal girls frequently are nonspecific but include foreign bodies or infections attributable to group A streptococci, herpes simplex virus, *Neisseria gonorrhoeae, Chlamydia trachomatis, Trichomonas vaginalis,* or enteric bacteria, including *Shigella* species.

Etiology

The microbiologic cause of BV has not been delineated fully. Typical microbiologic findings in vaginal specimens show an increase in concentrations of *Gardnerella vaginalis,* genital mycoplasmas, anaerobic bacteria (eg, *Prevotella* species and *Mobiluncus* species), *Ureaplasma* species, *Mycoplasma* species, and a marked decrease in concentration of hydrogen peroxide–producing *Lactobacillus* species.

Epidemiology

BV is the most prevalent cause of vaginal discharge in sexually active adolescents and adult women. BV can accompany other conditions associated with vaginal discharge, such as trichomoniasis or cervicitis caused by other pathogens, such as *Neisseria gonorrhoeae* and *Chlamydia trachomatis.* Although evidence of sexual transmission of BV is inconclusive, correct and consistent use of condoms reduces the risk of acquisition. An increased prevalence of BV is associated with increasing number of sexual partners, a new sex partner, lack of condom use, and douching. Women who never have been sexually active also can be affected. Preexisting BV may be a risk factor for pelvic inflammatory disease. BV increases the risk of complications after gynecologic surgery, complications during pregnancy, and acquisition of many other sexually transmitted infections.

Incubation Period

Unknown.

Diagnostic Tests

The clinical diagnosis of BV requires the presence of 3 or more of the following symptoms or signs (Amsel criteria):

- Homogenous, thin gray or white, noninflammatory vaginal discharge that coats the vaginal walls
- Vaginal fluid pH greater than 4.5
- A fishy odor (amine test) of vaginal discharge before or after addition of 10% potassium hydroxide (ie, the "whiff test")
- Presence of "clue cells" (squamous vaginal epithelial cells covered with bacteria, which cause a stippled or granular appearance and ragged "moth-eaten" borders) on microscopic examination of at least 20% of vaginal epithelial cells.

A Gram stain of vaginal secretions is an alternative means of establishing the diagnosis and is considered by some experts the gold standard. A paucity of large gram-positive bacilli consistent with decreased lactobacilli and a predominance of gram-negative and gram-variable rods and cocci (eg, *G vaginalis, Prevotella* species, *Porphyromonas* species, and *Peptostreptococcus* species) with or without the presence of curved gram-negative rods (*Mobiluncus* species) are characteristic. Douching, recent intercourse, menstruation, and coexisting infection can alter findings on Gram stain. Culture of vaginal fluid is not recommended. Sexually active women should be evaluated for coinfection with other sexually transmitted infections, and hepatitis B and human papillomavirus immunization series should be documented.

Treatment

All nonpregnant patients who are symptomatic should be treated after discussion of patient preference for oral versus intravaginal treatment, possible adverse effects, and need to evaluate for other coinfections. Nonpregnant patients with symptoms should be treated with metronidazole for 7 days, tinidazole for 2 days, metronidazole gel intravaginally for 5 days, or clindamycin cream intravaginally, at bedtime, for 7 days. Clindamycin cream can weaken latex condoms and diaphragms for up to 5 days after completion of therapy. Approximately 30% of appropriately treated females have a recurrence within 3 months. Early relapse and relapses can occur. Retreatment with the same topical regimen is reasonable. For patients with multiple recurrences, metronidazole gel, twice weekly for 4 to 6 months, may be considered. Follow-up visits on completion of therapy for BV are unnecessary if symptoms resolve. Routine treatment of male sexual partners is not recommended.

Pregnant or breastfeeding women with symptoms of BV should be treated, regardless of history of prior risk factors for adverse pregnancy outcomes. Asymptomatic pregnant women with a history of adverse pregnancy outcomes (eg, previous preterm birth, premature rupture of membranes, chorioamnionitis) may be considered for treatment. Metronidazole is the preferred treatment.

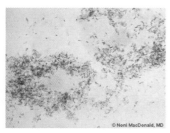

Image 13.1
Clue cells are squamous epithelial cells covered with bacteria found in bacterial vaginosis. Copyright Noni MacDonald, MD.

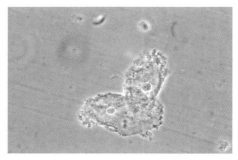

Image 13.2
This photomicrograph reveals bacteria adhering to vaginal epithelial cells known as clue cells. Clue cells are epithelial cells that have had bacteria adhere to their surface, obscuring their borders, and imparting a stippled appearance. The presence of such clue cells is a sign that the patient has bacterial vaginosis. Courtesy of Centers for Disease Control and Prevention/ M Rein.

14

Bacteroides and *Prevotella* Infections

Clinical Manifestations

Bacteroides and *Prevotella* organisms from the oral cavity can cause chronic sinusitis, chronic otitis media, dental infection, peritonsillar abscess, cervical adenitis, retropharyngeal space infection, aspiration pneumonia, lung abscess, pleural empyema, or necrotizing pneumonia. Species from the gastrointestinal tract are recovered in patients with peritonitis, intra-abdominal abscess, pelvic inflammatory disease, postoperative wound infection, or vulvovaginal and perianal infections. Soft tissue infections include synergistic bacterial gangrene and necrotizing fasciitis. Invasion of the bloodstream from the oral cavity or intestinal tract can lead to brain abscess, meningitis, endocarditis, arthritis, or osteomyelitis. Skin involvement can lead to omphalitis in newborn infants; cellulitis at the site of fetal monitors, human bite wounds, or burns; infections adjacent to the mouth or rectum; and decubitus ulcers. Neonatal infections, including conjunctivitis, pneumonia, bacteremia, or meningitis, rarely occur. Most *Bacteroides* and *Prevotella* infections are polymicrobial.

Etiology

Most *Bacteroides* and *Prevotella* organisms associated with human disease are pleomorphic, non–spore-forming, facultatively anaerobic, gram-negative bacilli.

Epidemiology

Bacteroides species and *Prevotella* species are part of the normal flora of the mouth, gastrointestinal tract, and female genital tract. Members of the *Bacteroides fragilis* group predominate in the gastrointestinal tract flora; members of the *Prevotella melaninogenica* (formerly *Bacteroides melaninogenicus*) and *Prevotella oralis* (formerly *Bacteroides oralis*) groups are found in the oral cavity. These species cause infection as opportunists, usually after an alteration of the body's physical barrier and in conjunction with other endogenous flora. Endogenous infection results from aspiration, spillage from the bowel, or damage to mucosal surfaces from trauma, surgery, or chemotherapy. Mucosal injury or granulocytopenia predispose to infection. Except in infections resulting from human bites, no evidence of person-to-person transmission exists.

Incubation Period

Variable depending on inoculum and site of involvement; usually 1 to 5 days.

Diagnostic Tests

Anaerobic culture media are necessary for recovery of *Bacteroides* or *Prevotella* species. Because infections usually are polymicrobial, aerobic cultures also should be obtained. A putrid odor suggests anaerobic infection. Use of an anaerobic transport tube or a sealed syringe is recommended for collection of clinical specimens.

Treatment

Abscesses should be drained when feasible; abscesses involving the brain, liver, and lungs may resolve with effective antimicrobial therapy. Necrotizing soft tissue lesions should be debrided surgically, and can require repeated procedures.

The choice of antimicrobial agent(s) is based on anticipated or known in vitro susceptibility testing. Bacteroides infections of the mouth and respiratory tract generally are susceptible to penicillin G, ampicillin, and extended-spectrum penicillins, such as ticarcillin or piperacillin. Clindamycin is active against virtually all mouth and respiratory tract *Bacteroides* and *Prevotella* isolates and is recommended by some experts as the drug of choice for anaerobic infections of the oral cavity and lungs. Some species of *Bacteroides* and almost 50% of *Prevotella* species produce beta-lactamase. A beta-lactam penicillin active against *Bacteroides* species combined with a beta-lactamase inhibitor (eg, piperacillin-tazobactam) can be useful to treat these infections. *Bacteroides* species of the gastrointestinal tract usually are resistant to penicillin G but are susceptible to metronidazole, beta-lactam plus beta-lactamase inhibitors, and sometimes clindamycin. More than 80% of isolates are susceptible to cefoxitin and meropenem. Cefuroxime, cefotaxime, and ceftriaxone are not reliably effective.

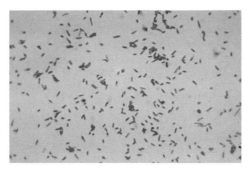

Image 14.1
This photomicrograph shows *Bacteroides fragilis* after being cultured in a thioglycollate medium for 48 hours. *B fragilis* is a gram-negative rod that constitutes 1% to 2% of the normal colonic bacterial microflora in humans. It is associated with extraintestinal infections such as abscesses and soft tissue infections, as well as diarrheal diseases. Courtesy of Centers for Disease Control and Prevention/Dr V.R. Dowell, Jr.

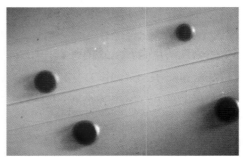

Image 14.2
Prevotella melaninogenica pigmented colonies. Courtesy of Centers for Disease Control and Prevention.

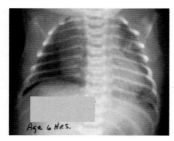

Image 14.3
Bacteroides fragilis pneumonia in a newborn (*B fragilis* isolated from the placenta and blood culture from the newborn). Anaerobic cultures were obtained because of a fecal odor in the amniotic fluid.

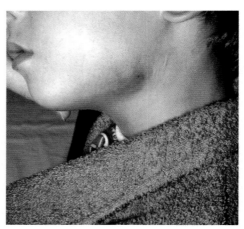

Image 14.4
Prevotella melaninogenica (previously *Bacteroides melaninogenica*) and group A alphahemolytic streptococcus cultured from a submandibular subcutaneous abscess aspirate from a 12-year-old boy. There was no apparent dental, pharyngeal, or middle ear infection.

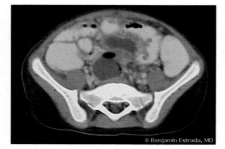

Image 14.5
Bacteroides fragilis abdominal abscess in a 9-year-old male. Copyright Benjamin Estrada, MD.

15

Balantidium coli Infections
(Balantidiasis)

Clinical Manifestations

Most human infections are asymptomatic. Acute symptomatic infection is characterized by rapid onset of nausea, vomiting, abdominal discomfort or pain, and bloody or watery mucoid diarrhea. In many patients, the course is chronic with intermittent episodes of diarrhea, anorexia, and weight loss. Rarely, organisms spread to mesenteric nodes, pleura, or liver. Inflammation of the gastrointestinal tract and local lymphatic vessels can result in bowel dilation, ulceration, and secondary bacterial invasion. Colitis produced by *Balantidium coli* often is indistinguishable from colitis produced by *Entamoeba histolytica*. Fulminant disease can occur in malnourished or otherwise debilitated or immunocompromised patients.

Etiology

B coli, a ciliated protozoan, is the largest pathogenic protozoan.

Epidemiology

Pigs are the primary host reservoir of *B coli*, but other sources have been reported. Infections occur in most areas of the world but are rare in industrialized countries. Cysts excreted in feces can be transmitted directly from hand to mouth or indirectly through fecally contaminated water or food. Excysted trophozoites infect the colon. A person is infectious as long as cysts are excreted in stool. Cysts are viable in the environment for months.

Incubation Period

Unknown, but may be several days.

Diagnostic Tests

Diagnosis is established by scraping lesions via sigmoidoscopy, histologic examination of intestinal biopsy specimens, or ova and parasite examination of stool. The diagnosis usually is established by demonstrating trophozoites (or less frequently, cysts) in stool or tissue specimens. Stool examination is not sensitive, and repeated stool examination is necessary to diagnose infection, because shedding of organisms can be intermittent. Microscopic examination of fresh diarrheal stools must be performed promptly.

Treatment

The drug of choice is a tetracycline, which should not be given to children younger than 8 years or during pregnancy unless the benefits of therapy are greater than the risks of dental staining. Alternative drugs are metronidazole and iodoquinol. Successful use of nitazoxanide also has been reported.

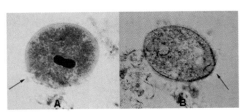

Image 15.1
Balantidium coli trophozoites are characterized by their large size (40–>70 μm); the presence of cilia on the cell surface, which are particularly visible in B; a cytostome (arrows); a bean-shaped macronucleus that is often visible (A); and a smaller, less conspicuous micronucleus. Courtesy of Centers for Disease Control and Prevention.

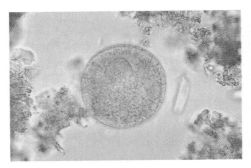

Image 15.2
Balantidium coli cyst in stool preparation. Courtesy of Centers for Disease Control and Prevention/Dr L.L.A. Moore, Jr.

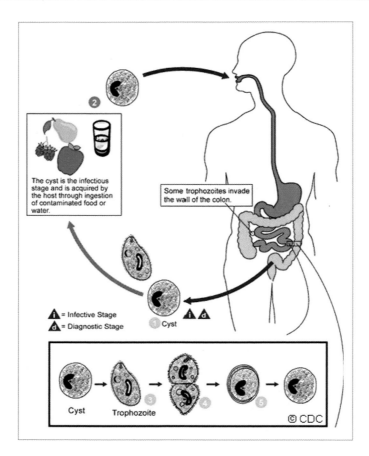

The cyst is the infectious stage and is acquired by the host through ingestion of contaminated food or water.

Some trophozoites invade the wall of the colon.

$\blacktriangle$ i = Infective Stage
$\blacktriangle$ d = Diagnostic Stage

① Cyst

Cyst   Trophozoite

© CDC

Image 15.3

Cysts are the parasite stage responsible for transmission of balantidiasis (1). The host most often acquires the cyst through ingestion of contaminated food or water (2). Following ingestion, excystation occurs in the small intestine, and the trophozoites colonize the large intestine (3). The trophozoites reside in the lumen of the large intestine of humans and animals, where they replicate by binary fission, during which conjugation may occur (4). Trophozoites undergo encystation to produce infective cysts (5). Some trophozoites invade the wall of the colon and multiply. Some return to the lumen and disintegrate. Mature cysts are passed with feces (1). Courtesy of Centers for Disease Control and Prevention/ Alexander J. da Silva, PhD/Melanie Moser.

16

Baylisascaris Infections

Clinical Manifestations

Baylisascaris procyonis, a raccoon roundworm, is a rare cause of acute eosinophilic meningo-encephalitis. In a young child, acute central nervous system (CNS) disease (eg, altered mental status and seizures) accompanied by peripheral and/or cerebrospinal fluid (CSF) eosinophilia occurs 2 to 4 weeks after infection. Severe neurologic sequelae or death are usual outcomes. *B procyonis* also is a rare cause of extraneural disease in older children and adults. Ocular larva migrans can result in diffuse unilateral subacute neuroretinitis; direct visualization of worms in the retina sometimes is possible. Visceral larval migrans can present with nonspecific signs, such as macular rash, pneumonitis, and hepatomegaly. Similar to visceral larva migrans caused by *Toxocara,* subclinical or asymptomatic infection is thought to be the most common infection.

Etiology

B procyonis is a 10- to 25-cm roundworm (nematode) with a life cycle usually limited to its definitive host, the raccoon, and to soil. Domestic dogs and some exotic pets, such as kinkajous and ringtails, can serve as definitive hosts and a potential source of human disease.

Epidemiology

B procyonis is distributed focally throughout the United States; in endemic regions, an estimated 22% to 80% of raccoons harbor this intestinal parasite. Embryonated eggs containing infective larvae are ingested from the soil by raccoons, rodents, and birds. When infective eggs or an infected host is eaten by a raccoon, the larvae grow to maturity in the small intestine where adult female worms shed millions of eggs per day. The eggs are 60 to 80 μm in size and have an outer shell that permits long-term viability in soil. Cases of raccoon infection have been reported in the Midwest, Northeast, West Coast, and more recently in the South.

Risk factors for *Baylisascaris* infection include contact with raccoon latrines and uncovered sand boxes, geophagia/pica, age younger than 4 years and, in older children, developmental delay and exposure to kinkajous and other related pets that may harbor this organism. Nearly all reported cases have been in males.

Diagnostic Tests

Baylisascaris infection is confirmed by identification of larvae in biopsy specimens. Serologic assays (serum, CSF) are available in research laboratories. A presumptive diagnosis can be made on the basis of clinical (meningoencephalitis, diffuse unilateral subacute neuroretinitis, pseudotumor), epidemiologic (raccoon exposure), and laboratory (blood and CSF eosinophilia) findings. Neuroimaging results can be normal initially, but as larvae grow and migrate through CNS tissue, focal abnormalities are found in periventricular white matter and elsewhere. In ocular disease, ophthalmologic examination can reveal characteristic chorioretinal lesions or rarely larvae. Because eggs are not shed in human feces, stool examination is not helpful. The disease is not transmitted from person to person.

Treatment

No drug has been demonstrated to be effective. On the basis of CNS and CSF penetration and in vitro activity, albendazole, in conjunction with high-dose corticosteroids, has been advocated most widely. Some experts advocate use of additional anthelmintic agents. Limited data are available regarding safety and efficacy of these therapies in children. Preventive therapy with albendazole should be considered for children with a history of ingestion of soil potentially contaminated with raccoon feces. Worms localized to the retina may be killed by direct photocoagulation.

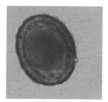

Image 16.1
Unembryonated egg of *Baylisascaris procyonis.*
B procyonis eggs are 80 to 85 μm by 65 to 70
μm in size, thick-shelled, and usually slightly oval
in shape. They have a similar morphology to
fertile eggs of *Ascaris lumbricoides,* although
eggs of *A lumbricoides* are smaller (55–75 μm by
35–50 μm). The definitive host for *B procyonis* is
the raccoon, although dogs may also serve as
definitive hosts. As humans do not serve as
definitive hosts for *B procyonis,* eggs are not
considered a diagnostic finding and are not
excreted in human feces. Courtesy of Cheryl
Davis, MD, Western Kentucky University, KY.

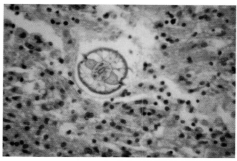

Image 16.2
Baylisascaris procyonis larva in cross-section
(at midbody level) (diameter, 60 μm) recovered
from the cerebrum of a rabbit with neural larval
migrans. Characteristic features include a centrally located (slightly compressed) intestine,
flanked on either side by large triangular-shaped
excretory columns. Prominent lateral cuticular
alae are visible on opposite sides of the body
(hematoxylin-eosin stain). Courtesy of Gavin.

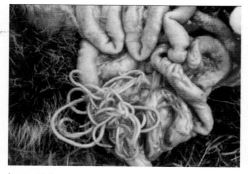

Image 16.3
Baylisascaris is raccoon roundworm, which may
cause ocular and neural larval migrans, and
encephalitis in humans. Photo used with permission of Michigan DNR Wildlife Disease Lab.

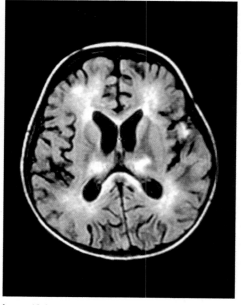

Image 16.4
Neuroimaging of human *Baylisascaris procyonis*
neural larval migrans. Axial T2-weighted magnetic resonance image (at the level of the lateral
ventricles) demonstrates abnormal patchy hyper-
intense signal of periventricular white matter and
basal ganglia. Courtesy of Gavin.

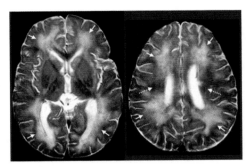

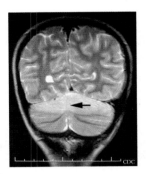

Image 16.5

Biopsy-proven *Baylisascaris procyonis* encephalitis in a 13-month-old boy. Axial T2-weighted magnetic resonance images obtained 12 days after symptom onset show abnormal high signal throughout most of the central white matter (arrows) compared with the dark signal expected at this age (broken arrows). Courtesy of Sorvillo F, Ash LR, Berlin OG, Morse SA. Baylisascaris procynois: an emerging helminthic zoonosis. *Emerg Infect Dis.* 2002;8(4):355–359.

Image 16.6

Coronal T2-weighted magnetic resonance imaging of the brain in a 4-year-old child with *Baylisascaris procyonis* eosinophilic meningitis. Arrow shows diffuse edema of the superior cerebellar hemispheres (scale bar increments = cm). Courtesy of Centers for Disease Control and Prevention/*Emerging Infectious Diseases* and Poulomi J. Pai.

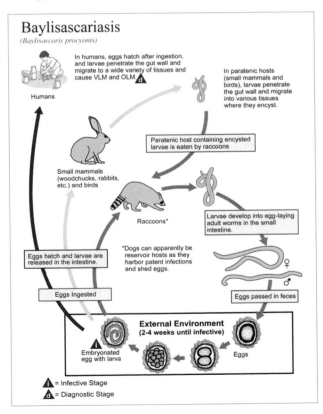

Image 16.7

This illustration depicts the life cycle of *Baylisascaris procyonis,* the causal agent of baylisascariasis. Courtesy of Centers for Disease Control and Prevention/Alexander J. da Silva, PhD/Melanie Moser.

17

Blastocystis hominis Infections

Clinical Manifestations

The importance of *Blastocystis hominis* as a cause of gastrointestinal tract disease is controversial. The asymptomatic carrier state is well documented. *B hominis* has been associated with symptoms of bloating, flatulence, mild to moderate diarrhea without fecal leukocytes or blood, abdominal pain, nausea, and poor weight gain. When *B hominis* is identified in stool from symptomatic patients, other causes of this symptom complex, particularly *Giardia intestinalis* and *Cryptosporidium parvum,* should be investigated before assuming that *B hominis* is the cause of the illness.

Etiology

B hominis previously has been classified as a protozoan, but molecular studies have characterized it as a stramenopile (a eukaryote). Multiple forms include vacuolar, which is observed most commonly in clinical specimens; granular; ameboid; and cystic.

Epidemiology

B hominis is recovered from 1% to 20% of stool specimens examined for ova and parasites. Because transmission is believed to be fecal-oral, presence of the organism may be a marker of other pathogens spread by fecal contamination. Transmission from animals occurs.

Incubation Period

Unknown.

Diagnostic Tests

Stool specimens should be preserved in polyvinyl alcohol and stained with trichrome or iron-hematoxylin before microscopic examination. The parasite can be found in small or large numbers. The presence of 5 or more organisms per high-power (x400 magnification) field can indicate heavy infection that, to some experts, suggests causation when other enteropathogens are absent. Other experts consider 10 or more organisms per 10 oil immersion fields (x1,000 magnification) to represent heavy infection.

Treatment

Some experts recommend treatment only for patients with persistent symptoms and in whom no other pathogens are found. Randomized controlled treatment trials for both nitazoxanide and metronidazole have demonstrated benefit in symptomatic patients. Other experts believe that *B hominis* does not cause symptomatic disease and recommend only a careful search for other causes of symptoms.

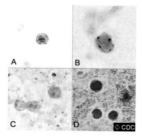

Image 17.1
A–D: *Blastocystis hominis* cyst-like forms (trichrome stain). The sizes vary from 4 to 10 μm. The vacuoles stain variably from red to blue. The nuclei in the peripheral cytoplasmic rim are clearly visible, staining purple (B) (4 nuclei). Specimens A–C contributed by Ray Kaplan, MD, SmithKline Beecham Diagnostic Laboratories, Atlanta, GA; D courtesy of Centers for Disease Control and Prevention.

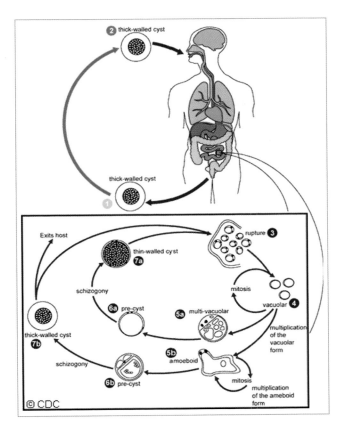

Image 17.2

Knowledge of the life cycle and transmission is still under investigation; therefore, this is a proposed life cycle for *Blastocystis hominis*. The classic form found in human stools is the cyst, which varies tremendously in size from 6 to 40 μm (1). The thick-walled cyst present in the stools (1) is believed to be responsible for external transmission, possibly by the fecal-oral route through ingestion of contaminated water or food (2). The cysts infect epithelial cells of the digestive tract and multiply asexually (3, 4). Vacuolar forms of the parasite give origin to multi-vacuolar (5a) and ameboid (5b) forms. The multi-vacuolar develops into a pre-cyst (6a) that gives origin to a thin-walled cyst (7a) thought to be responsible for autoinfection. The ameboid form gives origin to a pre-cyst (6b), which develops into a thick-walled cyst by schizogony (7b). *B hominis* stages were reproduced from Singh M, Suresh K, Ho LC, Ng GC, Yap EH. Elucidation of the life cycle of the intestinal protozoan *Blastocystis hominis. Parasitol Res.* 1995;81:449. Permission granted by Springer Science + Business Media.

18

Blastomycosis

Clinical Manifestations

Infections can be acute, chronic, or fulminant but are asymptomatic in up to 50% of infected people. The most common manifestation of blastomycosis in children is pulmonary disease, with fever, chest pain, and nonspecific symptoms, such as fatigue and myalgia. Rarely, patients may develop acute respiratory distress syndrome. Typical radiographic patterns include patchy pneumonitis, a mass-like infiltrate, or nodules. Disseminated blastomycosis, which can occur in up to 25% of cases, most commonly involves the skin, osteoarticular structures, and the genitourinary tract. Cutaneous manifestations can be verrucous, nodular, ulcerative, or pustular. Abscesses usually are subcutaneous but can involve any organ. Central nervous system infection is rare, as is intrauterine or congenital infection.

Etiology

Blastomycosis is caused by *Blastomyces dermatitidis*, a dimorphic fungus existing in the yeast form at 37°C (98°F), in infected tissues, and in a mycelial form at room temperature and in soil. Conidia, produced from hyphae of the mycelial form, are infectious.

Epidemiology

Infection is acquired through inhalation of conidia from soil. Person-to-person transmission does not occur. Blastomycosis is endemic in certain areas of the United States, with most cases occurring in the Ohio and Mississippi river valleys, the southeastern states, and states that border the Great Lakes. Sporadic cases also have been reported in Hawaii, Israel, India, Africa, and Central and South America. Blastomycosis can occur in immunocompetent and immunocompromised hosts.

Incubation Period

2 weeks to 3 months.

Diagnostic Tests

Definitive diagnosis of blastomycosis is based on identification of characteristic thick-walled, broad-based, single budding yeast cells either by culture or histopathology. The organism can be seen in sputum, tracheal aspirates, cerebrospinal fluid, urine, or material from lesions processed with 10% potassium hydroxide or a silver stain. Children with pneumonia who are unable to produce sputum may require bronchoalveolar lavage or open biopsy to establish the diagnosis. Organisms can be cultured on brain-heart infusion media and Sabouraud dextrose agar at room temperature. Chemiluminescent DNA probes are available for identification of *B dermatitidis*. Because serologic tests (immunodiffusion and complement fixation) lack adequate sensitivity, every effort should be made to obtain appropriate specimens for culture.

Treatment

Amphotericin B is the treatment of choice for severe infection. Liposomal amphotericin B is recommended for central nervous system infection. Oral itraconazole or fluconazole can be used for mild or moderate infections, either alone or after a short course of amphotericin B. Although itraconazole is indicated for treatment of nonmeningeal, non–life-threatening infections in adults, the safety and efficacy of this agent in children with blastomycosis has not been established; however, its use in children in this setting has been recommended. Therapy usually is continued for at least 6 months for pulmonary and extrapulmonary disease.

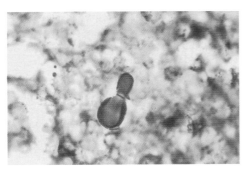

Image 18.1
Histopathology of blastomycosis. Yeast cell of
Blastomyces dermatitidis undergoing broad-base
budding (methenamine silver stain). Courtesy of
Centers for Disease Control and Prevention/
Libero Ajello, MD.

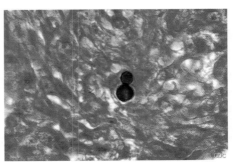

Image 18.2
This photomicrograph depicts the fungal agent
Blastomyces dermatitidis (hematoxylin-eosin
stain). Courtesy of Centers for Disease Control
and Prevention/Libero Ajello, MD.

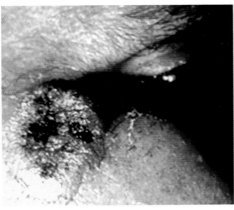

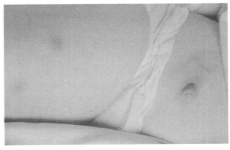

Image 18.4
Nodular skin lesions of blastomycosis, one of
which is a bullous lesion on top of a nodule.
Aspiration of the bulla revealed yeast forms of
Blastomyces dermatitidis. Courtesy of Centers
for Disease Control and Prevention.

Image 18.3
Cutaneous blastomycosis (face). Cutaneous
lesions are nodular, verrucous, or ulcerative as in
this man. Most cutaneous lesions are due to
hematogenous spread from a pulmonary infection. Courtesy of Edgar O. Ledbetter, MD, FAAP.

19

Borrelia Infections

(Relapsing Fever)

Clinical Manifestations

Two types of relapsing fever occur in humans: tickborne and louseborne. Both are characterized by sudden onset of high fever, shaking chills, sweats, headache, muscle and joint pain, and nausea. A fleeting macular rash of the trunk and petechiae of the skin and mucous membranes sometimes occur. Findings and complications can differ between types of relapsing fever and include hepatosplenomegaly, jaundice, thrombocytopenia, iridocyclitis, cough with pleuritic pain, pneumonitis, meningitis, and myocarditis. Mortality rates are 10% to 70% in untreated louseborne relapsing fever (possibly related to comorbidities in refugee-type settings where this disease typically is found) and 4% to 10% in untreated tickborne relapsing fever. Death occurs predominantly in people with underlying illnesses or extremes of age. Early treatment reduces mortality. Untreated, an initial febrile period of 2 to 7 days terminates spontaneously by crisis. This is followed by an afebrile period of days to weeks, then by one relapse or more (0–13 for tickborne, 1–5 for louseborne). Relapses typically become shorter and milder progressively as afebrile periods lengthen. Infection during pregnancy often is severe and can result in preterm birth, abortion, stillbirth, or neonatal infection.

Etiology

Relapsing fever is caused by certain spirochetes of the genus *Borrelia*. *Borrelia recurrentis* is the only species that causes louseborne (epidemic) relapsing fever, and there is no animal reservoir of *B recurrentis*. Worldwide, at least 14 *Borrelia* species cause tickborne (endemic) relapsing fever, including *Borrelia hermsii*, *Borrelia turicatae,* and *Borrelia parkeri* in North America.

Epidemiology

Louseborne epidemic relapsing fever has been reported in Ethiopia, Eritrea, Somalia, and the Sudan, especially in refugee and displaced populations. Epidemic transmission occurs when body lice *(Pediculus humanus)* become infected by feeding on humans with spirochetemia; infection is transmitted when infected lice are crushed and their body fluids contaminate a bite wound or skin abraded by scratching.

Endemic tickborne relapsing fever is distributed widely throughout the world, is transmitted by soft-bodied ticks (*Ornithodoros* species), and occurs sporadically and in small clusters, often within families. Ticks become infected by feeding on rodents or other small mammals and transmit infection via their saliva and other fluids when they take subsequent blood meals. Ticks serve as reservoirs of infection. Soft-bodied ticks inflict painless bites and feed briefly (10–30 minutes), usually at night, so people often are unaware of bites.

Most tickborne relapsing fever in the United States is caused by *B hermsii*. Infection typically results from tick exposures in rodent-infested cabins in western mountainous areas, including state and national parks. *B turicatae* infections occur less frequently; most cases have been reported from Texas and often are associated with tick exposures in rodent-infested caves.

Infected body lice and ticks remain alive and infectious for several years without feeding. Relapsing fever is not transmitted person to person, but perinatal transmission from an infected mother to her infant does occur.

Incubation Period

7 days (range 2–18).

Diagnostic Tests

Spirochetes can be observed by dark field microscopy and in Wright-, Giemsa-, or acridine orange-stained preparations of thin or dehemoglobinized thick smears of peripheral blood or in stained buffy-coat preparations. Organisms often can be detected in blood obtained during febrile episodes. Spirochetes can be cultured from blood in Barbour-Stoenner-Kelly medium or by intraperitoneal inoculation of immature laboratory mice. Serum antibodies to *Borrelia* species can be detected by enzyme immunoassay and Western immunoblot analysis at some reference and commercial specialty laboratories; these tests are not standardized and are affected by antigenic variations among and within *Borrelia* species and strains. Serologic cross-reactions occur with other spirochetes, including *Borrelia burgdorferi, Treponema pallidum,* and *Leptospira* species.

Treatment

Treatment of tickborne relapsing fever with a 5- to 10-day course of a tetracycline, usually doxycycline, produces prompt clearance of spirochetes and remission of symptoms. For children younger than 8 years of age and for pregnant women, penicillin or erythromycin is the preferred drug. Penicillin G procaine or intravenous penicillin G is recommended as initial therapy for people who are unable to take oral therapy, although low-dose penicillin G has been associated with a higher frequency of relapse. A Jarisch-Herxheimer reaction (an acute febrile reaction accompanied by headache, myalgia, and an aggravated clinical picture lasting less than 24 hours) commonly is observed during the first few hours after initiating antimicrobial therapy. Because this reaction sometimes is associated with transient hypotension attributable to decreased effective circulating blood volume (especially in louseborne relapsing fever), patients should be hospitalized and monitored closely, particularly during the first 4 hours of treatment. However, the Jarisch-Herxheimer reaction in children typically is mild and usually can be managed with antipyretic agents alone.

Single-dose treatment using a tetracycline, penicillin, erythromycin, or chloramphenicol is effective for curing louseborne relapsing fever.

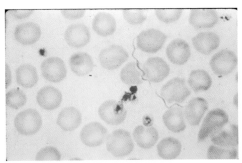

Image 19.1
Relapsing fever. Thin smear of peripheral blood showing a spirochete of *Borrelia* (Wright stain). Courtesy of Gary Overturf, MD.

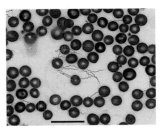

Image 19.2
Borrelia hermsii in a thin smear of mouse blood stained with Wright-Giemsa and visualized with oil immersion bright-field microscopy (x600) for the confirmation of infection with relapsing fever spirochetes in humans and other animals (scale bar = 20 mm). Courtesy of Schwan TG, Policastro PF, Miller Z, Thompson RL, Damrow T, Keirans JE. Tickborne relapsing fever caused by Borrelia hermsii, Montana. *Emerg Infect Dis.* 2003;9(9):1151–1154.

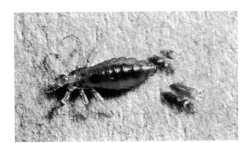

Image 19.3
This image depicts an adult female body louse, *Pediculus humanus,* and 2 larval young. *P humanus* has been shown to serve as a vector for diseases such as typhus due to *Rickettsia prowazekii,* trench fever caused by *Rochalimaea quintana,* and relapsing fever due to *Borrelia recurrentis.* Courtesy of World Health Organization.

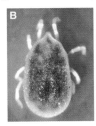

Image 19.4
An *Ornithodoros hermsi* nymph. The length of the soft bodied tick is 3.0 μm, excluding the legs. It is responsible for transmitting endemic relapsing fever. Courtesy of Schwan TG, Policastro PF, Miller Z, Thompson RL, Damrow T, Keirans JE. Tick-borne relapsing fever caused by Borrelia hermsii, Montana. *Emerg Infect Dis.* 2003;9(9):1151–1154.

20

Brucellosis

Clinical Manifestations

Onset of brucellosis in children can be acute or insidious. Manifestations are nonspecific and include fever, night sweats, weakness, malaise, anorexia, weight loss, arthralgia, myalgia, abdominal pain, and headache. Physical findings may include lymphadenopathy, hepatosplenomegaly, and arthritis. Abdominal pain and peripheral arthritis are reported more frequently in children than in adults. Neurologic deficits, ocular involvement, epididymoorchitis, liver or spleen abscesses, anemia, thrombocytopenia, and pancytopenia also are reported. Serious complications include meningitis, endocarditis, and osteomyelitis. Chronic disease is less common among children than among adults, although rate of relapse is similar.

Etiology

Brucella bacteria are aerobic small, nonmotile, gram-negative coccobacilli. The species that are known to infect humans are *Brucella abortus, Brucella melitensis, Brucella suis* and, rarely, *Brucella canis.* Three recently identified species, *Brucella ceti, Brucella pinnipedialis,* and *Brucella inopinata,* are potential human pathogens.

Epidemiology

Brucellosis is a zoonotic disease of wild and domestic animals. It is transmissible to humans by direct or indirect exposure to aborted fetuses or tissues or fluids of infected animals. Transmission occurs by inoculation through mucous membranes or cuts and abrasions in the skin, inhalation of contaminated aerosols, or ingestion of undercooked meat or unpasteurized dairy products. People in occupations such as farming, ranching, and veterinary medicine as well as abattoir workers, meat inspectors, and laboratory personnel are at increased risk. Clinicians should alert the laboratory if they anticipate *Brucella* may grow from microbiologic specimens so that appropriate laboratory precautions can be taken. In the United States, 100 to 200 cases of brucellosis are reported annually: 3% to 10% of cases occur in children and result from ingestion of unpasteurized dairy products. Although human-to-human transmission is rare, in utero and breast milk transmission has been reported.

Incubation Period

Variable but usually 3 to 4 weeks after exposure.

Diagnostic Tests

A definitive diagnosis is established by recovery of *Brucella* species from blood, bone marrow, or other tissue specimens. A variety of media will support growth of *Brucella* species, but cultures should be incubated for a minimum of 4 weeks. Newer BACTEC systems have greater reliability and can detect *Brucella* species within 5 to 7 days. In patients with a clinically compatible illness, serologic testing can confirm the diagnosis with a fourfold or greater increase in antibody titers between acute and convalescent serum specimens collected at least 2 weeks apart. The serum agglutination test, the gold standard test for diagnosis, will detect antibodies against *B abortus, B suis,* and *B melitensis; B canis* requires specific antigen testing. Most patients with active infection will have a titer of 1:160 or greater within 2 to 4 weeks of clinical disease onset. Immunoglobulin (Ig) M is produced within 7 days, followed by a gradual increase in *Brucella* antigen-specific IgG. Low IgM titers may persist for months or years. Increased concentrations of IgG agglutinins are found in acute infection, chronic infection, and relapse. When interpreting serum agglutination test results, the possibility of cross-reactions of *Brucella* antibodies with antibodies against other gram-negative bacteria, such as *Yersinia enterocolitica* serotype 09, *Francisella tularensis,* and *Vibrio cholerae,* should be considered. Enzyme immunoassay is a sensitive method for determining IgG, IgA, and IgM anti-*Brucella* antibody titers. Until better standardization is established, enzyme immunoassay should be used only for suspected cases with negative serum agglutination test results or for evaluation of patients with suspected chronic brucellosis, reinfection, or complicated cases.

Treatment

Oral doxycycline or tetracycline is the drug of choice and should be administered for a minimum of 6 weeks. However, oral trimethoprim-sulfamethoxazole for at least 4 to 6 weeks is appropriate therapy for younger children. To decrease the rate of relapse, combination therapy with a tetracycline (or trimethoprim-sulfamethoxazole if tetracyclines are contraindicated) and rifampin is recommended. Because of the potential emergence of rifampin resistance, rifampin monotherapy is not recommended. Prolonged antimicrobial therapy is imperative for achieving a cure. Relapses generally are associated with premature discontinuation of therapy.

For treatment of serious infections or complications, including endocarditis, meningitis, spondylitis and osteomyelitis, gentamicin for the first 7 to 14 days of therapy, in addition to a tetracycline and rifampin for a minimum of 6 weeks (or trimethoprim-sulfamethoxazole, if tetracyclines are not used), are recommended. For life-threatening complications of brucellosis, such as meningitis or endocarditis, the duration of therapy often is extended for 4 to 6 months. Surgical intervention should be considered in patients with complications, such as deep tissue abscesses, endocarditis, mycotic aneurysm, and foreign body infections.

The benefit of corticosteroids for people with neurobrucellosis is unproven.

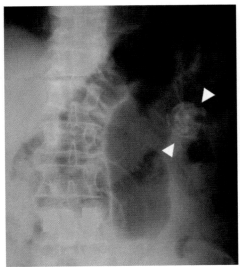

Image 20.1
A calcified *Brucella* granuloma in the spleen of a man with fever of several years' duration. *Brucella* organisms that survive the action of polymorphonuclear leukocytes are ingested by macrophages and become localized in the organs of the reticuloendothelial system.

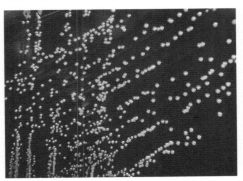

Image 20.2
Brucella melitensis colonies. *Brucella* spp colony characteristics: Fastidious organism and colonies usually are not visible at 24 hours. *Brucella* grows slowly on most standard laboratory media (eg, sheep blood, chocolate, and trypticase soy agars). Pinpoint, smooth, translucent, non-hemolytic colonies are shown at 48 hours of incubation. Courtesy of Centers for Disease Control and Prevention/Larry Stauffer, Oregon State Public Health Laboratory.

21

Burkholderia Infections

Clinical Manifestations

Burkholderia cepacia complex has been associated with severe pulmonary infections in patients with cystic fibrosis, significant bacteremia in preterm infants after prolonged hospitalization, and infection in children with chronic granulomatous disease, hemoglobinopathies, or malignant neoplasms. Health care–associated infections include wound and urinary tract infections and pneumonia. In patients with cystic fibrosis pulmonary infections occur late in the course of disease, typically after respiratory epithelial damage caused by *Pseudomonas aeruginosa* infection. Patients with *B cepacia* complex infection can become chronically infected and experience a change in the rate of pulmonary decompensation, exhibit a more rapid decline in pulmonary function, or experience an unexpectedly rapid deterioration in clinical status resulting in death. In patients with chronic granulomatous disease, pneumonia is the most common manifestation of *B cepacia* complex infection; lymphadenitis also occurs. Disease onset is insidious, with low-grade fever early in the course and systemic symptoms occurring 3 to 4 weeks later. Pleural effusion is common, and lung abscess can occur.

Burkholderia pseudomallei is the cause of **melioidosis**, which is endemic in Southeast Asia and northern Australia but also is found in other tropical and subtropical areas, including the Indian Subcontinent and South and Central America. Melioidosis can occur in the United States, usually among travelers returning from areas with endemic disease. Melioidosis can be asymptomatic, manifest as a localized infection, or present as fulminant septicemia. Pericarditis, septic arthritis, prostatic abscess, and brain abscess associated with nonsepticemic melioidosis also have been reported. Acute suppurative parotitis is a frequent manifestation that occurs in children in Thailand. Localized infection usually is nonfatal and most commonly manifests as pneumonia, but skin, soft tissue, and skeletal infections also occur. In severe cutaneous infection, necrotizing fasciitis has been reported. In dissemi-nated infection, hepatic and splenic abscesses can occur, and relapses are common without prolonged therapy.

Etiology

Burkholderia organisms are nutritionally diverse, oxidase- and catalase-producing, non–lactose-fermenting, gram-negative bacilli. *B cepacia* complex comprises at least 10 species (*B cepacia*, *Burkholderia multivorans*, *Burkholderia cenocepacia*, *Burkholderia stabilis*, *Burkholderia vietnamiensis*, *Burkholderia dolosa*, *Burkholderia ambifaria*, *Burkholderia anthina*, *Burkholderia pyrrocinia*, and *Burkholderia ubonensis*). Other species of *Burkholderia* include *Burkholderia gladioli*, *Burkholderia mallei* (the agent responsible for glanders), *Burkholderia thailandensis*, *Burkholderia oklahomensis*, and *B pseudomallei*.

Epidemiology

Burkholderia species are waterborne and soil-borne organisms that can survive for prolonged periods in a moist environment. Epidemiologic studies of recreational camps and social events attended by people with cystic fibrosis from different geographic areas have demonstrated person-to-person spread of *B cepacia* complex. The source for acquisition of *B cepacia* complex by patients with chronic granulomatous disease has not been identified. Health care–associated spread of *B cepacia* complex most often is associated with contamination of disinfectant solutions used to clean reusable patient equipment, such as bronchoscopes and pressure transducers, or to disinfect skin. Contaminated medical products, including mouthwash and inhaled medications, have been identified as a cause of multistate outbreaks of colonization and infection. *B gladioli* also has been isolated from sputum from people with cystic fibrosis and can be mistaken for *B cepacia*. The clinical significance of *B gladioli* is unknown.

In areas with highly endemic infection, *B pseudomallei* is acquired early in life, with the highest seroconversion rates between 6 and 42 months of age. Disease can be acquired by direct inhalation of aerosolized organisms or dust particles containing organisms, by percutaneous or wound inoculation with contaminated soil or water, or by ingestion of contaminated soil or water. Symptomatic infection can occur in infants. Risk factors for disease include frequent contact with soil and water as well as underlying chronic disease, such as diabetes mellitus and renal insufficiency, with most people presenting with melioidosis in areas with endemic disease. *B pseudomallei* also has been reported to cause pulmonary infection in people with cystic fibrosis and people traveling to areas with endemic infection as well as septicemia in children with chronic granulomatous disease.

Incubation Period

Median of 9 days (range 1–21); can be prolonged (years) for melioidosis.

Diagnostic Tests

Isolation of *B cepacia* complex from patients is diagnostic. In cystic fibrosis lung infection, culture of sputum on selective agar is recommended to decrease the potential for overgrowth by mucoid *Pseudomonas aeruginosa*. Definitive diagnosis of melioidosis is made by isolation of *B pseudomallei* from blood or other infected sites. The likelihood of successfully isolating the organism is increased by culture of sputum, throat, rectum, and ulcer or skin lesion specimens. A positive result by the indirect hemagglutination assay for a traveler who has returned from an area with endemic infection may support the diagnosis of melioidosis, but definitive diagnosis still requires isolation of *B pseudomallei* from an infected site.

Treatment

Meropenem is the agent most active against most *B cepacia* complex isolates, although other drugs that may be effective include imipenem, trimethoprim-sulfamethoxazole, ceftazidime, doxycycline, and chloramphenicol. Most experts recommend combinations of antimicrobial agents that provide synergistic activity against *B cepacia* complex. Nearly all *B cepacia* complex isolates are intrinsically resistant to aminoglycosides and colistin. The drugs of choice for initial treatment of melioidosis include ceftazidime and meropenem or imipenem for a minimum of 10 to 14 days. After acute therapy is completed, eradication therapy with trimethoprim-sulfamethoxazole and doxycycline for 12 to 24 weeks is recommended to reduce recurrence.

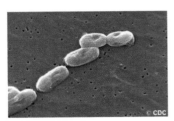

Image 21.1
Scanning electron micrograph of *Burkholderia cepacia*. *Burkholderia* infections often have an insidious onset, and *B cepacia* is a nosocomial pathogen. Courtesy of Centers for Disease Control and Prevention/Janice Haney Carr.

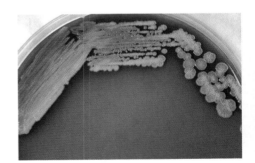

Image 21.2
This photograph depicts the colonial morphology displayed by gram-negative *Burkholderia pseudomallei* bacteria, which was grown on a medium of chocolate agar, for a 72-hour period, at a temperature of 37°C. Courtesy of Centers for Disease Control and Prevention/Dr Todd Parker, Audra Marsh.

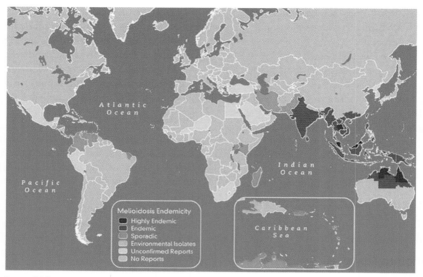

Image 21.3

Endemicity of melioidosis infection. Courtesy of Centers for Disease Control and Prevention National Center for Emerging and Zoonotic Infectious Diseases Division of Global Migration and Quarantine.

22

Human Calicivirus Infections (Norovirus and Sapovirus)

Clinical Manifestations

Abrupt onset of vomiting accompanied by watery diarrhea, abdominal cramps, and nausea are characteristic of human calicivirus (HuCV) infections. Mild to moderate diarrhea without vomiting is common in children. Symptoms last from 24 to 60 hours. Systemic manifestations, including myalgia, malaise, and headache, may accompany gastrointestinal tract symptoms.

Etiology

Caliciviruses are 20- to 40-nm, nonenveloped, single-stranded RNA viruses of the family *Caliciviridae*. This family is divided into 5 genera (*Lagovirus, Nebovirus, Vesivirus, Sapovirus,* and *Norovirus*), with the noroviruses and sapoviruses associated with disease in humans. HuCVs are diverse genetically and antigenically, but for epidemiologic purposes, they are classified into genogroups and genotypes.

Epidemiology

Although noroviruses and sapoviruses include some viruses found in animals, humans are considered the primary reservoir for HuCVs that cause human disease. HuCVs have a worldwide distribution, with multiple antigenic types circulating simultaneously in the same region. The most commonly detected HuCVs are noroviruses, which are a major cause of sporadic cases and outbreaks of acute gastroenteritis in the United States. The norovirus genogroup 2 type 4 (GII.4) has been predominant during the past decade in the United States, Europe, and Oceania. Sapovirus infections are reported mainly among children with sporadic acute diarrhea, although sapoviruses increasingly have been recognized as a cause of outbreaks. Asymptomatic norovirus excretion is common across all age groups, with the highest prevalence in children. Outbreaks with high incidences tend to occur in closed populations, such as nursing homes, child care centers, and cruise ships. Transmission is by person-to-person spread via the fecal-oral route or through contaminated food or water. Norovirus is recognized as the most common cause of foodborne illness and foodborne disease outbreaks in the United States. Common-source outbreaks have been described after ingestion of ice, shellfish, and a variety of ready-to-eat foods, including salads and bakery products, usually contaminated by infected food handlers. Transmission via vomitus has been documented, and exposure to contaminated surfaces and aerosolized vomitus has been implicated in some outbreaks. Viral excretion peaks 4 days after exposure and may persist for as long as 3 weeks. Prolonged excretion can occur in immunocompromised hosts. Infection occurs year-round.

Incubation Period

12 to 48 hours.

Diagnostic Tests

Commercial assays for diagnosis of individual cases are not available in the United States. The following tests are available in some research and reference laboratories: electron microscopy for detection of viral particles in stool, enzyme immunoassay for detection of viral antigen in stool or antibody in serum, and reverse transcriptase PCR assay for detection of viral RNA in stool. Laboratory and epidemiologic support for investigation of suspected calicivirus outbreaks is available at the Centers for Disease Control and Prevention.

Treatment

Supportive therapy includes oral or intravenous rehydration solutions to replace and maintain fluid and electrolyte balance.

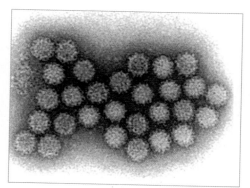

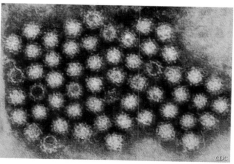

Image 22.1

This is a norovirus in a stool specimen from a patient with acute gastroenteritis, visualized by negative contrast staining and transmission electron microscopy. Particles frequently appear in clumps. Noroviruses are small, round-structured viruses (particle size 28–32 nm) with a rough surface that contrasts with the smooth edge of astroviruses and picornaviruses, which also can be found in stool specimens. Copyright David O. Matson, MD, PhD, FAAP.

Image 22.2

This transmission electron micrograph revealed some of the ultrastructural morphology displayed by norovirus virions, or virus particles. Noroviruses belong to the genus *Norovirus* and the family Caliciviridae. They are a group of related, single-stranded RNA, nonenveloped viruses that cause acute gastroenteritis in humans. Courtesy of Centers for Disease Control and Prevention/ Charles D. Humphrey.

23

Campylobacter Infections

Clinical Manifestations

Predominant symptoms of *Campylobacter* infections include diarrhea, abdominal pain, malaise, and fever. Stools can contain visible or occult blood. In neonates and young infants, bloody diarrhea without fever can be the only manifestation of infection. Fever can be pronounced in children and results in febrile seizures that can have onset before gastrointestinal tract symptoms. Abdominal pain can mimic that produced by appendicitis or intussusception. Mild infection lasts 1 or 2 days and resembles viral gastroenteritis. Most patients recover in less than 1 week, but 10% to 20% have a relapse or a prolonged or severe illness. Severe or persistent infection can mimic acute inflammatory bowel disease. Bacteremia is uncommon but can occur in children, including neonates. Immunocompromised hosts can have prolonged, relapsing, or extraintestinal infections, especially with *Campylobacter fetus* and other *Campylobacter* species. Immunoreactive complications, such as acute idiopathic polyneuritis (Guillain-Barré syndrome), Miller Fisher syndrome (ophthalmoplegia, areflexia, ataxia), reactive arthritis, Reiter syndrome (arthritis, urethritis, and bilateral conjunctivitis), myocarditis, pericarditis, and erythema nodosum, can occur during convalescence.

Etiology

Campylobacter species are motile, comma-shaped, gram-negative bacilli. There are 21 species within the genus *Campylobacter*, but *Campylobacter jejuni* and *Campylobacter coli* are the species isolated most commonly from patients with diarrhea. *C fetus* predominantly causes systemic illness in neonates and debilitated hosts. Other *Campylobacter* species, including *Campylobacter upsaliensis*, *Campylobacter lari*, and *Campylobacter hyointestinalis*, can cause similar diarrheal or systemic illnesses in children.

Epidemiology

Data from the Foodborne Diseases Active Surveillance Network (**www.cdc.gov/foodnet**) indicate a 30% decrease in the incidence of infections since 1996 but little change in incidence since 2004. The highest rates of infection occur in children younger than 4 years. In susceptible people, as few as 500 organisms can cause infection.

The gastrointestinal tracts of domestic and wild birds and animals are reservoirs of infection. *C jejuni* and *C coli* have been isolated from feces of 30% to 100% of healthy chickens, turkeys, and water fowl. Poultry carcasses usually are contaminated. Many farm animals and meat sources can harbor the organism, and pets (especially young animals), including dogs, cats, hamsters, and birds, are potential sources of infection. Transmission of *C jejuni* and *C coli* occurs by ingestion of contaminated food or by direct contact with fecal material from infected animals or people. Improperly cooked poultry, untreated water, and unpasteurized milk have been the main vehicles of transmission. *Campylobacter* infections usually are sporadic; outbreaks are rare but have occurred among school children who drank unpasteurized milk. Person-to-person spread occurs occasionally, particularly among very young children, and outbreaks of diarrhea in child care centers have been reported but are uncommon. Person-to-person transmission also has occurred in neonates of infected mothers and has resulted in health care–associated outbreaks in nurseries. In neonates, *C jejuni* and *C coli* usually cause gastroenteritis, whereas *C fetus* often causes septicemia or meningitis. Enteritis occurs in people of all ages. Excretion of *Campylobacter* organisms typically lasts 2 to 3 weeks without treatment.

Incubation Period

2 to 5 days but can be longer.

Diagnostic Tests

C jejuni and *C coli* can be cultured from feces, and *Campylobacter* species, including *C fetus*, can be cultured from blood. Laboratory identification of *C jejuni* and *C coli* in stool specimens requires selective media, microaerophilic conditions, and an incubation temperature of 42°C to 43°C. Unless the laboratory uses a non-selective isolation technique, many *Campylobacter* species other than *C jejuni* and *C coli* will not be detected. *C upsaliensis, C hyointestinalis,* and *C fetus* may not be isolated because of susceptibility to antimicrobial agents present in routinely used *Campylobacter* selective media. The presence of motile curved, spiral, or S-shaped rods resembling *Vibrio cholerae* by stool phase contrast or darkfield microscopy can provide rapid, presumptive evidence for *Campylobacter* species infection. This is less sensitive than culture. *C jejuni* and *C coli* can be detected directly in stool specimens by commercially available enzyme immunoassays, which provide rapid and reliable methods for laboratory diagnosis of enteric infections with *C jejuni* and *C coli.*

Treatment

Rehydration is the mainstay for all children with diarrhea. Azithromycin and erythromycin shorten the duration of illness and excretion of organisms, and prevent relapse when given early in the illness. Treatment with azithromycin or erythromycin usually eradicates the organism from stool within 2 to 3 days. A fluoroquinolone, such as ciprofloxacin, may be effective, but resistance to ciprofloxacin is common (22% of *C coli* isolates and 23% of *C jejuni* isolates in the United States in 2009). If antimicrobial therapy is given for treatment of gastroenteritis, the recommended duration is 3 to 5 days. Antimicrobial agents for bacteremia should be selected on the basis of antimicrobial susceptibility tests. *C fetus* generally is susceptible to aminoglycosides, extended-spectrum cephalosporins, meropenem, imipenem, ampicillin, and erythromycin.

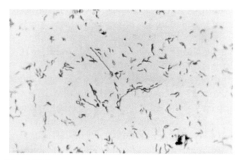

Image 23.1

This photomicrograph depicts findings observed in a 48-hour culture of *Campylobacter jejuni* bacteria revealing characteristic thin-, comma-, or gull winged–shaped forms displayed by this bacterium. *C jejuni* is a slender, curved, motile rod that is microaerophilic (ie, it has a reduced requirement for oxygen). It is a relatively fragile organism, being sensitive to environmental stresses such as drying, heating, disinfectants, and acidic conditions. Courtesy of Centers for Disease Control and Prevention/Robert Weaver, PhD.

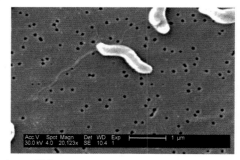

Image 23.2

This scanning electron micrograph depicts a number of gram-negative *Campylobacter jejuni* bacteria (magnification x20,123). The *C jejuni* bacterium is fragile. It cannot tolerate drying and can be killed by oxygen. It grows only if there is less than the atmospheric amount of oxygen present. Freezing reduces the number of *Campylobacter* bacteria present on raw meat. Courtesy of Centers for Disease Control and Prevention/ Dr Patricia Fields/Dr Collette Fitzgerald.

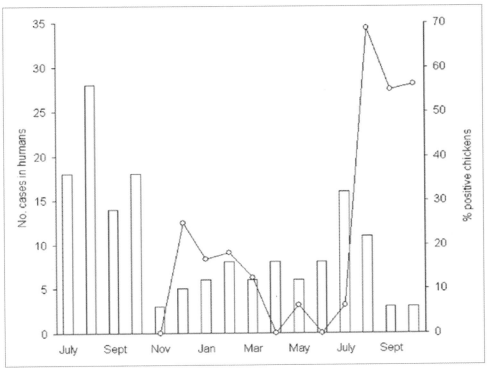

Image 23.3

Monthly distribution of the number of sporadic cases of *Campylobacter* infections in humans from July 2000 to October 2001 (columns) and of the prevalence of *Campylobacter* in whole retail chickens from November 2000 to October 2001 (line graph), Quebec. Courtesy of Michaud S, Ménard S, Arbeit RD. Campylobacteriosis, Eastern Townships, Québec. *Emerg Infect Dis*. 2004;10(10):1844–1847.

24

Candidiasis

(Moniliasis, Thrush)

Clinical Manifestations

Mucocutaneous infection results in oro-pharyngeal (thrush) or vaginal or cervical candidiasis; intertriginous lesions of the gluteal folds, buttocks, neck, groin, and axilla; paronychia; and onychia. Dysfunction of T lymphocytes, other immunologic disorders, and endocrinologic diseases are associated with chronic mucocutaneous candidiasis. Chronic or recurrent oral candidiasis can be the presenting sign of HIV infection or primary immunodeficiency. Esophageal and laryngeal candidiasis can occur in immuno-compromised patients. Disseminated or invasive candidiasis occurs in very low birth weight newborn infants and in immunocompromised or debilitated hosts, can involve virtually any organ or anatomic site, and rapidly can be fatal. Candidemia can occur with or without systemic disease in patients with indwelling central vascular catheters, especially patients receiving prolonged intravenous infusions with parenteral alimentation or lipids. Peritonitis can occur in patients undergoing peritoneal dialysis, especially in patients receiving prolonged broad-spectrum antimicrobial therapy. Candiduria can occur in patients with indwelling urinary catheters, focal renal infection, or disseminated disease.

Etiology

Candida species are yeasts that reproduce by budding. *Candida albicans* and several other species form long chains of elongated yeast forms called pseudohyphae. *C albicans* causes most infections, but in some regions and patient populations, the non-*albicans Candida* species now account for more than half of invasive infections. Other species, including *Candida tropicalis, Candida parapsilosis, Candida glabrata, Candida krusei, Candida guilliermondii, Candida lusitaniae,* and *Candida dubliniensis,* also can cause serious infections, especially in immunocompromised and debilitated hosts. *C parapsilosis* is second only to *C albicans* as a cause of systemic candidiasis in very low birth weight neonates.

Epidemiology

Like other *Candida* species, *C albicans* is present on skin and in the mouth, intestinal tract, and vagina of immunocompetent people. Vulvovaginal candidiasis is associated with pregnancy, and newborn infants can acquire the organism in utero, during passage through the vagina, or postnatally. Mild mucocutaneous infection is common in healthy infants. Person-to-person transmission occurs rarely. Invasive disease typically occurs in people with impaired immunity, with infection usually arising endogenously from colonized sites. Factors such as extreme prematurity, neutropenia, or treatment with corticosteroids or cytotoxic chemotherapy increases the risk of invasive infection. People with diabetes mellitus generally have localized mucocutaneous lesions. An estimated 5% to 20% of newborn infants weighing less than 1,000 g at birth develop invasive candidiasis. Patients with neutrophil defects, such as chronic granulomatous disease or myeloperoxidase deficiency, also are at increased risk. Patients undergoing intravenous alimentation or receiving broad-spectrum antimicrobial agents, especially extended-spectrum cephalosporins, carbapenems, and vancomycin, or requiring long-term indwelling central venous or peritoneal dialysis catheters have increased susceptibility to infection. Postsurgical patients can be at risk, particularly after cardiothoracic or abdominal procedures.

Incubation Period

Unknown.

Diagnostic Tests

The presumptive diagnosis of mucocutaneous candidiasis or thrush usually can be made clinically, but other organisms or trauma also can cause clinically similar lesions. Yeast cells and pseudohyphae can be found in *C albicans*–infected tissue and are identifiable by microscopic examination of scrapings prepared with Gram, calcofluor white, or fluorescent antibody stains or suspended in 10% to 20% potassium hydroxide. Endoscopy is useful for diagnosis of esophagitis. Ophthalmologic examination can reveal typical retinal lesions that can result from candidemia. Lesions in the brain, kidney, liver, or spleen can be detected by ultrasonography, computed tomography, or magnetic resonance imaging; however, these lesions typically do not appear by imaging until 2 to 4 weeks into illness or after neutropenia has resolved.

A definitive diagnosis of invasive candidiasis requires isolation of the organism from a normally sterile body site (eg, blood, cerebrospinal fluid, bone marrow) or demonstration of organisms in a tissue biopsy specimen. Negative cultures do not exclude invasive infection in immunocompromised hosts; in some settings, blood culture is only 50% sensitive. Recovery of the organism is expedited using blood culture systems that are biphasic or that use a lysis-centrifugation method. Special fungal culture media are not needed to grow *Candida* species. A presumptive species identification of *C albicans* can be made by demonstrating germ tube formation, and molecular fluorescence in situ hybridization testing rapidly can distinguish *C albicans* from non-*albicans Candida* species.

Treatment

Mucous Membrane and Skin Infections.
Oral candidiasis in immunocompetent hosts is treated with oral nystatin suspension or clotrimazole troches applied to lesions. Troches should not be used in infants. Fluconazole may be more effective than oral nystatin or clotrimazole troches and may be considered if other treatments fail. Fluconazole can be beneficial for immunocompromised patients with oropharyngeal candidiasis. Voriconazole or posaconazole are alternative drugs. Although cure rates with fluconazole are greater than with nystatin, relapse rates are comparable.

Esophagitis caused by *Candida* species is treated with oral or intravenous fluconazole or oral itraconazole solutions for 14 to 21 days after clinical improvement. Alternatively, intravenous amphotericin B, voriconazole, caspofungin, micafungin, or anidulafungin (for people 18 years of age and older) can be used for refractory, azole-resistant, or severe esophageal candidiasis. Duration of treatment depends on severity of illness, age, and degree of immunocompromise.

Skin infections are treated with topical nystatin, miconazole, clotrimazole, naftifine, ketoconazole, econazole, or ciclopirox. Nystatin usually is effective and is the least expensive of these drugs.

Vulvovaginal candidiasis is treated effectively with many topical formulations, including clotrimazole, miconazole, butoconazole, terconazole, and tioconazole. Such topically applied azole drugs are more effective than nystatin. Oral azole agents (fluconazole, itraconazole, and ketoconazole) also are effective and should be considered for recurrent or refractory cases.

For chronic mucocutaneous candidiasis, fluconazole, itraconazole, and voriconazole are effective drugs. Low-dose amphotericin B administered intravenously is effective in severe cases. Relapses are common once therapy is terminated, and treatment should be viewed as a lifelong process, hopefully using only intermittent pulses of antifungal agents. Invasive infections in patients with this condition are rare.

Keratomycosis is treated with corneal baths of amphotericin B in conjunction with systemic therapy. Patients with cystitis caused by *Candida,* especially patients with neutropenia, patients with renal allographs, and patients undergoing urologic manipulation, should be treated with fluconazole for 7 days because of the concentrating effect of fluconazole in the urinary tract. An alternative is 7 days of low-dose amphotericin B intravenously. Repeated bladder irrigations with amphotericin B (50 µg/mL of sterile water) have been used to treat patients with candidal cystitis, but this does not treat disease beyond the bladder and is not recommended routinely. A urinary catheter in a patient with candidiasis should be removed or replaced promptly.

Invasive Disease. Treatment of invasive candidiasis in neonates and adults without neutropenia should include prompt removal of any infected vascular or peritoneal catheters and replacement, if necessary, when infection is controlled. Avoidance or reduction of systemic immunosuppression also is advised when feasible. Immediate replacement of a catheter over a wire in the same catheter site is not recommended.

Amphotericin B deoxycholate is the drug of choice for treating neonates with systemic candidiasis; if urinary tract involvement and meningitis are excluded, lipid formulations can be considered. Echinocandins should be used with caution in neonates, because dosing and safety have not been established. Treatment for neonates is at least 3 weeks. In clinically stable children and adults without neutropenia, fluconazole or an echinocandin (caspofungin, micafungin, anidulafungin) is the recommended treatment. In nonneutropenic patients with candidemia and no metastatic complications, treatment is 2 weeks after documented clearance of *Candida* from the bloodstream and resolution of clinical illness.

In critically ill neutropenic patients, an echinocandin or a lipid formulation of amphotericin B is recommended because of the fungicidal nature of these agents when compared with fluconazole, which is fungistatic. In less seriously ill neutropenic patients, fluconazole is the alternative treatment for patients who have not had recent azole exposure, but voriconazole can be considered. The duration of treatment for candidemia without metastatic complications is 2 weeks after documented clearance of *Candida* organisms from the bloodstream and resolution of neutropenia.

Most *Candida* species are susceptible to amphotericin B, although *C lusitaniae* and some strains of *C glabrata* and *C krusei* have decreased susceptibility or resistance. Among patients with persistent candidemia despite appropriate therapy, investigation for a deep focus of infection should be conducted. Short-course therapy (ie, 7–10 days) can be used for intravenous catheter-associated infections if the catheter is removed promptly, there is rapid resolution of candidemia once treatment is initiated, and there is no evidence of infection beyond the bloodstream. Lipid-associated preparations of amphotericin B can be used as an alternative to amphotericin B deoxycholate in patients who experience significant toxicity during therapy. Published reports in adults and anecdotal reports in preterm infants indicate

that lipid-associated amphotericin B preparations have failed to eradicate renal candidiasis, because these large-molecule drugs may not penetrate well into the renal parenchyma. Flucytosine is not recommended routinely for use with amphotericin B deoxycholate. Fluconazole may be appropriate for patients with impaired renal function or for patients with meningitis. However, data on fluconazole use for *Candida* meningitis are limited. Fluconazole is not an appropriate choice for therapy before the infecting *Candida* species has been identified, because *C krusei* is resistant to fluconazole, and more than 50% of *C glabrata* isolates also can be resistant. Although voriconazole is effective against *C krusei*, it is often ineffective against *C glabrata*. The echinocandins (caspofungin, micafungin, and anidulafungin) all are active in vitro against *Candida* species and are appropriate first-line drugs for *Candida* infections in severely ill or neutropenic patients. The echinocandins should be used with caution against *C parapsilosis* infection because some decreased in vitro susceptibility has been reported. If an echinocandin is initiated empirically and *C parapsilosis* is isolated in a recovering patient, then the echinocandin can be continued. Echinocandins are not recommended for treatment of central nervous system infections.

Ophthalmologic evaluation is recommended for all patients with candidemia. Evaluation should occur once candidemia is controlled, and in patients with neutropenia, evaluation should be deferred until recovery of the neutrophil count.

Chemoprophylaxis. Invasive candidiasis in neonates is associated with prolonged hospitalization and neurodevelopmental impairment or death in almost 75% of affected infants with extremely low birth weight (ELBW [less than 1,000 g]). The poor outcomes, despite prompt diagnosis and therapy, make prevention of invasive candidiasis in this population desirable. Four prospective randomized controlled trials and 10 retrospective cohort studies of fungal prophylaxis in neonates with birth weight less than 1,000 g or less than 1,500 g have demonstrated significant reduction of *Candida* colonization, rates of invasive candidiasis, and *Candida*-related mortality in nurseries with a moderate or high incidence of invasive candidiasis. Besides birth weight, other risk factors for invasive candidiasis in neonates include inadequate infection-prevention practices and injudicious use of antimicrobial agents. Adherence to optimal infection control practices, including "bundles" for intravascular catheter insertion and maintenance and antimicrobial stewardship, can diminish infection rates and should be optimized before implementation of chemoprophylaxis as standard practice in a neonatal intensive care unit. On the basis of current data, fluconazole is the preferred agent for prophylaxis, because it has been shown to be effective and safe. Fluconazole prophylaxis is recommended for ELBW infants cared for in neonatal intensive care units with moderate (5%–10%) or high (≥10%) rates of invasive candidiasis.

Fluconazole can decrease the risk of mucosal (eg, oropharyngeal and esophageal) candidiasis in patients with advanced HIV disease. However, an increased incidence of infections attributable to *C krusei* (which intrinsically is resistant to fluconazole) has been reported in non–HIV-infected patients receiving prophylactic fluconazole. Adults undergoing allogenic hematopoietic stem cell transplantation had significantly fewer *Candida* infections when given fluconazole, but limited data are available for children. Prophylaxis should be considered for children undergoing allogenic hematopoietic stem cell transplantation during the period of neutropenia. Prophylaxis is not recommended routinely for other immunocompromised children, including children with HIV infection.

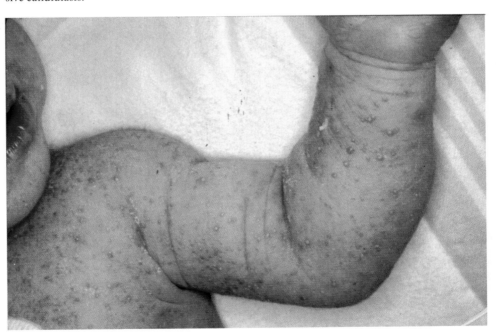

Image 24.1
Congenital neonatal candidiasis. Copyright James Brien, DO.

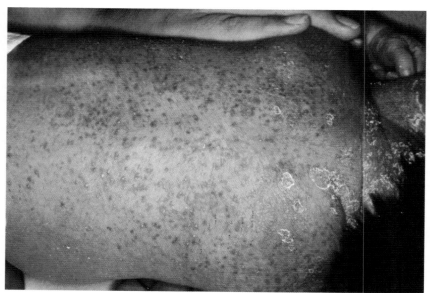

Image 24.2
Congenital neonatal candidiasis. Copyright James Brien, DO.

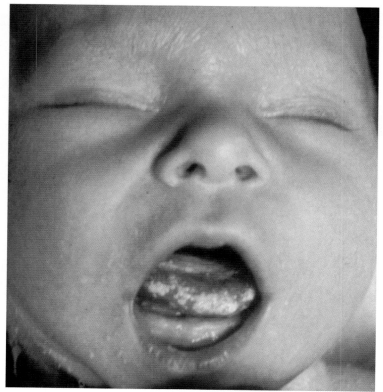

Image 24.3
Thrush in a 1-week-old. Copyright James Brien, DO.

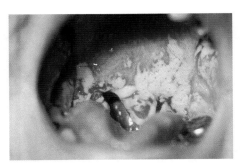

Image 24.4
Oral thrush covering the soft palate and uvula. Courtesy of Centers for Disease Control and Prevention.

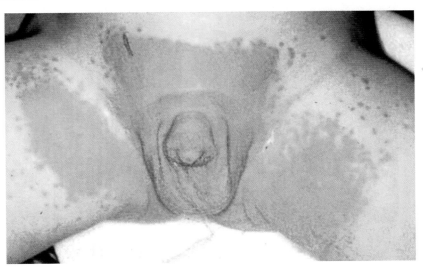

Image 24.5
Candida (monilia) rash with typical satellite lesions in an infant boy.

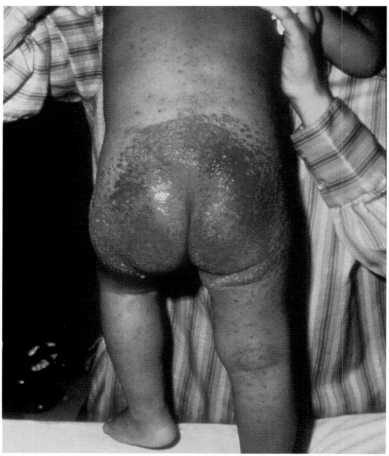

Image 24.6
Severe *Candida* diaper dermatitis with satellite lesions. Courtesy of George Nankervis, MD.

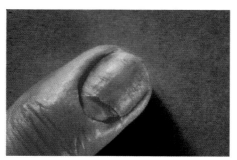

Image 24.7
Candidiasis of the fingernail bed. Courtesy of
Centers for Disease Control and Prevention/
Sherry Brinkman.

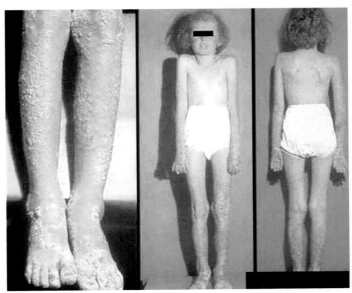

Image 24.8
Chronic mucocutaneous candidiasis in an immunodeficient preadolescent girl. Copyright James Brien, DO.

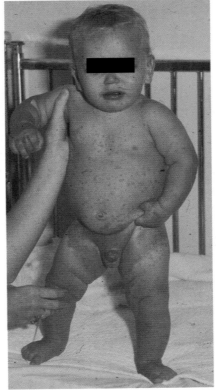

Image 24.9
A 7-month-old white male with mucocutaneous candidiasis, generalized. Courtesy of Larry Frenkel, MD.

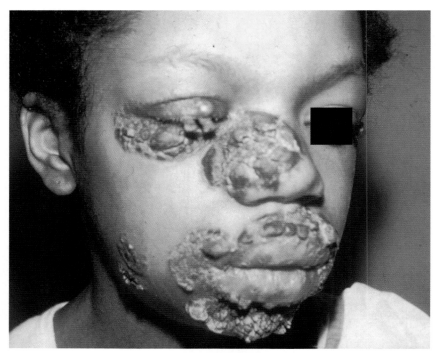

Image 24.10

An immunocompromised 5-year-old male with multiple *Candida* granulomatous lesions, a rare response to an invasive cutaneous infection. These crusted, verrucous plaques and horn-like projections require systemic candicidal agents for eradication or palliation. Courtesy of George Nankervis, MD.

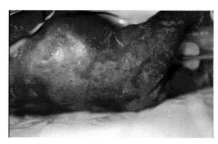

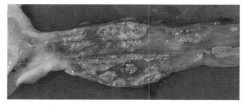

Image 24.12

Candida esophagitis with abscesses and ulceration of the mucosa. Courtesy of Dimitris P. Agamanolis, MD.

Image 24.11

Photograph of a very low birth weight neonate who developed invasive fungal dermatitis of the back caused by *Candida albicans*. This is an uncommon presentation that often is accompanied by disseminated infection. The diagnosis is established by skin biopsy that reveals invasion of the yeast into the dermis and culture that grows the yeast on routine culture media within 2 to 4 days. Courtesy of Carol Baker, MD.

25

Cat-Scratch Disease
(Bartonella henselae)

Clinical Manifestations

The predominant manifestation of cat-scratch disease (CSD) in an immunocompetent person is regional lymphadenopathy. Fever and mild systemic symptoms occur in approximately 30% of patients. A skin papule or pustule often is found at the presumed site of inoculation and usually precedes development of lymphadenopathy by approximately 2 weeks (range, 7–60 days). Lymphadenopathy involves nodes that drain the site of inoculation, typically axillary, but cervical, submental, epitrochlear, or inguinal nodes can be involved. The skin overlying affected lymph nodes typically is tender, warm, erythematous, and indurated. Most CSD lymph nodes will resolve spontaneously within 4 to 6 weeks, but approximately 25% of affected nodes suppurate spontaneously. Most people with CSD are afebrile or have low-grade fever with mild systemic symptoms such as malaise, anorexia, fatigue, and headache. Inoculation of the eyelid conjunctiva can result in Parinaud oculoglandular syndrome, which consists of conjunctivitis and ipsilateral preauricular lymphadenopathy. Less common manifestations of *Bartonella henselae* infection (approximately 25% of cases) most likely reflect bloodborne disseminated disease and include fever of unknown origin, conjunctivitis, uveitis, neuroretinitis, encephalopathy, aseptic meningitis, osteolytic lesion, hepatitis, granulomata in the liver and spleen, glomerulonephritis, pneumonia, thrombocytopenic purpura, erythema nodosum, and endocarditis. Neuroretinitis is characterized by unilateral painless vision impairment, papillitis, macular edema, and lipid exudates (macular star).

Etiology

B henselae, the causative organism of CSD, is a fastidious, slow-growing, gram-negative bacillus that also is the causative agent of bacillary angiomatosis (vascular proliferative lesions of skin and subcutaneous tissue) and bacillary peliosis (reticuloendothelial lesions in visceral organs, primarily the liver). The latter 2 manifestations of infection are reported primarily in patients with HIV infection. *B henselae* is related closely to *Bartonella quintana,* the agent of louseborne trench fever and a causative agent of bacillary angiomatosis and bacillary peliosis.

Epidemiology

CSD is a common infection, although its true incidence is unknown. *B henselae* is one of the most common causes of benign regional lymphadenopathy in children. Cats are the natural reservoir for *B henselae,* with a seroprevalence of 13% to 90% of domestic and stray cats in the United States. Other animals, including dogs, can be infected and occasionally are associated with human infection. Cat-to-cat transmission occurs via the cat flea *(Ctenocephalides felis)* with infection resulting in bacteremia that usually is asymptomatic in infected cats and lasts weeks to months. Fleas acquire the organism when feeding on a bacteremic cat and then shed infectious organisms in their feces. The bacteria are transmitted to humans by inoculation through a scratch or bite or hands contaminated by flea feces touching an open wound or the eye. Kittens (more often than cats) and animals that are from shelters or adopted as strays are more likely to be bacteremic. Most reported cases occur in people younger than 20 years of age, with most patients having a history of recent contact with apparently healthy cats, typically kittens. Person-to-person transmission does not occur.

Incubation Period

From scratch to primary cutaneous lesion; 7 to 12 days; from primary lesion to lymphadenopathy; 5 to 50 days (median, 12).

Diagnostic Tests

B henselae is a fastidious organism; recovery by routine culture rarely is achieved. Specialized laboratories experienced in isolating *Bartonella* organisms are recommended for processing of cultures. The indirect immunofluorescent antibody (IFA) assay for detection of serum antibodies to antigens of *Bartonella* species is useful for diagnosis of CSD. The IFA test is available at many commercial laboratories and through the Centers for Disease Control and Prevention (CDC). PCR assays are available in some commercial and research laboratories and at the CDC for testing of tissue or body fluids, such as pleural or cerebrospinal fluid. If tissue (eg, lymph node) specimens are available, bacilli occasionally may be visualized using Warthin-Starry silver stain; however, this test is not specific for *B henselae*. Early histologic changes in lymph node specimens consist of lymphocytic infiltration with epithelioid granuloma formation. Later changes consist of polymorphonuclear leukocyte infiltration with granulomas that become necrotic and resemble granulomas from patients with tularemia, brucellosis, and mycobacterial infections.

Treatment

Management of localized CSD primarily is aimed at relief of symptoms because infection usually is self-limited, resolving spontaneously in 2 to 4 months. However, some experts recommend a 5-day course of azithromycin orally to speed recovery. Painful suppurative nodes can be treated with needle aspiration; incision and drainage should be avoided, and surgical excision generally is unnecessary.

Antimicrobial therapy may hasten recovery in acutely or severely ill patients with systemic symptoms, particularly people with hepatic or splenic involvement or painful adenitis, and is recommended for all immunocompromised patients. Reports suggest that several oral antimicrobial agents (azithromycin, ciprofloxacin, trimethoprim-sulfamethoxazole, and rifampin) and parenteral gentamicin are effective, but the role of antimicrobial therapy remains unclear. The optimal duration of therapy is not known but may be several weeks for systemic disease.

Antimicrobial therapy for patients with bacillary angiomatosis and bacillary peliosis has been shown to be beneficial and is recommended. Azithromycin or doxycycline is effective for treatment of these conditions; therapy should be administered for several months to prevent relapse in immunocompromised people.

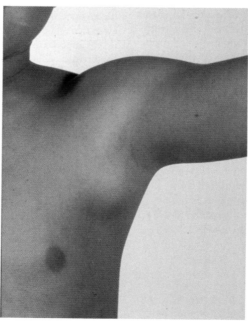

Image 25.1
Cat-scratch disease in the axilla. Copyright James Brien, DO.

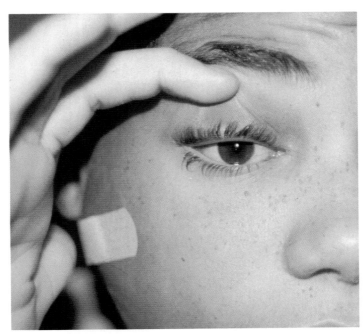

Image 25.2
Eyelid erythema and preauricular adenopathy typical of occuloglandular syndrome of cat-scratch disease. Copyright James Brien, DO.

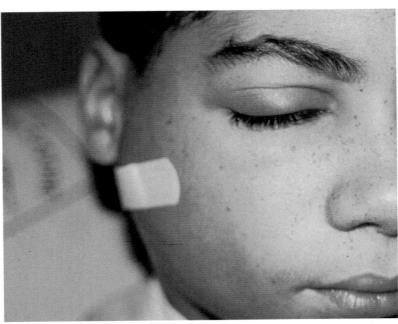

Image 25.3
Same patient as in Image 25.2. Copyright James Brien, DO.

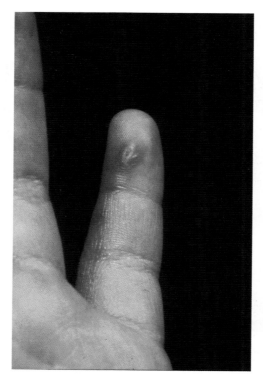

Image 25.4
Inoculation granulomas of cat-scratch disease on the finger. Copyright James Brien, DO.

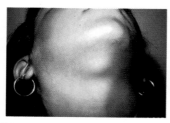

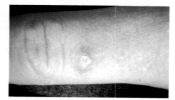

Image 25.6
Cat-scratch granuloma of the finger of a 6-year-old white male. This is a typical inoculation site lesion, which was noted about 10 days before the development of regional lymphadenopathy.

Image 25.5
Submental lymphadenitis due to cat-scratch disease.

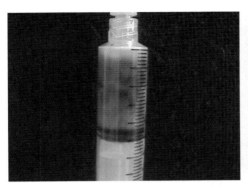

Image 25.7
Sanguinopurulent exudate aspirated from the axillary node of a patient with cat-scratch disease. Copyright Michael Rajnik, MD, FAAP.

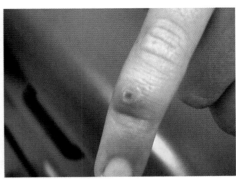

Image 25.8
Cat-scratch disease granuloma of the finger in a 12-year-old white male with epitrochlear node involvement (see Image 25.9). Copyright Michael Rajnik, MD, FAAP.

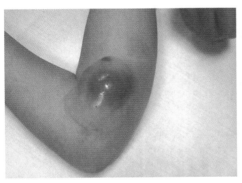

Image 25.9
Epitrochlear suppurative adenitis of cat-scratch disease in the child in Image 25.8 with a cat-scratch granuloma of the finger. Copyright Michael Rajnik, MD, FAAP

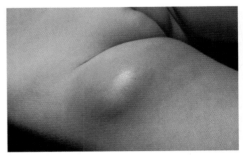

Image 25.10
Inguinal lymphadenitis due to cat-scratch disease in a 3-year-old white female. Copyright Ed Fajardo, MD.

26

Chancroid

Clinical Manifestations

Chancroid is an acute ulcerative disease of the genitalia. An ulcer begins as an erythematous papule that becomes pustular and erodes over several days, forming a sharply demarcated, somewhat superficial lesion with a serpiginous border. The base of the ulcer is friable and can be covered with a gray or yellow, purulent exudate. Single or multiple ulcers can be present. Unlike a syphilitic chancre, which is painless and indurated, the chancroid ulcer often is painful and nonindurated and can be associated with a painful, unilateral inguinal suppurative adenitis (bubo). Without treatment, the ulcer(s) can resolve in several weeks.

In most males, chancroid manifests as a genital ulcer with or without inguinal tenderness; edema of the prepuce is common. In females, most lesions are at the vaginal introitus and symptoms include dysuria, dyspareunia, vaginal discharge, pain on defecation, or anal bleeding. Constitutional symptoms are unusual.

Etiology

Chancroid is caused by *Haemophilus ducreyi*, which is a gram-negative coccobacillus.

Epidemiology

Chancroid is a sexually transmitted infection associated with poverty, prostitution, and illicit drug use. Chancroid is rare in the United States, and when it does occur, it usually is associated with sporadic outbreaks. Coinfection with syphilis or herpes simplex virus (HSV) occurs in as many as 10% of patients. Chancroid is a well-established cofactor for transmission of HIV. Because sexual contact is the only known route of transmission, the diagnosis of chancroid in infants and young children is strong evidence of sexual abuse.

Incubation Period

3 to 10 days.

Diagnostic Tests

Chancroid usually is diagnosed on the basis of clinical findings (one or more painful genital ulcers with tender suppurative inguinal adenopathy) and by excluding other genital ulcerative diseases, such as syphilis, HSV infection, or lymphogranuloma venereum. Confirmation is made by isolation of *Haemophilus ducreyi* from a genital ulcer or lymph node aspirate, although sensitivity is less than 80%. Because special culture media and conditions are required for isolation, laboratory personnel should be informed of the suspicion of chancroid. Buboes almost always are sterile. Fluorescent monoclonal antibody stains and PCR assays can provide a diagnosis but are not available in most clinical laboratories.

Treatment

Recommended regimens include azithromycin or ceftriaxone. Alternatives include erythromycin or ciprofloxacin. Ciprofloxacin is not approved by the US Food and Drug Administration for people younger than 18 years for this indication and should not be administered to pregnant or lactating women. Patients with HIV infection and uncircumcised males may need prolonged therapy. *H ducreyi* strains with intermediate resistance to ciprofloxacin or erythromycin have been reported worldwide.

Clinical improvement occurs 3 to 7 days after initiation of therapy, and healing is complete in approximately 2 weeks. Adenitis often is slow to resolve and can require needle aspiration or surgical incision. Patients should be reexamined 3 to 7 days after initiating therapy to verify healing. Slow clinical improvement and relapses can occur after therapy, especially in HIV-infected people. Close clinical follow-up is recommended; re-treatment with the original regimen usually is effective in patients who experience a relapse.

Patients should be evaluated for other sexually transmitted infections at the time of diagnosis.

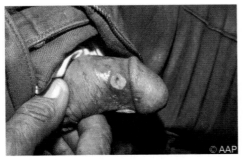

Image 26.1
Ulcerative chancroid lesions with inflammation of the shaft and glans penis caused by *Haemophilus ducreyi*. Chancroid lesions are irregular in shape, painful, and soft (non-indurated) to touch. Courtesy of Hugh Moffet, MD.

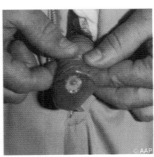

Image 26.2
Chancroid ulcer on the glans penis. Coinfection with syphilis or herpes simplex virus occurs in as many as 10% of patients. Courtesy of Hugh Moffet, MD.

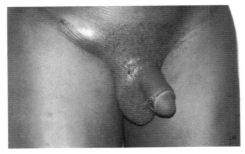

Image 26.3
This adolescent black male presented with a chancroid lesion of the groin and penis affecting the ipsilateral inguinal lymph nodes. First signs of infection typically appear 3 to 5 days after exposure, although symptoms can take up to 2 weeks to appear. Courtesy of Centers for Disease Control and Prevention/J. Pledger.

27

Chlamydophila (formerly Chlamydia) pneumoniae

Clinical Manifestations

Patients can be asymptomatic or mildly to moderately ill with a variety of respiratory tract diseases caused by *Chlamydophila pneumoniae*, including pneumonia, acute bronchitis, prolonged cough and, less commonly, nonexudative pharyngitis, laryngitis, otitis media, and sinusitis. In some patients, a sore throat precedes the onset of cough by a week or more. *C pneumoniae* can present as severe community-acquired pneumonia in immunocompromised hosts and has been associated with acute respiratory tract exacerbation in patients with cystic fibrosis and in acute chest syndrome in children with sickle cell disease. Chest radiographs may reveal an infiltrate(s) of a variety of patterns ranging from bilateral infiltrates to a single patchy subsegmental infiltrate. Illness can be prolonged, with cough often persisting 2 to 6 weeks or longer. The clinical course can be biphasic, culminating in atypical pneumonia.

Etiology

C pneumoniae is an obligate intracellular bacterium that is distinct antigenically, genetically, and morphologically from other *Chlamydia* species and is grouped in the genus *Chlamydophila*. All isolates of *C pneumoniae* appear to be closely related by serology.

Epidemiology

C pneumoniae infection is presumed to be transmitted from person to person via infected respiratory tract secretions. It is unknown whether there is an animal reservoir. The disease occurs worldwide, but in tropical and less developed areas, disease occurs earlier in life than in industrialized countries in temperate climates. In the United States, approximately 50% of adults have *C pneumoniae*–specific serum antibody by 20 years of age, indicating prior infection by the organism. Initial infection peaks between 5 and 15 years of age. Recurrent infection is common, especially in adults. Clusters of infection have been reported in groups of children and young adults. There is no evidence of seasonality.

Incubation Period

Mean, 21 days.

Diagnostic Tests

No reliable diagnostic test to identify the organism is available commercially, and none has been approved by the US Food and Drug Administration for use in the United States. Serologic testing has been the primary laboratory means of diagnosis of *C pneumoniae* infection. Microimmunofluorescent antibody test is the most sensitive and specific serologic test for acute infection. A fourfold increase in immunoglobulin (Ig) G titer between acute and convalescent sera or an IgM titer of 16 or greater is evidence of acute infection; use of acute and convalescent titers is preferable over an IgM titer. Use of a single IgG titer in diagnosis of acute infection is not recommended. In primary infection, IgM antibody appears approximately 2 to 3 weeks after onset of illness, but a single IgM antibody titer for diagnosis can be either falsely positive (cross-reactivity with other *Chlamydia* species) or falsely negative. Early antimicrobial therapy also may suppress antibody response. Because of difficulty of accurately detecting *C pneumoniae* by culture, serologic testing, or immunohistochemistry testing, several PCR tests, including multiplex, hybridization probe methods, and fluorescent probe-based methods, have been developed. Sensitivity and specificity of these different PCR techniques remains unknown. Currently, PCR testing for *C pneumoniae* is not available commercially.

Treatment

Most respiratory tract infections thought to be caused by *C pneumoniae* are treated empirically. For suspected *C pneumoniae* infections, treatment with macrolides (eg, erythromycin, azithromycin, or clarithromycin) is recommended. Tetracycline or doxycycline may be used in children older than 8 years. Newer fluoroquinolones (levofloxacin and moxifloxacin) are alternative drugs for patients who are unable to tolerate macrolide antibiotics. Duration of therapy typically is 10 to 14 days; azithromycin is 5 days.

28

Chlamydophila (formerly Chlamydia) psittaci

(Psittacosis, Ornithosis)

Clinical Manifestations

Psittacosis (ornithosis) is an acute respiratory tract infection with systemic symptoms including fever, nonproductive cough, headache, and malaise. Less common manifestations are pharyngitis, diarrhea, and altered mental status. Extensive interstitial pneumonia can occur, with radiographic changes characteristically more severe than would be expected from physical examination findings. Endocarditis, myocarditis, pericarditis, thrombophlebitis, nephritis, hepatitis, and encephalitis are rare complications.

Etiology

Chlamydophila psittaci is an obligate intracellular bacterial pathogen that is distinct antigenically, genetically, and morphologically from *Chlamydia* species and, following reclassification, is grouped in the genus *Chlamydophila*.

Epidemiology

Birds are the major reservoir of *C psittaci*. The term psittacosis commonly is used, although the term ornithosis more accurately describes the potential for nearly all domestic and wild birds to spread this infection, not just psittacine birds (eg, parakeets, parrots, and macaws). In the United States, psittacine birds, pigeons, and turkeys are important sources of human disease. Importation and illegal trafficking of exotic birds is associated with an increased incidence of human disease, because shipping, crowding, and other stress factors may increase shedding of the organism among birds. Infected birds, whether asymptomatic or obviously ill, can transmit the organism. Infection usually is acquired by inhaling aerosolized excrement or secretions from the eyes or beaks of birds. Handling of plumage and mouth-to-beak contact are the modes of exposure described most frequently. Excretion of *C psittaci* from birds may be intermittent or continuous for weeks or months. Pet owners; workers at poultry slaughter plants, poultry farms, pet shops; and laboratory personnel working with *C psittaci* are at increased risk of infection. Psittacosis is worldwide in distribution and tends to occur sporadically.

Incubation Period

5 to 14 days but may be longer.

Diagnostic Tests

A confirmed case of psittacosis requires a clinically compatible illness and laboratory confirmation by one of the following: (1) isolation of *C psittaci* from respiratory tract specimens or blood, or (2) fourfold or greater increase in immunoglobulin G (IgG) by complement fixation (CF) or microimmunofluorescence (MIF) between acute- and convalescent-phase serum obtained at least 2 to 4 weeks apart. A probable case of psittacosis requires a clinically compatible illness and either (1) supportive serologic test results (eg, *C psittaci* IgM ≥32 in at least 1 serum specimen obtained after onset of symptoms), or (2) detection of *C psittaci* DNA in a respiratory tract specimen by PCR assay. For serologic testing, MIF is more sensitive and specific than CF for *C psittaci*; however, both tests can cross-react with other chlamydial species and should be interpreted cautiously. Treatment with antimicrobial agents may suppress the antibody response; in such cases, a third serum sample obtained 4 to 6 weeks after the acute sample may be useful in confirming the diagnosis. Culturing the organism is difficult and should be attempted only by experienced personnel in laboratories where strict measures prevent the spread of the organism.

Treatment

Tetracycline or doxycycline for a minimum of 10 days is the drug of choice but should not be given routinely to children younger than 8 years or to pregnant women. Therapy should continue 10 to 14 days after fever abates, and with severe infection, intravenous doxycycline may be considered. Erythromycin and azithromycin are alternative agents and are recommended for younger children and pregnant women.

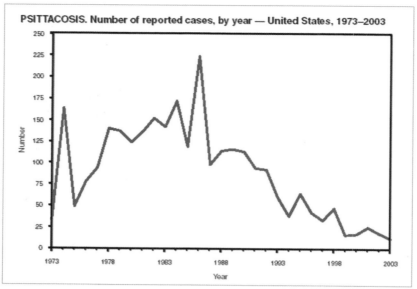

Image 28.1
Graphic demonstration of the number of US cases of psittacosis reported per year (1973–2003).
Courtesy of *Morbidity and Mortality Weekly Report.*

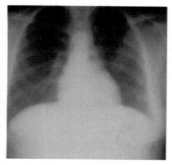

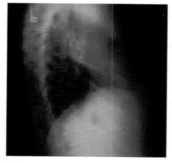

Image 28.2
Chlamydophila psittaci pneumonia in a 16-year-old girl with a cough of 3 weeks' duration. The family had several parrots in the home that were purchased from a roadside stand near the Texas-Mexico border. Interstitial pneumonia most prominent in the lower lobe of the left lung is shown. Complement fixation titer for *C psittaci,* 1:128. Copyright David Waagner.

Image 28.3
Lateral chest radiograph of the patient in Image 28.2. Most domestic and wild birds can transmit *Chlamydophila psittaci.* Copyright David Waagner.

29

Chlamydia trachomatis

Clinical Manifestations

Chlamydia trachomatis is associated with a range of clinical manifestations, including neonatal conjunctivitis, pneumonia in young infants, genital tract infection, lymphogranuloma venereum (LGV), and trachoma. **Neonatal conjunctivitis** is characterized by ocular congestion, edema, and discharge developing a few days to several weeks after birth and lasting for 1 to 2 weeks. In contrast to trachoma, scars and pannus formation are rare. **Pneumonia** usually is an afebrile illness of insidious onset occurring between 2 and 19 weeks after birth. A repetitive staccato cough, tachypnea, and rales in an afebrile 6-week-old infant are characteristic but not always present. Wheezing is uncommon. Hyperinflation usually accompanies infiltrates by chest radiograph. Nasal stuffiness and otitis media may occur. Untreated disease can recur. Severe chlamydial pneumonia has occurred occasionally in infants and some immunocompromised adults.

Genitourinary tract manifestations of chlamydial infection, such as vaginitis in prepubertal girls; urethritis, cervicitis, endometritis, salpingitis, and perihepatitis (Fitz-Hugh-Curtis syndrome) in postpubertal females; urethritis and epididymitis in males; and Reiter syndrome (arthritis, urethritis, and bilateral conjunctivitis) can occur. Infection can persist for months to years. Reinfection is common. In postpubertal females, chlamydial infection can progress to pelvic inflammatory disease and result in ectopic pregnancy or infertility. **LGV** classically is an invasive lymphatic infection with an initial ulcerative lesion on the genitalia accompanied by tender, suppurative, inguinal or femoral lymphadenopathy that typically is unilateral. However, anorectal infection is and can cause hemorrhagic proctocolitis or stricture among women and men who engage in anal intercourse. The proctocolitis can resemble inflammatory bowel disease.

Trachoma is a chronic follicular keratoconjunctivitis with neovascularization of the cornea that results from repeated and chronic infection. Blindness secondary to extensive local scarring and inflammation occurs in 1% to 15% of people with trachoma. Trachoma is rare in the United States.

Etiology

C trachomatis is an obligate intracellular bacterium with at least 18 serologic variants (serovars) divided between biologic variants (biovars): oculogenital (serovars A–K) and LGV (serovars L1, L2, and L3). Trachoma usually is caused by serovars A through C, and genital and perinatal infections are caused by B and D through K.

Epidemiology

C trachomatis is the most frequent reportable sexually transmitted infection (STI) in the United States, with high rates among sexually active adolescents and young adults. A significant proportion of patients are asymptomatic, thereby providing an ongoing reservoir for infection. Prevalence of the organism consistently is highest among adolescent females and among 15- to 24-year-old females recently screened in prenatal clinics was 7%. Oculogenital serovars of *C trachomatis* can be transmitted from the genital tract of infected mothers to their infants during birth. Acquisition occurs in approximately 50% of infants born vaginally to infected mothers and in some infants born by cesarean delivery with intact membranes. The risk of neonatal conjunctivitis is 25% to 50%, and the risk of pneumonia is 5% to 20% in infants who contract *C trachomatis*. The nasopharynx is the anatomic site most commonly infected.

Genital tract infection in adolescents and adults is transmitted sexually. The possibility of sexual abuse should be considered in prepubertal children beyond infancy who have vaginal, urethral, or rectal chlamydial infection. Nasopharyngeal cultures may remain positive for as long as 28 months, but spontaneous resolution of vaginal and rectal infection occurs by 16 to 18 months. Infection is not known to be communicable among infants and children.

LGV biovars are worldwide in distribution but particularly are prevalent in tropical and subtropical areas. Although disease is rare in the United States, outbreaks of LGV have been reported in Europe, and cases have been reported in the United States in men who have sex with men. Infection often is asymptomatic in women. Perinatal transmission is rare. LGV is infectious during active disease.

Incubation Period

Variable, depending on the type of infection, but usually 1 week.

Diagnostic Tests

Nucleic acid amplification tests (NAATs) tests largely have replaced tissue culture isolation and nonamplified direct detection methods because of the generally better sensitivity and high specificity of NAATs. High sensitivity of NAATs enables testing of urine and vaginal swabs. However, commercially available NAATs, such as PCR, transcription-mediated amplification, and strand-displacement amplification tests, vary in specimen types and populations for which manufacturers have obtained approval from the US Food and Drug Administration (FDA). In addition, evaluation of NAATs still is limited for pediatric patients.

For **postpubertal individuals,** commercial NAATs have been approved by the FDA for testing of endocervical and male intraurethral swab and male or female urine specimens. Certain NAATs also have been approved for testing of vaginal swab specimens collected by a clinician or by the patient. NAATs have not been approved by the FDA for use with rectal specimens, but some laboratories have met Clinical Laboratory Improvement Amendments requirements and have validated NAATs of rectal swab specimens from males who engage in receptive rectal sexual exposure. Testing of pharyngeal specimens is not recommended.

NAATs have not been approved by the FDA for testing of conjunctival specimens from infants with suspected C trachomatis **conjunctivitis** or for testing of nasopharyngeal swab, tracheal aspirate, or lung biopsy specimens from infants with suspected C trachomatis pneumonia.

Tissue culture has been recommended for C trachomatis testing of specimens when evaluating a **child for possible sexual abuse**; culture of the organism may be the only acceptable diagnostic test in certain legal juris-

dictions. NAATs are not approved by the FDA for this indication. Test specificity, which is of critical concern because of the potential legal consequences of positive test results, has been high in limited evaluations of NAATs for this indication. Some experts and expert groups recommend that a positive NAAT result be followed by additional testing with a second NAAT that detects a different target and that specimens be saved according to forensic standards to permit additional evaluation.

Serum anti–C trachomatis antibody concentrations are difficult to determine, and only a few clinical laboratories perform this test. In children with pneumonia, an acute microimmunofluorescent serum titer of C trachomatis–specific immunoglobulin (Ig) M of 1:32 or greater is diagnostic. Diagnosis of LGV can be made by serologic testing. However, most available serologic tests in the United States are based on enzyme immunoassays and might not provide a quantitative "titer-based" result.

Diagnosis of **genitourinary tract** chlamydial disease in a child, adolescent, or adult should prompt investigation for other STIs, including syphilis, gonorrhea, and HIV infection. In the case of an infant, evaluation of the mother also is advisable.

Diagnosis of ocular **trachoma** usually is made clinically in countries with endemic infection.

Treatment

- Infants with **chlamydial conjunctivitis** or **pneumonia** are treated with oral erythromycin base or ethylsuccinate for 14 days. Limited data on azithromycin therapy for treatment of C trachomatis infections in infants suggest that a single daily dose for 3 days may be effective. Oral sulfonamides may be used to treat chlamydial conjunctivitis after the immediate neonatal period for infants who do not tolerate erythromycin. Topical treatment is unnecessary. Because the efficacy of erythromycin therapy is approximately 80%, a second course may be required. A diagnosis of C trachomatis infection in an infant should prompt treatment of the mother and her sexual partner(s). The need for treatment of infants can be avoided by screening pregnant women to detect and treat *C trachomatis* infection before delivery.

An association between orally administered erythromycin and infantile hypertrophic pyloric stenosis (IHPS) has been reported in infants younger than 6 weeks. However, because confirmation of erythromycin as a contributor to cases of IHPS will require additional investigation and because alternative therapies are not as well studied, the American Academy of Pediatrics continues to recommend use of erythromycin for treatment of diseases caused by *C trachomatis*. Physicians who prescribe erythromycin to newborn infants should inform parents about the signs and potential risks of developing IHPS.

- Infants born to mothers known to have untreated chlamydial infection are at high risk of infection; however, prophylactic antimicrobial treatment is not indicated, because the efficacy of such treatment is unknown. Infants should be monitored clinically to ensure appropriate treatment if infection develops. If adequate follow-up cannot be ensured, some experts recommend that preemptive therapy be considered.
- For uncomplicated *C trachomatis* **anogenital tract infection in adolescents or adults,** oral doxycycline for 7 days or azithromycin in a single 1-g oral dose is recommended. Alternatives include oral erythromycin base, erythromycin ethylsuccinate for 7 days, ofloxacin (600 mg/day in 2 divided daily doses), or levofloxacin for 7 days. **For children who weigh less than 45 kg,** the recommended regimen is oral erythromycin for 14 days. **For children who weigh more than 45 kg but who are younger than 8 years,** the recommended regimen is azithromycin as a single dose. **For children older than 8 years,** the recommended regimen is azithromycin twice a day for 7 days. **For pregnant women,** the recommended treatment is azithromycin or amoxicillin for 7 days. Erythromycin base for 7 days is an alternative regimen. Doxycycline, ofloxacin, and levofloxacin are contraindicated during pregnancy.

Follow-up Testing. Repeat testing (preferably by NAAT) is recommended 3 weeks after treatment of pregnant women. Because these regimens for pregnant women may not be highly efficacious, a second course of therapy may be required. Nonpregnant adult or adolescent patients treated for uncomplicated *Chlamydia* infection with azithromycin or doxycycline do not need to be retested unless compliance is in question, symptoms persist, or reinfection is suspected. Previously infected adolescents are a high priority for repeat testing for *C trachomatis,* usually 3 to 6 months after initial infection. Women recently treated for chlamydial infection have a high risk of reinfection. Thus consideration should be given to retest all women treated for chlamydial infection whenever they next seek medical care within the following 3 to 12 months.

- For **LGV,** doxycycline for 21 days is the preferred treatment for children 8 years of age and older. Erythromycin base for 21 days is an alternative regimen; azithromycin once weekly for 3 weeks probably is effective.
- Treatment of **trachoma** is more difficult, and recommendations for therapy differ. The most widely used therapy is topical treatment with erythromycin, tetracycline, or sulfacetamide ointment. However, because of improved adherence and greater efficacy, the World Health Organization encourages use of azithromycin as a single dose or in 3 weekly doses as the first-line antimicrobial agent to treat trachoma.

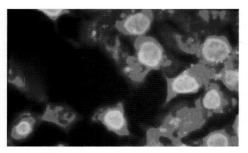

Image 29.1
Infected HeLa cells (fluorescent antibody stain). *Chlamydia trachomatis* is the most common reportable sexually transmitted infection in the United States, with high rates of infection among sexually active adolescents and young adults. Copyright Noni MacDonald, MD.

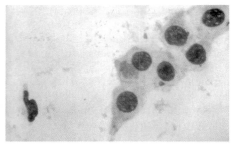

Image 29.2
Photomicrograph of *Chlamydia trachomatis* taken from a urethral scrape (iodine-stained inclusions in McCoy cell line, x200). Untreated, chlamydial infection can cause severe, costly reproductive and other health problems, including both short- and long-term consequences (eg, pelvic inflammatory disease, infertility, potentially fatal tubal pregnancy).

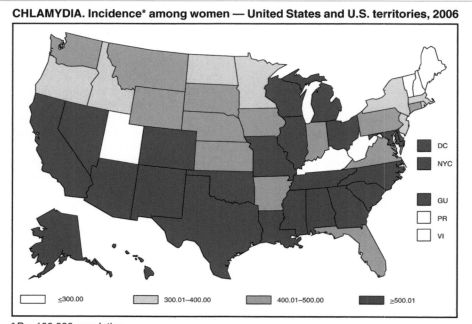

CHLAMYDIA. Incidence* among women — United States and U.S. territories, 2006

Legend:
- ☐ DC
- ☐ NYC
- ☐ GU
- ☐ PR
- ☐ VI

- ☐ ≤300.00
- ☐ 300.01–400.00
- ☐ 400.01–500.00
- ■ ≥500.01

* Per 100,000 population.

Chlamydia refers to genital infections caused by *Chlamydia trachomatis*. In 2006, the chlamydia rate among women in the United States and U.S. territories was 511.7 cases per 100,000 population.

Image 29.3
Map showing incidence of *Chlamydia trachomatis* genital infections in the United States in 2006. Courtesy of *Morbidity and Mortality Weekly Report*.

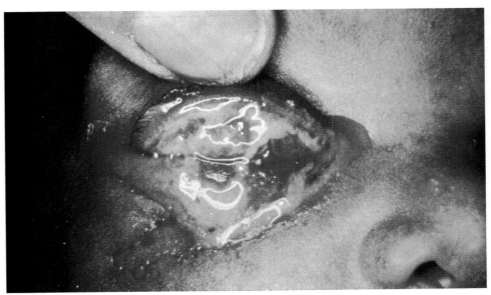

Image 29.4
Chlamydia trachomatis conjunctivitis. Courtesy of Gary Overturf, MD.

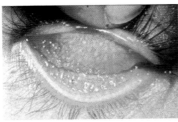

Image 29.5
Conjunctivitis in an infant due to *Chlamydia trachomatis.* The risk of neonatal conjunctivitis is 25% to 50% for infants of untreated, infected mothers. Copyright James Brien, DO.

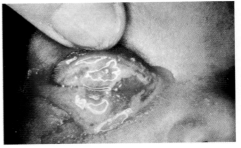

Image 29.6
Conjunctivitis due to *Chlamydia trachomatis,* the most common cause of ophthalmia neonatorum. This is the same infant as in Image 29.5. Copyright James Brien, DO.

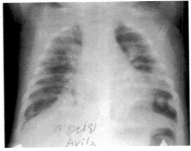

Image 29.7
Chlamydia trachomatis pneumonia, severe and bilateral, in a 5-week-old infant. Courtesy of Edgar O. Ledbetter, MD, FAAP.

30

Clostridium botulinum
(Botulism and Infant Botulism)

Clinical Manifestations

Botulism is a neuroparalytic disorder characterized by an acute, afebrile, symmetric, descending, flaccid paralysis. Paralysis is caused by blockade of neurotransmitter release at the voluntary motor and autonomic neuromuscular junctions. Four distinct, naturally occurring forms of human botulism exist: foodborne, wound, adult intestinal colonization, and infant. Fatal cases of iatrogenic botulism result from injection of excess therapeutic botulinum toxin. Onset of symptoms occurs abruptly within hours or evolves gradually over several days and includes diplopia, dysphagia, dysphonia, and dysarthria. Cranial nerve palsies are followed by symmetric, descending, flaccid paralysis of somatic musculature in patients who are fully alert. Classic infant botulism, which occurs predominantly in infants younger than 6 months is preceded by or begins with constipation and manifests as decreased movement, loss of facial expression, poor feeding, weak cry, diminished gag reflex, ocular palsies, loss of head control, and progressive descending generalized weakness and hypotonia. Sudden infant death can be caused by rapidly progressing botulism.

Etiology

Botulism results from absorption of botulinum toxin into the circulation from a wound or mucosal surface. Seven antigenic toxin types of Clostridium botulinum have been identified. Human botulism is caused by neurotoxins A, B, E and, rarely, F. Non-botulinum species of Clostridium rarely may produce these neurotoxins and cause disease. Almost all cases of infant botulism are caused by toxin types A and B. A few cases of types E and F have been reported from Clostridium butyricum (type E), C botulinum (type E), and Clostridium baratii (type F). C botulinum spores are ubiquitous in soils and dust worldwide.

Epidemiology

Foodborne botulism (in the United States annual average, 17 cases in 2006–2010; age range, 3–87 years) results when food contaminated with spores of C botulinum is preserved or stored improperly under anaerobic conditions that permit germination, multiplication, and toxin production. Illness follows ingestion of preformed botulinum toxin. Outbreaks have occurred after ingestion of restaurant-prepared foods, home-prepared foods, and commercially canned foods. Immunity to botulinum toxin does not develop after botulism. Botulism is not transmitted from person to person.

Infant botulism (in the United States annual average, 90 laboratory-confirmed cases in 2006–2010; age range, <1 to 60 weeks; median age, 15 weeks) results after ingested spores of C botulinum or related neurotoxigenic clostridial species germinate, multiply, and produce botulinum toxin in the intestine, probably through a mechanism of transient permissiveness of the intestinal microflora. Most cases occur in breastfed infants at the time of first introduction of nonhuman milk substances; the source of spores usually is not identified. Honey has been identified as an avoidable source. Manufacturers of light and dark corn syrups cannot ensure that any given product will be free of C botulinum spores, but no case of infant botulism has been proven to be attributable to consumption of contaminated corn syrup. Rarely, intestinal botulism can occur in older children and adults, usually after intestinal surgery and exposure to antimicrobial agents.

Wound botulism (in the United States annual average, 26 laboratory-confirmed cases in 2006–2010; age range, 23–66 years) results when C botulinum contaminates traumatized tissue, germinates, multiplies, and produces toxin. Gross trauma or crush injury can be a predisposing event. During the last decade, self-injection of contaminated black tar heroin has been associated with most cases.

Incubation Period

Foodborne botulism 12 to 48 hours (range, 6 hours–8 days); infant botulism 3 to 30 days from exposure to spore-containing material; wound botulism, 4 to 14 days from injury until symptoms.

Diagnostic Tests

A toxin neutralization bioassay in mice is used to detect botulinum toxin in serum, stool, gastric aspirate, or suspect foods. Enriched selective media is required to isolate *C botulinum* from stool and foods. In infant and wound botulism, the diagnosis is made by demonstrating *C botulinum* toxin or organisms in feces, wound exudate, or tissue specimens. To increase the likelihood of diagnosis, suspect foods should be collected and serum and stool or enema specimens should be obtained from all people with suspected foodborne botulism. In foodborne cases, serum specimens may be positive for toxin as long as 16 days after admission. Stool or enema and gastric aspirates are the best diagnostic specimens for culture. In infant botulism cases, toxin assay and culture of a stool or enema specimen is the test of choice. Organisms and toxin may persist in stool for up to 5 months. If constipation makes obtaining a stool specimen difficult, a small enema of sterile, nonbacteriostatic water should be used promptly. The most prominent electromyographic finding is an incremental increase of evoked muscle potentials at high-frequency nerve stimulation (20–50 Hz). This pattern may not be seen in infants, and its absence does not exclude the diagnosis.

Treatment

Meticulous Supportive Care. Neurologic recovery from botulism may take weeks to months. Therefore, an important aspect of therapy in all forms of botulism is meticulous supportive care, in particular respiratory and nutritional support.

Antitoxin for Infant Botulism. Human-derived antitoxin is given urgently on the basis of a clinically compatible illness. Botulism Immune Globulin for intravenous use (Baby-BIG) is licensed by the US Food and Drug Administration (FDA) for treatment of infant botulism caused by *C botulinum* type A or type B. BabyBIG is made and distributed by the California Department of Public Health. Baby-BIG has been shown to decrease significantly days of mechanical ventilation, days of intensive care unit stay, and overall hospital stays.

Antitoxin for Non-Infant Forms of Botulism. Immediate administration of antitoxin is the key to successful therapy, because antitoxin arrests the progression of paralysis. However, because botulinum neurotoxin binds irreversibly, administration of antitoxin does not reverse paralysis. On suspicion of botulism, antitoxin should be procured immediately through the state health department; all states maintain a 24-hour telephone service for reporting suspected foodborne botulism. In 2010, investigational HBAT replaced the licensed type AB antitoxin and the investigational type E antitoxin. HBAT is the only botulinum antitoxin now available in the United States for treatment of noninfant forms of botulism. HBAT contains antitoxin against all 7 (A–G) botulinum toxin types and has been "de-speciated" by enzymatic removal of the Fc immunoglobulin fragment. HBAT is provided under a Centers for Disease Control and Prevention–sponsored, FDA investigational new drug treatment protocol that includes specific, detailed instructions for intravenous administration of antitoxin.

Antimicrobial Agents. Antimicrobial therapy is not indicated in infant botulism. Aminoglycoside agents potentiate the paralytic effects of the toxin and should be avoided. Penicillin or metronidazole should be given to patients with wound botulism after antitoxin has been administered. The role of antimicrobial therapy in the adult intestinal colonization form of botulism is not established.

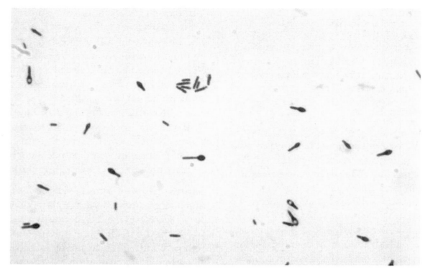

Image 30.1
A photomicrograph of spore forms of *Clostridium botulinum* type A Gram stain. These *C botulinum* bacteria were cultured in thioglycolate broth for 48 hours at 35°C.
The bacterium *C botulinum* produces a nerve toxin that causes the rare but serious paralytic illness botulism. Courtesy of Centers for Disease Control and Prevention/Dr George Lombard.

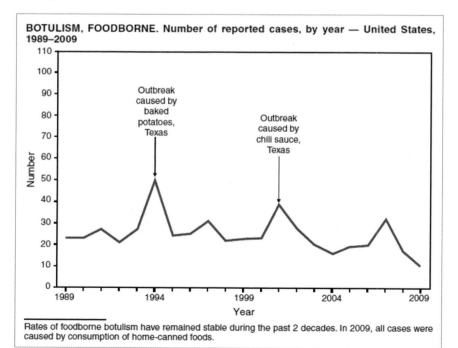

Image 30.2
Foodborne botulism cases per year in the United States, 1989–2009. Courtesy of *Morbidity and Mortality Weekly Report.*

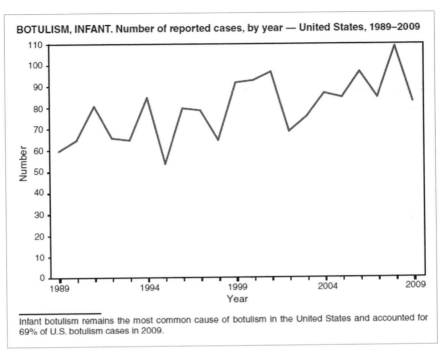

BOTULISM, INFANT. Number of reported cases, by year — United States, 1989–2009

Infant botulism remains the most common cause of botulism in the United States and accounted for 69% of U.S. botulism cases in 2009.

Image 30.3
Infant botulism, number of reported cases by year in the United States, 1989–2009.
Courtesy of *Morbidity and Mortality Weekly Report.*

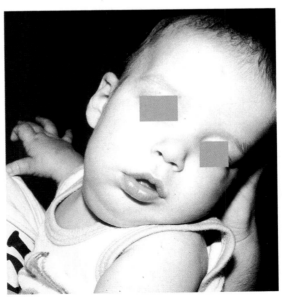

Image 30.4
Infantile botulism in a 4-month-old boy with a 6-day history of progressive weakness, constipation, decreased appetite, and weight loss. The infant had been afebrile, was breastfed, and had not received honey. He was intubated within 24 hours of admission and remained on a ventilator for 26 days. Stool specimens were positive for *Clostridium botulinum* type A. Copyright Larry I. Corman.

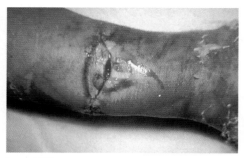

Image 30.5
Wound botulism in the compound fracture of the right arm of a 14-year-old boy. The patient fractured his right ulna and radius and subsequently developed wound botulism. Courtesy of Centers for Disease Control and Prevention.

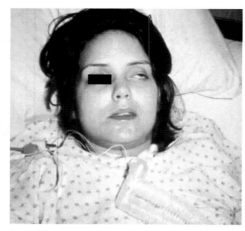

Image 30.6
Botulism with ocular muscle paralysis in a preadolescent female. She also had respiratory muscle weakness but did not require ventilatory support.

31

Clostridium difficile

Clinical Manifestations

Clostridium difficle is associated with several syndromes as well as with asymptomatic carriage. Mild to moderate illness is characterized by watery diarrhea, low-grade fever, and mild abdominal pain. Pseudomembranous colitis generally is characterized by diarrhea with mucus, abdominal cramps and pain, fever, and systemic toxicity. Occasionally, children have marked abdominal tenderness and distention with minimal diarrhea (toxic megacolon). The colonic mucosa often contains 2- to 5-mm, raised, yellowish plaques. Disease often begins while the child is hospitalized receiving antimicrobial therapy but can occur more than 2 weeks after cessation of therapy. Community-associated C difficle disease is less common but is increasing in frequency. The illness typically is associated with antimicrobial therapy or prior hospitalization. Complications, which usually occur in older adults, can include toxic megacolon, intestinal perforation, systemic inflammatory response syndrome, and death. Severe or fatal disease is more likely to occur in neutropenic children with leukemia, in infants with Hirschsprung disease, and in patients with inflammatory bowel disease. Colonization by toxin-producing strains without symptoms occurs in children younger than 5 years and is common in infants younger than 1 year.

Etiology

Clostridium difficile is a spore-forming, obligate anaerobic, gram-positive bacillus. Disease is related to A and B toxins produced by these organisms.

Epidemiology

C difficile can be isolated from soil and is found commonly in the hospital environment. C difficile is acquired from the environment or from stool of other colonized or infected people by the fecal-oral route. Intestinal colonization rates in healthy infants can be as high as 50% but usually are less than 5% in children older than 5 years and adults. Hospitals, nursing homes, and child care facilities are major reservoirs for C difficile. Risk factors for acqui-

sition include prolonged hospitalization and exposure to an infected person either in the hospital or the community. Risk factors for disease include antimicrobial therapy, repeated enemas, gastric acid suppression therapy, prolonged nasogastric tube intubation, gastrostomy and jejunostomy tubes, underlying bowel disease, gastrointestinal tract surgery, renal insufficiency, and humoral immunocompromise. C difficile colitis has been associated with almost every antimicrobial agent. A more virulent strain of C difficile with variations in toxin genes has emerged as a cause of outbreaks among adults and is associated with severe disease. Hospitalization of children for C difficile colitis is increasing.

Incubation Period

Unknown, but usually 5 to 10 days after initiation of antimicrobial therapy.

Diagnostic Tests

The diagnosis of C difficile disease is based on the presence of diarrhea and of C difficile toxins in a diarrheal stool specimen. Isolation of the organism from stool is not useful in an asymptomatic patient. Endoscopic findings of pseudomembranes and hyperemic, friable rectal mucosa suggest pseudomembranous colitis. The most common testing method for C difficile toxins is the commercially available enzyme immunoassay (EIA), which detects toxins A and B. Although EIAs are rapid and performed easily, their sensitivity is relatively low. Two-step testing algorithms that use the sensitive but nonspecific glutamine dehydrogenase EIA combined with confirmatory toxin testing of positive results also can be used. Molecular assays using nucleic acid amplification tests (NAATs) have been developed, are US Food and Drug Administration approved, and now are preferred. NAATs combine good sensitivity and specificity, provide results to clinicians in times comparable to EIAs, and are not required to be part of a 2- or 3-step algorithm. Many children's hospitals are converting to NAAT technology to diagnose C difficile infection. The predictive value of a positive test result in a child younger than 5 years is unknown, because asymptomatic carriage of toxigenic strains often occurs in these children. C difficile toxin degrades at room temperature and can be undetectable within 2 hours after collection of a stool specimen. Stool specimens that are not tested promptly or maintained at 4°C can yield false-negative results. Because colonization with *C difficile* in infants is common, testing for other causes of diarrhea always is recommended in these patients. None of the assays are recommended for test of cure.

Treatment

Precipitating antimicrobial therapy should be discontinued as soon as possible. Antimicrobial therapy for *C difficile* infection is indicated only for symptomatic patients. Strains of *C difficile* are susceptible to metronidazole and vancomycin. Metronidazole is the drug of choice for the initial treatment of children and adolescents with mild to moderate diarrhea and for first relapse. Oral vancomycin or vancomycin administered by enema plus intravenous metronidazole is indicated as initial therapy for patients with severe disease (hospitalized in an intensive care unit, pseudomem-

branous colitis by endoscopy, or underlying intestinal tract disease) and for patients who do not respond to oral metronidazole. Vancomycin for intravenous use can be prepared for oral use. Intravenously administered vancomycin is not effective for *C difficile* infection. Therapy with either metronidazole or vancomycin or the combination should be administered for at least 10 days. Up to 25% of patients experience a relapse after discontinuing therapy, but infection usually responds to a second course of the same treatment. Metronidazole should not be used for treatment of a second recurrence or for chronic therapy, because neurotoxicity is possible. Tapered or pulse regimens of vancomycin are recommended under this circumstance. Drugs that decrease intestinal motility should not be administered.

Investigational therapies include other antimicrobial agents, toxin binders, probiotics, and restoring intestinal tract flora (intestinal microbiota transplantation).

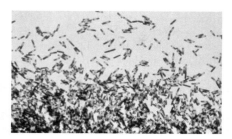

Image 31.1
Clostridium difficile is a gram-positive spore-forming bacteria that can be part of the normal intestinal flora in as many as 50% of children younger than 2 years. It is a cause of pseudomembranous colitis and antibiotic-associated diarrhea in older children and adults.

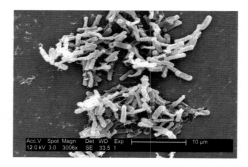

Image 31.2
This micrograph depicts gram-positive *Clostridium difficile* from a stool sample culture obtained using a .1 µm filter. People can become infected if they touch items or surfaces that are contaminated with *C difficile* spores and then touch their mouth or mucous membranes. Health care workers can spread the bacteria to other patients or contaminate surfaces through hand contact. Courtesy of Lois Higg/Centers for Disease Control and Prevention.

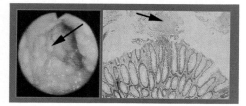

Image 31.3
The right-hand panel shows the typical pseudomembranes of *Clostridium difficile* colitis; the left-hand panel shows the histology, with the pseudomembrane structure at the top middle (arrows). Courtesy of Carol J. Baker, MD.

32

Clostridium perfringens Food Poisoning

Clinical Manifestations

Clostridium perfringens foodborne illness is characterized by a sudden onset of watery diarrhea and moderate to severe, crampy, midepigastric pain. Vomiting and fever are uncommon. Symptoms usually resolve within 24 hours. The short incubation period, short duration, and absence of fever in most patients differentiate *C perfringens* foodborne disease from shigellosis and salmonellosis, and the infrequency of vomiting and longer incubation period contrast with the clinical features of foodborne disease associated with heavy metals, *Staphylococcus aureus* enterotoxins, *Bacillus cereus* emetic toxin, and fish and shellfish toxins. Diarrheal illness caused by *B cereus* diarrheal enterotoxins can be indistinguishable from that caused by *C perfringens*. Enteritis necroticans (known locally as pigbel) results from necrosis of the midgut and is a cause of severe illness and death attributable to *C perfringens* food poisoning among children in Papua, New Guinea. Rare cases have been reported elsewhere associated with diabetes mellitus.

Etiology

Food poisoning is caused by a heat-labile enterotoxin produced in vivo by *C perfringens* type A; enteritis necroticans is caused by type C.

Epidemiology

C perfringens is a gram-positive, spore-forming bacillus that is ubiquitous in the environment and commonly is present in raw meat and poultry. At an optimum temperature, *C perfringens* has one of the fastest growth rates of any bacterium. Spores of *C perfringens* can survive cooking. Spores germinate and multiply during slow cooling and storage at temperatures from 20°C to 60°C (68°F–140°F). Illness results from consumption of food containing high numbers of organisms ($>10^5$ colony forming units/g) followed by enterotoxin production in the intestine. Beef, poultry, gravies, and dried or precooked foods are common sources. Infection usually is acquired at banquets or institutions (eg, schools and camps) or from food provided by caterers or restaurants where food is prepared in large quantities and kept warm for prolonged periods. Illness is not transmissible from person to person.

Incubation Period

6 to 24 hours, usually 8 to 12 hours.

Diagnostic Tests

Because the fecal flora of healthy people commonly includes *C perfringens,* counts of *C perfringens* spores of 10^6/g of feces or greater obtained within 48 hours of onset of illness are required to support the diagnosis in ill people. The diagnosis also can be supported by detection of *C perfringens* enterotoxin in stool by commercially available kits. *C perfringens* can be confirmed as the cause of an outbreak when the concentration of organisms is at least 10^5/g in the epidemiologically implicated food. Although *C perfringens* is an anaerobe, special transport conditions are unnecessary, because the spores are durable. Stool specimens, rather than rectal swab specimens, should be obtained.

Treatment

Oral rehydration or, occasionally, intravenous fluid and electrolyte replacement are indicated to prevent or treat dehydration. Antimicrobial agents are not indicated.

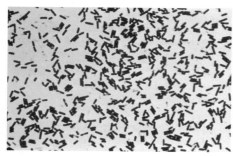

Image 32.1

This photomicrograph reveals numbers of *Clostridium perfringens* bacteria grown in Schaedler broth and subsequently stained using Gram stain (magnification x1,000). *C perfringens* is a spore-forming, heat-resistant bacterium that can cause foodborne disease. The spores persist in the environment and often contaminate raw food materials. These bacteria are found in mammalian feces and soil. Courtesy of Centers for Disease Control and Prevention/Don Stalons.

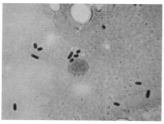

Image 32.2

Clostridium perfringens, an anaerobic, gram-positive, spore-forming bacillus causes a broad spectrum of pathology, including food poisoning. In Papua, New Guinea, *C perfringens* is a cause of severe illness and death called necrotizing enteritis necroticans (locally known as pigbel). Courtesy of Hugh Moffet, MD.

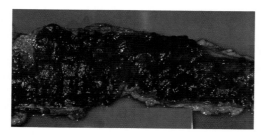

Image 32.3

Hemorrhagic necrosis of the intestine in a patient with *Clostridium perfringens* sepsis. Courtesy of Dimitris P. Agamanolis, MD.

33

Clostridial Myonecrosis

(Gas Gangrene)

Clinical Manifestations

Onset is heralded by acute pain at the site of the wound, followed by edema, exquisite tenderness, exudate, and progression of pain. Systemic findings initially include tachycardia disproportionate to the degree of fever, pallor, diaphoresis, hypotension, renal failure and, later, alterations in mental status. Crepitus is suggestive but not pathognomonic of *Clostridium* infection and is not present always. Diagnosis is based on clinical manifestations, including the characteristic appearance of necrotic muscle at surgery. Untreated gas gangrene can lead to disseminated myonecrosis, suppurative visceral infection, septicemia, and death within hours.

Etiology

Clostridial myonecrosis is caused by *Clostridium* species, most often *Clostridium perfringens,* which are large, gram-positive, spore-forming, anaerobic bacilli with a blunt end. Other *Clostridium* species (eg, *Clostridium sordellii, Clostridium septicum, Clostridium novyi*) also can be associated with myonecrosis. Disease manifestations are caused by potent clostridial exotoxins (eg, *C sordellii* with medical abortion and *C septicum* with malignancy). Mixed infection with other gram-positive and gram-negative bacteria is common.

Epidemiology

Clostridial myonecrosis usually results from contamination of open wounds involving muscle. The sources of *Clostridium* species are soil, contaminated objects, and human and animal feces. Dirty surgical or traumatic wounds with significant devitalized tissue and foreign bodies predispose to disease. Nontraumatic gas gangrene occurs rarely in immunocompromised people.

Incubation Period

From injury, 1 to 4 days.

Diagnostic Tests

Anaerobic cultures of wound exudate, involved soft tissue and muscle, and blood specimens should be performed. Because *Clostridium* species are ubiquitous, their recovery from a wound is not diagnostic unless typical clinical manifestations are present. A Gram-stained smear of wound discharge demonstrating characteristic gram-positive bacilli and absent or sparse polymorphonuclear leukocytes suggests clostridial infection. Tissue specimens (not swab specimens) are appropriate for anaerobic culture. Because some pathogenic *Clostridium* species are exquisitely oxygen sensitive, care should be taken to optimize anaerobic growth conditions. A radiograph of the affected site can demonstrate gas in the tissue, but this is a nonspecific finding. Occasionally, blood cultures are positive and are considered diagnostic.

Treatment

Prompt and complete surgical excision of necrotic tissue and removal of foreign material is essential. Management of shock, fluid and electrolyte imbalance, hemolytic anemia, and other complications is crucial. High-dose penicillin G should be administered intravenously. Clindamycin, metronidazole, meropenem, ertapenem, and chloramphenicol can be considered as alternative drugs for patients with a serious penicillin allergy or for treatment of polymicrobial infections. The combination of penicillin G and clindamycin may be superior to penicillin alone because of the theoretical benefit of clindamycin inhibiting toxin synthesis. Hyperbaric oxygen may be beneficial, but data from adequately controlled studies on its efficacy are not available.

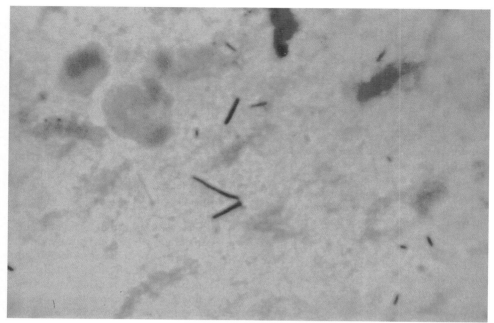

Image 33.1
Clostridial myonecrosis: tissue aspirate. Courtesy of Gary Overturf, MD.

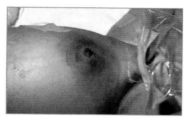

Image 33.2
Clostridial omphalitis in an infant with myonecrosis of the abdominal wall (periumbilical). Early and complete surgical excision of necrotic tissue and careful management of shock, fluid balance, and other complications are crucial for survival.

34

Coccidioidomycosis

Clinical Manifestations

Primary pulmonary infection is acquired by inhaling fungal spores and is asymptomatic or self-limited in 60% of children. Symptomatic disease can resemble influenza or community-acquired pneumonia, with malaise, fever, cough, myalgia, headache, and chest pain. Constitutional symptoms, including extreme fatigue and weight loss, are common and can persist for weeks or months. Acute infection can be associated only with cutaneous abnormalities, such as erythema multiforme, an erythematous maculopapular rash, and erythema nodosum. Chronic pulmonary lesions are rare, but up to 5% of infected people develop asymptomatic pulmonary radiographic residua (eg, cysts, nodules, or coin lesions). Nonpulmonary primary infection is rare and usually follows trauma associated with contamination of wounds by arthroconidia. Cutaneous lesions and soft tissue infections often are accompanied by regional lymphadenitis.

Disseminated infection occurs in less than 0.5% of infected people; common sites of dissemination include skin, bones and joints, central nervous system (CNS), and lungs. Dissemination is more common in infants than older children and adults. Meningitis almost invariably is fatal if untreated. Congenital infection is rare.

Etiology

Coccidioides species are dimorphic fungi. In soil, *Coccidioides* organisms exist in the mycelial phase as a mold growing in branching, septate hyphae. Infectious arthroconidia (ie, spores) become airborne and infect the host after inhalation. Using molecular markers, the genus *Coccidioides* now is divided into 2 species: *Coccidioides immitis*, confined mainly to California, and *Coccidioides posadasii*, encompassing southwestern United States, northern Mexico, and areas of Central and South America.

Epidemiology

Coccidioides species are found in soil in areas of the southwestern United States with endemic infection, including California, Arizona, New Mexico, west and south Texas, southern Nevada, and Utah; northern Mexico; and throughout certain parts of Central and South America. In areas with endemic coccidioidomycosis, clusters of cases can follow dust-generating events, such as storms, seismic events, archaeologic digging, or recreational activities. Most cases occur without a known preceding event. Infection is thought to provide lifelong immunity. Person-to-person transmission of coccidioidomycosis does not occur except for congenital infection following in utero exposure. Preexisting impairment of T-lymphocyte–mediated immunity is a major risk factor for severe primary coccidioidomycosis, disseminated disease, or relapse of past infection. Other people at risk of severe or disseminated disease include people of African or Filipino ancestry, women in the third trimester of pregnancy, people with diabetes or cardiopulmonary disease, and infants. Donor organ–derived coccidioidomycosis has occurred. In regions without endemic infection, careful travel histories should be obtained from people with symptoms or findings compatible with coccidioidomycosis.

Incubation Period

Typically 10 to 16 days (range, 7–28).

Diagnostic Tests

Diagnosis of coccidioidomycosis is best established using serologic, histopathologic, and culture methods. Serologic tests are useful to confirm the diagnosis and provide prognostic information. The immunoglobulin (Ig) M response can be detected by enzyme immunoassay (EIA) or immunodiffusion methods. In approximately 50% and 90% of primary infections, IgM is detected in the first and third weeks, respectively. IgG response can be detected by immunodiffusion, EIA, or complement fixation (CF) tests. Immunodiffusion and CF tests are highly specific. CF antibodies in serum usually are of low titer and are transient if the disease is asymptomatic or mild. Persistent high titers (≥1:16) occur with severe disease and almost always in disseminated infection. Cerebrospinal fluid (CSF) antibodies also are detectable by CF testing. Increasing serum and CSF titers indicate progressive disease, and decreasing titers usually suggest improvement. CF titers may not be reliable in immunocompromised patients. Because clinical laboratories use different diagnostic tests, positive results should be confirmed in a reference laboratory.

Spherules are as large as 80 μm in diameter and can be visualized with 100 to 400 × magnification in infected body fluid specimens (eg, pleural fluid, bronchoalveolar lavage) and biopsy specimens of skin lesions or organs. The presence of a mature spherule with endospores is pathognomonic of infection. Culture of organisms is possible but potentially hazardous to laboratory personnel, because spherules can convert to arthroconidia-bearing mycelia on culture plates.

Treatment

Antifungal therapy for uncomplicated primary infection in people without risk factors for severe disease is controversial. Although most cases will resolve without therapy, some experts believe that treatment may reduce illness duration or risk for severe complications. Most experts would treat people at risk of severe disease or people with severe primary infection. Severe primary infection is manifested by CF titers of 1:16 or greater, infiltrates involving more than half of one lung or portions of both lungs, weight loss of greater than 10%, marked chest pain, severe malaise, inability to work or attend school, intense night sweats, or symptoms that persist for more than 2 months. Fluconazole or itraconazole is recommended for 3 to 6 months. Repeated patient encounters every 1 to 3 months for up to 2 years, either to document radiographic resolution or to identify pulmonary or extrapulmonary complications, are recommended.

Amphotericin B is recommended as alternative therapy if lesions are progressing or are in critical locations, such as the vertebral column. In patients experiencing failure of conventional amphotericin B deoxycholate therapy or experiencing drug-related toxicities, lipid formulation of amphotericin B can be substituted.

Oral fluconazole is recommended for treatment of patients with CNS infections. Patients who respond to azole therapy should continue this treatment indefinitely. For CNS infections that are unresponsive to oral azoles or associated with severe basilar inflammation, intrathecal amphotericin B deoxycholate therapy (0.1–1.5 mg per dose) can be used to augment azole therapy. A subcutaneous reservoir can facilitate administration into the cisternal space or lateral ventricle. Consultation with a specialist for treatment of patients with CNS disease caused by *Coccidioides* species is recommended. The role of newer azole antifungal agents, such as voriconazole, posaconazole, and echinocandins, in treatment of coccidiomycosis has not been established.

The duration of antifungal therapy is variable and depends on the site(s) of involvement, clinical response, and mycologic and immunologic test results. In general, therapy is continued until clinical and laboratory evidence indicates that active infection has resolved. Treatment for disseminated coccidioidomycosis is at least 6 months but for some patients may be extended to 1 year. The required duration of treatment with azoles is uncertain, except for patients with CNS infection, osteomyelitis, underlying HIV infection, or solid organ transplant recipients, for whom suppressive therapy is lifelong. Women should be advised to avoid pregnancy while receiving fluconazole, which may be teratogenic.

Surgical debridement or excision of lesions in bone, pericardium, and lung has been advocated for localized, symptomatic, persistent, resistant, or progressive lesions. In some localized infections with sinuses, fistulae, or abscesses, amphotericin B has been instilled locally or used for irrigation of wounds.

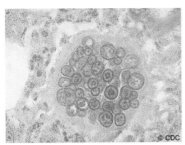

Image 34.1
Spherule with endospores of *Coccidioides immitis* (periodic acid-Schiff stain). Courtesy of Centers for Disease Control and Prevention.

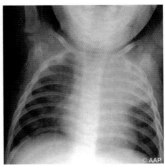

Image 34.2
Pneumonia due to *Coccidioides immitis* in the upper lobe of the left lung of a 5½-month-old infant. The organism was isolated from gastric aspirate, and complement fixation test result was elevated.

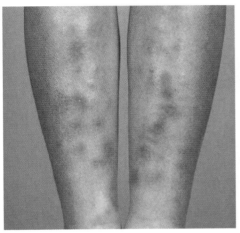

Image 34.3
Erythema nodosum in a preadolescent girl with primary pulmonary coccidioidomycosis.

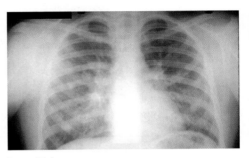

Image 34.4
Primary pulmonary coccidioidomycosis in an 11-year-old boy who recovered spontaneously. The acute disease is usually self-limited in otherwise healthy children. The patient also had erythema nodosum lesions over the tibial area.

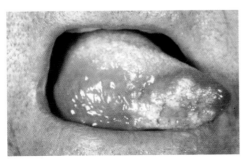

Image 34.5
Coccidioidomycosis of the tongue in an adult male. Courtesy of Edgar O. Ledbetter, MD, FAAP.

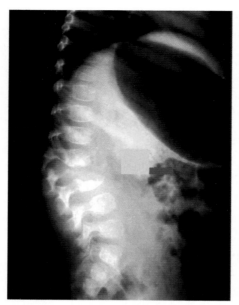

Image 34.6
Spondylitis due to *Coccidioides immitis* in a
2-year-old white male with disseminated disease.

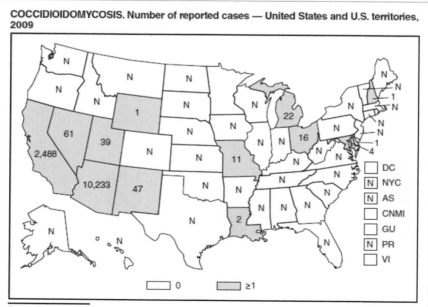

COCCIDIOIDOMYCOSIS. Number of reported cases — United States and U.S. territories, 2009

During 2009, coccidioidomycosis cases reported from Arizona increased. In June 2009, one of the major commercial laboratories in Arizona changed reporting practices to conform with the accepted laboratory case definition from the Council of State and Territorial Epidemiologists; this change might have resulted in an artifactual increase.

Image 34.7
Coccidioidomycosis. Number of reported cases—United States and US Territories, 2009. Courtesy of *Morbidity and Mortality Weekly Report.*

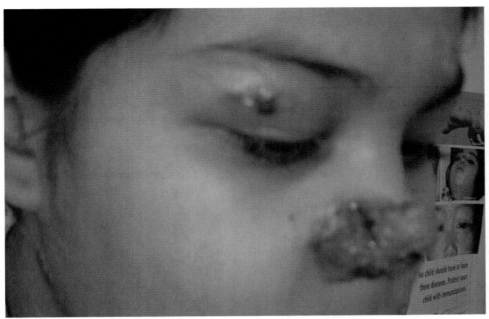

Image 34.8

A 15-year-old Hispanic female who originally presented with forehead lesions without other symptoms. At the third visit she had disseminated coccidioidomycosis disease and had developed extensive cutaneous lesions all over her body with severe nasal involvement. Courtesy of Sabiha Hussain, MD.

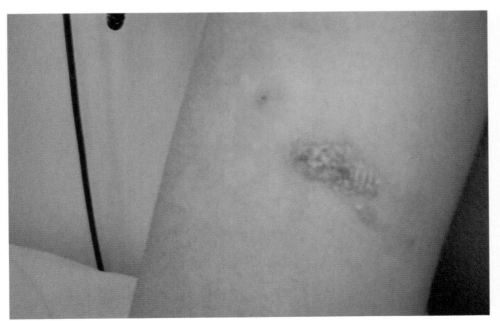

Image 34.9

A 15-year-old Hispanic female who originally presented with forehead lesions without other symptoms. At the third visit she had disseminated coccidioidomycosis disease and had developed extensive cutaneous lesions all over her body with severe nasal involvement. Courtesy of Sabiha Hussain, MD.

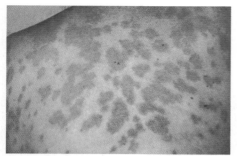

Image 34.10
Erythema nodosum lesions on skin of the back
due to hypersensitivity to antigens of *Coccidioi-des immitis.* Courtesy of Centers for Disease
Control and Prevention/Lucille K. Georg, MD.

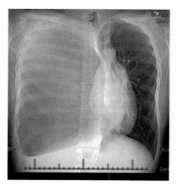

Image 34.11
Chest radiograph of a previously healthy 14-year-
old boy who had a several month history of intermittent fever, weight loss, and chest pain and
recent onset of exercise intolerance. His pyo-
pneumothorax was caused by *Coccidioides
immitis.* He lived in West Texas near the Mexican
border. Courtesy of Jeffrey R. Starke, MD.

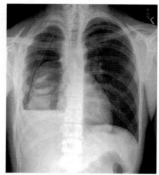

Image 34.12
A chest tube was inserted emergently in the
patient in 34.11, and his right lung was expanded.
Courtesy of Jeffrey R. Starke, MD.

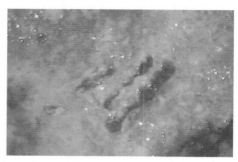

Image 34.13
After 7 days of hospitalization. The patient in
34.11 had a video-assisted thoracostomy followed by an open thoracotomy for decortication
procedure. This photograph demonstrated the
copious fluid, and thin and thick fibrinous exudate
of a chronic empyema found at surgery. Courtesy
of Jeffrey R. Starke, MD.

35

Coronaviruses, Including SARS

Clinical Manifestations

Human coronaviruses (HCoVs) 229E, OC43, NL63, and HKU1 are associated most frequently with the common cold, an upper respiratory tract infection characterized by rhinorrhea, nasal congestion, sore throat, sneezing, and cough that can be associated with fever. Symptoms are self-limiting and typically peak on day 3 or 4 of illness. HCoV infections also may be associated with acute otitis media or asthma exacerbations. Less frequently, HCoVs have been associated with lower respiratory tract infections, including bronchiolitis, croup (especially HCoV-NL63), and pneumonia, primarily in infants and immunocompromised children and adults.

SARS-CoV, the HCoV responsible for the 2002–2003 global outbreaks of severe acute respiratory syndrome (SARS), is associated with more severe symptoms. It disproportionately affects adults, who typically present with fever, myalgia, headache, malaise, and chills followed by a nonproductive cough and dyspnea generally 5 to 7 days later. Approximately 25% of infected adults develop watery diarrhea. Twenty percent develop worsening respiratory distress requiring intubation and ventilation. The overall associated mortality rate is approximately 10%, with most deaths occurring in the third week of illness; mortality approaches 50% in people older than 60 years. Typical laboratory abnormalities include increased lactate dehydrogenase and creatinine kinase concentrations. Most have progressive unilateral or bilateral ill-defined airspace infiltrates on chest imaging.

SARS-CoV infections in children are less severe than adults; notably, no infants or children died from SARS-CoV infection in the 2002–2003 outbreaks. Infants and children younger than 12 years who develop SARS typically present with fever, cough, and rhinorrhea. Associated lymphopenia is less severe, and radiographic changes are milder and generally resolve more quickly than in adolescents and adults. Adolescents who develop SARS have

clinical courses more closely resembling those of adult disease. They also are more likely to develop dyspnea, hypoxemia, and worsening chest radiographic findings.

Etiology

Coronaviruses are classified in the *Nidovirus* family. Coronaviruses are enveloped, nonsegmented, single-stranded, positive-sense RNA viruses named after their corona- or crown-like surface projections observed on electron microscopy that correspond to large surface spike proteins. Coronaviruses can infect humans as well as a variety of different animals. Three serologically and genetically distinct groups of coronaviruses have been described. HCoVs 229E and NL63 belong to group I, and HCoVs OC43, -HKU1, and SARS-CoV belong to group II. Serogroups I and II have been isolated from mammals and serogroup III has been isolated from birds.

Epidemiology

Coronaviruses were first recognized as animal pathogens in the 1930s. Thirty years later, 229E and OC43 were identified as human pathogens, along with other coronavirus strains. In 2003, SARS-CoV was identified as a novel virus responsible for the 2002–2003 global outbreaks of SARS, which lasted for 9 months, infected 8,096 people, and resulted in 774 deaths. Most experts believe SARS-CoV evolved from a natural reservoir of SARS-CoV–like viruses in bats through civet cats as intermediate hosts.

HCoVs other than SARS-CoV can be found worldwide. They cause most disease in the winter and spring months in temperate climates. Seroprevalence data suggest that exposure is common in early childhood, with approximately 90% of adults being seropositive for 229E, OC43, and NL63 and 60% being seropositive for HKU1. In contrast, SARS-CoV infection has not been detected in humans since early 2004.

The modes of transmission for HCoV other than SARS-CoV have not been well studied. However, it is likely that transmission occurs primarily via a combination of droplet and direct and indirect contact spread. For SARS-CoV, studies suggest that droplet and direct contact spread are likely the most common modes of transmission, although evidence of indirect contact spread and aerosol spread also exist.

HCoVs other than SARS-CoV are most likely to be transmitted during the first few days of illness, when symptoms and respiratory viral loads are at their highest. SARS-CoV is most likely to be transmitted during the second week of illness, when both symptoms and respiratory viral loads peak.

Incubation Period

Non-SARS HCoVs, 2 to 5 days; for SARS-CoV 2 to 10 days (median, 4).

Diagnostic Tests

Diagnostic laboratory and clinical guidance for SARS is available on the Centers for Disease Control and Prevention Web site (**www.cdc. gov/ncidod/sars/**). Specimens obtained from the upper and lower respiratory tract are appropriate for viral detection. Stool and serum samples also frequently are positive in patients with SARS-CoV. For 299E and OC43, specimens are most likely to be positive during the first few days of illness; whether this is also true for NL63 and HKU1 is unknown. For SARS-CoV, respiratory and stool specimens may not be positive until the second week of illness; serum samples are most likely positive in the first week. Compared with adults, infants and children with SARS-CoV infections are less likely to have positive specimens.

Treatment

Infections attributable to HCoVs generally are treated with supportive care. SARS-CoV infections are more serious. Steroids, type 1 interferons, convalescent plasma, ribavirin, and lopinavir/ritonavir all were used clinically to treat patients with SARS, albeit without benefit of controlled data documenting efficacy.

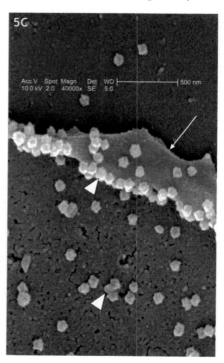

Image 35.2
This scanning electron micrograph (SEM) revealed the thickened, layered edge of SARS infected Vero E6 culture cells. The thickened edges of the infected cells were ruffled, and appeared to comprise layers of folded plasma membranes. Note the layered cell edge (arrows) seen by SEM. Virus particles (arrowheads) are extruded from the layered surfaces. Courtesy of Centers for Disease Control and Prevention/ Dr Mary Ng Mah Lee, National University of Singapore.

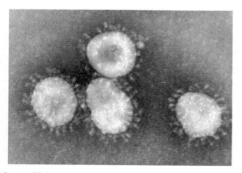

Image 35.1
Coronaviruses are a group of viruses that have a halo or crown-like (corona) appearance when viewed in an electron microscope. Severe acute respiratory syndrome (SARS) coronavirus was the etiologic agent of the 2003 SARS outbreak. Additional specimens are being tested to learn more about this coronavirus and its etiologic link with SARS. Courtesy of Centers for Disease Control and Prevention/Dr Fred Murphy.

36

Cryptococcus neoformans Infections

(Cryptococcosis)

Clinical Manifestations

Primary infection is acquired by inhalation of aerosolized fungal elements from contaminated soil and often is asymptomatic or mild. Pulmonary disease is characterized by cough, chest pain, and constitutional symptoms. Chest radiographs may reveal a solitary nodule or mass or focal or diffuse infiltrates. Hematogenous dissemination to the central nervous system (CNS), bones, skin, and other sites can occur, but dissemination is rare in children without defects in T-lymphocyte–mediated immunity (eg, children with leukemia, systemic lupus erythematosus, chronic mucocutaneous candidiasis, other congenital immunodeficiency, or AIDS or children who have undergone solid organ transplantation). Usually, several sites are infected, but manifestations of involvement at one site predominate. Cryptococcal meningitis, the most common and serious form of cryptococcal infection, often follows an indolent course. Findings are characteristic of meningitis, meningoencephalitis, or space-occupying lesions but can sometimes manifest only as behavioral changes. Cryptococcal fungemia without apparent organ involvement occurs in patients with HIV infection but is rare in children.

Etiology

Cryptococcus neoformans (var *neoformans* and var *grubii*) and *Cryptococcus gattii* are, with rare exception, the only 2 species of the genus *Cryptococcus* that are human pathogens.

Epidemiology

C neoformans var *neoformans* and *C neoformans* var *grubii* are isolated primarily from soil contaminated with pigeon or other bird guano and cause most human infections, especially infections in immunocompromised hosts. *C neoformans* infects 5% to 10% of adults with AIDS, but infection is rare in HIV-infected children. *C gattii* (formerly *C neoformans* var *gattii*) is associated with trees and soil around trees and has emerged as an outbreak-associated pathogen in British Columbia, Canada, and the Pacific Northwest region of the United States. *C gattii* causes disease in immunocompetent and immunocompromised people, but infection is rare in children. Person-to-person transmission does not occur.

Incubation Period

C neoformans, unknown; *C gattii,* 8 weeks to 13 months.

Diagnostic Tests

Definitive diagnosis requires isolation of the organism from body fluid or tissue specimens. Blood should be cultured by lysis-centrifugation. Media containing cycloheximide, which inhibits growth of *C neoformans,* should not be used. Sabouraud dextrose agar is useful for isolation of *Cryptococcus* from sputum, bronchopulmonary lavage, tissue, or cerebrospinal fluid (CSF) specimens. Use of Niger seed (birdseed) can increase the rate of detection in sputum and urine specimens. *C gattii* will turn CGB agar blue, but *C neoformans* leaves CGB agar green. In refractory or relapse cases, susceptibility testing can be helpful, although antifungal resistance is uncommon. A large quantity of CSF may be needed to recover the organism. In children with CNS disease, CSF cell count and protein and glucose concentrations can be normal. The latex agglutination test and enzyme immunoassay for detection of cryptococcal capsular polysaccharide antigen in serum or CSF specimens are excellent rapid diagnostic tests. Antigen is detected in CSF or serum specimens from more than 90% of patients with cryptococcal meningitis. In patients with cryptococcal meningitis, antigen test results can be negative when antigen concentrations are low or very high (prozone effect), if infection is caused by unencapsulated strains, or if the patient is less severely immunocompromised. Encapsulated yeast cells can be visualized using India ink or other stains of CSF and bronchoalveolar lavage specimens. Focal lesions (eg, skin) can be biopsied for fungal staining and culture.

Treatment

Amphotericin B deoxycholate in combination with oral flucytosine is indicated as initial therapy for patients with meningeal and other serious cryptococcal infections. Serum flucytosine concentrations should be maintained between 40 and 60 µg/mL. Patients with meningitis should receive combination therapy for at least 2 weeks followed by consolidation therapy with fluconazole for a minimum of 8 to 10 weeks or until CSF culture is sterile. Alternatively, the amphotericin B deoxycholate and flucytosine combination can be continued for 6 to 10 weeks. Lipid formulations of amphotericin B can be substituted for conventional amphotericin B in children with renal impairment. Amphotericin B alone is an acceptable alternative and is administered for 4 to 6 weeks. A lumbar puncture should be performed after 2 weeks of therapy to document microbiologic clearance. The 20% to 40% of patients in whom culture is positive after 2 weeks of therapy will require a more prolonged treatment course. When infection is refractory to systemic therapy, intraventricular amphotericin B can be administered. Monitoring of serum crypto-coccal antigen is not useful to monitor response to therapy in patients with cryptococcal meningitis. Patients with less severe disease can be treated with fluconazole or itraconazole, but data on use of these drugs for children with *C neoformans* infection are limited. Another potential treatment option for HIV-infected patients with less severe disease is combination therapy with fluconazole and flucytosine. This combination has superior efficacy to fluconazole alone, but toxicity associated with this regimen often limits its usefulness. Increased intracranial pressure occurs frequently despite microbiologic response and often is associated with clinical deterioration. Significant elevation of intracranial pressure should be managed with frequent repeated lumbar punctures or placement of a lumbar drain.

Children with HIV infection who have completed initial therapy for cryptococcosis should receive lifelong suppressive therapy with fluconazole. Oral itraconazole daily or amphotericin B deoxycholate 1 to 3 times weekly are alternatives.

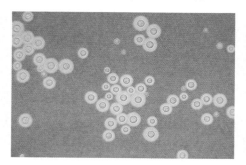

Image 36.1

This photomicrograph depicts *Cryptococcus neoformans* using a light India ink staining preparation. Courtesy of Centers for Disease Control and Prevention/Dr Leonor Haley.

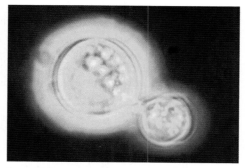

Image 36.2

Cryptococcus neoformans. Thin-walled encapsulated yeast in cerebrospinal fluid (India ink preparation, original magnification of cerebrospinal fluid x450).

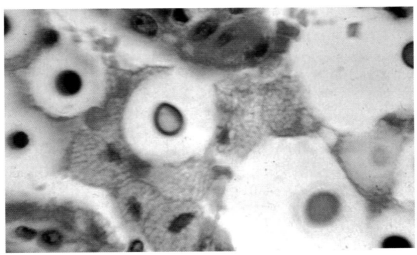

Image 36.3
Cryptococcosis of the liver (original magnification x810) in an immunodeficient patient with dissemi-nated disease. The mucinous capsules are prominent. Courtesy of Edgar O. Ledbetter, MD, FAAP.

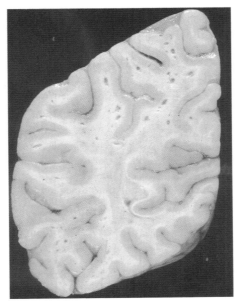

Image 36.4
Cryptococcus meningitis. Cystic lesions resulting from accumulation of organisms in perivascular spaces. Courtesy of Dimitris P. Agamanolis, MD.

37

Cryptosporidiosis

Clinical Manifestations

Frequent, nonbloody, watery diarrhea is the most common manifestation of cryptosporidiosis, although infection can be asymptomatic. Other symptoms include abdominal cramps, fatigue, fever, vomiting, anorexia, and weight loss. In infected immunocompetent adults and children, diarrheal illness is self-limited, usually lasting 6 to 14 days. Infected immunocompromised people, such as people with AIDS, might experience chronic, severe diarrhea, which can lead to malnutrition and weight loss and, as such, could be a significant contributing factor leading to death. Pulmonary, biliary tract, or disseminated infection occurs rarely in immunocompromised people.

Etiology

Cryptosporidium species are oocyst-forming coccidian protozoa. Oocysts are excreted in feces of an infected host and are transmitted via the fecal-oral route. *C hominis,* which predominantly infects humans, and *Cryptosporidium parvum,* which infects cattle, and other mammals, are the primary *Cryptosporidium* species that infect humans.

Epidemiology

Extensive waterborne disease outbreaks have been associated with contamination of drinking water and recreational water (eg, swimming pools, lakes, and interactive fountains). The incidence of cryptosporidiosis in the United States has been increasing since 2005. In children, the incidence of cryptosporidiosis is greatest during summer and early fall, corresponding to the outdoor swimming season. Because oocysts are chlorine tolerant, multistep treatment processes often are used to remove (eg, filter) and inactivate (eg, ultraviolet treatment) oocysts from contaminated water to protect public drinking water supplies. Typical filtration systems used for swimming pools are only partially effective in removing oocysts from contaminated water. As a result, *Cryptosporidium* species have become the leading cause of recreational water-associated outbreaks.

In addition to waterborne transmission, humans can acquire infections from livestock and animals found in petting zoos. Person-to-person transmission occurs and can cause outbreaks in child care centers, in which 20% to 70% of attendees reportedly have been infected. *Cryptosporidium* species also can cause traveler's diarrhea.

Incubation Period

Usually 3 to 14 days; oocyst shedding 2 weeks after symptom resolution except in immunocompromised people who may shed for months.

Diagnostic Tests

The detection of oocysts by microscopic examination of stool specimens is diagnostic. Routine laboratory examination of stool for ova and parasites might not include testing for *Cryptosporidium* species, so testing for the organism specifically should be requested. The direct immunofluorescent antibody method for detection of oocysts in stool is the current test of choice for diagnosis. Oocysts are small (4–6 μm in diameter) and can be missed in a rapid scan of a slide. Enzyme immunoassays and immune chromatography (point-of-care rapid tests) for detecting antigen in stool are available commercially, but confirmation of results by microscopy may be indicated.

At least 3 stool specimens collected on separate days should be examined before considering test results to be negative. Organisms can be identified by intestinal biopsy or sampling of intestinal fluid.

Treatment

Generally, immunocompetent people need no specific therapy. A 3-day course of nitazoxanide oral suspension is recommended for treatment of all people 1 year of age and older. In HIV-infected patients, improvement in CD4+ T-lymphocyte count associated with antiretroviral therapy can lead to symptom resolution. The duration of treatment in HIV-infected children can be up to 14 days. Nitazoxanide, paromomycin, or a combination of paromomycin and azithromycin may be effective, but few data regarding efficacy are available.

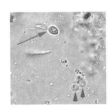

Image 37.1

Cryptosporidium spp oocysts are rounded and measure 4.2 to 5.4 μm in diameter. Sporozoites are sometimes visible inside the oocysts, indicating that sporulation has occurred. *Cryptosporidium* spp oocysts (pink arrows) in wet mount. A budding yeast (brown arrow) is in the same field. Courtesy of Centers for Disease Control and Prevention.

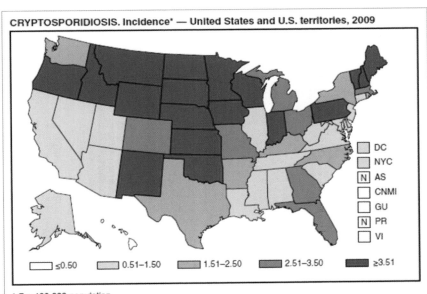

CRYPTOSPORIDIOSIS. Incidence* — United States and U.S. territories, 2009

DC
NYC
N AS
CNMI
GU
N PR
VI

≤0.50   0.51–1.50   1.51–2.50   2.51–3.50   ≥3.51

* Per 100,000 population.

Cryptosporidiosis is widespread geographically in the United States. Differences in reported incidence among states might reflect differences in risk factors, increased cases associated with outbreaks, or difference in the capacity to detect and report cases. Cryptosporidiosis incidence increases during summer, coinciding with increased use of recreational water.

Image 37.2

Cryptosporidiosis. Incidence—United States and US Territories, 2009. Courtesy of *Morbidity and Mortality Weekly Report.*

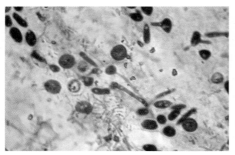

Image 37.3

This micrograph of a direct fecal smear is stained to detect *Cryptosporidium* sp, an intracellular protozoan parasite. Using a modified cold Kinyoun acid-fast staining technique and under an oil immersion lens, the *Cryptosporidium* sp oocysts, which are acid-fast, stain red, and the yeast cells, which are not acid-fast, stain green. Reprinted from Ma P, Soave R. Three-step stool examination for Cryptosporidiosis in 10 homosexual men with protracted watery diarrhea. *J Infect Dis.* 1983;147(5):824–828, with permission from Oxford University Press.

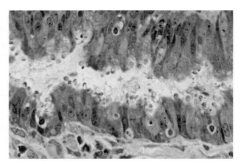

Image 37.4

Histopathology of cryptosporidiosis, intestine. Plastic-embedded, toluidine blue–stained section shows numerous *Cryptosporidium* organisms at luminal surfaces of epithelial cells. Courtesy of Centers for Disease Control and Prevention/Dr Edwin P. Ewing, Jr.

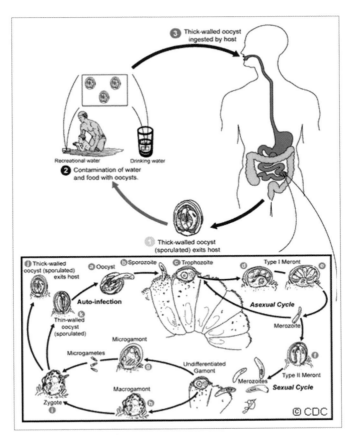

Image 37.5

Life cycle of *Cryptosporidium*.

Sporulated oocysts are excreted by the infected host through feces and possibly other routes such as respiratory secretions (1). Transmission of *C parvum* occurs mainly through contact with contaminated drinking or recreational water. Occasionally food sources may serve as vehicles for transmission. Many outbreaks in the US have occurred in water parks, community swimming pools, and child care centers. Zoonotic transmission of *C parvum* occurs through exposure to infected animals or to water contaminated by feces (2). Following ingestion (and possibly inhalation) by a suitable host (3), excystation (a) occurs. The sporozoites are released and parasitize epithelial cells (b, c) of the gastrointestinal tract or other tissues.

In these cells, the parasites undergo asexual multiplication (schizogony or merogony) (d, e, f) and then sexual multiplication (gametogony), producing microgamonts (male) (g) and macrogamonts (female) (h). On fertilization of the macrogamonts by the microgametes (i), oocysts (j, k) develop that sporulate in the infected host. Two different types of oocysts are produced: the thick-walled, which is commonly excreted from the host (j), and the thin-walled (k), which is primarily involved in autoinfection. Oocysts are infective on excretion, thus permitting direct and immediate fecal-oral transmission. Courtesy of Centers for Disease Control and Prevention/Alexander J. da Silva, PhD/Melanie Moser.

38

Cutaneous Larva Migrans

Clinical Manifestations

Nematode larvae produce pruritic, reddish papules at the site of skin entry, a condition referred to as creeping eruption. As the larvae migrate through skin advancing several millimeters to a few centimeters a day, intensely pruritic, serpiginous tracks or bullae are formed. Larval activity can continue for several weeks or months but eventually is self-limiting. An advancing serpiginous tunnel in the skin with an associated intense pruritus virtually is pathognomonic. Rarely, in infections with a large burden of parasites, pneumonitis (Löffler syndrome), which can be severe, and myositis may follow skin lesions. Occasionally, the larvae reach the intestine and may cause eosinophilic enteritis.

Etiology

Infective larvae of cat and dog hookworms (ie, *Ancylostoma braziliense* and *Ancylostoma caninum*) are usual causes. Other skin-penetrating nematodes are occasional causes.

Epidemiology

Cutaneous larva migrans is a disease of children, utility workers, gardeners, sunbathers, and others who come in contact with soil contaminated with cat and dog feces. In the United States, the disease is most prevalent in the Southeast. Most cases in the United States are imported by travelers returning from tropical and subtropical areas.

Diagnostic Tests

Because the diagnosis usually is made clinically, biopsies are not indicated. Biopsy specimens typically demonstrate an eosinophilic inflammatory infiltrate, but the migrating parasite is not visualized. Eosinophilia and increased immunoglobulin E serum concentrations occur in some cases. Larvae have been detected in sputum and gastric washings in patients with the rare complication of pneumonitis.

Treatment

The disease usually is self-limited, with spontaneous cure after several weeks or months. Orally administered albendazole or mebendazole is the recommended therapy.

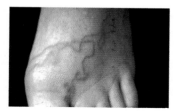

Image 38.1
Cutaneous larva migrans lesions of the foot of a 10-year-old girl. In the United States this dog and cat hookworm infection is most commonly seen in the southeastern states. These raised, serpiginous, pruritic, migrating eruptions may extend rapidly. Copyright Gary Williams, MD.

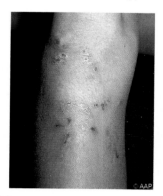

Image 38.2
Cutaneous larva migrans 48 hours after treatment. Orally administered albendazole or ivermectin is the recommended therapy.

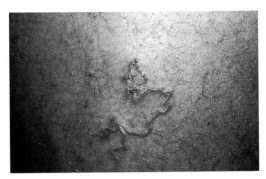

Image 38.3
Adult who noted a migrating skin lesion on left thigh for 2 weeks. Copyright Larry I. Corman.

39

Cyclosporiasis

Clinical Manifestations

Watery diarrhea is the most common symptom and can be profuse and protracted. Anorexia, nausea, vomiting, substantial weight loss, flatulence, abdominal cramping, myalgia, and prolonged fatigue also can occur. Low-grade fever occurs in approximately 50% of people. Biliary tract disease also has been reported. Infection usually is self-limited, but untreated people may have remitting, relapsing symptoms for weeks to months. Asymptomatic infection occurs most commonly in settings where cyclosporiasis is endemic.

Etiology

Cyclospora cayetanensis is a coccidian protozoan; oocysts (rather than cysts) are passed in stools and become infectious days to weeks following excretion.

Epidemiology

C cayetanensis is endemic in many resource-limited countries. In the United States, 10% of cases occur in people younger than 20 years, and a history of travel has been reported in approximately one-third of patients with cyclosporiasis. Both foodborne and waterborne outbreaks have been reported, with most cases occurring in May through July. Most of the outbreaks in the United States and Canada have been associated with consumption of imported fresh produce, including Guatemalan raspberries and Thai basil. Humans are the only known hosts for *C cayetanensis*. Direct person-to-person transmission is unlikely. The oocysts are resistant to most disinfectants used in food and water processing and can remain viable for prolonged periods in cool, moist environments.

Incubation Period

Approximately 7 days (range, 2–14).

Diagnostic Tests

Diagnosis is made by identification of oocysts (8–10 μm in diameter) in stool, intestinal fluid/aspirate, or intestinal biopsy specimens. Oocysts may be shed at low levels, even by people with profuse diarrhea. This makes repeated stool examinations, sensitive recovery methods (eg, concentration procedures), and detection methods that highlight the organism critical. Oocysts are autofluorescent and variably acid-fast after modified acid-fast staining of stool specimens (ie, oocysts that either have retained or not retained the stain can be visualized). Investigational molecular diagnostic assays (eg, PCR) are available at reference laboratories.

Treatment

Trimethoprim-sulfamethoxazole, typically for 7 to 10 days, is the drug of choice. People infected with HIV may need long-term maintenance therapy.

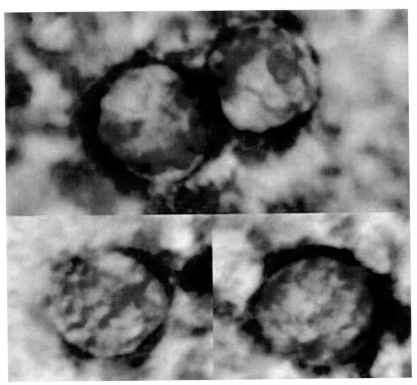

Image 39.1
Four *Cyclospora* oocysts from fresh stool fixed in 10% formalin and stained with safranin, showing the uniform staining of oocysts by this method. Courtesy of Centers for Disease Control and Prevention.

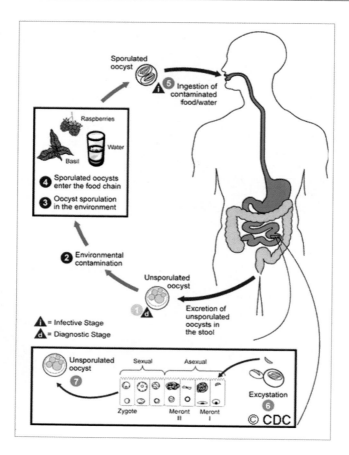

Image 39.2

Cyclospora cayetanensis. When freshly passed in stools, the oocyst is not infective (1) (thus direct fecal-oral transmission cannot occur; this differentiates *Cyclospora* from another important coccidian parasite, *Cryptosporidium*). In the environment (2), sporulation occurs after days or weeks at temperatures between 22°C to 32°C, resulting in division of the sporont into 2 sporocysts, each containing 2 elongate sporozoites (3). Fresh produce and water can serve as vehicles for transmission (4) and the sporulated oocysts are ingested (in contaminated food or water) (5). The oocysts excyst in the gastrointestinal tract, freeing the sporozoites, which invade the epithelial cells of the small intestine (6). Inside the cells they undergo asexual multiplication and sexual development to mature into oocysts, which will be shed in stools (7). The potential mechanisms of contamination of food and water are still under investigation. Some elements of this figure were created based on an illustration by Ortega YR, Sterling CR, Gilman RH. Cyclospora cayetanensis. *Adv Parasitol.* 1998;40:399–418. Courtesy of Centers for Disease Control and Prevention/Elsevier, with permission.

40

Cytomegalovirus Infection

Clinical Manifestations

Manifestations of acquired human cytomegalovirus (CMV) infection vary with the age and immunocompetence of the host. Asymptomatic infections are the most common, particularly in children. An infectious mononucleosis-like syndrome with prolonged fever and mild hepatitis, occurring in the absence of heterophile antibody production, can occur in adolescents and adults. Pneumonia, colitis, and retinitis may occur in immunocompromised hosts, including people receiving treatment for malignant neoplasms, people infected with HIV, and people receiving immunosuppressive therapy for organ or hematopoietic stem cell transplantation.

Congenital infection has a spectrum of manifestations but usually is not evident at birth (asymptomatic congenital CMV infection). Approximately 10% of infants with congenital CMV infection have involvement that is evident at birth (symptomatic congenital CMV disease), with manifestations including intrauterine growth restriction, jaundice, purpura, hepatosplenomegaly, microcephaly, intracerebral calcifications, and retinitis; developmental delay is common among these infants as they grow. Sensorineural hearing loss (SNHL) is the most common sequela following congenital infection, with the likelihood of SNHL being higher among infants with symptomatic infection noted at birth. Congenital CMV infection is the leading nongenetic cause of SNHL in children in the United States. Approximately 21% of all hearing loss at birth is attributable to congenital CMV infection; 25% of all hearing loss at 4 years of age is attributable to congenital CMV infection. Late-onset and progressive hearing losses occur following congenital CMV infection. Approximately 33% to 50% of SNHL attributable to congenital CMV infection is late-onset loss. Approximately 50% of children with SNHL will continue to have further deterioration or progression of their loss, and these children should be evaluated regularly for early detection and intervention as appropriate.

Infection acquired intrapartum from maternal cervical secretions or postpartum from human milk usually is not associated with clinical illness in term babies. In preterm infants, infection resulting from human milk or from transfusion from CMV-seropositive donors has been associated with systemic infections, including lower respiratory tract disease and interstitial pneumonia.

Etiology

Human CMV, also known as human herpesvirus 5, is a member of the herpesvirus family (*Herpesviridae*), subfamily (*Betaherpesvirinae*), and cytomegalovirus genus (*Cytomegalovirus*). The viral genome contains double-stranded DNA.

Epidemiology

CMV is highly species specific, and only human strains produce human disease. The virus is ubiquitous and has numerous strain types. Transmission occurs horizontally (by direct person-to-person contact with virus-containing secretions), vertically (from mother to infant before, during, or after birth), and via transfusions of blood, platelets, and white blood cells from infected donors. CMV also can be transmitted with organ or hematopoietic stem cell transplantation. Infections have no seasonal predilection. CMV persists in latent form after a primary infection or subclinical reactivation, and frequent and symptomatic reactivation can occur years later, particularly under conditions of immunosuppression. Reinfection with other strains of CMV can occur in seropositive hosts.

Horizontal transmission probably is the result of salivary exposure, but contact with infected urine also can have a role. Spread of CMV in households and child care centers is well documented. Excretion rates from urine or saliva in children 1 to 3 years of age who attend child care centers usually range from 30% to 40% but can be as high as 70%. Young children can transmit CMV to their parents, including mothers who may be pregnant, and other caregivers, including child care staff. In adolescents and adults, sexual transmission also occurs.

Seropositive healthy people have latent CMV in their leukocytes and tissues; hence, blood transfusions and organ transplantation can result in viral transmission. Severe CMV disease following transfusion or organ transplantation is more likely to occur if the recipient is immunosuppressed and seronegative or is a preterm infant. In contrast, among nonautologous hematopoietic stem cell transplant recipients, it is seropositive recipients who receive transplants from seronegative donors who are at greatest risk of disease when exposed after transplant. Latent CMV commonly will reactivate in immunosuppressed people and can result in disease if immunosuppression is severe (eg, in patients with AIDS or solid organ and hematopoietic stem cell transplant recipients).

Vertical transmission of CMV to an infant occurs in one of the following time periods: (1) in utero by transplacental passage during maternal viremia; (2) at birth during passage through an infected maternal genital tract; or (3) postnatally by ingestion of CMV-positive human milk. Approximately 1% of all live-born infants are infected in utero and excrete CMV at birth, making this the most common congenital viral infection. Congenital infection and associated disabilities can occur no matter in what trimester the mother is infected, but severe sequelae are associated most commonly with primary maternal infection acquired during the first half of gestation. In utero fetal infection can occur during the mother's primary infection or in a seropositive mother who acquires a different CMV strain or who reactivates her latent virus. Damaging fetal infections following nonprimary maternal infection have been reported, and the role of acquisition of a different viral strain in women with preexisting CMV antibody as a cause of symptomatic infection with sequelae in infants is an area of current research.

Cervical excretion is common among seropositive women, resulting in exposure of many infants to CMV at birth. Cervical excretion rates are highest among young mothers in lower socioeconomic groups. Similarly, although disease can occur in seronegative infants fed CMV-infected human milk, most infants who acquire CMV from ingestion of infected human milk do not develop clinical illness. Among infants who acquire infection from maternal cervical secretions or human milk, preterm infants are at greater risk of CMV illness and sequelae.

Incubation Period

Horizontally transmitted CMV infection unknown; 3 to 12 weeks and 1 to 4 months after blood transfusion or organ transplantation, respectively.

Diagnostic Tests

The diagnosis of CMV disease is confounded by the ubiquity of the virus, the high rate of asymptomatic excretion, the frequency of reactivated infections, development of serum immunoglobulin (Ig) M CMV-specific antibody in some episodes of reactivation, reinfection with different strains of CMV, and concurrent infection with other pathogens.

Virus can be isolated in cell culture from urine, pharynx, peripheral blood leukocytes, human milk, semen, cervical secretions, and other tissues and body fluids. Recovery of virus from a target organ provides strong evidence that the disease is caused by CMV infection. A presumptive diagnosis of CMV infection beyond the neonatal period can be made on the basis of a fourfold antibody titer increase in paired serum specimens or by demonstration of virus excretion. Techniques for detection of viral DNA in tissues and some fluids, such as cerebrospinal fluid, by PCR assay or hybridization are available. Detection of pp65 antigen or quantification of viral DNA (eg, by quantitative PCR assay) in white blood cells also may be used to detect infection in immunocompromised hosts.

Various immunofluorescent assays, indirect hemagglutination assays, latex agglutination assays, and enzyme immunoassays are available for detecting CMV-specific antibodies.

Amniocentesis has been used in several small series of patients to establish the diagnosis of intrauterine infection. Proof of congenital infection requires isolation of CMV from urine, stool, respiratory tract secretions, or CSF obtained within 2 to 4 weeks of birth. A positive PCR assay result from a neonatal dried blood spot confirms congenital infection, but a negative result does not exclude congenital infection because of poor test sensitivity. Differentiation between intrauterine and perinatal infection is difficult at later than 2 to 4 weeks of age unless clinical manifestations of the former (eg, chorioretinitis, intracranial calcifications) are present. A strongly positive CMV-specific IgM during early infancy is suggestive of congenital CMV infection, but IgM antibody assays vary in accuracy for identification of primary infection.

Treatment

Intravenous ganciclovir is approved for induction and maintenance treatment of retinitis caused by acquired or recurrent CMV infection in immunocompromised adult patients, including HIV-infected patients, and for prevention of CMV disease in adult transplant recipients. Valganciclovir, the oral prodrug of ganciclovir, also is approved for treatment (induction and maintenance) of CMV retinitis in immunocompromised adult patients, including HIV-infected patients, and for prevention of CMV disease in kidney, kidney-pancreas, or heart transplant recipients at high risk of CMV disease. Valganciclovir also is approved for prevention of CMV disease in kidney or heart transplant pediatric patients 4 months of age and older. Ganciclovir and valganciclovir also are used to treat CMV infections of other sites (esophagus, colon, lungs) and for preemptive treatment of immunosuppressed adults with CMV antigenemia or viremia. Oral ganciclovir is not available in the United States, but oral valganciclovir is available both in tablet and in powder for oral solution formulations.

Data in neonates with symptomatic congenital CMV disease involving the central nervous system (CNS) suggest possible benefit of 6 weeks of parenteral ganciclovir therapy for protecting against hearing deterioration and potentially in decreasing developmental impairment. Antiviral therapy is not recommended routinely in neonates and young infants because of possible toxicities, including neutropenia. If parenteral ganciclovir or oral valganciclovir are used in the management of neonates congenitally infected with CMV, their use should be limited to patients with symptomatic congenital CMV disease involving the CNS who are able to start treatment within the first month of life. Experts differ in opinion as to whether patients with isolated hearing loss should be classified as symptomatic with CNS involvement; however, patients with such limited involvement are not the group in which therapeutic benefit has been documented.

Preterm infants with perinatally acquired CMV infection can have symptomatic, end-organ disease (eg, pneumonitis, hepatitis, thrombocytopenia). Antiviral treatment has not been studied in this population. If such patients are treated with parenteral ganciclovir, a reasonable approach is to treat for 2 weeks and then reassess responsiveness to therapy. If clinical data suggest benefit of treatment, an additional 1 to 2 weeks of parenteral ganciclovir can be considered if symptoms and signs have not been resolved.

In hematopoietic stem cell transplant recipients, the combination of immune globulin intravenous (IGIV) or CMV immune globulin intravenous (CMV-IGIV) and ganciclovir administered intravenously has been reported to be synergistic in treatment of CMV pneumonia. Unlike CMV-IGIV, IGIV products have varying anti-CMV antibody concentrations from lot to lot, are not tested routinely, and do not have a specified titer of antibodies to CMV. Valganciclovir and foscarnet also have been approved for treatment and maintenance of CMV retinitis in adults with AIDS. Foscarnet is more toxic (with high rates of limiting nephrotoxicity) but may be advantageous for some patients with HIV infection.

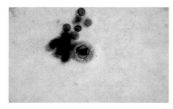

Image 40.1
Cells with intranuclear inclusions in the urine of infant with congenital cytomegalovirus disease.

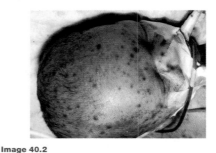

Image 40.2
A 1-day-old infant who was small for gestational age and had microcephaly, hepatomegaly, jaundice, and a "blueberry muffin" rash. The infant also developed thrombocytopenia and disseminated intravascular coagulation. The infant died at 48 hours of age. Kidney and lung tissue culture tested positive for cytomegalovirus. Courtesy of Larry I. Corman, MD.

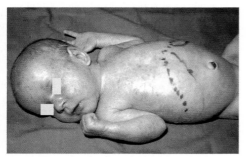

Image 40.3
Three-week-old infant with congenital cytomegalovirus infection with purpuric skin lesions and hepatosplenomegaly. Courtesy of Edgar O. Ledbetter, MD, FAAP.

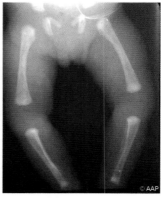

Image 40.4
Infant with lethal cytomegalovirus disease with radiographic changes in long bones of osteitis characterized by fine vertical metaphyseal striations. Courtesy of Edgar O. Ledbetter, MD, FAAP.

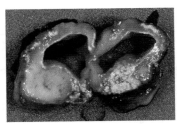

Image 40.5
Congenital cytomegalovirus encephalitis. Microcephaly and cerebral calcification. Courtesy of Dimitris P. Agamanolis, MD.

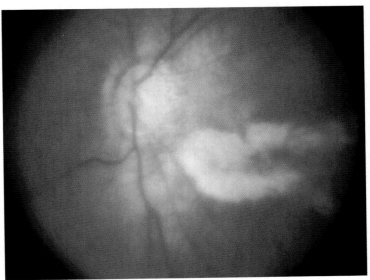

Image 40.6
Characteristic white perivascular infiltrates in the retina of an infant with congenital cytomegalovirus infection. Courtesy of George Nankervis, MD.

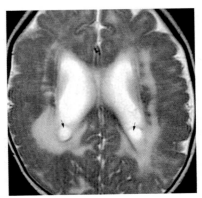

Image 40.7
Axial T2-weighted magnetic resonance image demonstrates periventricular germinolytic cysts (arrows). Also note the periventricular white matter hyperintensities that are representative of demyelination and gliosis.

41

Dengue

Clinical Manifestations

Dengue has a wide range of clinical presentations, from a mild viral syndrome to classic dengue fever and severe dengue (ie, dengue hemorrhagic fever or dengue shock syndrome). Approximately 5% of patients develop severe dengue, which is more common with second or other subsequent infections. Less common clinical syndromes include myocarditis, pancreatitis, hepatitis, and neuroinvasive disease.

Dengue is a dynamic disease beginning with a nonspecific, acute febrile illness lasting 2 to 7 days (febrile phase), progressing to severe disease during fever defervescence (critical phase) and ending in a convalescent phase. Fever can be biphasic and usually is accompanied by muscle, joint, and/or bone pain; headache; retro-orbital pain; facial erythema; oropharyngeal erythema; macular or maculopapular rash; leukopenia; and petechiae or other minor bleeding manifestations. Signs of progression to severe dengue occur in the late febrile phase and include persistent vomiting, abdominal pain, mucosal bleeding, difficulty breathing, early signs of shock, and a rapid decline in platelet count with an increase in hematocrit (hemoconcentration). Patients with nonsevere disease begin to improve during the critical phase, and people with clinically significant plasma leakage attributable to increased vascular permeability develop severe disease with pleural effusions and/or ascites, hypovolemic shock, and hemorrhage.

Etiology

Four related RNA viruses of the genus *Flavivirus*, dengue viruses (DENV)-1, -2, -3, and -4, cause symptomatic (~25%) and asymptomatic (~75%) infections. Infection with one DENV type produces lifelong immunity against that type. A person has a lifetime risk of up to 4 DENV infections.

Epidemiology

DENV primarily is transmitted to humans through the bite of infected *Aedes aegypti* mosquitoes. Humans are the main amplifying host of DENV and the main source of virus for *Aedes* mosquitoes. Because of the approximately 7 days of viremia, DENV can be transmitted following receipt of blood products, donor organs or tissue, percutaneous exposure to blood, and exposure in utero or at parturition.

Dengue is a major public health problem in the tropics and subtropics; an estimated 50 million cases occur annually, and 40% of the world's population lives in areas with DENV transmission. In the United States, dengue is endemic in Puerto Rico, the Virgin Islands, and American Samoa. In addition, millions of US travelers, including children, are at risk, because dengue is the leading cause of febrile illness among travelers returning from the Caribbean, Latin America, and South Asia. Outbreaks with local DENV transmission have occurred in Texas, Hawaii, and Florida in the last decade. However, although 16 states have *A aegypti* and 35 states have *A albopictus* mosquitoes, local dengue transmission is uncommon because of infrequent contact between people and infected mosquitoes. Dengue occurs in both children and adults and affects both sexes with no differences in infection rates or disease severity.

Incubation Period

3–14 days before symptom onset; infected people can transmit to mosquitoes 1–2 days before symptoms develop and throughout the viremic period.

Diagnostic Tests

Laboratory confirmation of a clinical diagnosis of dengue depends on when a serum sample is obtained during the course of illness and may require detection of anti-DENV immunoglobulin (Ig) M antibodies by enzyme immunosorbent assay, detection of DENV RNA by reverse-transcriptase PCR assay, or detection of DENV antigen by immunoassay. DENV RNA is detectable during the febrile phase, but anti-DENV IgM antibodies are not detectable until 4 to 5 days after illness onset. Other approaches are fourfold or greater increase in reciprocal IgG anti-DENV titer or hemagglutination inhibition titer to DENV antigens in acute- and convalescent-phase sera or IgM anti-DENV in cerebrospinal fluid. Diagnostic testing for DENV is available through commercial reference laboratories, some state public health laboratories, and the Dengue Branch of the Centers for Disease Control and Prevention.

Treatment

No specific antiviral therapy exists for dengue. During the febrile phase, patients should stay well hydrated and avoid use of aspirin, aspirin-containing drugs, and other nonsteroidal anti-inflammatory drugs to minimize the potential for bleeding. Additional supportive care is required if the patient becomes dehydrated or develops warning signs for severe disease at the time of fever defervescence.

Early recognition of shock and intensive supportive therapy can reduce risk of death from approximately 10% to less than 1% in severe dengue. During the critical phase, maintenance of fluid volume and hemodynamic status is central to management of severe cases. Reabsorption of extravascular fluid occurs during the convalescent phase with stabilization of hemodynamic status and diuresis. It is important to watch for signs of fluid overload, which may manifest as a decrease in the patient's hematocrit as a result of the dilutional effect of reabsorbed fluid.

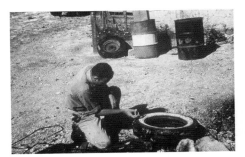

Image 41.1

This photograph depicts an entomologic field technician inspecting some discarded automobile tires for the presence of mosquitoes, primarily *Aedes aegypti*, which is a vector responsible for the transmission of Dengue fever to humans. Dengue fever is primarily a disease of the tropics, and the viruses that cause it are maintained in a cycle that involves humans, and *A aegypti*, a domestic, day-biting mosquito that prefers to feed on humans. Infection with dengue viruses produces a spectrum of clinical illness ranging from a nonspecific viral syndrome, to severe and fatal hemorrhagic disease. Important risk factors for Dengue fever include the strain and serotype of the infecting virus, as well as the age, immune status, and genetic predisposition of the patient. Courtesy of Centers for Disease Control and Prevention.

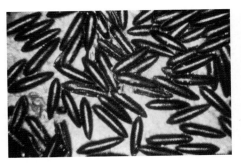

Image 41.2

This photograph shows numerous eggs of the dengue fever mosquito vector, *Aedes aegypti*. *A aegypti* mosquitoes deposit their eggs in any water-holding container located in or around houses. These containers include large uncovered jars for drinking water, and refuse receptacles such as bottles and food tins. Courtesy of Centers for Disease Control and Prevention.

42

Diphtheria

Clinical Manifestations

Respiratory tract diphtheria usually occurs as membranous nasopharyngitis or obstructive laryngotracheitis. Membranous pharyngitis associated with a bloody nasal discharge should suggest diphtheria. Local infections are associated with a low-grade fever and gradual onset of manifestations over 1 to 2 days. Less commonly, diphtheria presents as cutaneous, vaginal, conjunctival, or otic infection. Cutaneous diphtheria is more common in tropical areas and among the urban homeless. Extensive neck swelling with cervical lymphadenitis (bull neck) is a sign of severe disease. Life-threatening complications of respiratory diphtheria include upper airway obstruction caused by extensive membrane formation; myocarditis, which often is associated with heart block; and cranial and peripheral neuropathies. Palatal palsy, characterized by nasal speech, frequently occurs in pharyngeal diphtheria.

Etiology

Diphtheria is caused by toxigenic strains of *Corynebacterium diphtheriae*. In industrialized countries, toxigenic strains of *Corynebacterium ulcerans* are emerging as an important cause of a diphtheria-like illness. *C diphtheriae* is an irregularly staining, gram-positive, nonspore-forming, nonmotile, pleomorphic bacillus. *C diphtheriae* strains may be either toxigenic or nontoxigenic. Toxigenic strains express an exotoxin that consists of an enzymatically active A domain and a binding B domain, which promotes the entry of A into the cell. The toxin inhibits protein synthesis in cells, resulting in myocarditis, acute tubular necrosis, and delayed peripheral nerve conduction. Nontoxigenic strains of *C diphtheriae* can cause sore throat and, rarely, other invasive infections, including endocarditis.

Epidemiology

Humans are the sole reservoir of *C diphtheriae*. Organisms are spread by respiratory droplets and by contact with discharges from skin lesions. In untreated people, organisms can be present in discharges from the nose and throat and from eye and skin lesions for 2 to 6 weeks after infection. Patients treated with an appropriate antimicrobial agent usually are communicable for less than 4 days. Transmission results from intimate contact with patients or carriers. People who travel to areas where diphtheria is endemic or people who come into contact with infected travelers from such areas are at increased risk of being infected with the organism. Severe disease occurs more often in people who are unimmunized or inadequately immunized. Fully immunized people may be asymptomatic carriers or have mild sore throat. The incidence of respiratory diphtheria is greatest during autumn and winter, but summer epidemics can occur in warm climates in which skin infections are prevalent. Diphtheria remains endemic in the independent states of the former Soviet Union as well as in Africa, Latin America, Asia, the Middle East, and parts of Europe, where childhood immunization coverage with diphtheria toxoid–containing vaccines is suboptimal. No case of respiratory tract diphtheria has been reported in the United States since 2003. Cases of cutaneous diphtheria likely still occur in the United States, but they are not reportable.

Incubation Period

2 to 7 days; occasionally longer.

Diagnostic Tests

Specimens for culture should be obtained from the nose or throat or any mucosal or cutaneous lesion. Material should be obtained from beneath the membrane, or a portion of the membrane itself should be submitted for culture. Because special medium is required for isolation, laboratory personnel should be notified that *C diphtheriae* is suspected. Specimens collected for culture can be placed in any transport medium (eg, Amies, Stuart media) and transported at 4°C or in silica gel packs to a reference laboratory for culture. All *C diphtheriae* isolates should be sent through the state health department to the Centers for Disease Control and Prevention (CDC).

Treatment

Antitoxin. Because the condition of patients with diphtheria can deteriorate rapidly, a single dose of equine antitoxin should be administered on the basis of clinical diagnosis, even before culture results are available. Antitoxin is available through the CDC. To neutralize toxin from the organism as rapidly as possible, the preferred route of administration is intravenous. Before intravenous administration of antitoxin, tests for sensitivity to horse serum should be performed, initially with a scratch test of a 1:1,000 dilution of antitoxin in saline solution followed by an intradermal test if the scratch test result is negative. If the patient is sensitive to equine antitoxin, desensitization is necessary. Allergic reactions to horse serum can be expected in 5% to 20% of patients. The dose of antitoxin depends on the site and size of the diphtheria membrane, duration of illness, and degree of toxic effects; presence of soft, diffuse cervical lymphadenitis suggests moderate to severe toxin absorption. Antitoxin probably is of no value for cutaneous disease.

Antimicrobial Therapy. Erythromycin administered orally or parenterally for 14 days, penicillin G administered intramuscularly or intravenously for 14 days, or penicillin G procaine administered intramuscularly for 14 days constitute acceptable therapy. Antimicrobial therapy is required to stop toxin production, to eradicate *C diphtheriae*, and to prevent transmission, but it is not a substitute for antitoxin, which is the primary therapy. Elimination of the organism should be documented 24 hours after completion of treatment by 2 consecutive negative cultures from specimens taken 24 hours apart.

Immunization. Active immunization against diphtheria should be undertaken during convalescence from diphtheria; disease does not necessarily confer immunity.

Cutaneous Diphtheria. Thorough cleansing of the lesion with soap and water and administration of an appropriate antimicrobial agent for 10 days are recommended.

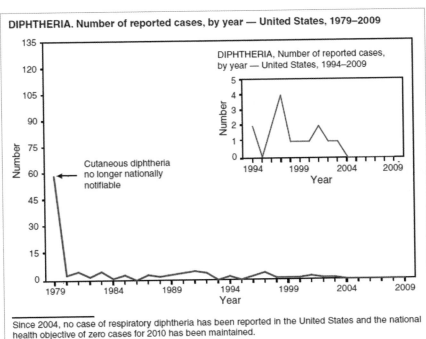

DIPHTHERIA. Number of reported cases, by year — United States, 1979–2009

DIPHTHERIA, Number of reported cases, by year — United States, 1994–2009

Cutaneous diphtheria no longer nationally notifiable

Since 2004, no case of respiratory diphtheria has been reported in the United States and the national health objective of zero cases for 2010 has been maintained.

Image 42.1
Diphtheria. Number of reported cases—United States and US territories, 1979–2009.
Courtesy of *Morbidity and Mortality Weekly Report.*

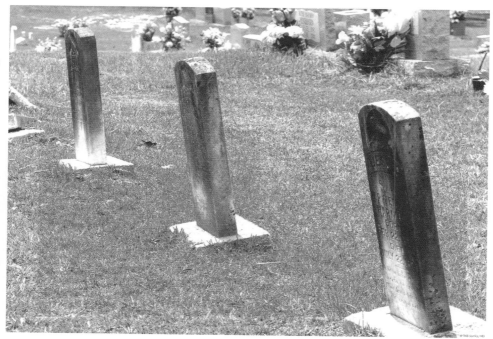

Image 42.2

Baby graves dating from the 1890s in a central Mississippi family cemetery. Diphtheria was a common cause of these infant deaths prior to the introduction of a toxoid vaccine around 1921. In the pre-antibiotic era treatment was limited to comfort care or tracheotomy. Vaccination of children and adults has reduced the number of diphtheria cases in the United States. However, reluctance to immunize children sets the stage for another generation of rows of tiny memories. Copyright Will Sorey, MD.

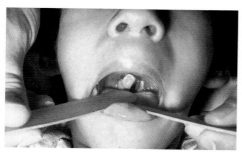

Image 42.3

Pharyngeal diphtheria with membranes covering the tonsils and uvula in a 15-year-old girl. Tonsillar and pharyngeal diphtheria may need to be differentiated from group A streptococcal pharyngitis, infectious mononucleosis, Vincent angina, acute toxoplasmosis, thrush, and leukemia, as well as other less common entities including tularemia and acute cytomegalovirus infection.

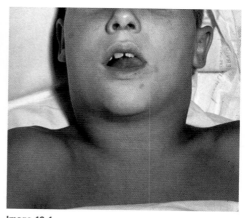

Image 42.4

Bull neck appearance of diphtheritic cervical lymphadenopathy in a 13-year-old boy.

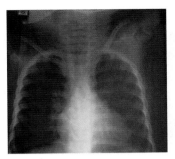

Image 42.5

Chest radiograph of a 2-year-old male with laryngotracheal diphtheria. Diphtheritic pneumonia was obscured by hyperaeration on chest radiograph at time of admission to hospital due to laryngotracheal membranous obstruction. Courtesy of Edgar O. Ledbetter, MD, FAAP.

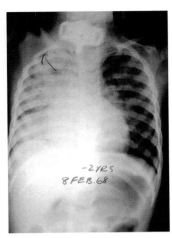

Image 42.6

Diphtheritic pneumonia 3 days after the admission radiograph in Image 42.5 following a tracheostomy complicated by early pneumothorax. Unfortunately, the tracheal membrane was not visualized at the time of tracheostomy and diphtheria antitoxin therapy was not prescribed. Courtesy of Edgar O. Ledbetter, MD, FAAP.

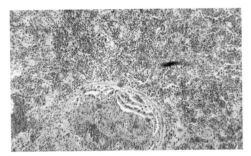

Image 42.7

Diphtheria pneumonia (hemorrhagic) with bronchiolar membranes (hematoxylin-eosin stain). From the patient in images 42.5 and 42.6. Courtesy of Edgar O. Ledbetter, MD, FAAP.

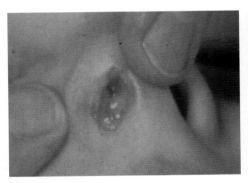

Image 42.8

Nasal membrane of diphtheria in a preschool-aged white male. Courtesy of George Nankervis, MD.

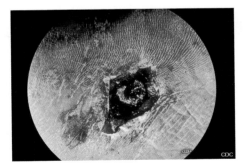

Image 42.9

This is a close-up of a diphtheria skin lesion caused by the organism *Corynebacterium diphtheriae*. Courtesy of Centers for Disease Control and Prevention/Brodsky, MD.

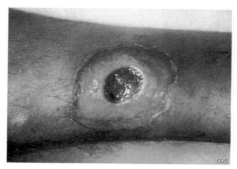

Image 42.10

A diphtheria skin lesion on the leg. *Corynebacterium diphtheriae* can not only affect the respiratory, cardiovascular, renal, and neurologic systems, but the cutaneous system as well, where it sometimes manifests as an open, isolated wound. Courtesy of Centers for Disease Control and Prevention.

43

Ehrlichia and *Anaplasma* Infections

(Human Ehrlichiosis and Anaplasmosis)

Clinical Manifestations

Previously referred to as ehrlichiosis, 2 distinct names—ehrlichiosis and anaplasmosis—now commonly are used to describe infections caused by bacteria of the genus *Ehrlichia* and genus *Anaplasma,* respectively. In the United States, human ehrlichiosis is caused by 3 different *Ehrlichia* species. Infection with *Anaplasma phagocytophilum* causes human granulocytic anaplasmosis (HGA) (Table 43.1). These 4 infections have similar signs, symptoms, and clinical courses. All are acute, systemic, febrile illnesses that have some clinical similarities to Rocky Mountain spotted fever (RMSF). However, *Ehrlichia* and *Anaplasma* species do not cause vasculitis or endothelial cell damage characteristic of rickettsial diseases.

Common systemic manifestations present in more than 50% of patients include fever, headache, chills, malaise, myalgia, and nausea. More variable symptoms include arthralgia, vomiting, diarrhea, cough, and confusion, usually present in 20% to 50% of patients. For *E chaffeensis,* rash is reported in approximately 60% of children, although it is reported less commonly in adults; rash is present in fewer than 10% of people with anaplasmosis. When present, rash is variable in appearance (usually involving the trunk and sparing the hands and feet) and location and typically develops approximately 1 week after onset of illness. More severe manifestations of these diseases include acute respiratory distress syndrome, encephalopathy, meningitis, disseminated intravascular coagulation, spontaneous hemorrhage, and renal failure. Significant laboratory findings can include leukopenia, lymphopenia, thrombocytopenia, and elevated serum hepatic transaminase concentrations. Cerebrospinal fluid abnormalities (ie, pleocytosis with a predominance of lymphocytes and increased total protein concentration) are common. Symptoms typically last 1 to 2 weeks, and recovery generally occurs without sequelae. Fatal infections have been reported more commonly for *E chaffeensis* infections (approximately 1%–3% case fatality) than for HGA (< 1% case fatality). Typically, *E chaffeensis* causes more severe disease than does *A phagocytophilum.* Secondary

Table 43.1

Human Ehrlichiosis and Anaplasmosis in the United States

Disease	Causal Agent	Major Target Cell	Tick Vector	Geographic Distribution
Ehrlichiosis caused by *Ehrlichia chaffeensis* (also known as human monocytic ehrlichiosis, or HME)	*E chaffeensis*	Usually monocytes	Lone star tick (*Amblyomma americanum*)	Predominantly southeast, south central, and Midwestern states
Anaplasmosis (also known as human granulocytic anaplasmosis, or HGA)	*Anaplasma phagocytophilum*	Usually granulocytes	Black-legged or deer tick (*Ixodes scapularis*) or Western black-legged tick (*Ixodes pacificus*)	Northeast and north central states and northern California
Ehrlichiosis caused by *Ehrlichia ewingii*	*E ewingii*	Usually granulocytes	Lone star tick (*A americanum*)	Southeast, south central, and Midwestern states
Ehrlichiosis caused by the *Ehrlichia muris*–like agent	*E muris*–like agent	Not determined	*I scapularis* is identified as a possible vector	Minnesota, Wisconsin

or opportunistic infections may occur in severe illnes, and people with underlying immunosuppression are at greater risk of severe disease. Fulminant disease has been reported in people who initially received trimethoprim-sulfamethoxazole before a correct diagnosis was confirmed.

Etiology

In the United States, ehrlichiosis and anaplasmosis are caused by at least 4 species of obligate intracellular bacteria with tropisms for different white blood cells. Ehrlichiosis results from infection with *E chaffeensis* (human monocytic ehrlichiosis), *E ewingii*, or *E muris*–like agent, and anaplasmosis is caused by *A phagocytophilum*. *Ehrlichia* and *Anaplasma* species are gram-negative cocci.

Epidemiology

Although the reported incidences of *E chaffeensis* and *A phagocytophilum* infections during 2007 each were only 3.0 cases per million population, the infections are under-recognized, and selected active surveillance programs have shown the incidence to be substantially higher in some areas with endemic infection. Recent surveillance data also show that the incidence of reported cases seems to be increasing. Most cases of *E chaffeensis* infection occur in people from the southeastern and south central United States. Cases attributable to the new *E muris*–like agent have been reported only from Minnesota and Wisconsin, but possibly occur with the same distribution as Lyme disease. Ehrlichiosis caused by *E chaffeensis* and *E ewingii* are associated with the bite of the lone star tick (*Amblyomma americanum*). However, the distribution of *A americanum* is expanding, and the geographic range of reported ehrlichiosis probably will expand in the future as well. Most cases of human anaplasmosis have been reported in the north central and northeastern United States, particularly Wisconsin, Minnesota, Connecticut, and New York, but cases in many other states, including California, have been identified. In most of the United States, *A phagocytophilum* is transmitted by the black-legged or deer tick (*Ixodes scapularis*) and probably for the *E muris*–like agent. In the western United States, the western black-legged tick (*Ixodes pacificus*) is the main vector for *A phagocytophilum*. Various mammalian wildlife reservoirs for the agents of human ehrlichiosis have been identified, including white-tailed deer, white-footed mice, and *Neotoma* wood rats. Reported cases of symptomatic ehrlichiosis characteristically are in older people, with age-specific incidences greatest in people older than 40 years. However, recent seroprevalence data indicate that exposure to *Ehrlichia* is common in children. Most human infections occur between April and September, and the peak occurrence is from May through July. Coinfections of anaplasmosis with other tick-borne diseases, including babesiosis and Lyme disease, have been described.

Incubation Period

Typically 5 to 10 days after a tick bite (median, 9).

Diagnostic Tests

Differences between ehrlichiosis and anaplasmosis compared with RMSF are (1) rash is present in more than 90% of patients with RMSF, (2) leukopenia and absolute lymphopenia and neutropenia are uncommon in RMSF, and (3) histopathologic vasculitis is a hallmark of RMSF but not ehrlichiosis and anaplasmosis. The Centers for Disease Control and Prevention (CDC) defines a confirmed case of human ehrlichiosis or anaplasmosis as

- A clinically compatible illness (fever plus one or more of the following: headache, myalgia, anemia, leukopenia, thrombocytopenia, or any elevation of serum hepatic transaminase concentrations) plus serologic evidence of a fourfold change in immunoglobulin (Ig) G–specific antibody titer by indirect immunofluorescent antibody (IFA) assay between paired serum specimens (one taken in the first week of illness and a second 2–4 weeks later)
- Detection of *Ehrlichia* or *Anaplasma* DNA in a clinical specimen via amplification of a specific target by PCR assay
- Demonstration of *Ehrlichia* or *Anaplasma* antigen in a biopsy/autopsy sample by immunohistochemical methods
- Isolation of *Ehrlichia* or *Anaplasma* bacteria from a clinical specimen in cell culture

The CDC further defines a probable case as serologic evidence of elevated IgG or IgM antibody reactive with *Ehrlichia* or *Anaplasma* antigen by IFA, enzyme immunosorbent assay (EIA), dot-EIA, or serologic assays in other formats, or identification of morulae in the cytoplasm of monocytes or granulocytes by microscopic examination. *E ewingii* and probably the *E muris*–like agent share some antigens with *E chaffeensis*, so most cases of *E ewingii* ehrlichiosis can be diagnosed serologically using *E chaffeensis* antigens. These tests are available in reference laboratories, in some commercial laboratories and state health departments, and at the CDC. Testing should be limited to patients with clinical presentations consistent with the illness. Examination of peripheral blood smears to detect morulae in peripheral blood monocytes or granulocytes is insensitive. Use of PCR assay to amplify nucleic acid from peripheral blood of patients in the acute phase of ehrlichiosis appears to be sensitive, specific, and promising for early diagnosis. PCR assay for both anaplasmosis and ehrlichiosis is available increasingly at many commercial laboratories. Broth isolation can be conducted on appropriate clinical samples sent to specialty research laboratories or the CDC.

Treatment

Doxycycline is the drug of choice for treatment of human ehrlichiosis and anaplasmosis, regardless of patient age. Ehrlichiosis and anaplasmosis can be severe or fatal in untreated patients or patients with predisposing conditions, and initiation of therapy early in the course of disease helps minimize complications of illness. Failure to respond to doxycycline within the first 3 days suggests infection with an agent other than *Ehrlichia* or *Anaplasma* species. Treatment should continue for at least 3 days after defervescence; the standard course of treatment is 7 to 14 days. Unequivocal evidence of clinical improvement generally is evident by 1 week, although some symptoms (eg, headache, weakness, malaise) can persist for weeks after adequate therapy. Severe or complicated disease may require longer treatment courses.

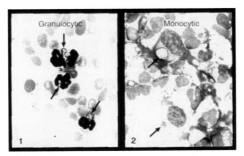

Image 43.1
Etiologic agents of ehrlichiosis. Photomicrographs of human white blood cells infected with the agent of human granulocytic ehrlichiosis (sometimes referred to as *Ehrlichia phagocytophila*) and the agent of human monocytic ehrlichiosis (*Ehrlichia chaffeensis*). Courtesy of Centers for Disease Control and Prevention.

EHRLICHIOSIS, HUMAN GRANULOCYTIC. Number of reported cases, by county — United States, 2006

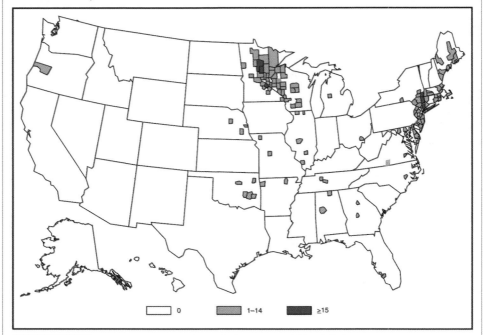

0   1–14   ≥15

As a result of recent taxonomic changes, human granulocytic enrlichiosis is now known as anaplasmosis (caused by *Anaplasma phagocytophilum*). Cases of this disease are reported primarily from the upper Midwest and coastal New England, reflecting the range of the primary tick vector species, *Ixodes scapularis*, and human population density.

Image 43.2
Reported granulocytic ehrlichiosis cases by county, 2006. Courtesy of *Morbidity and Mortality Weekly Report.*

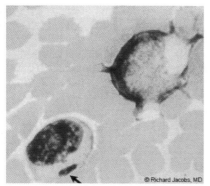

Image 43.3
The intracytoplasmic inclusion, or morula, of human monocytic ehrlichiosis in a cytocentrifuge preparation of cerebrospinal fluid from a patient with central nervous system involvement. Copyright Richard Jacobs, MD.

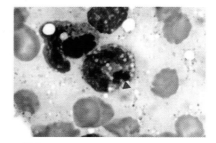

Image 43.4
Bone marrow examination (Wright stain, magnification x1,000). Intraleukocytic morulae of *Ehrlichia* can be seen (arrow) within monocytoid cells. Courtesy of Safdar N, Love RB, Maki DG. Severe *Ehrlichia chaffeensis* infection in a lung transplant recipient: a review of ehrlichiosis in the immunocompromised patient. *Emerg Infect Dis.* 2002;8(3):320–323.

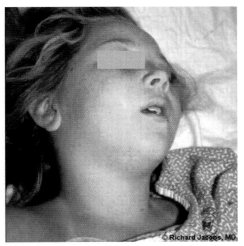

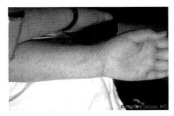

Image 43.6

The petechial and vasculitic rash of human monocytic ehrlichiosis in the patient in Image 43.5. Copyright Richard Jacobs, MD.

Image 43.5

Human monocytic ehrlichiosis (HME). A semi-comatose 16-year-old girl with leukopenia, lymphopenia, thrombocytopenia, and elevated transaminase levels. The HME PCR and serologic test results were positive for HME. Copyright Richard Jacobs, MD.

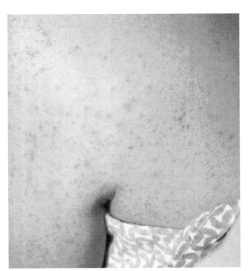

Image 43.7

The same characteristic rash of human monocytic ehrlichiosis in the patient in images 43.5 and 43.6. The differential diagnosis of this rash includes Rocky Mountain spotted fever, meningococcemia, and Stevens-Johnson syndrome. Other tick-borne diseases such as Lyme disease, babesiosis, Colorado tick fever, relapsing fever, and tularemia may need to be considered. Kawasaki disease also has caused some diagnostic confusion. Copyright Richard Jacobs, MD.

44

Enterovirus (Nonpoliovirus) and Parechovirus Infections

(Group A and B Coxsackieviruses, Echoviruses, Numbered Enteroviruses, and Human Parechoviruses)

Clinical Manifestations

Nonpolio enteroviruses are responsible for significant and frequent illnesses in infants and children and result in protean clinical manifestations. The most common manifestation is nonspecific febrile illness, which in very young infants can lead to evaluation for bacterial sepsis. Other manifestations can include the following: (1) respiratory: coryza, pharyngitis, herpangina, stomatitis, bronchiolitis, pneumonia, and pleurodynia; (2) skin: hand-foot-and-mouth disease, onychomadesis (periodic shedding of nails), and nonspecific exanthems; (3) neurologic: aseptic meningitis, encephalitis, and motor paralysis; (4) gastrointestinal/genitourinary: vomiting, diarrhea, abdominal pain, hepatitis, pancreatitis, and orchitis; (5) eye: acute hemorrhagic conjunctivitis and uveitis; (6) heart: myopericarditis; and (7) muscle: myositis. Neonates, especially those who acquire infection in the absence of serotype-specific maternal antibody, are at risk of severe disease, including sepsis, meningoencephalitis, myocarditis, hepatitis, coagulopathy, and pneumonitis. Infection with enterovirus 71 is associated with hand-foot-and-mouth disease, herpangina and, in a small proportion of cases, severe neurologic disease, including brainstem encephalomyelitis and paralytic disease, and secondary pulmonary edema/hemorrhage and cardiopulmonary collapse. Other noteworthy but not exclusive serotype associations include coxsackievirus A16 with hand-foot-and-mouth disease, coxsackievirus A24 variant and enterovirus 70 with acute hemorrhagic conjunctivitis, enterovirus 68 with respiratory illness, and coxsackieviruses B1 through B5 with pleurodynia and myopericarditis.

Patients with humoral and combined immune deficiencies can have persistent central nervous system (CNS) infections, a dermatomyositis-like syndrome, and/or disseminated infection.

Severe, multisystem disease is reported in hematopoietic stem cell transplant patients and children with malignancies.

As a group, human parechoviruses (formerly echoviruses 22 and 23, and others) appear to cause similar clinical diseases as enteroviruses, including febrile illnesses, exanthems, sepsis-like syndromes, and respiratory tract, gastrointestinal tract, and CNS infections. Neonates and young infants have presented with more severe clinical disease and long-term sequelae than have older children.

Etiology

The enteroviruses are RNA viruses. The nonpolio enteroviruses include more than 100 distinct serotypes formerly subclassified as group A coxsackieviruses, group B coxsackieviruses, echoviruses, and newer numbered enteroviruses. A new classification system groups these nonpolio enteroviruses into 4 species on the basis of genetic similarity, although traditional serotype names are retained for individual serotypes. Echoviruses 22 and 23 have been reclassified within a new genus *(Parechovirus)* and are termed human parechovirus (HPeV) 1 and 2, respectively.

Epidemiology

Humans are the only known reservoir for human enteroviruses, although some primates can become infected. Enterovirus infections are spread by fecal-oral and respiratory routes and from mother to infant prenatally, peripartum, and possibly postpartum via breastfeeding. Enteroviruses can survive on environmental surfaces for periods long enough to allow transmission from fomites. Hospital nursery and other institutional outbreaks can occur. Infection incidence, clinical attack rates, and disease severity typically are greatest in infants and young children, and infections occur more frequently in tropical areas and where poor hygiene and overcrowding are present. Most enterovirus infections in temperate climates occur in the summer and fall (June through October), but seasonal patterns are less evident in the tropics. Epidemics of enterovirus meningitis, enterovirus 71–associated hand-foot-and-mouth disease with neurologic and cardiopulmonary complications, and enterovirus 70– and coxsackievirus A24–associated acute hemorrhagic conjunctivitis occur. Fecal viral shedding can continue for several weeks or months after onset of infection, but respiratory tract shedding usually is limited to 1 to 3 weeks or less. Viral shedding can occur without signs of clinical illness.

Seroepidemiologic studies of human parechoviruses suggest that infection occurs commonly during early childhood. HPeV 1 has been noted to circulate throughout the year; other human parechoviruses occur more often during late spring and summer months.

Incubation Period

3 to 6 days; acute hemorrhagic conjunctivitis, 24 to 72 hours.

Diagnostic Tests

Enteroviruses can be detected by reverse-transcriptase PCR assay and culture from a variety of specimens, including stool, rectal swabs, throat swabs, conjunctival swabs, tracheal aspirates, urine, blood, and tissue biopsy specimens during acute illness and from cerebrospinal fluid (CSF) when meningitis is present. Patients with enterovirus 71 neurologic disease often have negative results of culture and PCR assay of CSF even when they have CSF pleocytosis; in these patients, results of PCR assay and culture of throat or rectal swab or vesicle fluid specimens more frequently are positive. PCR assays for detection of enterovirus RNA are available at many reference and commercial laboratories for CSF and other specimens. PCR assay is more rapid and more sensitive than isolation of enteroviruses in cell culture and can detect all enteroviruses, including serotypes that are difficult to culti-

vate in viral culture. Sensitivity of culture ranges from 0% to 80% depending on serotype and cell lines used. Culture usually requires 3 to 8 days to detect growth. Although used less frequently for diagnosis, acute infection with a known enterovirus serotype can be determined at reference laboratories by demonstration of a change in neutralizing or other serotype-specific antibody titer between acute and convalescent serum specimens or detection of serotype-specific immunoglobulin M. Serologic methods are insensitive, and commercially available assays may lack specificity.

Commercially available enteroviral PCR assays will not detect any of the human parechoviruses. However, the Centers for Disease Control and Prevention has developed PCR primers that detect all known parechoviruses, and this represents the best diagnostic modality currently available.

Treatment

No specific therapy is available for enteroviruses or parechoviruses. Immune globulin intravenous (IGIV) may be beneficial for chronic enteroviral meningoencephalitis in immunodeficient patients. IGIV also has been used in life-threatening neonatal infections, severe infections in people with malignancies, hematopoietic stem cell transplant recipients, people with suspected viral myocarditis, and people with enterovirus 71 neurologic disease, but proof of efficacy is lacking. Interferons occasionally have been used for treatment of enterovirus-associated myocarditis, without definitive proof of efficacy. The antiviral drug pleconaril has in vitro activity against enteroviruses but is not available. Pleconaril is being investigated in neonates with enteroviral sepsis syndrome.

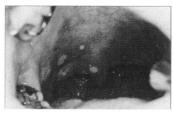

Image 44.1
A 4-year-old white female with pharyngeal inflammation and palatal lesions of hand-foot-and-mouth disease, a coxsackievirus A infection. Copyright Larry Frenkel, MD.

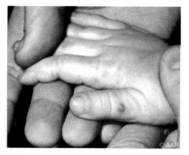

Image 44.3
Enterovirus infection in a preschool female. Hand-foot-and-mouth syndrome lesions are caused by coxsackievirus A16 and enterovirus 71.

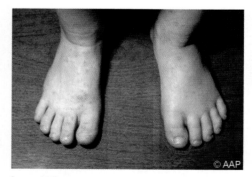

Image 44.5
Enterovirus infection (hand-foot-and-mouth disease) affecting the feet.

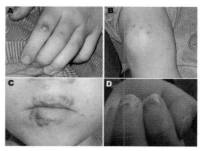

Image 44.2
Vesicular eruptions in hand (A), foot (B), and mouth (C) of a 6-year-old boy with coxsackievirus A6 infection. Several of his fingernails shed (D) 2 months after the pictures were taken. Courtesy of Österback R, Vuorinen T, Linna M, Susi P, Hyypiä T, Waris M. Coxackievirus A6 and hand, foot, and mouth disease, Finland. *Emerg Infect Dis.* 2009;15(9):1485–1488.

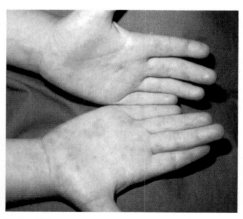

Image 44.4
Enterovirus infection (hand-foot-and-mouth disease) affecting the hands.

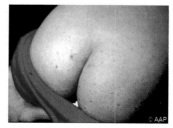

Image 44.6
Enterovirus infection (hand-foot-and-mouth disease). This rash, commonly seen over the buttocks, often appears macular, maculopapular, or papulovesicular and may be petechial.

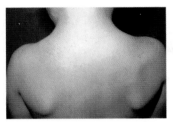

Image 44.7
Enterovirus infection (hand-foot-and-mouth disease). The rash may also be seen on the trunk.

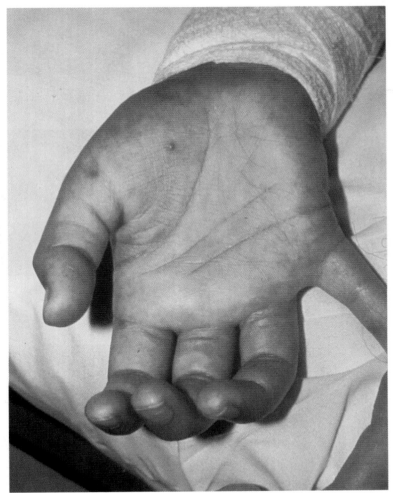

Image 44.8
Characteristic papulovesicular lesions on the palm of a 2-year-old male with hand-foot-and-mouth syndrome, a coxsackievirus A infection, most often A-16, or enterovirus 71. Courtesy of George Nankervis, MD.

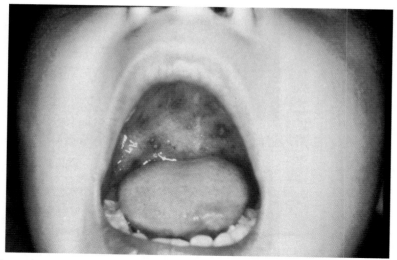

Image 44.9
Characteristic papulovesicular lesions of hand-foot-and-mouth disease in a 2-year-old male. Courtesy of George Nankervis, MD.

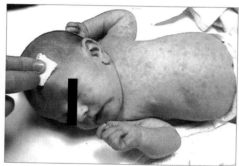

Image 44.10
Newborn with generalized enteroviral exanthem. Copyright Michael Rajnik, MD, FAAP.

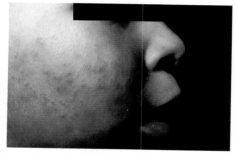

Image 44.11
Skin lesions on the side of young girl's face due to echovirus type 9. Courtesy of Centers for Disease Control and Prevention.

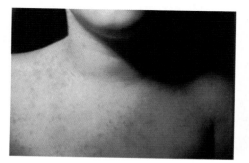

Image 44.12
Skin lesions on the neck and chest of a young girl due to echovirus type 9. Echoviruses comprise 1 of 5 serotypes, which make up the genus *Enterovirus,* and are associated with illnesses, including aseptic meningitis, nonspecific rashes, encephalitides, and myositis. Courtesy of Centers for Disease Control and Prevention.

45

Epstein-Barr Virus Infections

(Infectious Mononucleosis)

Clinical Manifestations

Infectious mononucleosis manifests typically as fever, pharyngitis with petechiae, exudative pharyngitis, lymphadenopathy, hepato-splenomegaly, and atypical lymphocytosis. The spectrum of manifestations ranges from asymptomatic to fatal infection. Infections commonly are unrecognized in infants and young children. Rash can occur and is more common in patients treated with ampicillin or amoxicillin as well as with other penicillins. Central nervous system (CNS) complications include aseptic meningitis, encephalitis, myelitis, optic neuritis, cranial nerve palsies, transverse myelitis, and Guillain-Barré syndrome. Hematologic complications include splenic rupture, thrombocytopenia, agranulocytosis, hemolytic anemia, and hemophagocytic lymphohistiocytosis (HLH) or hemophagocytic syndrome (HPS). Pneumonia, orchitis, and myocarditis are observed infrequently. Fatal disseminated infection or B-lymphocyte or T-lymphocyte lymphomas can occur in children with no detectable immunologic abnormality as well as in children with congenital or acquired cellular immune deficiencies.

Epstein-Barr virus (EBV) is associated with several other distinct disorders, including X-linked lymphoproliferative syndrome, post-transplantation lymphoproliferative disorders, Burkitt lymphoma, nasopharyngeal carcinoma, and undifferentiated B- or T-lymphocyte lymphomas of the CNS. X-linked lymphoproliferative syndrome occurs in people with an inherited, maternally derived, recessive genetic defect. The syndrome is characterized by several expressions, including occurrence of fatal EBV infections early in life among boys, nodular B-lymphocyte lymphomas often with CNS involvement, and profound hypogammaglobulinemia.

EBV-associated lymphoproliferative disorders result in a number of complex syndromes in patients who are immunocompromised, such as transplant recipients or people infected with HIV. The highest incidence of these disorders occurs in liver and heart transplant recipients, in whom the proliferative states range from benign lymph node hypertrophy to monoclonal lymphomas. Other EBV syndromes are of greater importance outside the United States, including Burkitt lymphoma (a B-lymphocyte tumor), found primarily in Central Africa, and nasopharyngeal carcinoma, found primarily in Southeast Asia and the Inuit population. EBV also has been associated with Hodgkin disease (B-lymphocyte tumor), non-Hodgkin lymphomas (B- and T-lymphocyte), gastric carcinoma "lymphoepitheliomas," and a variety of common epithelial malignancies.

Chronic fatigue syndrome is not related to EBV infection; however, fatigue lasting weeks to a few months, can occur in less than 10% of cases of classic infectious mononucleosis.

Etiology

EBV (also known as human herpesvirus 4) is a gammaherpesvirus of the *Lymphocryptovirus* genus and is the most common cause of infectious mononucleosis.

Epidemiology

Humans are the only known reservoir of EBV, and approximately 90% of US adults have been infected. Close personal contact usually is required for transmission. The virus is viable in saliva for several hours outside the body, but the role of fomites in transmission is unknown. EBV also can be transmitted by blood transfusion or transplantation. Infection commonly is contracted early in life. Endemic infectious mononucleosis is common in group settings of adolescents, such as in educational institutions. No seasonal pattern has been documented. Intermittent excretion in saliva may be lifelong after infection.

Incubation Period

Infectious mononucleosis, an estimated 30 to 50 days.

Diagnostic Tests

Routine diagnosis depends on serologic testing. Nonspecific tests for heterophile antibody, including the Paul-Bunnell test and slide agglutination reaction test, are available most commonly. The heterophile antibody response primarily is immunoglobulin (Ig) M, which appears during the first 2 weeks of illness and gradually disappears over a 6-month period. The results of heterophile antibody tests often are negative in children younger than 4 years with EBV infection, but heterophile antibody tests identify approximately 85% of cases of classic infectious mononucleosis in older children and adults during the second week of illness. An absolute increase in atypical lymphocytes during the second week of illness with infectious mononucleosis is a characteristic but nonspecific finding. However, the finding of greater than 10% atypical lymphocytes together with a positive heterophile antibody test result is considered diagnostic of acute infection.

Multiple specific serologic antibody tests for EBV infection are available in diagnostic virology laboratories (Table 45.1). The most commonly performed test is IgG against the viral capsid antigen (VCA). Because VCA IgG occurs in high titer early in infection and persists for life, testing of acute and convalescent serum specimens may not be useful for establishing the presence of active infection. Testing for presence of VCA IgM and the absence of antibodies to EBV nuclear antigen (EBNA) is useful for identifying active and recent infections. Because serum antibody against EBNA is not present until several weeks to months after onset of infection, a positive anti-EBNA antibody test excludes an active primary infection. Testing for antibodies against early antigen is not useful for interpretation of serologic results because of the unreliability of the assays that are used.

Serologic tests for EBV are useful particularly for evaluating patients who have heterophile-negative infectious mononucleosis. Testing for other agents, especially cytomegalovirus, *Toxoplasma* species, human herpesvirus 6, and HIV, also may be indicated for some of these patients. Diagnosis of the entire range of EBV-associated illness requires use of molecular and antibody techniques, particularly for patients with immune deficiencies.

Isolation of EBV from oropharyngeal secretions by culture in cord blood cells is possible, but techniques for performing this procedure usually are not available in routine diagnostic laboratories. PCR assay for detection of EBV DNA in serum, plasma, and tissue and reverse-transcriptase PCR assay for detection of EBV RNA in lymphoid cells or tissue are useful in evaluation of immunocompromised patients.

Treatment

Patients with suspected EBV infections should not be given ampicillin or amoxicillin as these drugs cause nonallergic morbilliform rashes in a high proportion of patients. Although therapy with short-course corticosteroids may have a beneficial effect on acute symptoms, because of potential adverse effects, their use should be considered only for patients with impending airway obstruction, massive splenomegaly, myocarditis, hemolytic anemia, or HLH. The duration of corticosteroid therapy is 7 days with subsequent tapering. Life-threatening HLH has been treated with cytotoxic agents and immunomodulators, including cyclosporin and corticosteroids. Acyclovir has no proven value in treatment. Decreasing immunosuppressive therapy is beneficial for patients with EBV-induced post-transplant lymphoproliferative disorders, whereas an antiviral drug, such as valacyclovir or ganciclovir, sometimes is used in patients with active replicating EBV infection with or without passive antibody therapy provided by immune globulin intravenous.

Contact sports should be avoided until the patient is recovered fully from infectious mononucleosis and the spleen no longer is palpable. In the first 3 weeks following the onset of symptoms, the risk of splenic rupture is related primarily to splenic fragility; thus, both strenuous and contact sports must be avoided. Following the initial 3-week period, clearance for contact sport participation is dependent on resolution of symptoms and of splenomegaly. Imaging modalities, such as ultrasonography, offer greater sensitivity and accuracy than palpation and may be useful in determining whether an athlete can safely return to contact sport participation.

Table 45.1
Serum Epstein-Barr Virus (EBV) Antibodies in EBV Infection

Infection	VCA IgG	VCA IgM	EA (D)	EBNA
No previous infection	−	−	−	−
Acute infection	+	+	+/−	−
Recent infection	+	+/−	+/−	+/−
Past infection	+	−	+/−	+

Abbreviations: EA (D), early antigen diffuse staining; EBNA, EBV nuclear antigen; VCA IgG, immunoglobulin (Ig) G class antibody to viral capsid antigen; VCA IgM, IgM class antibody to VCA.

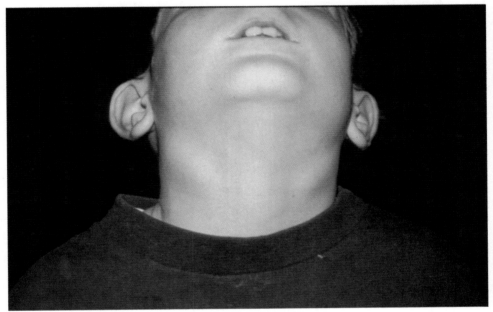

Image 45.1
Mononucleosis. This boy with acute EBV infection has the typical marked bilateral tender cervical lymphadenopathy without external signs of inflammation, such as erythema or warmth. Courtesy of James Brien, DO.

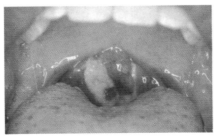

Image 45.2
Epstein-Barr virus disease with pharyngeal and tonsillar exudate. Copyright James Brien, DO.

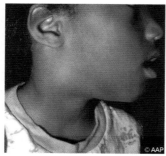

Image 45.3
Cervical lymphadenopathy in a 7-year-old girl with infectious mononucleosis.

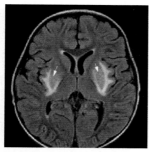

Image 45.5
Epstein-Barr virus encephalitis. Axial fluid attenuated inversion recovery magnetic resonance image shows basal ganglia hyperintensity (arrows).

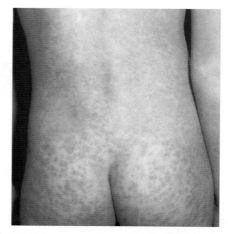

Image 45.4
This morbilliform rash arose in a patient with infectious mononucleosis after amoxicillin was prescribed. This is a nonallergic cutaneous eruption. Courtesy of Centers for Disease Control and Prevention/Dr Thomas F. Sellers, Emory University.

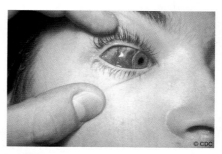

Image 45.6
A conjunctival hemorrhage of the right eye of a patient with infectious mononucleosis. At times, noninfectious conjunctivitis, as well as other corneal abnormalities, may manifest because of the body's systemic response to viral infections such as infectious mononucleosis. Courtesy of Centers for Disease Control and Prevention/Dr Thomas F. Sellers, Emory University.

46

Escherichia coli and Other Gram-Negative Bacilli
(Septicemia and Meningitis in Neonates)

Clinical Manifestations

Neonatal septicemia or meningitis caused by *Escherichia coli* and other gram-negative bacilli cannot be differentiated clinically from septicemia or meningitis caused by other organisms. The early signs of sepsis can be subtle and similar to signs observed in noninfectious processes. Signs of septicemia include fever, temperature instability, heart rate abnormalities, grunting respirations, apnea, cyanosis, lethargy, irritability, anorexia, vomiting, jaundice, abdominal distention, and diarrhea. Meningitis, especially early in the course, can occur without overt signs suggesting central nervous system involvement. Some gram-negative bacilli, such as *Citrobacter koseri, Chronobacter* (formerly *Enterobacter) sakazakii, Serratia marcescens,* and *Salmonella* species, are associated with brain abscesses in infants with meningitis caused by these organisms.

Etiology

E coli strains with the K1 capsular polysaccharide antigen cause approximately 40% of cases of *E coli* septicemia and 80% of cases of *E coli* meningitis. Other important gram-negative bacilli causing neonatal septicemia include non-K1 strains of *E coli* and *Klebsiella* species, *Enterobacter* species, *Proteus* species, *Citrobacter* species, *Salmonella* species, *Pseudomonas* species, *Acinetobacter* species, and *Serratia* species. Nonencapsulated strains of *Haemophilus influenzae* and anaerobic gram-negative bacilli are rare causes.

Epidemiology

The source of *E coli* and other gram-negative bacterial pathogens in neonatal infections during the first several days of life typically is the maternal genital tract. Reservoirs for gram-negative bacilli also can be present within the health care environment. Acquisition of gram-negative organisms can occur through person-to-person transmission from hospital nursery personnel and from nursery environmental sites, such as sinks, countertops, powdered infant formula, and respiratory therapy equipment, especially among very preterm infants who require prolonged neonatal intensive care management. Predisposing factors in neonatal gram-negative bacterial infections include maternal intrapartum infection, gestation less than 37 weeks, low birth weight, and prolonged rupture of membranes. Metabolic abnormalities (eg, galactosemia), fetal hypoxia, and acidosis have been implicated as predisposing factors. Neonates with defects in the integrity of skin or mucosa (eg, myelomeningocele) or abnormalities of gastrointestinal or genitourinary tracts are at increased risk of gram-negative bacterial infections. In neonatal intensive care units, systems for respiratory and metabolic support, invasive or surgical procedures, indwelling vascular lines, and frequent use of broad-spectrum antimicrobial agents enable selection and proliferation of strains of gram-negative bacilli that are resistant to multiple antimicrobial agents.

Multiple mechanisms of resistance in gram-negative bacilli can be present simultaneously. Resistance resulting from production of chromosomally encoded or plasmid-derived AmpC beta-lactamases or from plasmid-mediated extended-spectrum beta-lactamases (ESBLs), occurring primarily in *E coli* and *Klebsiella* species but reported in many other gram-negative species, has been associated with nursery outbreaks, especially in very low birth weight infants. Organisms that produce ESBLs typically are resistant to penicillins, cephalosporins, and monobactams and can be resistant to aminoglycosides. Carbapenem-resistant strains have emerged among *Enterobacteriaceae,* especially *Klebsiella pneumoniae.*

Incubation Period

Birth to several weeks after birth or longer in very low birth weight, preterm infants with prolonged hospitalizations.

Diagnostic Tests

Diagnosis is established by growth of *E coli* or other gram-negative bacilli from blood, cerebrospinal fluid (CSF), or other usually sterile site cultures. Special laboratory procedures are required to detect some multiply drug-resistant gram-negative organisms.

Treatment

Initial empirical treatment for suspected early-onset gram-negative septicemia in neonates is ampicillin and an aminoglycoside. An alternative regimen of ampicillin and an extended-spectrum cephalosporin (such as cefotaxime) can be used, but rapid emergence of cephalosporin-resistant organisms, especially *Enterobacter* species, *Klebsiella* species, and *Serratia* species, and increased risk of colonization or infection with ESBL-producing *Enterobacteriaceae* can occur when use is routine. Hence, routine use of an extended-spectrum cephalosporin is not recommended unless bacterial meningitis is suspected.

The proportion of *E coli* bloodstream infections with onset within 72 hours of life that are resistant to ampicillin is high among very low birth weight infants. These *E coli* infections almost invariably are susceptible to gentamicin. Once the causative agent and its in vitro antimicrobial susceptibility pattern are known, nonmeningeal infections should be treated with ampicillin, an appropriate aminoglycoside, or an extended-spectrum cephalosporin (such as cefotaxime). Many experts would treat nonmeningeal infections caused by *Enterobacter* species, *Serratia* species, or *Pseudomonas* species and some other less commonly occurring gram-negative bacilli with a beta-lactam antimicrobial agent and an aminoglycoside. For ampicillin-susceptible CSF isolates of *E coli*, meningitis can be treated with ampicillin or cefotaxime; meningitis caused by an ampicillin-resistant isolate is treated with cefotaxime with or without an aminoglycoside. Combination therapy with beta-lactam and aminoglycoside antimicrobial agents is used for empirical therapy and until CSF is sterile. Some experts continue combination therapy for a longer duration. Expert advice from an infectious disease specialist can be helpful for management of meningitis.

The drug of choice for treatment of infections caused by ESBL-producing organisms is meropenem, which is active against gram-negative aerobic organisms with chromosomally mediated ampC beta-lactamases or ESBL-producing strains, except carbapenemase-producing strains, especially some *Klebsiella pneumoniae* isolates. Expert advice from an infectious disease specialist can help in management of ESBL-producing gram-negative infections in neonates.

All infants with gram-negative meningitis should undergo repeat lumbar puncture to ensure sterility of the CSF after 24 to 48 hours of therapy. If CSF remains culture positive, choice and doses of antimicrobial agents should be evaluated and another lumbar puncture should be performed. Duration of therapy is based on clinical and bacteriologic response of the patient and the site(s) of infection; the usual duration of therapy for uncomplicated bacteremia is 10 to 14 days, and for meningitis, minimum duration is 21 days.

All infants with gram-negative meningitis should undergo careful follow-up examinations, including testing for hearing loss, neurologic abnormalities, and developmental delay.

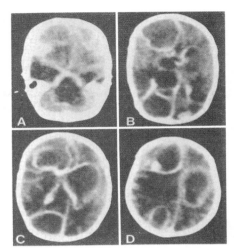

Image 46.1
Computed tomography scan of the head of a neonate 3 weeks after therapy for *Escherichia coli* meningitis demonstrating widespread destruction of cerebral cortex secondary to vascular thrombosis. Infant was blind, deaf, globally intellectually disabled, and had diabetes insipidus.

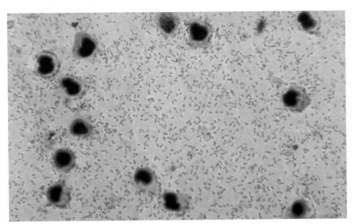

Image 46.2
Gram stain of *Escherichia coli* in the cerebrospinal fluid of a neonate with meningitis.

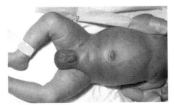

Image 46.3
Icteric premature infant with septicemia and perineal and abdominal wall cellulitis due to *Escherichia coli*.

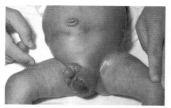

Image 46.4

Infant with *Escherichia coli* septicemia and perineal cellulitis, scrotal necrosis, and abdominal wall abscesses below the navel that required surgical drainage and antibiotics.

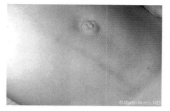

Image 46.5

A 1-year-old boy with gram-negative meningitis with tache cérébrale. Copyright Martin G. Myers, MD.

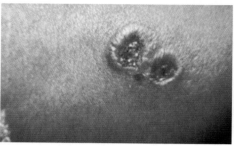

Image 46.6

Bullous, necrotic, umbilicated lesions in an infant with septicemia due to *Pseudomonas aeruginosa*.

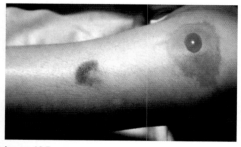

Image 46.7

Skin lesions due to *Pseudomonas aeruginosa* in a child with neutropenia and septicemia.

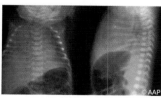

Image 46.9

Sepsis and pneumonia with empyema due to *Escherichia coli*. This newborn died at 12 hours of age.

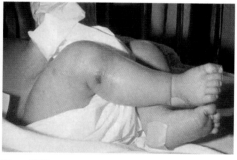

Image 46.8

Sepsis due to *Pseudomonas aeruginosa* with early ecthyma gangrenosum.

47

Escherichia coli Diarrhea

(Including Hemolytic Uremic Syndrome)

Clinical Manifestations

At least 5 pathotypes of diarrhea-producing *Escherichia coli* strains have been identified. Clinical features of disease caused by each pathotype are summarized as follows (Table 47.1):

- Shiga toxin-producing *E coli* (STEC) organisms are associated with diarrhea, hemorrhagic colitis, and hemolytic uremic syndrome (HUS). The term thrombotic thrombocytopenic purpura sometimes is used incorrectly for adults with STEC-associated HUS. STEC O157:H7 is the most consistently virulent STEC serotype, but other serotypes increasingly are being associated with illness. STEC illness typically begins with nonbloody diarrhea caused by virulent STEC serotypes, including O157:H7. Stools usually become bloody after 3 or 4 days. Severe abdominal pain is typical; fever occurs in less than one-third of cases. Severe infection can result in hemorrhagic colitis. In people with presumptive diagnoses of intussusception, appendicitis, inflammatory bowel disease, or ischemic colitis, disease caused by *E coli* O157:H7 and other STEC should be considered.
- Diarrhea caused by enteropathogenic *E coli* (EPEC) is watery. Although usually mild, diarrhea can result in dehydration and even death. Illness occurs almost exclusively in children younger than 2 years and predominantly in resource-limited countries, either sporadically or in epidemics. Chronic EPEC diarrhea can result in growth retardation.
- Diarrhea caused by enterotoxigenic *E coli* (ETEC) is a 1- to 5-day, self-limited illness of moderate severity, typically with watery stools and abdominal cramps. ETEC is common in infants in resource-limited countries and in travelers to those countries. ETEC infection rarely is diagnosed in the United States. Outbreaks and studies with small numbers of patients have demonstrated that ETEC infection occurs among nontravelers in the United States.

- Diarrhea caused by enteroinvasive *E coli* is similar clinically to diarrhea caused by *Shigella* species. Although dysentery can occur, diarrhea usually is watery without blood or mucus. Patients often are febrile, and stools can contain leukocytes.
- Enteroaggregative *E coli* (EAEC) organisms cause watery diarrhea and are common in people of all ages in industrialized as well as resource-limited countries. EAEC has been associated with prolonged diarrhea (14 days or longer). Asymptomatic infection can be accompanied by subclinical inflammatory enteritis, which can cause growth disturbances.

Sequelae of STEC Infection. HUS is a serious sequela of STEC enteric infection. *E coli* O157:H7 is the STEC serotype most commonly associated with HUS, defined by the triad of microangiopathic hemolytic anemia, thrombocytopenia, and acute renal dysfunction. HUS occurs in up to 15% of STEC-infected children. The illness is serious and typically develops 7 days (up to 3 weeks) after onset of diarrhea. More than 50% of children require dialysis, and 3% to 5% die. Patients with HUS can develop neurologic complications (eg, seizures, coma, or cerebral vessel thrombosis). Children presenting with an elevated white blood cell count ($>20 \times 10^9$ per mL) or hematocrit less than 23% and with oligoanuria are at higher risk of poor outcome. One or more years after HUS, patients with normal creatinine clearance and without proteinuria or hypertension have a good prognosis.

Etiology

Five pathotypes of diarrhea-producing *E coli* are defined by pathogenic and clinical characteristics. Each pathotype comprises characteristic serotypes, indicated by somatic (O) and flagellar (H) antigens. Some serotypes are found in more than one pathotype group.

Epidemiology

Transmission of most diarrhea-associated *E coli* strains is from food or water contaminated with human or animal feces or from infected symptomatic people. STEC is shed in feces of cattle and, to a lesser extent, sheep, deer, and other ruminants. Human infection is acquired via contaminated food or water or via direct contact with an infected person, a fomite, or a carrier animal or its environment. Many food vehicles have caused *E coli* O157 outbreaks, including undercooked ground beef (a major source), raw leafy greens, and unpasteurized milk. Outbreak investigations also have implicated petting zoos, drinking water, and ingestion of recreational water. The infectious dose is low; thus, person-to-person transmission is common in households and has occurred in child care centers. Less is known about the epidemiology of STEC strains other than O157:H7. Among children younger than 5 years, the incidence of HUS is highest in 1-year-old children and lowest in infants. An outbreak in Germany of HUS and bloody diarrhea caused by a virulent *E coli* strain O104:H4 with virulence profiles combining STEC and EAEC loci infected a large number of children and adults, with a high proportion of patients developing HUS.

With the exception of EAEC, non-STEC pathotypes most commonly are associated with disease in resource-limited countries, where food and water supplies commonly are contaminated and facilities and supplies for hand hygiene are suboptimal. Diarrhea attributable to ETEC occurs in people of all ages but especially is frequent and severe in infants in resource-limited countries. ETEC is a major cause of travelers' diarrhea. EAEC increasingly is recognized as a cause of diarrhea in the United States.

Incubation Period

E coli O157:H7, 3 to 4 days (range, 1–8); most other diarrhea-causing *E coli,* 10 hours to 6 days

Diagnostic Tests

Diagnosis of infection caused by diarrhea-associated *E coli* other than STEC is difficult, because tests are not widely available to distinguish these pathotypes from normal *E coli* strains present in stool flora. Several sensitive, specific, and rapid enzyme immunoassays (EIA) for detection of Shiga toxins in stool or broth culture of stool specimens are available commercially. These tests are necessary to detect non-O157 STEC infections. All stool specimens submitted for routine testing from patients with acute community-acquired diarrhea (regardless of patient age, season, or presence or absence of blood in the stool) should be cultured simultaneously for *E coli* O157:H7 and tested with an assay that detects Shiga toxins produced by O157 STEC. Serotyping with specific antisera then can confirm the isolates as *E coli* O157:H7.

STEC also should be sought in stool specimens from all patients diagnosed with postdiarrheal HUS. However, the absence of STEC does not preclude the diagnosis of probable STEC-associated HUS, because HUS typically is diagnosed a week or more after onset of diarrhea, when the organism may not be detectable by conventional methods. Additional methods used in reference and research laboratories include DNA probes and PCR assay. Serologic diagnosis using EIA to detect serum antibodies to *E coli* O157 and O111 lipopolysaccharides is available at the Centers for Disease Control and Prevention for outbreak investigations.

Treatment

Orally administered electrolyte-containing solutions usually are adequate to prevent or treat dehydration and electrolyte abnormalities. Antimotility agents should not be administered to children with inflammatory or bloody diarrhea. Careful monitoring of patients with hemorrhagic colitis (including complete blood cell count with smear, blood urea nitrogen, and creatinine concentrations) is recommended to detect changes suggestive of HUS. If patients have no laboratory evidence of hemolysis, thrombocytopenia, or nephropathy 3 days after resolution of diarrhea, their risk of developing HUS is low.

Antimicrobial Therapy. A meta-analysis did not find that children with hemorrhagic colitis caused by STEC have a greater risk of developing HUS if treated with an antimicrobial agent. However, a controlled trial has not been performed, and a beneficial effect of antimicrobial treatment has not been proven. Most experts advise not prescribing antimicrobial therapy for children with *E coli* O157:H7 enteritis or a clinical or epidemiologic picture strongly suggestive of STEC infection. For an episode of severe watery diarrhea in a traveler to a resource-limited country, therapy can be helpful. Azithromycin or a fluoroquinolone have been the most reliable agents for therapy, although fluoroquinolones are not approved in people younger than 18 years for this indication. Whenever possible, an antimicrobial agent should be chosen on the basis of results of susceptibility testing.

Table 47.1
Classification of *Escherichia coli* Associated With Diarrhea

Pathotype	Epidemiology	Type of Diarrhea	Mechanism of Pathogenesis
Shiga toxin-producing *E coli* (STEC)	Hemorrhagic colitis and hemolytic uremic syndrome in all ages	Bloody or nonbloody	Shiga toxin production, large bowel attachment, coagulopathy
Enteropathogenic *E coli* (EPEC)	Acute and chronic endemic and epidemic diarrhea in infants	Watery	Small bowel adherence and effacement
Enterotoxigenic *E coli* (ETEC)	Infant diarrhea in resource-limited countries and travelers' diarrhea in all ages	Watery	Small bowel adherence, heat stable/heat-labile enterotoxin production
Enteroinvasive *E coli* (EIEC)	Diarrhea with fever in all ages	Bloody or nonbloody; dysentery	Adherence, mucosal invasion and inflammation of large bowel
Enteroaggregative *E coli* (EAEC)	Acute and chronic diarrhea in all ages	Watery, occasionally bloody	Small and large bowel adherence, enterotoxin and cytotoxin production

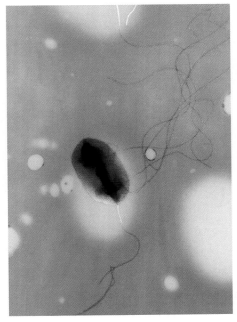

Image 47.1
Transmission electron micrograph of *Escherichia coli* O157:H7. Courtesy of Centers for Disease Control and Prevention/Peggy S. Hayes.

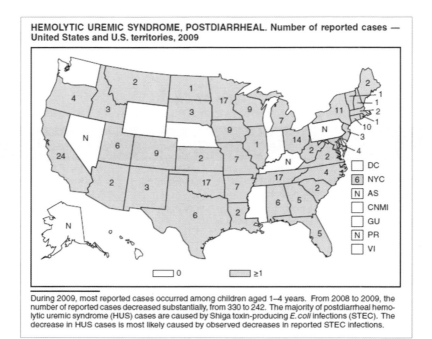

HEMOLYTIC UREMIC SYNDROME, POSTDIARRHEAL. Number of reported cases — United States and U.S. territories, 2009

During 2009, most reported cases occurred among children aged 1–4 years. From 2008 to 2009, the number of reported cases decreased substantially, from 330 to 242. The majority of postdiarrheal hemolytic uremic syndrome (HUS) cases are caused by Shiga toxin-producing *E. coli* infections (STEC). The decrease in HUS cases is most likely caused by observed decreases in reported STEC infections.

Image 47.2
Hemolytic uremic syndrome, postdiarrheal. Number of reported cases—United States and US territories, 2009. Courtesy of *Morbidity and Mortality Weekly Report.*

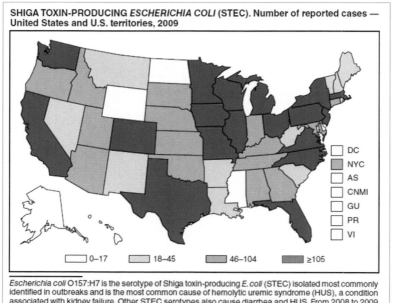

SHIGA TOXIN-PRODUCING *ESCHERICHIA COLI* (STEC). Number of reported cases — United States and U.S. territories, 2009

Escherichia coli O157:H7 is the serotype of Shiga toxin-producing *E. coli* (STEC) isolated most commonly identified in outbreaks and is the most common cause of hemolytic uremic syndrome (HUS), a condition associated with kidney failure. Other STEC serotypes also cause diarrhea and HUS. From 2008 to 2009 the number of reported STEC cases decreased from 5,309 to 4,643.

Image 47.3
Shiga toxin–producing *Escherichia coli*. Number of reported cases—United States and US territories, 2009. Courtesy of *Morbidity and Mortality Weekly Report.*

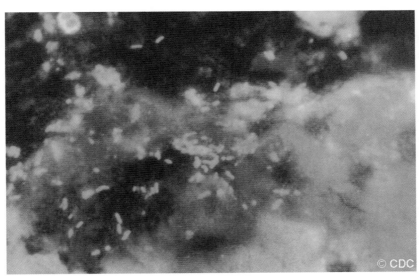

Image 47.4

Escherichia coli in the intestine from an 8-month-old child suffering from chronic diarrhea (fluorescent antibody stain). In a small number of individuals (mostly children <5 years and the elderly), *E coli* can cause hemolytic uremic syndrome, in which the red blood cells are destroyed and the kidneys fail. Courtesy of Centers for Disease Control and Prevention.

48

Fusobacterium Infections

(Including Lemierre Disease)

Clinical Manifestations

Fusobacterium necrophorum and *Fusobacterium nucleatum* can be isolated from oropharyngeal specimens in healthy people, are frequent components of human dental plaque, and may lead to periodontal disease. Invasive disease attributable to *Fusobacterium* species has been reported following otitis media, tonsillitis, gingivitis, and oropharyngeal trauma. Ten percent of cases of invasive *Fusobacterium* infections are associated with Epstein-Barr virus infection.

Invasive infection with *Fusobacterium* species can lead to life-threatening disease. Otogenic infection is the most frequent primary source in children younger than 5 years and can be complicated by meningitis and thrombosis of dural venous sinuses. Invasive infection following tonsillitis was described early in the 20th century and was referred to as postanginal sepsis or Lemierre disease. Lemierre disease occurs most often in adolescents and young adults and can include internal jugular vein thrombophlebitis or thrombosis (JVT), evidence of septic embolic lesions in lungs or other sterile sites, and isolation of *Fusobacterium* species from blood or other normally sterile sites. Lemierre-like syndromes also have been reported following infection with *Arcanobacterium haemolyticum*, *Bacteroides* species, and anaerobic streptococcal species; other anaerobic bacteria; and methicillin-susceptible and resistant strains of *Staphylococcus aureus*. Fever and sore throat are followed by severe neck pain (anginal pain) that can be accompanied by unilateral neck swelling, trismus, and dysphagia. People with classic Lemierre disease have a sepsis syndrome with multiple organ dysfunction, disseminated intravascular coagulation, empyema, pyogenic arthritis, or osteomyelitis. Persistent headache or other neurologic signs indicate the presence of cerebral venous sinus thrombosis (eg, cavernous sinus thrombosis), meningitis, or brain abscess.

JVT can be completely vaso-occlusive. Some children with JVT associated with Lemierre disease have evidence of thrombophilia at diagnosis, which can include presence of antiphospholipid antibodies, abnormal levels of factor VIII, and factor V Leiden. These findings often resolve over several months and can indicate response to the inflammatory, prothrombotic process associated with infection rather than an underlying hypercoagulable state.

Etiology

Fusobacterium species are anaerobic, non–spore-forming, gram-negative bacilli. Human infection usually results from *F necrophorum* subspecies *funduliforme*, but infections with other species including *F nucleatum*, *Fusobacterium gonidiaformans*, *Fusobacterium naviforme*, *Fusobacterium mortiferum*, and *Fusobacterium varium* have been reported. Infection with *Fusobacterium* species, alone or in combination with other oral anaerobic bacteria, can result in Lemierre disease.

Epidemiology

Fusobacterium species commonly are found in soil and in the respiratory tracts of animals, including cattle, dogs, fowl, goats, sheep, and horses, and can be isolated from the oropharynx of healthy people. *Fusobacterium* infections are most common in adolescents and young adults, but infections, including fatal cases of Lemierre disease, have been reported in infants and young children. Children with sickle cell disease may be at greater risk of infection, particularly osteomyelitis.

Incubation Period

Unknown.

Diagnostic Tests

Fusobacterium species can be isolated using conventional liquid anaerobic blood culture media. Colonies are cream to yellow colored, smooth, and round with a narrow zone of hemolysis on blood agar. Many strains fluoresce chartreuse green under ultraviolet light. Most *Fusobacterium* organisms are indole positive. Sequencing of the 16S rRNA gene and phylogenetic analysis can identify anaerobic bacteria to the genus or taxonomic group level and frequently to the species level.

Febrile children and adolescents, especially those with sore throat or neck pain who are sufficiently ill to warrant a blood culture, should have an anaerobic blood culture in addition to aerobic blood culture performed to detect invasive *Fusobacterium* species infection. Computed tomography and magnetic resonance imaging are more sensitive than ultrasonography to document thrombosis and thrombophlebitis of the internal jugular vein early in the course of illness.

Treatment

Fusobacterium species are susceptible to metronidazole, clindamycin, chloramphenicol, carbapenems, cefoxitin, and ceftriaxone. Metronidazole is the treatment preferred by many experts, because the drug has excellent activity against all *Fusobacterium* species and good tissue penetration. However, metronida-

zole lacks activity against microaerophilic streptococci that can coinfect some patients. Tetracyclines have limited activity. Up to 50% of *F nucleatum* and 20% of *F necrophorum* isolates produce beta-lactamases, rendering them resistant to penicillin, ampicillin, and some cephalosporins.

Because *Fusobacterium* infections often are polymicrobial, multiple antimicrobial agents frequently are necessary. Therapy with a penicillin-beta-lactamase inhibitor combination (eg, piperacillin-tazobactam) or a carbapenem or combination therapy with metronidazole in addition to other agents active against aerobic oral and respiratory tract pathogens is recommended. Duration of antimicrobial therapy depends on the anatomic location and severity of infection but usually is weeks. Surgical intervention involving debridement or incision and drainage of abscesses may be necessary. In cases with extensive thrombosis, anticoagulation therapy may decrease the risk of clot extension and shorten recovery time.

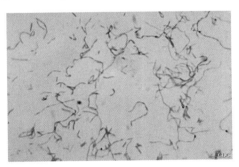

Image 48.1
This photomicrograph shows *Fusobacterium nucleatum* after being cultured in a thioglycollate medium for 48 hours. Courtesy of Centers for Disease Control and Prevention.

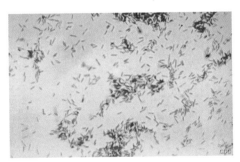

Image 48.2
This is a photomicrograph of *Fusobacterium russii* cultured in a thioglycollate medium for 48 hours. Like the genus *Bacteroides*, *Fusobacterium* are anaerobic, gram-negative bacteria that are normal inhabitors of the oral cavity, intestine, and female genital tract. *Fusobacterium* spp are associated most commonly with head and neck infections, pulmonary infections, and wound infections. Courtesy of Centers for Disease Control and Prevention/V. R. Dowell, Jr, MD.

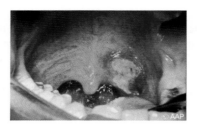

Image 48.3

Vincent stomatitis has been confused with diphtheria, though this infection is usually a mixed infection, including fusiform and spirochetal anaerobic bacteria including *Fusobacterium,* and is associated with severe pain and halitosis. Note ulceration of the soft palate with surrounding erythema. Courtesy of Edgar O. Ledbetter, MD, FAAP.

49

Giardia intestinalis (formerly *Giardia lamblia* and *Giardia duodenalis*) Infections

(Giardiasis)

Clinical Manifestations

Symptomatic infection with *Giardia intestinalis* causes a broad spectrum of clinical manifestations. Children can have occasional days of acute watery diarrhea with abdominal pain, or they may experience a protracted, intermittent, often debilitating disease characterized by passage of foul-smelling stools associated with flatulence, abdominal distention, and anorexia. Anorexia combined with malabsorption can lead to significant weight loss, failure to thrive, and anemia. Humoral immunodeficiencies predispose to chronic symptomatic *G intestinalis* infections. Asymptomatic infection is common; approximately 50% to 75% of infected people reported during outbreaks occurring in child care settings and in the community were asymptomatic.

Etiology

G intestinalis is a flagellate protozoan that exists in trophozoite and cyst forms; the infective form is the cyst. Infection is limited to the small intestine and biliary tract.

Epidemiology

Giardiasis is the most common intestinal parasitic infection of humans identified in the United States and globally with a worldwide distribution. Approximately 20,000 cases are reported in the United States each year, with highest incidence reported among children 1 to 9 years of age, adults 35 to 44 years of age, and residents of northern states. Peak onset of illness occurs annually during early summer through early fall. Humans are the principal reservoir of infection, but *Giardia* can infect dogs, cats, beavers, rodents, sheep, cattle, non-human primates, and other animals. People become infected directly from an infected person or through ingestion of fecally contaminated water or food. Most community-wide epidemics have resulted from a contaminated water supply. From 1971 to 2006, 123 drinking water outbreaks resulting in 28,127 cases of giaridiasis were reported in the United States. In 2007 and 2008, there were 2 *Giardia*-associated drinking water outbreaks involving 81 people. Outbreaks resulting from person-to-person transmission occur in child care centers or institutional care settings, where staff and family members in contact with infected children or adults become infected. Outbreaks associated with food or food handlers, although less common, also have been reported. Surveys conducted in the United States have identified overall prevalence rates of *Giardia* organisms in stool specimens that range from 5% to 7%, with variations depending on age, geographic location, and seasonality. Duration of cyst excretion is variable but can range from weeks to months. Giardiasis is communicable for as long as the infected person excretes cysts.

Incubation Period

1 to 3 weeks.

Diagnostic Tests

Commercially available, sensitive, and specific enzyme immunoassay (EIA) and direct fluorescence antibody (DFA) assays are becoming the standard for diagnosis of giaridiasis in the United States. EIA has a sensitivity of up to 95% and a specificity of 98% to 100% when compared with microscopy. DFA assay has the advantage that organisms are visualized. Traditionally, diagnosis has been based on the microscopic identification of trophozoites or cysts in stool specimens. However, this requires an experienced microscopist, and sensitivity can be suboptimal if the specimen contains low numbers of organisms. Stool needs to be examined as soon as possible or placed immediately in a preservative, such as neutral-buffered 10% formalin or polyvinyl alcohol. A single direct smear examination of stool has a sensitivity of 75% to 95%. Sensitivity is higher for diarrheal stool specimens, because they contain higher concentrations of organisms. Sensitivity of microscopy is increased by examining 3 or more specimens collected every other day. When giardiasis is suspected clinically but the organism is not found on repeated stool examination, examination of duodenal contents obtained by direct aspiration or by using a commercially available string test (Enterotest) may be diagnostic. Rarely, duodenal biopsy is required for diagnosis.

Treatment

Some infections are self-limited and treatment is not required. Dehydration and electrolyte abnormalities can occur and should be corrected. Tinidazole, metronidazole, and nitazoxanide are the drugs of choice. A 5- to 10-day course of metronidazole has an efficacy of 80% to 100% in pediatric patients. A 1-time dose of tinidazole, a nitroimidazole for children 3 years of age and older, has a median efficacy of 91% in pediatric patients (range, 80%–100%) and has fewer adverse effects than does metronidazole. A 3-day course of nitazoxanide oral suspension has similar efficacy to metronidazole and has the advantage(s) of treating other intestinal parasites and of being approved for use in children 1 year of age and older. Quinacrine and an oral suspension of furazolidone are alternatives but are used more often for combination therapy for refractory disease.

Symptom recurrence after completing antimicrobial treatment can be attributable to reinfection, post-*Giardia* lactose intolerance (occurs in 20%–40% of patients), immunosuppresion, insufficient treatment, or drug resistance. If reinfection is suspected, a second course of the same drug should be effective. Treatment with a different class of drug is recommended for resistant giardiasis.

Patients who are immunocompromised because of hypogammaglobulinemia or lymphoproliferative disease are at higher risk of giardiasis, and it is more difficult to treat in these patients. Patients with AIDS often respond to standard therapy; however, in some cases, additional treatment is required. If giardiasis is refractory to standard treatment among HIV-infected patients with AIDS, high doses, longer treatment duration, or combination therapy may be appropriate.

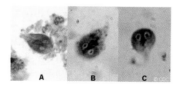

Image 49.1
Three trophozoites of *Giardia intestinalis* (A, trichrome stain. B and C, iron hematoxylin stain). Each cell has 2 nuclei with a large, central karyosome. Cell length: 9 to 21 μm. Trophozoites are usually seen in fresh diarrheal stool or in duodenal mucus. Courtesy of Centers for Disease Control and Prevention.

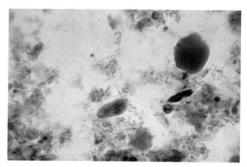

Image 49.2
Photomicrograph of a *Giardia lamblia* cyst seen using a trichrome stain. *G lamblia* is the protozoan organism that causes the disease giardiasis, a diarrheal disorder directly affecting the small intestine. Courtesy of Centers for Disease Control and Prevention.

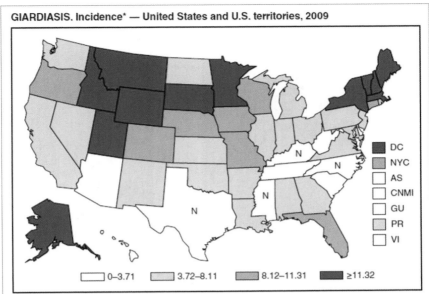

GIARDIASIS. Incidence* — United States and U.S. territories, 2009

DC
NYC
AS
CNMI
GU
PR
VI

0–3.71   3.72–8.11   8.12–11.31   ≥11.32

* Per 100,000 population.

Giardiasis is widespread geographically in the United States, with increased reporting in certain states and regions. Whether this difference is of true biologic significance or reflects differences in giardiasis case detection and reporting among states is unclear. Giardiasis was not a reportable disease in Indiana before 2009.

Image 49.3

Giardiasis. Incidence—United States and US territories, 2009. Courtesy of *Morbidity and Mortality Weekly Report.*

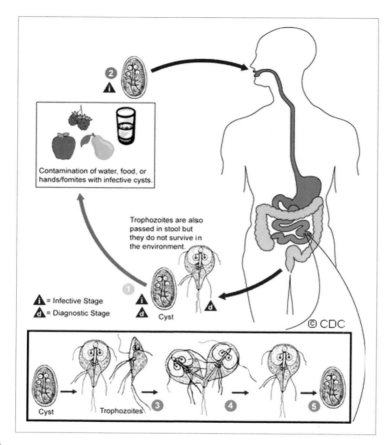

Image 49.4

Cysts are resistant forms and are responsible for transmission of giardiasis. Both cysts and trophozoites can be found in the feces (diagnostic stages) (1). The cysts are hardy and can survive several
months in cold water. Infection occurs by the ingestion of cysts in contaminated water or food, or
by the fecal-oral route (hands or fomites) (2). In the small intestine, excystation releases trophozoites
(each cyst produces 2 trophozoites) (3). Trophozoites multiply by longitudinal binary fission, remaining
in the lumen of the proximal small bowel where they can be free or attached to the mucosa by a ventral sucking disk (4). Encystation occurs as the parasites transit toward the colon. The cyst is the stage
found most commonly in non-diarrheal feces (5). Because the cysts are infectious when passed in
the stool or shortly afterward, person-to-person transmission is possible. While animals are infected
with *Giardia*, their importance as a reservoir is unclear. Courtesy of Centers for Disease Control and
Prevention/Alexander J. da Silva, PhD/Melanie Moser.

50

Gonococcal Infections

Clinical Manifestations

Gonococcal infections in children and adolescents occur in 3 distinct age groups.

- Infection in **neonates** usually involves the eyes. Other possible manifestations of neonatal gonococcal infection include scalp abscess (which can be associated with fetal scalp monitoring) and disseminated disease with bacteremia, arthritis, or meningitis.
- In children beyond the newborn period, including **prepubertal children,** gonococcal infection may occur in the genital tract and almost always is transmitted sexually. Vaginitis is the most common manifestation in prepubertal females. Gonococcal urethritis is possible but uncommon in the prepubertal male. Anorectal and tonsillopharyngeal infection also can occur in prepubertal children and often is asymptomatic.
- In **sexually active adolescents,** as in adults, gonococcal infection of the genital tract in females often is asymptomatic, and common clinical syndromes are urethritis, endocervicitis, and salpingitis. In males, infection often is symptomatic, and the primary site involved is the urethra. Infection of the rectum and pharynx can occur alone or with genitourinary tract infection in either sex. Rectal and pharyngeal infections often are asymptomatic. Extension from primary genital mucosal sites can lead to epididymitis in males and to bartholinitis, pelvic inflammatory disease (PID) with resultant tubal scarring, and perihepatitis (Fitz-Hugh-Curtis syndrome) in females. Even asymptomatic infection in females can progress to PID, with tubal scarring that can result in ectopic pregnancy or infertility. Infection involving other mucous membranes can produce conjunctivitis, pharyngitis, or proctitis. Hematogenous spread from mucosal sites can involve skin and joints (arthritis-dermatitis syndrome) and occurs in up to 3% of untreated people with mucosal gonorrhea. Bacteremia can result in a maculopapular rash with necrosis, tenosynovitis, and migratory arthritis. Arthritis may be reactive (sterile) or septic in nature. Meningitis and endocarditis occur rarely.

Etiology

Neisseria gonorrhoeae is a gram-negative, oxidase-positive diplococcus.

Epidemiology

Gonococcal infections occur only in humans. The source of the organism is exudate and secretions from infected mucosal surfaces; *N gonorrhoeae* is communicable as long as a person harbors the organism. Transmission results from intimate contact, such as sexual acts, parturition and, rarely, household exposure in prepubertal children. Sexual abuse should be considered strongly when genital, rectal, or pharyngeal colonization or infection is diagnosed in prepubertal children beyond the newborn period. In 2010, a total of 309,341 cases of gonorrhea were reported in the United States, a rate of 99 cases per 100,000 population. *N gonorrhoeae* is the second most commonly reported notifiable disease in the United States, with *Chlamydia trachomatis* genital tract infection being the most commonly reported. Reported incidence of infection is highest in females 15 through 24 years of age and in males 20 through 24 years of age. In 2009, gonorrhea rates remained highest among black people. Similar to recent years, the rate among black people was 20.5 times higher than the rate among white people. Rates among white people were 1.5 times higher than rates among people of Asian/Pacific Island ancestry. Concurrent infection with *C trachomatis* is common.

Incubation Period

2 to 7 days.

Diagnostic Tests

Microscopic examination of Gram-stained smears of exudate from the conjunctivae, vagina of prepubertal girls, male urethra, skin lesions, synovial fluid and, when clinically warranted, cerebrospinal fluid (CSF) may be useful in the initial evaluation. Identification of gram-negative intracellular diplococci in these smears can be helpful, particularly if the organism is not recovered in culture. However, because of low sensitivity, a negative gram stain result should not be considered sufficient for ruling out infection.

N gonorrhoeae can be isolated from normally sterile sites, such as blood, CSF, or synovial fluid, using nonselective chocolate agar with incubation in 5% to 10% carbon dioxide. Selective media that inhibit normal flora and nonpathogenic *Neisseria* organisms are used for cultures from nonsterile sites, such as the cervix, vagina, rectum, urethra, and pharynx. Specimens for *N gonorrhoeae* culture from mucosal sites should be inoculated immediately onto appropriate agar, because the organism is extremely sensitive to drying and temperature changes.

Caution should be exercised when interpreting the significance of isolation of *Neisseria* organisms, because *N gonorrhoeae* can be confused with other *Neisseria* species that colonize the genitourinary tract or pharynx. At least 2 confirmatory bacteriologic tests involving different biochemical principles should be performed by the laboratory. Interpretation of culture of *N gonorrhoeae* from the pharynx of young children necessitates particular caution because of the high carriage rate of nonpathogenic *Neisseria* species and the serious implications of such a culture result.

Nucleic acid amplification tests (NAATs) are highly sensitive and specific when used on male urethral swab, female endocervical or vaginal swab, and male or female urine specimens. These tests include PCR, transcription-mediated amplification, and strand-displacement assay. Use of urine specimens increases feasibility of initial testing and follow-up of populations such as adolescents. These techniques also permit dual testing of urine for *C trachomatis* and *N gonorrhoeae*.

Culture is the most widely used test for identifying *N gonorrhoeae* from nongenital sites, and specimens also should be sent for antimicrobial susceptibility testing to aid in management should infection persist following initial therapy. NAATs are not approved by the US Food and Drug Administration (FDA) for use on rectal or pharyngeal swabs; some commercial and public health laboratories offer NAATs of rectal and pharyngeal swab specimens following in-house validation testing. Some NAATs have the potential to cross-react with nongonococcal *Neisseria* that commonly are found in the throat. A limited number of nonculture tests are approved by the FDA for conjunctival specimens.

Sexual Abuse. In all prepubertal children beyond the newborn period and in adolescents who have gonococcal infection but report no prior sexual activity, sexual abuse must be considered to have occurred until proven otherwise. Cultures should be performed on genital, rectal, and pharyngeal swab specimens for all patients before antimicrobial treatment is given. All gonococcal isolates from such patients should be preserved. Nonculture gonococcal tests, including Gram stain, DNA probes, enzyme immunoassays, or NAATs of oropharyngeal, rectal, or genital tract swab specimens in children cannot be relied on as the sole method for diagnosis of gonococcal infection for this purpose, because false-positive results can occur. Detection of gonorrhea in a child requires an evaluation for other sexually transmitted infections, such as *C trachomatis* infection, syphilis, and HIV infection. Completion of the series of vaccines for hepatitis B and human papillomavirus (HPV) should be documented, then offered if not completed and if appropriate for those 9 years of age or older.

Treatment

Increases in the prevalence of fluoroquinolone resistance among gonococcal isolates in the United States resulted in new treatment recommendations in 2007. Because of the high prevalence of penicillin-, tetracycline-, and fluoroquinolone-resistant *N gonorrhoeae*, an extended-spectrum cephalosporin (eg, ceftriaxone, cefixime) is recommended as initial therapy for children and adults. Antimicrobial resistance is widespread in many parts of the world, so treatment recommendations can vary depending on where infection was acquired.

Ceftriaxone is recommended for gonococcal infections of all sites in children and adults in the United States. Cefixime is recommended for uncomplicated gonococcal vaginal, cervical, urethral, and rectal infections in a prepubertal child. Cefotaxime also can be used for gonococcal ophthalmia, scalp abscesses, and disseminated gonococcal infection in newborn infants.

All patients with presumed or proven gonorrhea should be evaluated for concurrent syphilis, HIV, and *C trachomatis* infections. Completion of the series of vaccines for hepatitis B and HPV should be documented and then recommended if not completed and if appropriate for the age of the child. All patients beyond the neonatal period with gonorrhea should be treated presumptively for *C trachomatis* infection. A single dose of ceftriaxone, spectinomycin, or azithromycin is not effective treatment for concurrent infection with syphilis.

Test-of-cure samples are not required in adolescents or adults with uncomplicated gonorrhea who are asymptomatic after being treated with one of the recommended antimicrobial regimens. However, because reinfection by a new or untreated partner is not uncommon, clinicians may consider advising sexually active adolescents and adults with gonorrhea to be retested 3 months after treatment. Children treated with ceftriaxone do not require follow-up cultures unless they remain in an at-risk environment, but if treated with other regimens, then follow-up culture is indicated. Patients who have symptoms that persist after treatment or whose symptoms recur shortly after treatment should be reevaluated by culture for *N gonorrhoeae,* and any gonococci isolated should be tested for antimicrobial susceptibility. Treatment failures have been reported more frequently from Asian countries. In addition to submission of clinical specimens for culture and susceptibility testing, a history of recent travel or sexual activity in Asian countries should be elicited in people with treatment failure.

Specific recommendations for management and antimicrobial therapy are as follows:

Neonatal Disease. Infants with clinical evidence of ophthalmia neonatorum, scalp abscess, or disseminated infections attributable to *N gonorrhoeae* should be hospitalized. Cultures of blood, eye discharge, and other potential sites of infection, such as CSF, should be performed on specimens from infants to confirm the diagnosis and to determine antimicrobial susceptibility. Tests for concomitant infection with *C trachomatis,* congenital syphilis, and HIV infection should be performed. Results of the maternal test for hepatitis B surface antigen should be confirmed. The mother and her partner(s) also need appropriate examination and management for *N gonorrhoeae.*

Nondisseminated Neonatal Infections. Recommended antimicrobial therapy, including that for ophthalmia neonatorum, is ceftriaxone given once. Infants with gonococcal ophthalmia should receive eye irrigations with saline solution immediately and at frequent intervals until discharge is eliminated. Topical antimicrobial treatment alone is inadequate and unnecessary. Infants with gonococcal ophthalmia should be hospitalized and evaluated for disseminated infection (eg, sepsis, arthritis, meningitis).

Disseminated Neonatal Infections. Recommended therapy for arthritis and septicemia is ceftriaxone for 7 days. If meningitis is documented, treatment should be continued for a total of 10 to 14 days.

Special Problems in Treatment of Children (Beyond the Neonatal Period) and Adolescents. Patients with uncomplicated infections of the vagina, endocervix, urethra, or anorectum and a history of severe adverse reactions to cephalosporins (anaphylaxis, Stevens-Johnson syndrome, and toxic epidermal necrolysis) should be treated with a single dose of spectinomycin, if available (spectinomycin currently is not available in the United States). Because data are limited regarding alternative regimens for treating gonorrhea among people who have documented severe cephalosporin allergy, consultation with an expert in infectious diseases is recommended. Patients with uncomplicated pharyngeal gonococcal infection should be treated with a single dose of ceftriaxone. A single dose of ceftriaxone is not effective treatment for concurrent infection with syphilis and spectinomycin is not active against *Treponema pallidum.*

Children or adolescents with HIV infection should receive the same treatment for gonococcal infection as children without HIV infection.

Acute PID. *N gonorrhoeae* and *C trachomatis* are implicated in many cases of PID; most cases have a polymicrobial etiology. No reliable clinical criteria distinguish gonococ-cal from nongonococcal-associated PID. Hence, broad-spectrum treatment regimens are recommended.

Acute Epididymitis. Sexually transmitted organisms, such as *N gonorrhoeae* or *C trachomatis,* can cause acute epididymitis

in sexually active adolescents and young adults but rarely if ever cause acute epididymitis in prepubertal children. The recommended regimen for sexually transmitted epididymitis is ceftriaxone plus doxycycline.

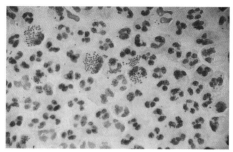

Image 50.1

This photomicrograph reveals gram-negative diplococci in a specimen obtained from a patient with acute gonococcal urethritis. Courtesy of Centers for Disease Control and Prevention/Joe Miller.

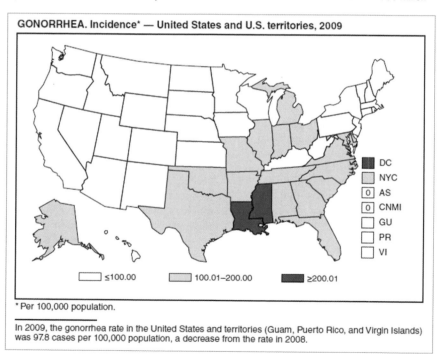

Image 50.2

Gonorrhea. Incidence—United States and US territories, 2009. Courtesy of *Morbidity and Mortality Weekly Report.*

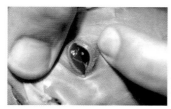

Image 50.3

An infant with gonococcal ophthalmia. In-hospital evaluation and treatment is recommended for infants with gonococcal ophthalmia. Copyright Martin G. Myers.

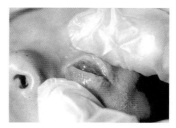

Image 50.4

An 8-day-old neonate with gonococcal ophthalmia. Copyright Martin G. Myers.

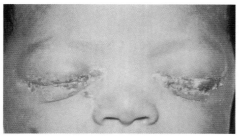

Image 50.5

This was a newborn with gonococcal ophthalmia neonatorum caused by a maternally transmitted gonococcal infection. Unless preventive measures are taken, it is estimated that gonococcal ophthalmia neonatorum will develop in 28% of infants born to women with gonorrhea. It affects the corneal epithelium causing microbial keratitis, ulceration, and perforation. Courtesy of Centers for Disease Control and Prevention/J. Pledger.

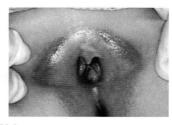

Image 50.6

Profuse, purulent vaginal discharge in an 18-month-old girl who has gonococcal vulvovaginitis. In preadolescent children, this infection is almost always associated with sexual abuse. Identification of the species of cultured gonococci is imperative in suspected cases of sexual abuse.

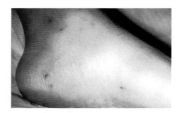

Image 50.8

Adolescent with septic arthritis of left ankle with petechial and necrotic skin lesions on the feet. Blood cultures were positive for *Neisseria gonorrhoeae*.

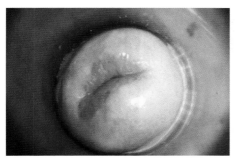

Image 50.7

This colposcopic view of this patient's cervix revealed an eroded ostium due to *Neisseria gonorrhoeae* infection. A chronic *N gonorrhoeae* infection can lead to complications that can be apparent, such as this cervical inflammation, and some can be quite insipid, giving the impression that the infection has subsided while treatment is still needed. Courtesy of Centers for Disease Control and Prevention.

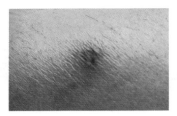

Image 50.9
Close-up view of necrotic gonococcal skin lesion from the patient in Image 50.8.

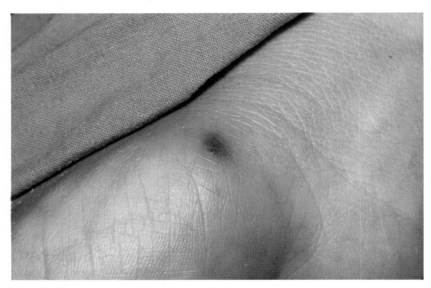

Image 50.10
Disseminated gonococcal infection. Courtesy of Gary Overturf, MD.

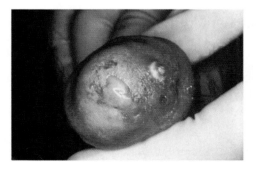

Image 50.11
This male presented with purulent penile discharge due to gonorrhea with an overlying penile pyodermal lesion. Pyoderma involves the formation of a purulent skin lesion as in this case located on the glans penis, and overlying the sexually transmitted infection gonorrhea. Courtesy of Centers for Disease Control and Prevention/Joe Miller.

51

Granuloma Inguinale
(Donovanosis)

Clinical Manifestations

Initial lesions of this sexually transmitted infection are single or multiple subcutaneous nodules that progress to form painless, highly vascular, beefy red and friable, granulomatous ulcers without regional adenopathy. Lesions usually involve genitalia, but anal infections occur in 5% to 10% of patients; lesions at distant sites (eg, face, mouth, or liver) are rare. Subcutaneous extension into the inguinal area results in induration that can mimic inguinal adenopathy (ie, "pseudobubo"). Fibrosis manifests as sinus tracts, adhesions, and lymphedema, resulting in extreme genital deformity. Urethral obstruction can occur.

Etiology

The disease, donovanosis, is caused by *Klebsiella granulomatis* (formerly known as *Calymmatobacterium granulomatis*), an intracellular gram-negative bacillus.

Epidemiology

Indigenous granuloma inguinale occurs rarely in the United States and most resource-rich countries. Cases still are reported in Papua, New Guinea, and parts of India, southern Africa, central Australia and, to a much lesser extent, the Caribbean and parts of South America, most notably Brazil. The highest incidence of disease occurs in tropical and subtropical environments. The incidence of infection seems to correlate with sustained high temperatures and high relative humidity. Infection usually is acquired by sexual intercourse, most commonly with a person with active infection but possibly also from a person with asymptomatic rectal infection. Young children can acquire infection by contact with infected secretions. The period of communicability extends throughout the duration of active lesions or rectal colonization.

Incubation Period

8 to 80 days.

Diagnostic Tests

The causative organism is difficult to culture, and diagnosis requires microscopic demonstration of dark-staining intracytoplasmic Donovan bodies on Wright or Giemsa staining of a crush preparation from subsurface scrapings of a lesion or tissue. The microorganism also can be detected by histologic examination of biopsy specimens. Lesions should be cultured for *Haemophilus ducreyi* to exclude chancroid. Granuloma inguinale often is misdiagnosed as carcinoma, which can be excluded by histologic examination of tissue or by response of the lesion to antimicrobial agents.

Treatment

Doxycycline is the treatment of choice. Doxycycline should not be given to children younger than 8 years or to pregnant women. Trimethoprim-sulfamethoxazole is an alternative regimen, except in pregnant women. Ciprofloxacin, which is not recommended for use in pregnant or lactating women or children younger than 18 years, is effective. Gentamicin can be added if no improvement is evident in several days. Erythromycin or azithromycin is an alternative therapy for pregnant women or women who are infected with HIV. Antimicrobial therapy is continued for at least 3 weeks or until the lesions have resolved. Partial healing usually is noted within 7 days of initiation of therapy. Relapse can occur, especially if the antimicrobial agent is stopped before the primary lesion has healed completely. Complicated or long-standing infection can require surgical intervention.

Patients should be evaluated for other sexually transmitted infections, such as gonorrhea, syphilis, chancroid, chlamydia, hepatitis B virus, and HIV infections. Immunization status for hepatitis B and human papillomavirus should be reviewed and documented and then recommended if not complete and appropriate for age.

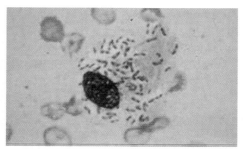

Image 51.1
Giemsa-stained Donovan bodies of granuloma inguinale. Courtesy of Robert Jerris, MD.

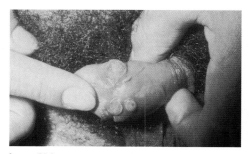

Image 51.2
This patient's penile lesions were due to gram-negative *Klebsiella granulomatis,* formerly known as *Calymmatobacterium granulomatis. K granulomatis* cause donovanosis, or granuloma inguinale, a sexually transmitted infection that is a slowly progressive, ulcerative condition of the skin and lymphatics of the genital and perianal area. A definitive diagnosis is achieved when a tissue smear tests positive for the presence of Donovan bodies. Courtesy of Centers for Disease Control and Prevention/Joe Miller/Dr Cornelia Arevalo, Venezuela.

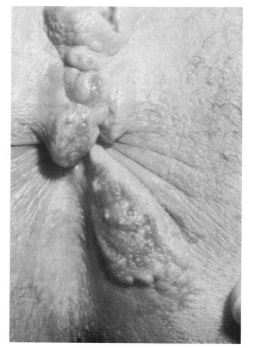

Image 51.3
This 19-year-old white female presented with a perianal granuloma inguinale lesion of about 8 months' duration. A genital ulcerative disease caused by the intracellular gram-negative bacterium *Klebsiella granulomatis,* granuloma inguinale, also known as donovanosis, occurs rarely in the United States. Courtesy of Centers for Disease Control and Prevention/Joe Miller/Dr Cornelia Arevalo, Venezuela.

52

Haemophilus influenzae Infections

Clinical Manifestations

Haemophilus influenzae type b (Hib) causes pneumonia, bacteremia, meningitis, epiglottitis, septic arthritis, cellulitis, otitis media, purulent pericarditis, and other less common infections, such as endocarditis, endophthalmitis, osteomyelitis, peritonitis, and gangrene. Non-type b encapsulated strains can cause disease similar to type b infections. Nontypable strains more commonly cause infections of the respiratory tract (eg, otitis media, sinusitis, pneumonia, conjunctivitis) and, less often, bacteremia, meningitis, chorioamnionitis, and neonatal septicemia.

Etiology

H influenzae is a pleomorphic gram-negative coccobacillus. Encapsulated strains express 1 of 6 antigenically distinct capsular polysaccharides (a through f); nonencapsulated strains lack capsule genes and are designated nontypable.

Epidemiology

The major reservoir of Hib is young infants and toddlers, who carry the organism in the upper respiratory tract, which is the natural habitat of *H influenzae* in humans. The mode of transmission is person-to-person by inhalation of respiratory tract droplets or by direct contact with respiratory tract secretions. In neonates, infection is acquired intrapartum by aspiration of amniotic fluid or by contact with genital tract secretions containing the organism. Pharyngeal colonization by *H influenzae* is relatively common, especially with nontypable and nontype b capsular type strains.

Before introduction of effective Hib conjugate vaccines, Hib was the most common cause of bacterial meningitis in children in the United States. The peak incidence of invasive Hib infections occurred between 6 and 18 months of age. In contrast, the peak age for Hib epiglottitis was 2 to 4 years of age.

Unimmunized children younger than 4 years are at increased risk of invasive Hib disease. Factors that predispose to invasive disease

include sickle cell disease, asplenia, HIV infection, certain immunodeficiency syndromes, and malignant neoplasms. Historically, invasive Hib was more common in boys; black, Alaska Native, Apache, and Navajo children; child care attendees; children living in crowded conditions; and children who were not breastfed.

Since introduction of Hib conjugate vaccines in the United States, the incidence of invasive Hib disease has decreased by 99% to fewer than 2 cases per 100,000 children younger than 5 years. In the United States, invasive Hib disease occurs primarily in underimmunized children and among infants too young to have completed the primary immunization series. Hib remains an important pathogen in many resource-limited countries where Hib vaccines are not available routinely. The epidemiology of invasive *H influenzae* disease in the United States has shifted in the postvaccination era. Nontypable *H influenzae* now causes most invasive *H influenzae* disease in all age groups. From 1999 through 2008, the annual incidence of invasive nontypable *H influenzae* disease was 1.73/100,000 in children younger than 5 years and 4.08/100,000 in adults 65 years and older.

Nontypable *H influenzae* causes approximately 30% to 50% of episodes of acute otitis media and sinusitis in children and is a common cause of recurrent otitis media. These infections are twice as frequent in boys and peak in the late fall.

Incubation Period

Unknown.

Diagnostic Tests

The diagnosis of invasive disease is established by growth of *H influenzae* from cerebrospinal fluid (CSF), blood, synovial fluid, pleural fluid, or pericardial fluid. Gram stain of an infected body fluid specimen can facilitate presumptive diagnosis. All *H influenzae* isolates associated with invasive infection should be serotyped. Although the potential for suboptimal sensitivity and specificity exists with slide agglutination serotyping (SAST) depending on reagents used, SAST or genotyping by PCR is an acceptable method for capsule typing. If PCR capsular typing is not available locally, isolates can be submitted to the state health department or to a reference laboratory for testing.

Otitis media attributable to *H influenzae* is diagnosed by culture of tympanocentesis fluid; cultures of other respiratory tract swab specimens (eg, throat, ear drainage) are not indicative of middle-ear culture results.

Treatment

Initial therapy for children with meningitis possibly caused by Hib is cefotaxime or ceftriaxone intravenously. Meropenem is an alternative empirical agent. Ampicillin can be substituted if the Hib isolate is susceptible to ampicillin. Treatment of other invasive *H influenzae* infections is similar. Therapy is continued at least 10 days by the intravenous route and longer in complicated infections. Dexamethasone may be beneficial for treatment of infants and children with Hib meningitis to diminish the risk of hearing loss, if

given before or concurrently with the first dose of antimicrobial agent(s). Epiglottitis is a medical emergeny since an airway must be established promptly. Pleural or pericardial fluid should be drained.

For empirical treatment of acute otitis media in children younger than 2 years or in children 2 years of age or older with severe disease, oral amoxicillin is recommended. Duration of therapy is 5 to 10 days. The 5- to 7-day course is considered for children 2 years of age and older. In the United States, approximately 30% to 40% of *H influenzae* isolates produce beta-lactamase, necessitating a beta-lactamase–resistant agent, such as amoxicillin-clavulanate; a cephalosporin, such as cefdinir, cefuroxime, or cefpodoxime; or azithromycin for children with allergy to beta-lactam antibiotics. In vitro susceptibility testing of isolates from middle-ear fluid specimens help guide therapy in complicated or persistent cases.

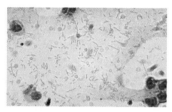

Image 52.1
Gram stain of cerebrospinal fluid (culture positive for *Haemophilus influenzae* type b).

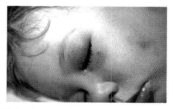

Image 52.2
A 16-month-old female with periorbital and facial cellulitis caused by *Haemophilus influenzae* type b. The patient had no history of trauma. Copyright Martin G. Myers, MD.

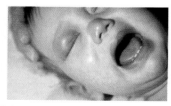

Image 52.3
A 10-month-old white male with periorbital cellulitis due to *Haemophilus influenzae* type b. Copyright Martin G. Myers, MD.

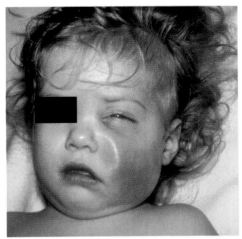

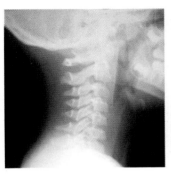

Image 52.5
Acute epiglottitis due to *Haemophilus influenzae* type b proven by blood culture. The swollen inflamed epiglottis looks like the shadow of a thumb on the lateral neck radiograph.

Image 52.4
A classic presentation of *Haemophilus influenzae* type b facial cellulitis in a 10-month-old white female. This once common infection has been nearly eliminated among children who have been immunized with the Hib vaccine.

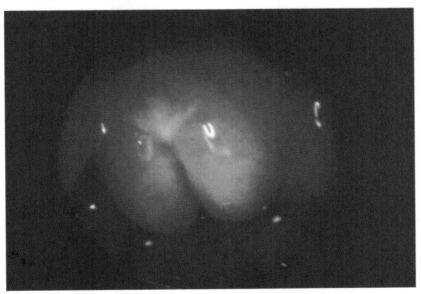

Image 52.6
Acute *Haemophilus influenzae* type b epiglottitis with striking erythema and swelling of the epiglottis.

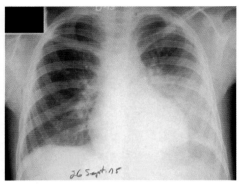

Image 52.7
Haemophilus influenzae type b pneumonia, bilateral, in a patient with acute epiglottitis (proved by blood culture). This is the same patient as in Image 52.5.

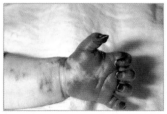

Image 52.9
Haemophilus influenzae type b sepsis with gangrene of the hand. Copyright Neal Halsey, MD.

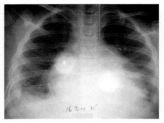

Image 52.8
Haemophilus influenzae type b bilateral pneumonia, empyema, and purulent pericarditis. Pericardiostomy drainage is important in preventing cardiac restriction.

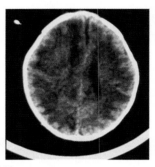

Image 52.10
Magnetic resonance imaging showing cerebral infarction in a patient who had *Haemophilus influenzae* type b (Hib) meningitis. The routine administration of Hib vaccine has virtually eliminated this type of devastating illness in the United States.

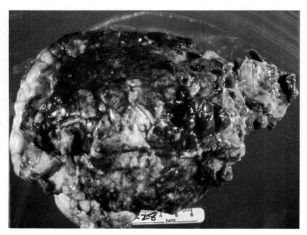

Image 52.11
Haemophilus influenzae meningitis in a 4-month-old infant who was evaluated in the morning for a well-child visit with normal clinical findings. By afternoon the child had necrosis of the hands and feet and died 12 hours later. This is the brain of the infant 24 hours after the well-child visit. No immunologic deficit was diagnosed. Copyright Jerri Ann Jenista, MD.

53

Hantavirus Pulmonary Syndrome

Clinical Manifestations

Hantaviruses in humans cause 2 distinct syndromes: hantavirus pulmonary syndrome (HPS), a noncardiogenic pulmonary edema observed in the New World, and hemorrhagic fever with renal syndrome (HFRS), which occurs worldwide. The prodromal illness of HPS is 3 to 7 days and is characterized by fever; chills; headache; myalgia of the shoulders, lower back, and thighs; nausea; vomiting; diarrhea; dizziness; and sometimes cough. Respiratory tract symptoms or signs usually do not occur for the first 3 to 7 days, at which time pulmonary edema and severe hypoxemia appear abruptly after the onset of cough and dyspnea. The disease then progresses over a number of hours. In severe cases, persistent hypotension caused by myocardial dysfunction is present. In fatal cases, death occurs in 1 to 2 days following hospitalization.

Extensive bilateral interstitial and alveolar pulmonary edema and pleural effusions are the result of a diffuse pulmonary capillary leak and appear to be caused by immune response to hantavirus in endothelial cells of the microvasculature. Endotracheal intubation and assisted ventilation usually are required for only 2 to 4 days, with resolution heralded by onset of diuresis and rapid clinical improvement.

The severe myocardial depression is different from that of septic shock; cardiac indices and stroke volume index are low, pulmonary wedge pressure is normal, and systemic vascular resistance is increased. Poor prognostic indicators include persistent hypotension, marked hemoconcentration, a cardiac index of less than 2, and abrupt onset of lactic acidosis with a serum lactate concentration of greater than 4 mmol/L (36 mg/dL).

The mortality rate for patients with HPS is 30% to 40%. Asymptomatic and mild forms of disease are rare. Limited information suggests that clinical manifestations and prognosis are similar in adults and children. Serious sequelae are uncommon.

Etiology

Hantaviruses are RNA viruses of the Bunyaviridae family. Within the Hantavirus genus, Sin Nombre virus (SNV) is the major cause of HPS in the 4-corners region of the United States (Arizona, Colorado, New Mexico, Utah). Bayou virus, Black Creek Canal virus, Monongahela virus, and New York virus are responsible for sporadic cases in Louisiana, Texas, Florida, New York, and other areas of the eastern United States (Utah, Colorado, Arizona, and New Mexico). Hantavirus serotypes associated with an HPS syndrome in South America and Panama include Andes virus, Oran virus, Laguna Negra virus, and Choclo virus. During the past decade, Chile and Argentina have reported most of the HPS cases in the Americas.

Epidemiology

Rodents, the natural hosts for hantaviruses, acquire a lifelong, asymptomatic, chronic infection with prolonged viruria and virus in saliva, urine, and feces. Humans acquire infection through direct contact with infected rodents, rodent droppings, or nests or inhalation of aerosolized virus particles from rodent urine, droppings, or saliva. Rarely, infection can be acquired from rodent bites or contamination of broken skin with excreta. Person-to-person transmission of hantaviruses has not been demonstrated in patients in the United States but has been reported in Chile and Argentina. At-risk activities include handling or trapping rodents; cleaning or entering closed, rarely used rodent-infested structures; cleaning feed storage or animal shelter areas; hand plowing; and living in a home with an increased density of mice in or around the home. For backpackers or campers, sleeping in a structure also inhabited by rodents has been associated with HPS. Weather conditions resulting in exceptionally heavy rainfall and improved rodent food supplies can result in a large increase in the rodent population. Increased rodent population results in more frequent contact between humans and infected mice and may account for increased human incidence. Most cases occur during spring and summer, and geographic location is determined by the habitat of the rodent carrier.

SNV is transmitted by the deer mouse, *Peromyscus maniculatus;* Black Creek Canal virus is transmitted by the cotton rat, *Sigmodon hispidu;* Bayou virus is transmitted by the rice rat, *Oryzomys palustris;* and New York virus is transmitted by the white-footed mouse, *Peromyscus leucopus.*

Incubation Period

1 to 6 weeks after exposure to infected rodents, their saliva, or excreta.

Diagnostic Tests

Characteristic laboratory findings include leukocytosis with immature granulocytes, more than 10% immunoblasts, thrombocytopenia, and increased hematocrit. In fatal cases, SNV has been identified by immunohistochemical staining of capillary endothelial cells of the lungs and almost every organ in the body. SNV RNA has been detected by reverse transcriptase PCR assay of peripheral blood mononuclear cells and other clinical specimens from the early phase of the disease. Viral RNA is not detected readily in bronchoalveolar lavage fluids.

Hantavirus-specific immunoglobulin (Ig) M and IgG antibodies are present at the onset of clinical disease. IgG could be negative in rapid fatal cases. A rapid diagnostic test can facilitate immediate appropriate supportive therapy and early transfer to a tertiary care facility. Enzyme immunoassay (available through many state health departments and the Centers for Disease Control and Prevention) and Western blot are assays that use recombinant antigens and have a high degree of specificity for detection of IgG and IgM antibody. Viral culture is not useful for diagnosis.

Treatment

Patients with suspected HPS should be transferred immediately to a tertiary care facility. Supportive management of pulmonary edema, severe hypoxemia, and hypotension during the first 24 to 48 hours is critical for recovery. Extracorporeal membrane oxygenation may provide particularly important short-term support for the severe capillary leak syndrome in the lungs. Ribavirin is active in vitro against hantaviruses, including SNV. However, 2 clinical studies (1 open-label study and 1 randomized, placebo-controlled, double-blind study) found that intravenous ribavirin probably is ineffective in treatment of HPS in the cardiopulmonary stage. Steroids are being evaluated in South American trials.

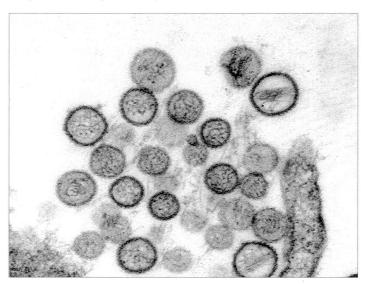

Image 53.1

Transmission electron micrograph of Sin Nombre virus, a frequent cause of hantavirus pulmonary syndrome. Courtesy of Centers for Disease Control and Prevention/Cynthia Goldsmith.

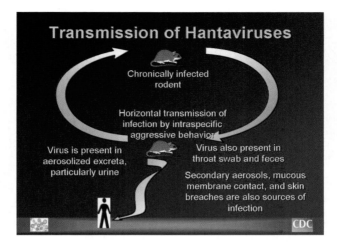

Image 53.2
Transmission of Hantaviruses: The virus is horizontally transmitted between rodents through intraspecific aggressive behaviors, such as biting. The virus is transmitted to humans from aerosolized rodent excreta, particularly urine. Transmission to humans also can occur from inhalation of secondary aerosols, and from rodent bites or other direct contact of infectious material with mucous membranes or broken skin. Courtesy of Centers for Disease Control and Prevention.

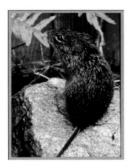

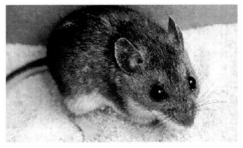

Image 53.4
Deer mouse (*Peromyscus maniculatus*). The deer mouse is a carrier of Sin Nombre virus, an etiologic agent of hantavirus pulmonary syndrome. Courtesy of Centers for Disease Control and Prevention.

Image 53.3
The cotton rat *(Sigmodon hispidus)* is the primary rodent host for the Black Creek Canal virus. Infected rodents show no visible evidence of acute or chronic infection. Courtesy of Centers for Disease Control and Prevention.

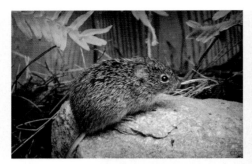

Image 53.5
This photograph depicts a cotton rat, *Sigmodon hispidus*, whose habitat includes the southeastern United States, and way down into Central and South America. Its body is larger than the deer mouse, *Peromyscus maniculatus*, and measures about 5 to 7 inches, which includes the head and body; the tail measures an additional 3 to 4 inches. Its hair is longer and coarser than *Peromyscus maniculatus*, and is a grayish-brown color, sometimes grayish-black. The cotton rat prefers overgrown areas with shrubs and tall grasses. The cotton rat is a hantavirus carrier that becomes a threat when it enters human habitation in rural and suburban areas. Hantavirus pulmonary syndrome (HPS) is a deadly disease transmitted by infected rodents through urine, droppings, or saliva. Humans can contract the disease when they breathe in aerosolized virus. All hantaviruses known to cause HPS are carried by New World rats and mice of the family Muridae, subfamily Sigmodontinae. Courtesy of Centers for Disease Control and Prevention/ James Guthany.

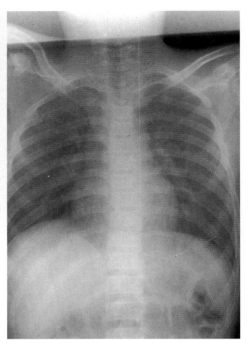

Image 53.6
Early hantavirus pulmonary syndrome.

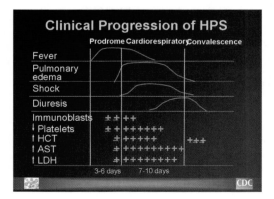

Image 53.7
Clinical Course of Hantavirus Pulmonary Syndrome (HPS): Clinical course of HPS starts with a febrile prodrome that may ultimately lead to hypotension and end-organ failure. The onset of the immune response precedes severe organ failure, which is thought to be immunopathologic in nature. Hypotension does not result in shock until the onset of respiratory failure, but this may reflect the severe physiological impact of lung edema. Courtesy of Centers for Disease Control and Prevention.

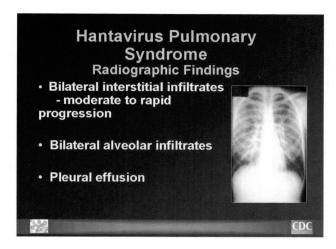

Image 53.8
Radiographic Findings of Hantavirus Pulmonary Syndrome (HPS): Findings usually include interstitial edema, Kerley B lines, hilar indistinctness, and peribronchial cuffing with normal cardiothoracic ratios. HPS begins with minimal changes of interstitial pulmonary edema and rapidly progresses to alveolar edema with severe bilateral involvement. Pleural effusions are common and are often large enough to be evident radiographically. Courtesy of Centers for Disease and Control and Prevention.

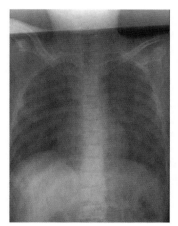

Image 53.9
Hantavirus pulmonary syndrome (early in course) in a 16-year-old male.

54

Helicobacter pylori Infections

Clinical Manifestations

Helicobacter pylori causes chronic active gastritis and results in duodenal and, to a lesser extent, gastric ulcers. Persistent infection with *H pylori* increases the risk of gastric cancer. *H pylori* infection can be asymptomatic or can result in gastroduodenal inflammation that can manifest as epigastric pain, nausea, vomiting, hematemesis, and guaiac-positive stools. Symptoms can resolve within a few days or wax and wane despite persistence of the organism for years or for life. *H pylori* infection is not associated with secondary gastritis (eg, autoimmune or chemical with nonsteroidal anti-inflammatory agents).

Etiology

H pylori is a gram-negative, spiral, curved, or U-shaped microaerophilic bacillus that has 2 to 6 sheathed flagella at one end. The organism is catalase, oxidase, and urease positive.

Epidemiology

H pylori has been isolated from humans and other primates. An animal reservoir for human transmission has not been demonstrated. Organisms are transmitted from infected humans by fecal-oral, gastro-oral, and oral-oral routes. Infection rates are low in children in resource-rich countries except in children from lower socioeconomic groups. Most infections are acquired in the first 5 years of life and can reach prevalence rates of up to 80% in resource-limited countries. Approximately 70% of infected people are asymptomatic, 20% of people have macroscopic (ie, visual) and microscopic findings of ulceration, and an estimated 1% have features of neoplasia.

Incubation Period

Unknown.

Diagnostic Tests

H pylori infection can be diagnosed by culture of gastric biopsy tissue on nonselective media (eg, chocolate agar) or selective media at 37°C (98°F) under microaerobic conditions for 3 to 7 days. Organisms usually can be visualized on histologic sections using several stains. Because of production of urease by organisms, urease testing of a gastric specimen can give a rapid and specific microbiologic diagnosis. Each of these tests requires endoscopy and biopsy. Noninvasive, commercially available tests include breath tests that detect labeled carbon dioxide in expired air after oral administration of isotopically labeled urea (13°C or 14°C); these tests are expensive and are not useful in young children. The first *H pylori* breath test for children 3 to 17 years of age was approved in 2012. A stool antigen test (monoclonal antibody test) also is available commercially and can be used for children of any age. Each of these commercially available tests (ie, breath or stool tests) has a high sensitivity and specificity.

Treatment

Treatment is recommended for infected patients who have peptic ulcer disease, gastric mucosa-associated lymphoid tissue-type lymphoma, or early gastric cancer. Screening for and treatment of infection, if found, also is recommended for children with one or more primary relatives with gastric cancer, children who are in a high-risk group for gastric cancer (eg, immigrants from resource-limited countries or countries with high rates of gastric cancer), or children who have unexplained iron-deficiency anemia. Treatment is recommended if infection is found at the time of diagnostic endoscopy for gastrointestinal tract symptoms. Eradication therapy for *H pylori* consists of at least 7 to 14 days of therapy; eradication rates are higher for regimens of 14 days. Effective treatment regimens include 2 antimicrobial agents (eg, clarithromycin plus either amoxicillin or metronidazole) plus a proton-pump inhibitor (lansoprazole, omeprazole, esomeprazole, pantoprazole, rabeprazole). These regimens are effective in eliminating the organism, healing the ulcer, and preventing recurrence.

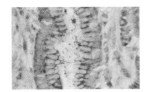

Image 54.1
Histology of the gastric mucosa demonstrates the characteristic curved organisms in the gastric glands.

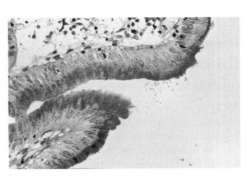

Image 54.2
A biopsy of gastric mucosa stained with Warthin-starry silver stain showing *Helicobacter pylori* organisms.

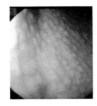

Image 54.3
Helicobacter pylori infection is a known risk factor for gastritis and duodenal ulcers in children and adults. Rarely, and primarily in older adulthood, *H pylori* also is associated with a gastric lymphoma of the mucosal-associated lymphoid tissue (MALToma). The gold standard for the diagnosis of *H pylori* infection of the stomach is endoscopy with biopsy. Endoscopy may show a nodular gastritis of the antrum.

55

Hemorrhagic Fevers Caused by Arenaviruses

Clinical Manifestations

Arenaviruses are responsible for several hemorrhagic fevers (HFs): Bolivian, Argentine, Brazilian, Venezuelan, Lassa, Chapare, and Lujo. Lymphocytic choriomeningitis virus (LCMV) also is an arenavirus but induces generally less severe disease, although it could be responsible for HFs in immunosuppressed patients; LCMV is discussed in a separate chapter. Disease associated with arenaviruses ranges in severity from mild, acute, febrile infections to severe illnesses in which vascular leak, shock, and multiorgan dysfunction are prominent features. Fever, headache, myalgia, conjunctival suffusion, bleeding, and abdominal pain are common early symptoms in all infections. Thrombocytopenia, axillary petechiae, and encephalopathy usually are present in Argentine HF, Bolivian HF, and Venezuelan HF, and exudative pharyngitis often occurs in Lassa fever. Mucosal bleeding occurs in severe cases as a consequence of vascular damage, thrombocytopenia, and platelet dysfunction. Proteinuria is common, but renal failure is unusual. Increased serum concentrations of aspartate transaminase can indicate a severe or fatal outcome of Lassa fever. Shock develops 7 to 9 days after onset of illness in more severely ill patients with these infections. Upper and lower respiratory tract symptoms can develop in people with Lassa fever. Encephalopathic signs such as tremor, alterations in consciousness, and seizures can occur in South American HFs and in severe cases of Lassa fever.

Etiology

Arenaviruses are RNA viruses. The major New World arenavirus hemorrhagic fevers occurring in the Western hemisphere are Argentine HF caused by Junin virus, Bolivian HF caused by Machupo virus, and Venezuelan HF caused by Guanarito virus. A fourth arenavirus, Sabia virus, caused 2 unrelated cases of naturally occurring HF in Brazil and 2 laboratory-acquired cases. Chapare virus has been isolated from a human fatal case in Bolivia. The Old World complex of arenaviruses includes Lassa virus, which causes Lassa fever in West Africa, and Lujo virus, described in southern Africa during an outbreak characterized by fatal human-to-human transmission, and usually produces less severe infections. Several other arenaviruses are known only from their rodent reservoirs in the Old and New World.

Epidemiology

Arenaviruses are maintained in nature by association with specific rodent hosts, in which they produce chronic viremia and viruria. The principal routes of infection are inhalation and contact of mucous membranes and skin (eg, through cuts, scratches, or abrasions) with urine and salivary secretions from these persistently infected rodents. All arenaviruses are infectious as aerosols, and arenaviruses causing HF should be considered highly hazardous to people working with any of the viruses in the laboratory. Laboratory-acquired infections have been documented with Lassa, Machupo, Junin, and Sabia viruses. The geographic distribution and habitats of the specific rodents that serve as reservoir hosts largely determine the areas with endemic infection and populations at risk. Before a vaccine became available in Argentina, several hundred cases of Argentine HF occurred yearly in agricultural workers and inhabitants of the Argentine pampas. The vaccine is not licensed in the United States. Epidemics of Bolivian HF occurred in small towns between 1962 and 1964; sporadic disease activity in the countryside has continued since then. Venezuelan HF first was identified in 1989 and occurs in rural north-central Venezuela. Lassa fever is endemic in most of West Africa, where rodent hosts live in proximity with humans, causing thousands of infections annually. Lassa fever has been reported in the United States in people who have traveled to West Africa.

Incubation Period

From 6 to 17 days.

Diagnostic Tests

Viral nucleic acid can be detected in acute disease by reverse transcriptase PCR assay. These viruses can be isolated from the blood of acutely ill patients as well as from various tissues obtained postmortem, but isolation should be attempted only under Biosafety Level 4 conditions. Virus antigen is detectable by enzyme immunoassay in acute specimens and postmortem tissues. Virus-specific immunoglobulin (Ig) M antibodies are present in the serum during acute stages but may be undetectable in rapidly fatal cases. The IgG antibody response is delayed. Diagnosis can be made retrospectively by immunohistochemistry in tissues obtained from autopsy.

Treatment

Intravenous ribavirin substantially decreases the mortality rate in patients with severe Lassa fever, particularly if they are treated during the first week of illness. For Argentine HF, transfusion of immune plasma in defined doses of neutralizing antibodies is the standard specific treatment when administered during the first 8 days from onset of symptoms. Intravenous ribavirin initiated 8 days or more after onset of Argentine HF symptoms does not reduce mortality; whether ribavirin treatment initiated early in the course of the disease has a role in the treatment of Argentine HF remains to be seen. Intravenous ribavirin is not available commercially in the United States.

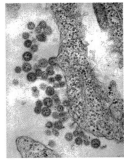

Image 55.1
Electron photomicrograph of the Machupo virus. Machupo virus is a member of the Arenavirus family, isolated in the Beni province of Bolivia in 1963; viral hemorrhagic fever. Courtesy of Centers for Disease Control and Prevention/ Dr W. Winn.

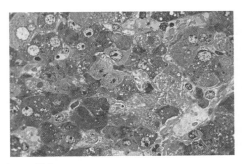

Image 55.2
This photomicrograph shows hepatitis caused by the Lassa virus, using toluidine-blue azure II stain. The Lassa virus, which can cause altered liver morphology with hemorrhagic necrosis and inflammation, is a member of the family *Arenaviridae,* and is a single-stranded RNA, zoonotic, or animal-borne pathogen. Courtesy of Centers for Disease Control and Prevention/ Dr Fred Murphy; Sylvia Whitfield.

56

Hemorrhagic Fevers and Related Syndromes Caused by Viruses of the Family Bunyaviridae

Clinical Manifestations

These vectorborne infections are severe febrile diseases in which shock and bleeding can be significant and multisystem involvement can occur. In the United States, one of these infections causes an illness marked by acute respiratory and cardiovascular failure.

Hemorrhagic fever with renal syndrome (HFRS) is a complex, multiphasic disease characterized by vascular instability and varying degrees of renal insufficiency. Fever, flushing, conjunctival injection, abdominal pain, and lumbar pain are followed by hypotension, oliguria and, subsequently, polyuria. Petechiae are frequent, but more serious bleeding manifestations are rare. Shock and acute renal insufficiency may occur. Nephropathia epidemica (attributable to Puumala virus) occurs in Europe and presents as a milder disease with acute influenza-like illness, abdominal pain, and proteinuria. Acute renal dysfunction also occurs, but hypotensive shock or requirement for dialysis is rare. However, more severe forms of HFRS (ie, attributable to Dobrava virus) also occur in Europe.

Crimean-Congo hemorrhagic fever (CCHF) is a multisystem disease characterized by hepatitis and profuse bleeding. Fever, headache, and myalgia are followed by signs of a diffuse capillary leak syndrome with facial suffusion, conjunctivitis, and proteinuria. Petechiae and purpura often appear on the skin and mucous membranes. A hypotensive crisis often occurs after the appearance of frank hemorrhage from the gastrointestinal tract, nose, mouth, or uterus.

Rift Valley fever (RVF), in most cases, is a self-limited febrile illness. Occasionally, hemorrhagic fever with shock and icterus, encephalitis, or retinitis develops.

Etiology

Bunyaviridae are segmented, single-stranded RNA viruses with different geographic distributions depending on their vector or reservoir. Hemorrhagic fever syndromes are associated with viruses from 3 genera: hantaviruses, nairoviruses (CCHF virus), and phleboviruses (RVF and sandfly fever viruses). Old World hantaviruses (Hantaan, Seoul, Dobrava, and Puumala viruses) cause HFRS, and New World hantaviruses (Sin Nombre and related viruses) cause hantavirus pulmonary syndrome.

Epidemiology

The epidemiology of these diseases mainly is a function of the distribution and behavior of their reservoirs and vectors. All genera except hantaviruses are associated with arthropod vectors, and hantavirus infections are associated with exposure to infected rodents.

Classic HFRS occurs throughout much of Asia and Eastern and Western Europe, with up to 100,000 cases per year. The most severe form of the disease is caused by the prototype Hantaan virus and Dobrava viruses in rural Asia and Europe, respectively; Puumala virus is associated with milder disease (nephropathia epidemica) in Western Europe. Seoul virus is distributed worldwide in association with *Rattus* species and can cause a disease of variable severity. Person-to-person transmission never has been reported with HFRS.

CCHF occurs in much of sub-Saharan Africa, the Middle East, areas in West and Central Asia, and the Balkans. CCHF virus is transmitted by ticks and occasionally by contact with viremic animals at slaughter. Health care–associated transmission of CCHF is a frequent and serious hazard.

RVF occurs throughout sub-Saharan Africa and has caused large epidemics in Egypt in 1977 and 1993–1995, Mauritania in 1987, Saudi Arabia and Yemen in 2000, Kenya in 1997 and 2006–2007, Madagascar in 1990 and 2008, and South Africa in 2010. The virus is arthropodborne and is transmitted from domestic livestock to humans by mosquitoes. The virus also can be transmitted by aerosol and by direct contact with infected aborted tissues or freshly slaughtered infected animal carcasses. Person-to-person transmission has not been reported, but laboratory-acquired cases are well documented.

Incubation Period

CCHF and RVF, 2 to 10 days; HFRS usually are longer, 7 to 42 days.

Diagnostic Tests

CCHF and RVF viruses can be cultivated readily (restricted to Biosafety Level 4 laboratories) from blood and tissue specimens of infected patients. Detection of viral antigen by enzyme immunoassay (EIA) is a useful alternative. Serum immunoglobulin (Ig) M and IgG virus-specific antibodies typically develop early in convalescence in CCHF and RVF but could be absent in rapidly fatal cases of CCHF. In HFRS, IgM and IgG antibodies usually are detectable at the time of onset of illness or within 48 hours, when it is too late for virus isolation and antigen detection. IgM antibodies or rising IgG titers in paired serum specimens, as demonstrated by EIA, are diagnostic; neutralizing antibody tests provide greater

virus strain specificity but rarely are tested. PCR assay performed with appropriate safety precautions is a useful complement to serodiagnostic assays on samples obtained during the acute phase of CCHF, RVF, or HFRS. Diagnosis can be made retrospectively by immunohistochemistry assay of tissues obtained from necropsy.

Treatment

Ribavirin administered intravenously to patients with HFRS within the first 4 days of illness seems effective in decreasing renal dysfunction, vascular instability, and mortality. However, intravenous ribavirin is not available commercially in the United States. Supportive therapy for HFRS should include (1) avoidance of transporting patients, (2) treatment of shock, (3) monitoring of fluid balance, (4) dialysis for complications of renal failure, (5) control of hypertension during the oliguric phase, and (6) early recognition of possible myocardial failure with appropriate therapy. Oral and intravenous ribavirin given to patients with CCHF has been associated with milder disease although no controlled studies have been performed.

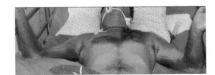

Image 56.2
Intubated patient with Crimean-Congo hemorrhagic fever, Republic of Georgia, 2009, showing massive ecchymoses on the upper extremities that extend to the chest. Courtesy of Zakhashvili K, Tsertsvadze N, Chikviladze T, et al. Crimean-Congo hemorrhagic fever in man, Republic of Georgia, 2009 [letter]. *Emerg Infect Dis.* 2010; 16(8):1326–1328.

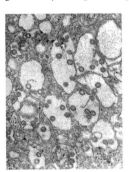

Image 56.1
Electron micrograph of the Rift Valley fever (RVF) virus. RVF virus is a member of the genus *Phlebovirus* in the family Bunyaviridae, first reported in livestock in Kenya around 1900. Courtesy of Centers for Disease Control and Prevention/Dr Fred Murphy.

57

Hepatitis A

Clinical Manifestations

Hepatitis A characteristically is an acute, self-limited illness associated with fever, malaise, jaundice, anorexia, and nausea. Symptomatic hepatitis A virus (HAV) infection occurs in approximately 30% of infected children younger than 6 years; few of these children will have jaundice. Among older children and adults, infection usually is symptomatic and typically lasts several weeks, with jaundice occurring in 70% or more. Signs and symptoms typically last less than 2 months, although 10% to 15% of symptomatic people have prolonged or relapsing disease lasting as long as 6 months. Fulminant hepatitis is rare but is more common in people with underlying liver disease. Chronic infection does not occur.

Etiology

HAV is an RNA virus classified as a member of the picornavirus family.

Epidemiology

The most common mode of transmission is person to person, resulting from fecal contamination and oral ingestion (ie, the fecal-oral route). In resource-limited countries where infection is endemic, most people are infected during the first decade of life. In the United States, hepatitis A was one of the most frequently reported vaccine-preventable diseases in the prevaccine era, but incidence of disease attributable to HAV has declined significantly since hepatitis A vaccine was licensed in 1995. These declining rates have been accompanied by a shift in age-specific rates. Historically, the highest rates occurred among children 5 to 14 years of age, and the lowest rates occurred among adults older than 40 years. Beginning in the late 1990s, national age-specific rates declined more rapidly among children than among adults; as a result, in recent years, rates have been similar among all age groups. In addition, the previously observed unequal geographic distribution of hepatitis A incidence in the United States, with the highest rates of dis-

ease occurring in a limited number of states and communities, has disappeared after introduction of targeted immunization in 1999.

Recognized risk factors for HAV infection include close personal contact with a person infected with HAV, international travel, household or personal contact with a child who attends a child care center, household or personal contact with a newly arriving international adoptee, a recognized foodborne outbreak, men who have sex with men, and use of illegal drugs. Transmission by blood transfusion or from mother to newborn infant (ie, vertical transmission) is limited to case reports. In approximately two-thirds of reported cases, the source cannot be determined. Fecal-oral spread from people with asymptomatic infections, particularly young children, likely accounts for many of these cases with an unknown source.

Common-source foodborne outbreaks occur; waterborne outbreaks are rare. Health care–associated transmission is unusual, but outbreaks have occurred in neonatal intensive care units from neonates infected through transfused blood who subsequently transmitted HAV to other neonates and staff.

Patients infected with HAV are most infectious during the 1 to 2 weeks before onset of jaundice or elevation of liver enzymes, when concentration of virus in the stool is highest. The risk of transmission subsequently diminishes and is minimal by 1 week after onset of jaundice. However, HAV can be detected in stool for longer periods, especially in neonates and young children.

Incubation Period

15 to 50 days, average 28 days.

Diagnostic Tests

Serologic tests for HAV-specific total (ie, immunoglobulin [Ig] G and IgM) antibody (anti-HAV) are available commercially. The presence of serum IgM anti-HAV indicates current or recent infection, although false-positive results may occur. IgM anti-HAV is detectable in up to 20% of vaccinees when measured 2 weeks after hepatitis A immunization. In most infected people, serum IgM anti-HAV becomes detectable 5 to 10 days before onset of symptoms and declines to undetectable concentrations within 6 months after infection. However, people who test positive for IgM anti-HAV more than 1 year after infection have been reported. IgG anti-HAV is detectable shortly after appearance of IgM. A positive total anti-HAV (ie, IgM and IgG) test result and a negative IgM anti-HAV test result indicate past infection and immunity.

Treatment

Supportive care.

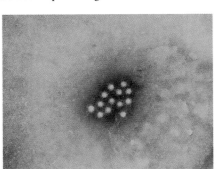

Image 57.1
An electron micrograph of the hepatitis A virus, an RNA virus classified as a member of the picornavirus group. Courtesy of Centers for Disease Control and Prevention/Betty Partin.

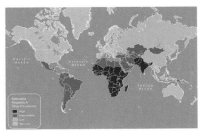

Image 57.2
Estimated prevalence of hepatitis A virus. Courtesy of Centers for Disease Control and Prevention.

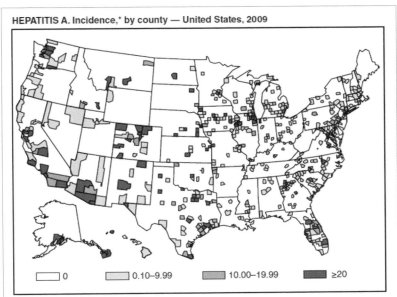

HEPATITIS A. Incidence,* by county — United States, 2009

| 0 | 0.10–9.99 | 10.00–19.99 | ≥20 |

* Per 100,000 population.

In 1999, routine hepatitis A vaccination was recommended for children living in 11 states with consistently elevated rates of disease. Since then, rates of infection with hepatitis A virus (HAV) have declined in all regions, with the greatest decline occurring in western states. HAV infection rates are now the lowest ever reported and similar in all regions. As of 2006, hepatitis A vaccine is now recommended for children in all states.

Image 57.3
Hepatitis A incidence by county, 2009. Courtesy of *Morbidity and Mortality Weekly Report.*

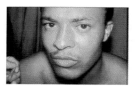

Image 57.4

Hepatitis A infection has caused this man's skin and the whites of his eyes to turn yellow. Other symptoms of hepatitis A can include loss of appetite, abdominal pain, nausea or vomiting, fever, headaches, and dark urine. Courtesy of Centers for Disease Control and Prevention.

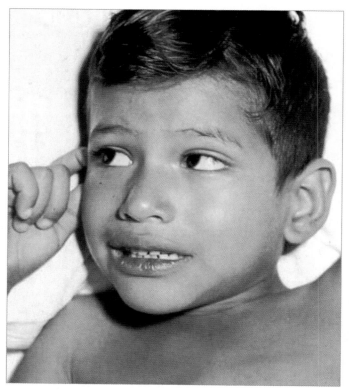

Image 57.5

Acute hepatitis A infection with scleral icterus in a 10-year-old male.

58

Hepatitis B

Clinical Manifestations

People acutely infected with hepatitis B virus (HBV) can be asymptomatic or symptomatic. The likelihood of developing symptoms of acute hepatitis is age dependent: less than 1% of infants younger than 1 year, 5% to 15% of children 1 through 5 years of age, and 30% to 50% of people older than 5 years are symptomatic, although few data are available for adults older than 30 years. When symptomatically infected, the spectrum of signs and symptoms is varied and includes subacute illness with nonspecific symptoms (eg, anorexia, nausea, or malaise), clinical hepatitis with jaundice, or fulminant hepatitis. Extrahepatic manifestations, such as arthralgia, arthritis, macular rashes, thrombocytopenia, polyarteritis nodosa, glomerulonephritis, or papular acrodermatitis (Gianotti-Crosti syndrome), can occur early in the course of illness and can precede jaundice. Acute HBV infection cannot be distinguished from other forms of acute viral hepatitis on the basis of clinical signs and symptoms or nonspecific laboratory findings.

Chronic HBV infection is defined as presence of any one of the following: hepatitis B surface antigen (HBsAg), nucleic acid, HBV DNA, or hepatitis B e antigen (HBeAg) in serum for at least 6 months or by presence of any one of the following: HBsAg, nucleic acid, HBV DNA, or HBeAg in serum from a person who tests negative for antibody of the immunoglobulin (Ig) M subclass to hepatitis B core antigen (IgM anti-HBc).

Age at the time of acute infection is the primary determinant of risk of progressing to chronic infection. More than 90% of infants infected perinatally or in the first year of life will develop chronic HBV infection. Between 25% and 50% of children infected between 1 and 5 years of age become chronically infected, whereas 5% to 10% of acutely infected older children and adults develop chronic HBV infection. Patients who develop acute HBV infection while immunosuppressed or with an underlying chronic illness (eg, end-stage renal

disease) have an increased risk of developing chronic infection. In the absence of treatment, up to 25% of infants and children who acquire chronic HBV infection will die prematurely from HBV-related hepatocellular carcinoma or cirrhosis. Risk factors for developing hepatocellular carcinoma include duration of infection, degree of histologic injury, replicative state of the virus (HBV DNA levels), presence of cirrhosis, and concomitant infection with hepatitis C virus (HCV) or HIV.

The clinical course of untreated chronic HBV infection varies according to the population studied, reflecting differences in age at acquisition, rate of loss of HBeAg, and possibly HBV genotype. Perinatally infected children usually have normal alanine aminotransferase (ALT) concentrations and minimal or mild liver histologic abnormalities, with detectable HBeAg and high HBV DNA concentrations (≥20,000 IU/mL) for years to decades after initial infection ("immune tolerant phase"). Chronic HBV infection acquired during later childhood or adolescence usually is accompanied by more active liver disease and increased serum transaminase concentrations. Patients with detectable HBeAg (*HBeAg-positive chronic hepatitis B*) usually have high concentrations of HBV DNA and HBsAg in serum and are more likely to transmit infection. Because HBV-associated liver injury is thought to be immune-mediated in people coinfected with HIV and HBV, the return of immune competence with antiretroviral treatment of HIV infection can lead to a reactivation of HBV-related liver inflammation and damage. Over time (years to decades), HBeAg becomes undetectable in many chronically infected people. This transition often is accompanied by development of antibody to HBeAg (anti-HBe) and decreases in serum HBV DNA and serum transaminase concentrations and can be preceded by a temporary exacerbation of liver disease. These patients have *inactive chronic infection* but still may have exacerbations of hepatitis. Serologic reversion (reappearance of HBeAg) is more common if loss of HBeAg is not accompanied by development of anti-HBe; reversion with loss of anti-HBe also can occur.

Some patients who lose HBeAg may continue to have ongoing histologic evidence of liver damage and moderate to high concentrations of HBV DNA *(HBeAg-negative chronic hepatitis B)*. Patients with histologic evidence of chronic HBV infection, regardless of HBeAg status, remain at higher risk of death attributable to liver failure compared with HBV-infected people with no histologic evidence of liver inflammation and fibrosis. Other factors that may influence natural history of chronic infection include gender, race, alcohol use, and coinfection with HCV, hepatitis D virus, or HIV.

Resolved hepatitis B is defined as clearance of HBsAg, normalization of serum transaminase concentrations, and development of antibody to HBsAg (anti-HBs). Chronically infected adults clear HBsAg and develop anti-HBs at the rate of 1% to 2% annually; during childhood, the annual clearance rate is less than 1%. Reactivation of resolved chronic infection is possible if these patients become immunosuppressed.

Etiology

Hepatitis B virus is a DNA-containing, 42-nm-diameter hepadnavirus. Important components of the viral particle include an outer lipoprotein envelope containing HBsAg and an inner nucleocapsid consisting of hepatitis B core antigen. Viral polymerase activity can be detected in preparations of plasma containing HBV.

Epidemiology

HBV is transmitted through infected blood or body fluids. Although HBsAg has been detected in multiple body fluids, including human milk and saliva, only blood; serum; semen; vaginal secretions; and cerebrospinal, synovial, pleural, pericardial, peritoneal, and amniotic fluids are considered the most potentially infectious. People with chronic HBV infection are the primary reservoirs for infection. Common modes of transmission include percutaneous and permucosal exposure to infectious body fluids; sharing or using non-sterilized needles, syringes, or glucose monitoring equipment or devices; sexual contact with an infected person; perinatal exposure to

an infected mother; and household exposure to a person with chronic HBV infection. Transmission by transfusion of contaminated blood or blood products is rare in the United States because of routine screening of blood donors and viral inactivation of certain blood products before administration.

Perinatal transmission of HBV is highly efficient and usually occurs from blood exposures during labor and delivery. In utero transmission of HBV accounts for less than 2% of perinatal infections in most studies. Without postexposure prophylaxis, the risk of an infant acquiring HBV from an infected mother as a result of perinatal exposure is 70% to 90% for infants born to mothers who are HBsAg and HBeAg positive; the risk is 5% to 20% for infants born to HBsAg-positive but HBeAg-negative mothers.

Person-to-person spread of HBV can occur in settings involving interpersonal contact over extended periods, such as in a household with a person with chronic HBV infection (eg, an adoptee). In regions of the world with a high prevalence of chronic HBV infection, transmission between children in household settings accounts for a substantial amount of transmission. The precise mechanisms of transmission from child to child are unknown; however, frequent interpersonal contact of nonintact skin or mucous membranes with blood-containing secretions, open skin lesions, or blood-containing saliva are potential means of transmission. Transmission from sharing inanimate objects, such as razors or toothbrushes, also can occur. HBV can survive in the environment for up to 7 days but is inactivated by commonly used disinfectants, including household bleach diluted 1:10 with water. HBV is not transmitted by the fecal-oral route.

Transmission among children born in the United States is unusual because of high coverage with hepatitis B vaccine starting at birth. The risk of HBV transmission is higher in children who have not completed a vaccine series, children undergoing hemodialysis, institutionalized children with developmental disabilities, and children emigrating from countries with endemic HBV (eg, Southeast Asia, China, Africa).

Acute HBV infection is reported most commonly among adults 30 through 49 years of age in the United States. Since 1990, the incidence of acute HBV infection has declined in all age categories, with a 98% decline in children younger than 19 years and a 93% decline in young adults 20 through 29 years of age, with most of the decline among people 20 through 24 years of age. Among acute hepatitis B patients interviewed in 2009, groups at highest risk included users of injection drugs, people with multiple heterosexual partners, men who have sex with men, and people who reported surgery during the 6 weeks to 6 months before onset of symptoms. Others at increased risk include people with occupational exposure to blood or body fluids, staff of institutions and nonresidential child care programs for children with developmental disabilities, patients undergoing hemodialysis, and sexual or household contacts of people with an acute or chronic infection. Approximately 60% of infected people do not have a readily identifiable risk. HBV infection in adolescents and adults is associated with other sexually transmitted infections, including syphilis and HIV. Outbreaks in nonhospital health care settings, including assisted-living facilities and nursing homes, highlighted the increased risk among people with diabetes mellitus undergoing assisted blood glucose monitoring.

The prevalence of HBV infection and patterns of transmission vary markedly throughout the world (Table 58.1). Approximately 45% of people worldwide live in regions of high HBV endemicity, where the prevalence of chronic HBV infection is greater than 8%. Historically in these regions, most new infections occurred as a result of perinatal or early childhood infections. In regions of intermediate HBV endemicity, where the prevalence of HBV infection is 2% to 7%, multiple modes of transmission (ie, perinatal, household, sexual, injection drug use, and health care–associated) contribute to the burden of infection. In countries of low endemicity, where chronic HBV infection prevalence is less than 2% (including the United States) and where routine immunization has been adopted, new infections are among unimmunized age groups.

Incubation Period

Acute infection, 45 to 160 days (average, 90 days).

Diagnostic Tests

Serologic antigen tests are available commercially to detect HBsAg and HBeAg. Serologic assays also are available for detection of anti-HBs, anti-HBc, IgM anti-HBc, and anti-HBe (Table 58.2 and Image 58.1). In addition, nucleic acid amplification testing, gene-amplification techniques (eg, PCR assay, branched DNA methods), and hybridization assays are available to detect and quantify HBV DNA. HBsAg is detectable during acute infection. If infection is self-limited, HBsAg disappears in most patients within a few weeks to several months after infection, followed by appearance of anti-HBs. The time between disappearance of HBsAg and appearance of anti-HBs is termed the *window period* of infection. During the window period, the only marker of acute infection is IgM anti-HBc, which is highly specific for establishing the diagnosis of acute infection. However, IgM anti-HBc usually is not present in infants infected perinatally. People with chronic HBV infection have circulating HBsAg and anti-HBc; on rare occasions, anti-HBs also is present. Both anti-HBs and anti-HBc are detected in people with resolved infection, whereas anti-HBs alone is present in people immunized with hepatitis B vaccine. Transient HBsAg antigenemia can occur following hepatitis B vaccine, with HBsAg being detected as early as 24 hours after and up to 2 to 3 weeks following administration of the vaccine. The presence of HBeAg in serum correlates with higher concentrations of HBV and greater infectivity. Tests for HBeAg and HBV DNA are useful in selection of candidates to receive antiviral therapy and to monitor response to therapy.

Treatment

No specific therapy for *acute* HBV infection is available, and acute HBV infection usually does not warrant referral to a hepatitis specialist. Hepatitis B immune globulin and corticosteroids are not effective treatment.

Table 58.1
Estimated International HBsAg Prevalence[a]

Region	Estimated HBsAg Prevalence (%)
North America	0.1
Mexico and Central America	0.3
South America	0.7
Western Europe	0.7
Australia and New Zealand	0.9
Caribbean (except Haiti)	1.0
Eastern Europe and North Asia	2.8
South Asia	2.8
Middle East	3.2
Haiti	5.6
East Asia	7.4
Southeast Asia	9.1
Africa	9.3
Pacific Islands	12.0

Abbreviation: HBsAg, hepatitis B surface antigen.

[a]From Centers for Disease Control and Prevention. A comprehensive immunization strategy to eliminate transmission of hepatitis B virus infection in the United States. Recommendations of the Advisory Committee on Immunization Practices (ACIP). Part II: immunization of adults. *MMWR Recomm Rep.* 2006;55(RR-16):1–33.

Table 58.2
Diagnostic Tests for Hepatitis B Virus (HBV) Antigens and Antibodies

Factors to Be Tested	HBV Antigen or Antibody	Use
HBsAg	Hepatitis B surface antigen	Detection of acutely or chronically infected people; antigen used in hepatitis B vaccine
Anti-HBs	Antibody to HBsAg	Identification of people who have resolved infections with HBV; determination of immunity after immunization
HBeAg	Hepatitis B e antigen	Identification of infected people at increased risk of transmitting HBV
Anti-HBe	Antibody to HBeAg	Identification of infected people with lower risk of transmitting HBV
Anti-HBc (total)	Antibody to HBcAg[a]	Identification of people with acute, resolved, or chronic HBV infection (not present after immunization); passively transferred maternal anti-HBc is detectable for as long as 24 months among infants born to HBsAg-positive women
IgM anti-HBc	IgM antibody to HBcAg	Identification of people with acute or recent HBV infections (including HBsAg-negative people during the "window" phase of infection)

Abbreviations: HBcAg, hepatitis B core antigen; IgM, immunoglobulin M.

[a]No test is available commercially to measure HBcAg.

Children and adolescents who have chronic HBV infection are at risk of developing serious liver disease, including primary hepatocellular carcinoma, with advancing age and should receive hepatitis A vaccine. Children with chronic HBV infection should be screened periodically for hepatic complications using serum liver transaminase tests, alpha-fetoprotein concentration, and abdominal ultrasonography. Patients with persistently elevated serum ALT concentrations (exceeding twice the upper limit of normal) and patients with an increased serum alpha-fetoprotein concentration or abnormal findings on abdominal ultrasonography should be referred to a specialist in management of chronic HBV infection for further management and treatment.

The goal of treatment in chronic HBV infection is to prevent progression to cirrhosis, hepatic failure, and hepatocellular carcinoma. Children without necroinflammatory liver disease and children with immunotolerant chronic HBV infection (ie, normal ALT concentrations despite presence of HBV DNA) usually do not warrant antiviral therapy. Treatment response is measured by biochemical, virologic, and histologic response. An important consideration in the choice of treatment is to avoid selection of antiviral-resistant mutations.

The US Food and Drug Administration (FDA) has approved 3 nucleoside analogues (eg, entecavir, lamivudine, and telbivudine), 2 nucleotide analogues (tenofovir and adefovir), and 2 interferon-alfa drugs (interferon alfa-2b and pegylated interferon alfa-2a) for treatment of chronic HBV infection in adults. Tenofovir, entecavir, and pegylated interferon alfa-2a are preferred in adults as first-line therapy. Of these, FDA licensure in the pediatric population is as follows: interferon, 1 year and older; lamivudine, 3 years and older; adefovir, 12 years and older; telbivudine, 16 years and older; and entecavir, 16 years and older.

The optimal agent and duration of therapy for chronic HBV infection in children remain unclear. Consultation with health care professionals with expertise in treating chronic hepatitis B in children is recommended.

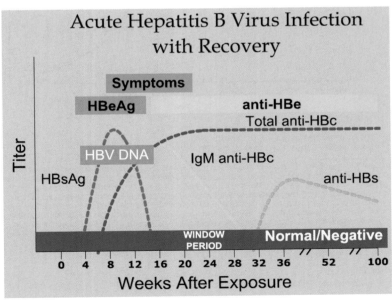

Image 58.1
Virologic and serologic response following acute hepatitis B virus infection. From Centers for Disease Control and Prevention. Viral Hepatitis Resource Center. Online Serology Training: Hepatitis B. Available at: http://www.cdc.gov/hepatitis/Resources/Professionals/Training/Serology/training. htm#one.

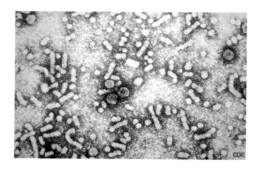

Image 58.2

This electron micrograph reveals the presence of hepatitis B virus (HBV). Infectious HBV virions are also known as Dane particles. These particles measure 42 nm in their overall diameter and contain a DNA-based core that is 27 nm in diameter.

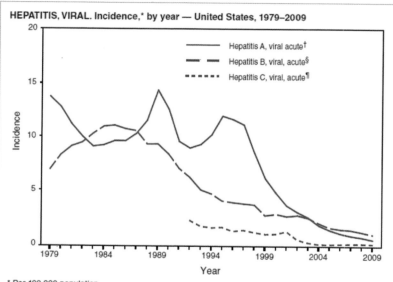

* Per 100,000 population.
† Hepatitis A vaccine was first licensed in 1995.
§ Hepatitis B vaccine was first licensed in June 1982.
¶ An anti-hepatitis C virus (HCV) antibody test first became available in May 1990.

Hepatitis A incidence continues to decline and in 2009 was the lowest ever recorded. This reduction in incidence is attributable, at least in part, to routine vaccination of children. Hepatitis A incidence has declined >90% since 1995. Routine hepatitis B vaccination of infants has reduced rates of hepatitis B infection by >95% in children. Rates also have declined among adults, but cases continue to occur among adults with high-risk behaviors. Outbreaks in health-care settings such as long-term–care facilities and nursing homes caused by failure to adhere to infection-control practices account for a substantial number of new cases among the elderly population. Incidence of acute hepatitis C has declined approximately 90% since 1992; however, a substantial burden of disease remains as a result of the estimated 3.2 million U.S. residents with chronic hepatitis C virus infection.

Image 58.3

Viral hepatitis incidence by year in the United States (1976–2006). Courtesy of *Morbidity and Mortality Weekly Report.*

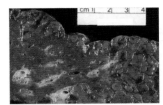

Image 58.4
Section of liver damaged by hepatitis B virus. Note the enlarged cells and blistering of the capsular surface. Copyright Anthony Demetris, MD, Director, Division of Transplantation Pathology, University of Pittsburgh Medical Center.

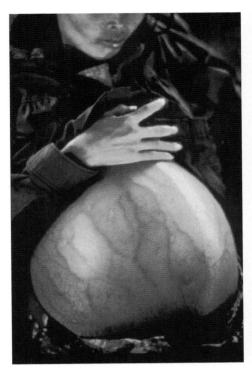

Image 58.5
This female Cambodian patient presented with a distended abdomen due to a hepatoma resulting from chronic hepatitis B infection. Copyright Dr Patricia F. Walker.

59

Hepatitis C

Clinical Manifestations

Signs and symptoms of hepatitis C virus (HCV) infection are indistinguishable from those of hepatitis A or hepatitis B virus (HBV) infections. Acute disease tends to be mild and insidious in onset, and most infected people, including children, are asymptomatic. Jaundice occurs in fewer than 20% of patients, and abnormalities in liver transaminase concentrations generally are less pronounced than abnormalities in patients with HBV infection. Persistent infection with HCV occurs in up to 80% of infected children, even in the absence of biochemical evidence of liver disease. Although chronic hepatitis develops in approximately 70% to 80% of infected adults, limited data indicate that chronic hepatitis and cirrhosis occur less commonly in children, in part because of the usually indolent nature of infection in pediatric patients. Infection with HCV is the leading indication for liver transplantation among adults in the United States.

Etiology

HCV is a small, single-stranded RNA virus and is a member of the Flavivirus family. Multiple HCV genotypes and subtypes exist.

Epidemiology

The incidence of acute symptomatic HCV infection in the United States was 0.2 per 100,000 in 2005; after asymptomatic infection and underreporting were considered, approximately 20,000 new cases were estimated to have occurred. For all age groups, the incidence of HCV infection decreased in the United States during the 1990s and has remained stable since then. Nevertheless, a large burden of disease still exists because HCV can establish chronic infection and because of high incidence of acute HCV infection throughout the 1980s. The prevalence of HCV infection in the general population is about 1.3%, equating to an estimated 3.2 million people. Seroprevalences vary among populations according to their associated risk factors. Worldwide, the prevalence of chronic HCV infection is highest in Africa.

HCV primarily is spread by parenteral exposure to blood of HCV-infected people. The common risk factors for acquiring HCV infection are injection drug use, having multiple sexual partners, or having received blood products before 1992. The current risk of HCV infection after blood transfusion in the United States is estimated to be 1 per 2 million units transfused because of exclusion of high-risk donors, of HCV-positive units after antibody testing, and screening of pools of blood units by some form of nucleic acid amplification test (NAAT). All intravenous and intramuscular immune globulin products available in the United States undergo an inactivation procedure for HCV or are documented to be HCV RNA negative.

Almost all HCV transmission is by parenteral or percutaneous routes. Approximately 60% of reported chronic HCV cases are in acknowledged injection drug users who have shared needles or injection paraphernalia and, to a lesser extent, in people who received transfusions before 1992; almost all of these infected people are outside the pediatric age range. Data from recent multicenter, population-based cohort studies indicate that approximately one-third of young injection drug users 18 to 30 years of age are infected with HCV. People with sporadic percutaneous exposures, such as health care professionals, represent approximately 1% of cases. Approximately half of the 18,000 people with hemophilia who received transfusions before adoption of heat treatment of clotting factors in 1987 are HCV seropositive. Also, more recently appreciated has been the number of infections acquired in the health care setting, especially nonhospital clinics, in which infection control and needle and intravenous hygienic procedures have not been strict. Prevalence is moderately high among people with frequent but smaller direct percutaneous exposures, such as patients receiving hemodialysis (10%–20%).

The increasing number of lifetime sex partners is associated directly with an increasing likelihood of being an intravenous drug user, and several prospective studies have not been able to demonstrate sexual transmission of HCV between heterosexual partners. However, the exception appears to be HCV transmission sexually between or to HIV-infected (presumably immunosuppressed) people. There have been an increasing number of reports of sexual transmission of HCV between HIV-infected men who have sex with men or of HIV-infected heterosexual women.

Transmission among family contacts is uncommon but can occur from direct or inapparent percutaneous or mucosal exposure to blood. Seroprevalence among pregnant women in the United States has been estimated at 1% to 2%. The risk of perinatal transmission averages 5% to 6%, and transmission occurs only from women who are HCV RNA positive at the time of delivery. Maternal coinfection with HIV has been associated with increased risk of perinatal transmission of HCV, which depends in part on the serologic concentration of HCV RNA in the mother. Serum antibody to HCV (anti-HCV) and HCV RNA have been detected in colostrum, but the risk of HCV transmission is similar in breastfed and bottle-fed infants.

All people with HCV RNA in their blood are considered to be infectious.

Incubation Period

6 to 7 weeks (range, 2 weeks–6 months); time from exposure to viremia, 1 to 2 weeks.

Diagnostic Tests

The 2 major types of tests available for laboratory diagnosis of HCV infections are immunoglobulin (Ig) G antibody enzyme immunoassays for HCV and NAATs to detect HCV RNA. Assays for IgM to detect early or acute infection are not available. Third-generation enzyme immunoassays are at least 97% sensitive and more than 99% specific. In June 2010, the US Food and Drug Administration (FDA) approved for use in people 15 years of age and older the OraQuick rapid blood test, which uses a test strip that produces a blue line within 20 minutes if anti-HCV antibodies are present. False-negative results early in the course of acute infection can result from any of the HCV sero-

logic tests because of the prolonged interval between exposure and onset of illness and seroconversion. Within 15 weeks after exposure and within 5 to 6 weeks after onset of hepatitis, 80% of patients will have positive test results for serum anti-HCV antibody. Among infants born to anti-HCV–positive mothers, passively acquired maternal antibody can persist for up to 18 months.

NAATs for qualitative detection of HCV RNA can be positive in serum or plasma within 1 to 2 weeks after exposure to the virus and weeks before onset of liver enzyme abnormalities or appearance of anti-HCV. Assays for detection of HCV RNA are used commonly to identify patients who have HCV infection, infants early in life (ie, perinatal transmission) when maternal antibody interferes with ability to detect antibody produced by the infant, and for monitoring patients receiving antiviral therapy. However, false-positive and false-negative results can occur from improper handling, storage, and contamination of test specimens.

Treatment

Patients diagnosed with HCV infection should be referred to a pediatric hepatitis specialist. Therapy is aimed at inhibiting HCV replication, eradicating infection, and improving the natural history of disease. Therapies are expensive and can have significant adverse reactions. Pegylated interferon-alfa in combination with ribavirin or interferon-alfa–2b with ribavirin is FDA-approved for treatment of HCV infection in children 3 to 17 years of age. Children have fewer adverse events compared with adults. Major adverse effects of therapy in pediatric patients include influenza-like symptoms, hematologic abnormalities, neuropsychiatric symptoms, thyroid abnormalities, ocular abnormalities including ischemic retinopathy and uveitis, and growth disturbances. Education of patients, their family members, and caregivers about adverse effects and their prospective management is an integral aspect of treatment.

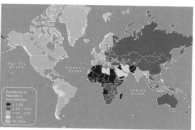

Image 59.1
Prevalence of chronic hepatitis C infection. Courtesy of Centers for Disease Control and Prevention.

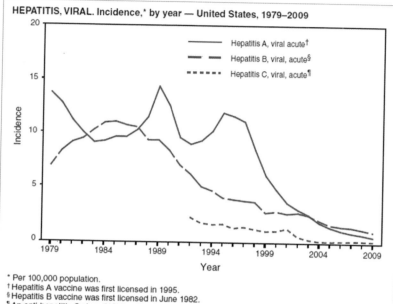

HEPATITIS, VIRAL. Incidence,* by year — United States, 1979–2009

* Per 100,000 population.
† Hepatitis A vaccine was first licensed in 1995.
§ Hepatitis B vaccine was first licensed in June 1982.
¶ An anti-hepatitis C virus (HCV) antibody test first became available in May 1990.

Hepatitis A incidence continues to decline and in 2009 was the lowest ever recorded. This reduction in incidence is attributable, at least in part, to routine vaccination of children. Hepatitis A incidence has declined >90% since 1995. Routine hepatitis B vaccination of infants has reduced rates of hepatitis B infection by >95% in children. Rates also have declined among adults, but cases continue to occur among adults with high-risk behaviors. Outbreaks in health-care settings such as long-term–care facilities and nursing homes caused by failure to adhere to infection-control practices account for a substantial number of new cases among the elderly population. Incidence of acute hepatitis C has declined approximately 90% since 1992; however, a substantial burden of disease remains as a result of the estimated 3.2 million U.S. residents with chronic hepatitis C virus infection.

Image 59.2
Viral hepatitis incidence by year in the United States (1976–2006). Courtesy of
Morbidity and Mortality Weekly Report.

60

Hepatitis D

Clinical Manifestations

Hepatitis D virus (HDV) causes infection only in people with acute or chronic hepatitis B virus (HBV) infection; HDV requires HBV as a helper virus and cannot produce infection in the absence of HBV. The importance of HDV infection lies in its ability to convert an asymptomatic or mild chronic HBV infection into fulminant or more severe or rapidly progressive disease. Acute coinfection with HBV and HDV usually causes an acute illness indistinguishable from acute HBV infection alone, except that the likelihood of fulminant hepatitis can be as high as 5%.

Etiology

HDV measures 36 to 43 nm in diameter and consists of an RNA genome and a delta protein antigen, each of which are coated with hepatitis B surface antigen (HBsAg).

Epidemiology

HDV infection is present worldwide, and an estimated 18 million people are infected. Over the past 20 years, HDV prevalence has decreased significantly in Europe. At least 8 genotypes of HDV have been described, each with a typical geographic pattern, with genotype I being the predominant type in Europe and North America. HDV can cause an infection at the same time as the initial HBV infection (coinfection) or it can infect a person already chronically infected with HBV (superinfection). Acquisition of HDV is by parenteral, percutaneous, or mucous membrane inoculation. HDV can be acquired from blood or blood products, through injection drug use, or by sexual contact, but only if HBV also is present. Transmission from mother to newborn infant is uncommon. Intrafamilial spread can occur among people with chronic HBV infection. High-prevalence areas include southern Italy and parts of Eastern Europe, South America, Africa, and the Middle East. In the United States, HDV infection is found most commonly in people who abuse injection drugs, people with hemophilia, and people who have emigrated from areas with endemic infection.

Incubation Period

Approximately 2 to 8 weeks; when HBV and HDV viruses infect simultaneously, 45 to 160 days; average, 90 days.

Diagnostic Tests

People with chronic HBV infection are at risk of HDV coinfection. Accordingly, their care should be supervised by an expert in hepatitis treatment, and consideration should be given to testing for anti-HDV immunoglobulin (Ig) G antibodies using a commercially available test if there is an elevation of transaminases. Anti-HDV may not be present until several weeks after onset of illness, and acute and convalescent sera can be required to confirm the diagnosis. Absence of IgM hepatitis B core antibody (anti-HBc), which is indicative of early HBV infection, suggests that the person has both chronic HBV infection and superinfection with HDV. Presence of anti-HDV IgG antibodies does not prove active infection and, thus, HDV RNA testing should be performed for diagnostic and therapeutic considerations. Presence of anti-HDV IgM is of lesser utility, because it is present in both acute and chronic HDV infections.

Treatment

HDV has proven difficult to treat. However, data suggest pegylated interferon-alpha may result in up to 40% of patients having a sustained response to treatment. Clinical trials suggest at least a year of therapy is associated with the best sustained responses, and longer courses may be warranted if the patient is able to tolerate the adverse events of therapy.

61

Hepatitis E

Clinical Manifestations

Hepatitis E virus (HEV) infection causes an acute illness with symptoms including jaundice, malaise, anorexia, fever, abdominal pain, and arthralgia. Disease is more common among adults than among children and is more severe in pregnant women, in whom mortality rates can reach 10% to 25% during the third trimester. Chronic HEV infection is rare and has been reported only in recipients of solid organ transplants and people with severe immunodeficiency.

Etiology

HEV is a spherical, nonenveloped, positive-strand RNA virus. HEV is classified in the genus *Hepevirus* of the family Hepeviridae. There are 4 major recognized genotypes with a single known serotype.

Epidemiology

Ingestion of fecally contaminated water is the most common route of HEV transmission, and large waterborne outbreaks have been reported in developing countries. Unlike the other agents of viral hepatitis, certain HEV genotypes (genotypes 3 and 4) also have zoonotic hosts, such as swine, and can be transmitted by eating uncooked pork. Person-to-person transmission appears to be much less efficient than with hepatitis A virus but occurs in sporadic and outbreaks settings. Sporadic HEV infection has been reported throughout the world and is common in Africa and the Indian subcontinent, where some studies have shown HEV to be the most common etiology of acute viral hepatitis. Mother-to-infant transmission of HEV occurs frequently and accounts for a significant proportion of fetal loss and infant mortality in countries with endemic infection. In the United States, serologic studies have demonstrated that approximately 20% of the population has immunoglobulin (Ig) G against HEV, with higher prevalence in areas with swine herds. However, symptomatic HEV infection in the United States is uncommon and generally occurs in people who acquire HEV genotype 1 infection after traveling to countries with endemic HEV.

Diagnostic Tests

Testing for IgM and IgG anti-HEV is available through some research and commercial reference laboratories. Because anti-HEV assays are not approved by the US Food and Drug Administration and their performance characteristics are not well defined, results should be interpreted with caution, particularly in cases lacking a discrete onset of illness associated with jaundice or with no recent history of travel to a country with endemic infection. Definitive diagnosis may be made by demonstrating viral RNA in serum or stool by means of reverse transcriptase PCR assay, which is available only in research settings (eg, with prior approval through the Centers for Disease Control and Prevention). Because virus circulates in the body for a relatively short period, the inability to detect HEV in serum or stool does not eliminate the possibility that the person was infected with HEV.

Treatment

Supportive.

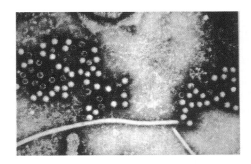

Image 61.1

This electron micrograph depicts hepatitis E viruses (HEV). HEV was classified as a member of the Caliciviridae family but have been reclassified in the genus *Hepevirus* of the family Hepeviridae. There are 4 major recognized genotypes with a single known serotype. HEV, the major etiologic agent of enterically transmitted non-A, non-B hepatitis worldwide, is a spherical, non-enveloped, single-stranded RNA virus that is approximately 32 to 34 nm in diameter. Courtesy of Centers for Disease Control and Prevention.

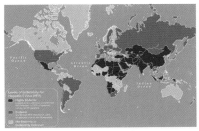

Image 61.2

Distribution of hepatitis E infection, 2010. Courtesy of Centers for Disease Control and Prevention.

62

Herpes Simplex

Clinical Manifestations

Neonatal. Herpes simplex virus (HSV) infection in newborns can manifest in 3 syndromes: (1) **disseminated disease** involving multiple organs, most prominently liver and lungs, but in 60% to 75% of cases also involving the central nervous system; (2) localized **central nervous system (CNS) disease**, with or without skin involvement (CNS disease); or (3) disease **localized to the skin, eyes, or mouth (SEM disease).** Approximately 25% of cases of neonatal HSV manifest as disseminated disease, 30% of cases manifest as CNS disease, and 45% of cases manifest as SEM disease. More than 80% of neonates with SEM disease have skin vesicles; those without vesicles have infection limited to the eyes or oral mucosa. Approximately two-thirds of neonates with disseminated or CNS disease have skin lesions, but these lesions may not be present at the time of initial presentation. Disseminated infection should be considered in neonates with sepsis syndrome, negative bacteriologic culture results, and severe liver dysfunction. HSV also should be considered as a causative agent in neonates with fever, a vesicular rash, or abnormal cerebrospinal fluid (CSF) findings, especially in the presence of seizures or during a time of year when enteroviruses are not circulating in the community. Although asymptomatic HSV infection is common in older children, it rarely, if ever, occurs in neonates.

Neonatal herpetic infections often are severe, with attendant high mortality and morbidity rates, even when antiviral therapy is administered. Recurrent skin lesions are common in surviving infants and can be associated with CNS sequelae, especially if recurrences are frequent during the first 6 months of life.

Initial signs of HSV infection most often develop within the first month of life. Infants with disseminated disease and SEM disease have an earlier age of onset, typically presenting between the first and second week of life; infants with CNS disease usually present with illness between the second and third week of life.

Children Beyond the Neonatal Period and Adolescents. Most primary HSV infections during childhood are asymptomatic. Gingivostomatitis, which is the most common clinical manifestation, is caused by HSV type 1 (HSV-1) and is characterized by fever, irritability, tender submandibular adenopathy, and an ulcerative enanthem involving the gingiva and mucous membranes of the mouth, often with perioral vesicular lesions.

Genital herpes, which is the most common manifestation of primary HSV infection in adolescents and adults, is characterized by vesicular or ulcerative lesions of the male or female genital organs, perineum, or both. Genital herpes usually is caused by HSV type 2 (HSV-2), but HSV-1 increasingly is becoming a common cause of genital herpes (20%–50% of all cases) in some populations. Most primary genital herpes infections are not recognized as such by the infected person or diagnosed by a health care professional.

Eczema herpeticum with vesicular lesions concentrated in the areas of eczematous involvement can develop in patients with atopic dermatitis who are infected with HSV.

In immunocompromised patients, severe local lesions and, less commonly, disseminated HSV infection with generalized vesicular skin lesions and visceral involvement can occur.

After primary infection, HSV persists for life in a latent form for life. The site of latency for virus-causing herpes labialis is the trigeminal ganglion, and the usual site of latency for genital herpes is the sacral dorsal root ganglia, although any of the sensory ganglia can be involved, depending on the site of primary infection. Reactivation of latent virus most commonly is asymptomatic. When symptomatic, recurrent herpes labialis HSV-1 manifests as single or grouped vesicles in the perioral region, usually on the vermilion border of the lips (typically called "cold sores" or "fever blisters"). Symptomatic recurrent genital herpes manifests as vesicular lesions on the penis, scrotum, vulva, cervix, buttocks, perianal areas, thighs, or back. Recurrences may be heralded by a prodrome of burning or itching at the site of an incipient recurrence, identification of which can be useful in instituting antiviral therapy early.

Conjunctivitis and keratitis can result from primary or recurrent HSV infection. Herpetic whitlow consists of single or multiple vesicular lesions on the distal parts of fingers. HSV infection can be a precipitating factor in erythema multiforme.

HSV encephalitis (HSE) occurs in children, adolescents, and adults and can result from primary or recurrent HSV-1 infection. Symptoms and signs usually include fever, alterations in the state of consciousness, personality changes, seizures, and focal neurologic findings. Encephalitis commonly has an acute onset with a fulminant course, leading to coma and death in untreated patients. HSE usually involves the temporal lobe, thus temporal lobe abnormalities on neuroimaging studies or electroencephalography in the context of a consistent clinical picture should increase the suspicion of HSE. CSF pleocytosis with a predominance of lymphocytes and some erythrocytes is usual. HSV infection also can cause meningitis with nonspecific clinical manifestations that usually are mild and self-limited. Such episodes of meningitis usually are associated with genital HSV-2 infection. A number of unusual CNS manifestations of HSV have been described, including Bell palsy, atypical pain syndromes, trigeminal neuralgia, ascending myelitis, postinfectious encephalomyelitis, and recurrent (Mollaret) meningitis.

Etiology

HSVs are enveloped, double-stranded, DNA viruses. Two distinct HSV types exist: HSV-1 and HSV-2. Infections with HSV-1 usually involve the face and skin above the waist; however, an increasing number of genital herpes cases are attributable to HSV-1. Infections with HSV-2 usually involve the genitalia and skin below the waist in sexually active adolescents and adults. However, either type of virus can be found at either site. HSV-2 is the most common cause of herpes simplex disease in neonates (~75% of cases). As with all human herpesviruses, HSV-1 and HSV-2 establish latency following primary infection, with periodic reactivation to cause recurrent symptomatic disease or asymptomatic viral shedding.

Epidemiology

HSV infections are ubiquitous and can be transmitted from people who are symptomatic or asymptomatic with either primary or recurrent infections.

Neonatal. The incidence of neonatal HSV infection is estimated to range from 1 in 3,000 to 1 in 20,000 live births. HSV is transmitted to a neonate most often during birth through an infected maternal genital tract but can be caused by an ascending infection through ruptured or apparently intact amniotic membranes. Intrauterine infections are uncommon. Other uncommon sources of neonatal infection include postnatal transmission from a parent or other caregiver, most often from a nongenital infection (eg, mouth or hands) or from another infected infant or caregiver in the nursery, probably via the hands of health care professionals.

The risk of HSV transmission to a neonate born to a mother who acquires primary genital infection near the time of delivery is estimated to be 25% to 60%. In contrast, the risk to a neonate born to a mother shedding HSV as a result of reactivation of infection acquired during the first half of pregnancy or earlier is approximately 2%. Distinguishing between primary and recurrent HSV infections in women by history or physical examination alone may be impossible, because primary and recurrent genital infections can be asymptomatic or associated with nonspecific symptoms and signs (eg, vaginal discharge, genital pain, or shallow ulcers). More than three-quarters of infants who contract HSV infection have been born to women with no history or clinical findings suggestive of genital HSV infection during or preceding pregnancy.

Children and Adolescents. More than 25% of US children have serologic evidence of HSV-1 infection by 7 years of age. Patients with primary gingivostomatitis or genital herpes usually shed virus for at least 1 week and occasionally for several weeks. Patients with symptomatic recurrences shed virus for a shorter period, typically 3 to 4 days. Intermittent asymptomatic reactivation of oral and genital herpes is common and likely occurs throughout the remainder of a person's life. The greatest density of virus is shed during symptomatic primary infections, and the lowest concentration of virus is shed during asymptomatic recurrent infections.

Infections with HSV-1 usually result from direct contact with virus shed from visible or microscopic orolabial lesions or from infected oral secretions. Infections with HSV-2 usually result from direct contact with virus shed from visible or microscopic genital lesions or in genital secretions during sexual activity. Genital infections caused by HSV-1 in children can result from autoinoculation of virus from the mouth, but sexual abuse always should be considered in prepubertal children with genital HSV-2 infections. Therefore, genital HSV isolates from children should be typed to differentiate between HSV-1 and HSV-2.

The incidence of HSV-2 infection correlates with the number of sexual partners and with acquisition of other sexually transmitted infections. After primary genital infection, which often is asymptomatic, some people experience frequent clinical recurrences, and others have no clinically apparent recurrences. Genital HSV-2 infection is more likely to recur than is genital HSV-1 infection.

Inoculation of abraded skin occurs from direct contact with HSV shed from oral, genital, or other skin sites. This contact can result in herpes gladiatorum among wrestlers, herpes rugbiaforum among rugby players, or herpetic whitlow of the fingers in any exposed person.

Incubation Period

For HSV infection occurring beyond the neonatal period, 2 days to 2 weeks.

Diagnostic Tests

HSV grows readily in cell culture. Special transport media are available that allow transport to local or regional laboratories for culture. Cytopathogenic effects typical of HSV infection usually are observed 1 to 3 days after cell inoculation. Methods of culture confirmation include fluorescent antibody staining, enzyme immunoassays (EIAs), and monolayer culture with typing. Cultures that remain negative by day 5 likely will continue to remain negative. PCR assay often can detect HSV DNA in CSF from neonates with CNS infection (neonatal HSV CNS disease) and from older children and adults with HSE and is the diagnostic method of choice for CNS HSV involvement. Viral cultures of CSF from a patient with HSE usually are negative.

For diagnosis of neonatal HSV infection, the following specimens should be obtained: (1) swab specimens from the mouth, nasopharynx, conjunctivae, and anus ("surface cultures") for HSV culture (all surface swab specimens can be obtained with a single swab and placed in 1 viral transport media tube); (2) specimens of skin vesicles and CSF for HSV culture and PCR; (3) whole blood sample for HSV PCR; and (4) whole blood sample for measuring alanine aminotransferase. Positive cultures obtained from any of the surface sites more than 12 to 24 hours after birth indicate viral replication and, therefore, are suggestive of infant infection rather than merely contamination after intrapartum exposure. As with any PCR assay, false-negative and false-positive results can occur. Rapid diagnostic techniques also are available, such as direct fluorescent antibody staining of vesicle scrapings or EIA detection of HSV antigens. These techniques are as specific but slightly less sensitive than culture. Typing HSV strains differentiates between HSV-1 and HSV-2 isolates.

HSV cell culture and PCR are the preferred tests for detecting HSV in genital ulcers or other mucocutaneous lesions consistent with genital herpes. The sensitivity of viral culture is low, especially for recurrent lesions, and declines rapidly as lesions begin to heal. PCR assays for HSV DNA are more sensitive and are increasingly used in many settings. Failure to detect HSV in genital lesions by culture or PCR does not indicate an absence of HSV infection, because viral shedding is intermittent.

Both type-specific and type-common antibodies to HSV develop during the first several weeks after infection and persist indefinitely. Although type-specific HSV-2 antibody usually indicates previous anogenital infection, the presence of HSV-1 antibody does not distinguish anogenital from orolabial infection reliably, because a substantial proportion of initial genital infections are caused by HSV-1 in some populations. Type-specific serologic tests can be useful in confirming a clinical diagnosis of genital herpes. Serologic testing is not useful in neonates.

Several glycoprotein G–based type-specific assays, including at least one that can be used as a point-of-care test, are available. The sensitivities and specificities of these tests for detection of HSV-2 immunoglobulin G antibody vary from 90% to 100%; false-negative results can occur, especially early after infection, and false-positive results can occur, especially in patients with low likelihood of HSV infection.

Treatment

Acyclovir is the drug of choice for many HSV infections (Table 62.1). Valacyclovir is an L-valyl ester of acyclovir that is metabolized to acyclovir after oral administration, resulting in higher serum concentrations than are achieved with oral acyclovir and similar serum concentrations as are achieved with intravenous administration of acyclovir. Famciclovir is converted rapidly to penciclovir after oral administration.

Neonatal. Parenteral acyclovir is the treatment of choice for neonatal HSV infections. Parenteral acyclovir should be administered to all neonates with HSV infection, regardless of manifestations and clinical findings. Approximately 50% of infants surviving neonatal HSV experience cutaneous recurrences. Use of oral acyclovir suppressive therapy for the 6 months following treatment of acute neonatal HSV disease has been shown to improve neurodevelopmental outcomes in infants with HSV

Table 62.1
Recommended Therapy for Herpes Simplex Virus Infections

Infection	Drug[a]
Neonatal	Parenteral acyclovir
Keratoconjunctivitis	Trifluridine[a] **OR** Iododeoxyuridine **OR** Vidarabine
Genital	Acyclovir **OR** Famciclovir[b] **OR** Valacyclovir
Mucocutaneous (immunocompromised or primary gingivostomatitis)	Acyclovir **OR** Famciclovir **OR** Valacyclovir
Acyclovir-resistant (severe infections, immunocompromised)	Parenteral foscarnet
Encephalitis	Parenteral acyclovir

[a]Treatment of herpes simplex virus ocular infection should involve an ophthalmologist.
[b]Famciclovir and valacyclovir are approved by the US Food and Drug Administration for treatment of adults.

CNS disease and to prevent skin recurrences in infants with any disease classification of neonatal HSV.

Infants with ocular involvement attributable to HSV infection should receive a topical ophthalmic drug as well as parenteral antiviral therapy.

Genital Infection

Primary. Many patients with first-episode herpes initially have mild clinical manifestations but can go on to develop severe or prolonged symptoms. Therefore, most patients with initial genital herpes should receive antiviral therapy. In adults, acyclovir and valacyclovir decrease the duration of symptoms and viral shedding in primary genital herpes. Valacyclovir and famciclovir do not seem to be more effective than acyclovir but offer the advantage of less frequent dosing. Intravenous acyclovir is indicated for patients with a severe or complicated primary infection that requires hospitalization.

Recurrent. Antiviral therapy for recurrent genital herpes can be administered either episodically to ameliorate or shorten the duration of lesions or continuously as suppressive therapy to decrease the frequency of recurrences. Oral acyclovir therapy initiated within 1 day of lesion onset or during the prodrome that precedes some outbreaks shortens the mean clinical course by approximately 1 day. If episodic therapy is used, a prescription for the medication should be provided with instructions to initiate treatment immediately when symptoms begin.

In adults with frequent genital HSV recurrences, daily oral acyclovir suppressive therapy is effective for decreasing the frequency of symptomatic recurrences and improving quality of life. After approximately 1 year of continuous daily therapy, acyclovir should be discontinued and the recurrence rate should be assessed. The safety of systemic valacyclovir and famciclovir therapy in pregnant women has not been established. Acyclovir may be administered orally to pregnant women with first-episode genital herpes or severe recurrent herpes and should be given intravenously to

pregnant women with severe HSV infection. Pregnant women or women of childbearing age with genital herpes should be encouraged to inform their health care professionals and those who will care for the newborn infant.

Mucocutaneous

Immunocompromised Hosts. Intravenous acyclovir is effective for treatment and prevention of mucocutaneous HSV infections. Acyclovir-resistant strains of HSV have been isolated from immunocompromised people receiving prolonged treatment with acyclovir. Under these circumstances, progressive disease may be observed despite acyclovir therapy. Foscarnet is the drug of choice for disease caused by acyclovir-resistant HSV isolates.

Immunocompetent Hosts. Limited data are available on effects of acyclovir on the course of primary or recurrent nongenital mucocutaneous HSV infections in immunocompetent hosts. Therapeutic benefit has been noted in a limited number of children with primary gingivostomatitis treated with oral acyclovir. Slight therapeutic benefit of oral acyclovir therapy has been demonstrated among adults with recurrent herpes labialis.

Other HSV Infections

Central Nervous System. Patients with HSE should be treated for 21 days with intravenous acyclovir. Patients who are comatose or semicomatose at initiation of therapy have a poorer outcome. For people with Bell's palsy, the combination of acyclovir and prednisone may be considered.

Ocular. Treatment of eye lesions should be undertaken in consultation with an ophthalmologist. Several topical drugs, such as 1% trifluridine, 0.1% iododeoxyuridine, and 3% vidarabine, have proven efficacy for superficial keratitis. Topical corticosteroids, by themselves, are contraindicated in suspected HSV conjunctivitis; however, ophthalmologists may choose to use corticosteroids in conjunction with antiviral drugs to treat locally invasive infections.

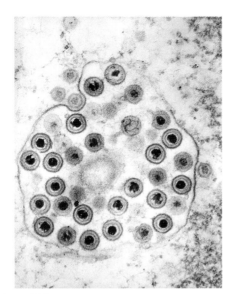

Image 62.1
This negatively stained transmission electron micrograph reveals the presence of numerous herpes simplex virions, members of the Herpesviridae virus family. Courtesy of Centers for Disease Control and Prevention/Dr Fred Murphy; Sylvia Whitfield.

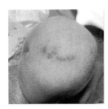

Image 62.3
Erythema toxicum neonatorum presents as blotchy, 2- to 3-cm erythematous macules, each of which has a single 1- to 4-mm central papule, vesicle, or pustule. Lesions are not present at birth but appear in the first 24 to 48 hours thereafter. The condition may be confused with neonatal herpes simplex infection. The condition occurs in about 50% of healthy term infants; preterm infants are affected less often. Individual lesions resolve in 4 to 5 days, with new lesions appearing for up to 10 days. A Wright-stained preparation of the pustule contents reveals numerous eosinophils. If obtained, a complete blood count may demonstrate eosinophilia. The condition is benign and self-limited, and no treatment is necessary. Courtesy of H. Cody Meissner, MD, FAAP.

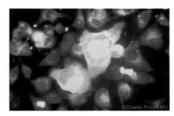

Image 62.2
Herpes simplex virus (direct fluorescent antibody stain). Copyright Charles Prober, MD.

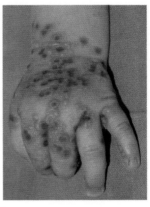

Image 62.4
Children who have atopic dermatitis are prone to recurrent skin infections, particularly with *Staphylococcus aureus* and herpes simplex virus (HSV), for several reasons. Exacerbations of eczema disrupt the skin's protective barrier. Eczema herpeticum results when areas of active dermatitis are infected by HSV.

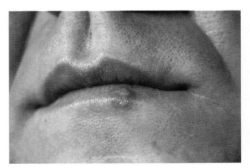

Image 62.5
This is a close-up of a herpes simplex lesion of the lower lip on the second day after onset. Also known as a cold sore, this lesion is caused by the contagious herpes simplex virus type 1 and should not be confused with a canker sore, which is not contagious. Courtesy of Centers for Disease Control and Prevention/Dr Hermann.

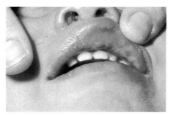

Image 62.6
Herpes simplex stomatitis, primary infection.

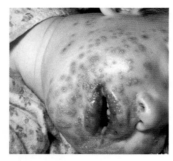

Image 62.8
Herpes simplex stomatitis, primary infection with extension to the face.

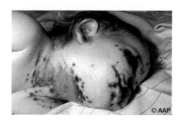

Image 62.10
Herpes simplex infection in a child with eczema and Stevens-Johnson syndrome. This is the same patient as in Image 62.9.

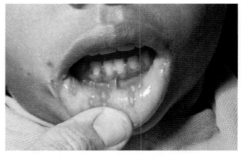

Image 62.7
Herpes simplex stomatitis, primary infection of the anterior oral mucous membranes. Tongue lesions also are common with primary herpes simplex virus infections.

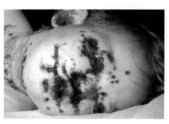

Image 62.9
Herpes simplex infection in a child with eczema with Kaposi varicelliform eruption and Stevens-Johnson syndrome.

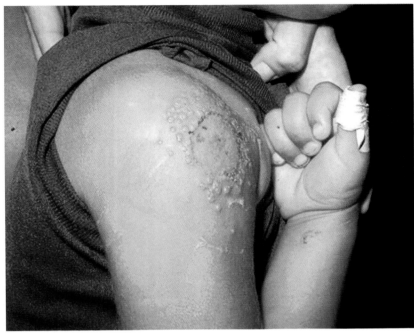

Image 62.11
Herpes simplex virus infection at a diphtheria, tetanus, and pertussis vaccine injection site reflecting self-inoculation. Courtesy of Edgar O. Ledbetter, MD, FAAP.

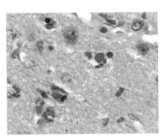

Image 62.12
Herpes simplex virus encephalitis. Viral intranuclear inclusions. Courtesy of Dimitris P. Agamanolis, MD.

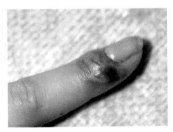

Image 62.13
An adolescent girl with herpetic whitlow secondary to orolabial lesions with self-inoculation. Copyright Martin G. Myers, MD.

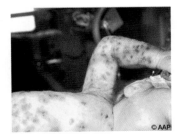

Image 62.14
Neonatal herpes simplex infection with disseminated vesicular lesions.

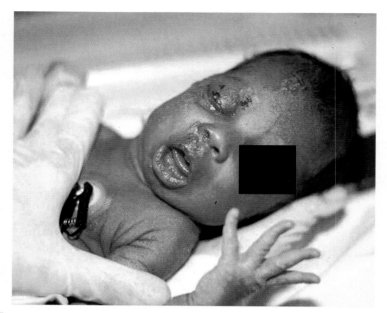

Image 62.15
Neonatal herpes skin lesions of the face. A 14-day-old premature infant developed vesicular lesions over the right eye and face on days 11 to 14 of life. Herpes simplex virus type 2 was recovered from viral culture of the vesicular fluid. Keratoconjunctivitis was diagnosed by ophthalmology and the infant was treated with topical antiviral eyedrops in addition to intravenous acyclovir. The child was born via a spontaneous vaginal delivery with a vertex presentation. Membranes had ruptured 8 hours prior to delivery. There was no history of genital herpes or fever blisters in either parent. The lesions were concentrated on the face and head, the presenting body parts in delivery. Copyright Barbara Jantausch, MD, FAAP.

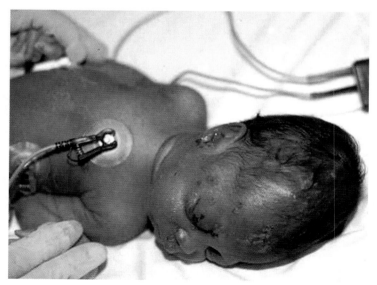

Image 62.16
Neonatal herpes skin lesions of the head and face. This is the same patient as shown in Image 62.15. Copyright Barbara Jantausch, MD, FAAP.

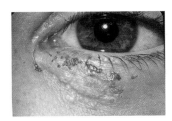

Image 62.17
A 15-year-old white female with recurrent facial and ocular herpes simplex virus infection. Copyright Larry Frenkel, MD.

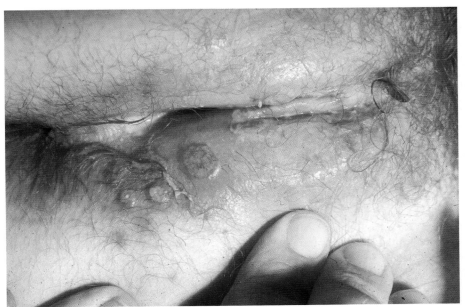

Image 62.18
A 15-year-old female with a primary herpes simplex infection of the genital area. Copyright Larry Frenkel, MD.

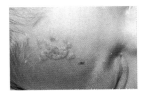

Image 62.19
Herpes simplex virus infection is characterized by clustered vesicles on an erythematous base. Copyright Daniel P. Krowchuk, MD, FAAP.

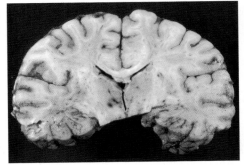

Image 62.20
Post-neonatal herpes simplex virus encephalitis. Hemorrhagic necrosis of the temporal lobes. Courtesy of Dimitris P. Agamanolis, MD.

63

Histoplasmosis

Clinical Manifestations

Histoplasma capsulatum causes symptoms in fewer than 5% of infected people. Clinical manifestations are classified according to site (pulmonary or disseminated), duration (acute, subacute, or chronic, and pattern (primary or reactivation) of infection. Most symptomatic patients have acute pulmonary histoplasmosis, a self-limited illness characterized by fever, chills, nonproductive cough, and malaise. Typical radiographic findings include diffuse interstitial or reticulonodular pulmonary infiltrates and hilar or mediastinal adenopathy. Most patients spontaneously recover 2 to 3 weeks after onset of symptoms. Exposure to a large inoculum of conidia can cause more severe pulmonary infection associated with high fever, hypoxemia, diffuse reticulonodular infiltrates, and acute respiratory distress syndrome. Chronic cavitary pulmonary histoplasmosis occurs most often in older adults and can mimic pulmonary tuberculosis. Mediastinal involvement, usually a complication of pulmonary histoplasmosis, includes mediastinal lymphadenitis, which can cause airway encroachment in young children. Inflammatory syndromes (pericarditis and rheumatologic syndromes) also can develop; erythema nodosum can occur in adolescents and adults. Primary cutaneous infections after trauma are rare.

Disseminated histoplasmosis can be either self-limited or progressive. Progressive disseminated histoplasmosis (PDH) can occur in otherwise healthy infants and children younger than 2 years. PDH can be a rapidly progressive illness following acute infection or a more chronic, slowly progressive disease. PDH in adults occurs most often in people with underlying immune deficiency (eg, HIV/AIDS, solid organ transplant, hematologic malignancy, tumor necrosis factor-α antagonists) or in people older than 65 years. Early manifestations of PDH in young children include prolonged fever, failure to thrive, and hepatosplenomegaly; if untreated, malnutrition, diffuse adenopathy, pneumonia, mucosal ulceration, pancytopenia, disseminated intravascular coagulopathy, and gastrointestinal tract bleeding can ensue. Central nervous system involvement is common. Chronic PDH generally occurs in adults with immune suppression and is characterized by prolonged fever, night sweats, weight loss, and fatigue; signs include hepatosplenomegaly, mucosal ulcerations, adrenal insufficiency, and pancytopenia.

Etiology

Histoplasma capsulatum var *capsulatum* is a dimorphic endemic fungus. It grows in the environment as a microconidia-bearing mold but converts to the yeast phase at body temperature. *H capsulatum* var *duboisii* is the cause of African histoplasmosis, and is found only in central and western Africa.

Epidemiology

H capsulatum is encountered in most parts of the world (including Africa, the Americas, Asia, and Europe) and is endemic in the eastern and central United States, particularly the Mississippi, Ohio, and Missouri River valleys. Infection is acquired through inhalation of conidia from soil, often contaminated with bat guano or bird droppings. The inoculum size, strain virulence, and immune status of the host affect severity of illness. Infections occur sporadically, in outbreaks when weather conditions (dry and windy) predispose to the spread of spores, or as point-source epidemics after exposure to activities that disturb contaminated soil. Recreational and occupational pursuits, such as playing in hollow trees, caving, mining, construction, excavation, demolition, farming, and cleaning of contaminated buildings, have been associated with histoplasmosis. Person-to-person transmission does not occur. Prior infection confers partial immunity; reinfection can occur but requires a larger inoculum.

Incubation Period

Variable, but usually 1 to 3 weeks.

Diagnostic Tests

Culture is the definitive method of diagnosis. *H capsulatum* from bone marrow, blood, sputum, and tissue specimens grows on standard mycologic media in 1 to 6 weeks. The lysis-centrifugation method is preferred for blood cultures. A DNA probe for *H capsulatum* permits rapid identification of cultured isolates. Demonstration of typical intracellular yeast forms by examination of stains of tissue, blood, bone marrow, or bronchoalveolar lavage specimens strongly supports the diagnosis of histoplasmosis when clinical, epidemiologic, and other laboratory studies are compatible.

Detection of *H capsulatum* antigen in serum, urine, a bronchoalveolar lavage specimen, or cerebrospinal fluid using a quantitative enzyme immunoassay is possible using a rapid, commercially available diagnostic test. Antigen detection in blood and urine specimens is most sensitive for severe, acute pulmonary infections and for progressive disseminated infections. Results often are transiently positive early in the course of acute, self-limited pulmonary infections. A negative test result does not exclude infection. If the result initially is positive, the antigen test also is useful for monitoring treatment response and, after treatment, identifying relapse. Cross-reactions occur in patients with blastomycosis, coccidioidomycosis, and paracoccidioidomycosis.

Serologic testing also is available and is most useful in patients with subacute or chronic pulmonary disease. A fourfold increase in either yeast-phase or mycelial-phase titers or a single titer of 1:32 or greater in either test is presumptive evidence of active or recent infection. Cross-reacting antibodies can result from *Blastomyces dermatitidis* and *Coccidioides* species infections. The immunodiffusion test is more specific than the complement fixation test, but the complement fixation test is more sensitive.

Treatment

Amphotericin B is recommended for severe or disseminated infections and itraconazole is recommended for mild to moderate infections that warrant antifungal therapy. Itraconazole is preferred over other azoles by most experts.

When used in adults, itraconazole is more effective, has fewer adverse effects, and is less likely to induce resistance than is fluconazole. Anecdotal experience has found itraconazole to be well tolerated and effective. Serum concentrations of itraconazole should be determined to ensure that effective, nontoxic levels are attained.

Immunocompetent children with uncomplicated acute pulmonary histoplasmosis rarely require antifungal therapy. If the patient is symptomatic for more than 4 weeks, itraconazole should be given for 6 to 12 weeks. For severe acute pulmonary infections, treatment with amphotericin B is recommended for 1 to 2 weeks followed by another 12 weeks of itraconazole. Methylprednisolone during the first 1 to 2 weeks of therapy can be used if respiratory complications develop.

All patients with chronic pulmonary histoplasmosis should be treated. Mild to moderate cases should be treated with itraconazole for 1 to 2 years. Severe cases initially should be treated with amphotericin B followed by itraconazole.

Mediastinal and inflammatory manifestations of infection generally are not treated with antifungals. However, mediastinal adenitis that causes obstruction of a bronchus, the esophagus, or another mediastinal structure may improve with a brief course of corticosteroids and itraconazole. Dense fibrosis of mediastinal structures without an associated granulomatous inflammatory component does not respond to antifungal therapy, and surgical intervention may be necessary.

For treatment of PDH in a nonimmunocompromised infant or child, amphotericin B is the drug of choice and is given for 4 to 6 weeks. Longer periods of therapy can be required for patients with severe disease, or underlying primary or acquired immunodeficiency.

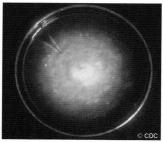

Image 63.1
Sabouraud dextrose agar plate culture of *Histoplasma capsulatum* showing typical fuzzy appearance of mold colony. Courtesy of Centers for Disease Control and Prevention.

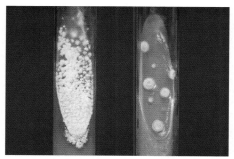

Image 63.2
These 2 slant cultures grew *Histoplasma capsulatum* colonies (left tube: Sabouraud agar; right tube: Sabhi agar). *H capsulatum* is the most common cause of fungal respiratory infections globally. While most infections are mild, 10% of cases can be life-threatening, such as inflammation of the pericardium and fibrosis of major blood vessels. Courtesy of Centers for Disease Control and Prevention/Dr Lenore Haley.

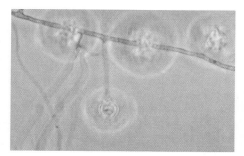

Image 63.3
This photomicrograph reveals a conidiophore of the fungus *Histoplasma capsulatum*. *H capsulatum* grows in soil and material contaminated with bat or bird droppings. Spores become airborne when contaminated soil is disturbed. Breathing the spores causes pulmonary histoplasmosis. Courtesy of Centers for Disease Control and Prevention/Dr Libero Ajello.

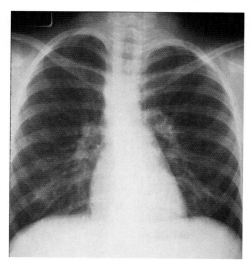

Image 63.4
Acute, primary histoplasmosis in a 13-year-old girl. Progressive disseminated histoplasmosis is unusual in otherwise healthy children.

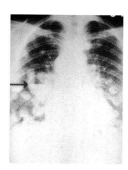

Image 63.5
Chest radiograph showing miliary densities in both lung fields plus a thin-walled cavity with a fluid level. Copyright American Society for Clinical Pathology.

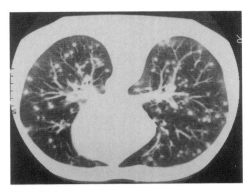

Image 63.6
Computed tomography scan of lungs showing classic snowstorm appearance of acute histoplasmosis. Courtesy of Centers for Disease Control and Prevention.

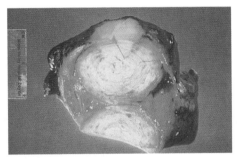

Image 63.8
Gross pathology specimen of lung showing cut surface of fibrocaseous nodule due to *Histoplasma capsulatum*. Copyright American Society for Clinical Pathology.

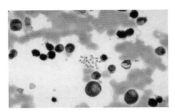

Image 63.7
Histoplasma capsulatum in peripheral blood smear. Copyright Martha Lepow.

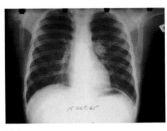

Image 63.9
A 10-year-old male with calcified left hilar lymph nodes secondary to histoplasmosis.

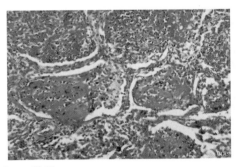

Image 63.10
This micrograph depicts the histopathologic changes associated with histoplasmosis of the lung. Courtesy of Centers for Disease Control and Prevention/Martin Hicklin, MD.

64

Hookworm Infections

(*Ancylostoma duodenale* and *Necator americanus*)

Clinical Manifestations

Patients with hookworm infection often are asymptomatic. Chronic hookworm infection, however, is a common cause of moderate and severe hypochromic, microcytic anemia in people living in tropical developing countries, and heavy infection can cause hypoproteinemia with edema. Chronic hookworm infection in children also can lead to physical growth delay, deficits in cognition, and developmental delay. After contact with contaminated soil, initial skin penetration of larvae, often involving the feet, can cause a stinging or burning sensation followed by pruritus and a papulovesicular rash that may persist for 1 to 2 weeks. Pneumonitis associated with migrating larvae is uncommon and usually mild, except in heavy infections. Colicky abdominal pain, nausea, and/or diarrhea and marked eosinophilia can develop 4 to 6 weeks after exposure. Blood loss secondary to hookworm infection develops 10 to 12 weeks after initial infection, and symptoms related to serious iron-deficiency anemia can develop in long-standing moderate or heavy hookworm infections. After oral ingestion of infectious *Ancylostoma duodenale* larvae, disease can quickly manifest with pharyngeal itching, hoarseness, nausea, and vomiting.

Etiology

Necator americanus is the major cause of hookworm infection worldwide, although *A duodenale* also is an important hookworm in some regions. Mixed infections are common. Both are roundworms (nematodes) with similar life cycles.

Epidemiology

Humans are the only reservoir. Hookworms are prominent in rural, tropical, and subtropical areas where soil contamination with human feces is common. Although the prevalence of both hookworm species is equal in many areas, *A duodenale* is the predominant species in the Mediterranean region, northern Asia, and selected foci of South America. *N americanus* is predominant in the Western hemisphere, sub-Saharan Africa, Southeast Asia, and a number of Pacific islands. Larvae and eggs survive in loose, sandy, moist, shady, well-aerated, warm soil (optimal temperature 23°C–33°C [73°F–91°F]). Hookworm eggs from stool hatch in soil in 1 to 2 days as rhabditiform larvae. These larvae develop into infective filariform larvae in soil within 5 to 7 days and can persist for weeks to months. Percutaneous infection occurs after exposure to infectious larvae. *A duodenale* transmission can occur by oral ingestion and possibly through human milk. Untreated infected patients can harbor worms for 5 years or longer.

Incubation Period

From exposure to noncutaneous symptoms is 4 to 12 weeks.

Diagnostic Tests

Microscopic demonstration of hookworm eggs in feces is diagnostic. Adult worms or larvae rarely are seen. Approximately 5 to 8 weeks are required after infection for eggs to appear in feces. A direct stool smear with saline solution or potassium iodide saturated with iodine is adequate for diagnosis of heavy hookworm infection; light infections require concentration techniques. Quantification techniques (eg, Kato-Katz, Beaver direct smear, or Stoll egg-counting techniques) to determine the clinical significance of infection and the response to treatment may be available from state or reference laboratories.

Treatment

Albendazole, mebendazole, and pyrantel pamoate all are effective treatments. Although data suggest that these drugs are safe in children younger than 2 years, the risks and benefits of therapy should be considered before administration. In 1-year-old children, the World Health Organization recommends reducing the albendazole dose to half of that given to older children. Reexamination of stool specimens 2 weeks after therapy to determine whether worms have been eliminated is helpful for assessing response to therapy. Re-treatment is indicated for persistent infection. Nutritional supplementation, including iron, is important when severe anemia is present. Severely affected children also may require blood transfusion.

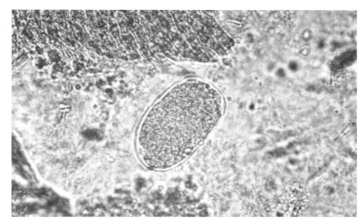

Image 64.1
Hookworm (*Necator americanus*) ova in stool preparation.

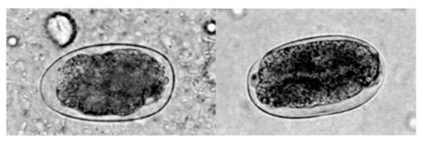

Image 64.2
Hookworm eggs examined on wet mount (eggs of *Ancylostoma duodenale* and *Necator americanus* cannot be distinguished morphologically). Diagnostic characteristics: 57 to 76 µm by 35 to 47 µm, oval or ellipsoidal, thin shell. The embryo (right) has begun cellular division and is at an early developmental stage (gastrula). Courtesy of Centers for Disease Control and Prevention.

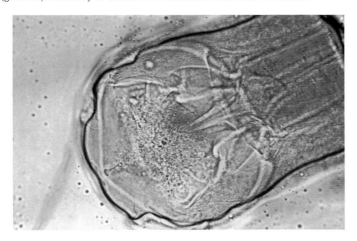

Image 64.3
This micrograph reveals the head of the hookworm *Necator americanus* and its mouth's cutting plates (magnification x400). The hookworm uses these sharp cutting teeth to grasp firmly to the intestinal wall, and while remaining fastened in place, ingests the host's blood, obtaining its nutrients in this fashion. Courtesy of Centers for Disease Control and Prevention/Dr Mae Melvin.

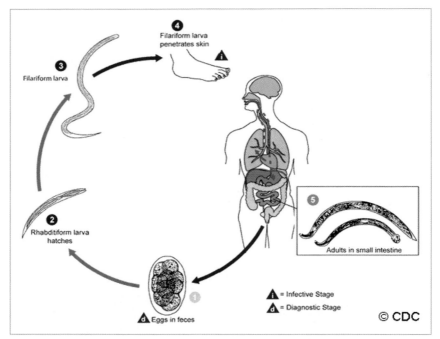

Image 64.4

Eggs are passed in the stool (1) and under favorable conditions (moisture, warmth, shade), larvae hatch in 1 to 2 days. The released rhabditiform larvae grow in feces or soil (2), and after 5 to 10 days (and 2 molts) they become filariform (third-stage) larvae that are infective (3). These infective larvae can survive 3 to 4 weeks in favorable environmental conditions. On contact with the human host, the larvae penetrate the skin and are carried through the veins to the heart and then to the lungs. They penetrate into the pulmonary alveoli, ascend the bronchial tree to the pharynx, and are swallowed (4). The larvae reach the small intestine, where they reside and mature into adults. Adult worms live in the lumen of the small intestine, where they attach to the intestinal wall with resultant blood loss by the host (5). Most adult worms are eliminated in 1 to 2 years, but longevity records can reach several years. Some *Ancylostoma duodenale* larvae, following penetration of the host skin, can become dormant (in the intestine or muscle). In addition, infection by *A duodenale* may also occur by the oral and transmammary route. *Necator americanus,* however, requires a transpulmonary migration phase. Courtesy of Centers for Disease Control and Prevention.

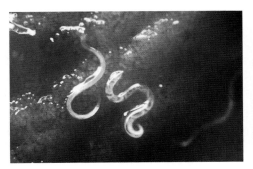

Image 64.5
This enlargement shows hookworms, *Ancylostoma caninum,* attached to the intestinal mucosa. Barely visible larvae penetrate the skin (often through bare feet), are carried to the lungs, go through the respiratory tract to the mouth, are swallowed, and eventually reach the small intestine. This journey takes about a week. Courtesy of Centers for Disease Control and Prevention.

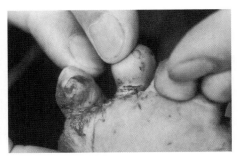

Image 64.6
This patient presented with a hookworm infection involving the toes of the right foot, which is also known as "ground itch." Usually the first sign of infection is itching and a rash at the site where skin touched contaminated soil or sand, which occurs when the larvae penetrate the skin, followed by anemia, abdominal pain, diarrhea, loss of appetite, and weight loss. Courtesy of Centers for Disease Control and Prevention.

65

Human Bocavirus

Clinical Manifestations

Human bocavirus (HBoV) first was identified in 2005 from a cohort of children with acute respiratory tract symptoms, including cough, rhinorrhea, wheezing, and fever. HBoV has been identified in 5% to 33% of all children with acute respiratory tract infections in various settings (eg, inpatient facilities, outpatient facilities, child care centers) using many different criteria to identify children for testing. The role of HBoV as a pathogen in human infection is confounded by simultaneous detection of other viral pathogens in patients from whom HBoV is identified, with coinfection rates as high as 80%. Current data have not proven that HBoV is a respiratory tract pathogen rather than simply a colonizing organism. HBoV has been detected in stool samples from children with acute gastroenteritis, but further studies are needed to determine the role of HBoV in gastroenteritis. Infection with HBoV appears to be ubiquitous, because nearly all children develop serologic evidence of previous HBoV infection by 5 years of age.

Etiology

HBoV is a nonenveloped, single-stranded DNA virus classified in the family Parvoviridae, genus *Bocaviru*. Three distinct genotypes have been described, although there are no data regarding antigenic variation or distinct serotypes.

Epidemiology

Detection of HBoV has been described only in humans. Transmission is presumed to be from respiratory tract secretions, although fecal-oral transmission may be possible on the basis of the finding of HBoV in stool specimens from children, including symptomatic children with diarrhea.

The frequent codetection of other viral pathogens of the respiratory tract in association with HBoV has led to speculation about the role played by HBoV: it may be a true copathogen, it can be shed for long periods after primary infection, or it may reactivate during subsequent viral infections. Extended and intermittent shedding of HBoV has been reported for up to 75 days after initial detection.

HBoV circulates worldwide and throughout the year. In temperate climates, seasonal clustering in the spring associated with increased transmission of other respiratory tract viruses has been reported.

Diagnostic Tests

Commercial molecular diagnostic assays for HBoV are available. HBoV PCR and detection of HBoV-specific antibody also are used by research laboratories to detect the presence of virus and infection, respectively.

Treatment

No specific therapy is available.

66

Human Herpesvirus 6 (Including Roseola) and 7

Clinical Manifestations

Clinical manifestations of primary infection with human herpesvirus 6 (HHV-6) include roseola (exanthem subitum) in approximately 20% of infected children, undifferentiated febrile illness without rash or localizing signs, and other acute febrile illnesses. HHV-6 infection often is accompanied by cervical and characteristic postoccipital lymphadenopathy, gastrointestinal tract or respiratory tract signs, and inflamed tympanic membranes. Fever usually is high (temperature >39.5°C [103.0°F]) and persists for 3 to 7 days. Approximately 20% of all emergency department visits for febrile children 6 through 12 months of age are attributable to HHV-6. Roseola is distinguished by the erythematous maculopapular rash that appears once fever resolves and can last hours to days. Febrile seizures are the most common complication and reason for hospitalization among children with primary HHV-6 infection. Approximately 10% to 15% of children with primary HHV-6 illnesses develop febrile seizures, predominantly between the ages of 6 and 18 months. Other neurologic manifestations that may accompany primary infection include a bulging fontanelle and encephalopathy or encephalitis. Hepatitis has been reported as a rare manifestation of initial illness. Congenital HHV-6 infection, which occurs in approximately 1% of newborn infants, generally is asymptomatic at birth. Whether clinical manifestations subsequently develop is not known.

The frequency and scope of the clinical manifestations occurring with human herpesvirus 7 (HHV-7) infection are unclear. Most primary infections with HHV-7 presumably are asymptomatic or mild and not distinctive. Some initial infections can present as typical roseola and may account for second or recurrent cases of roseola. Febrile illnesses associated with seizures also have been documented to occur during primary HHV-7 infection. Some investigators suggest that the association of HHV-7 with these clinical manifestations results from the ability of HHV-7 to reactivate HHV-6 from latency.

Following primary infection, HHV-6 and HHV-7 remain in a persistent or latent state and can reactivate. The clinical circumstances and manifestations of reactivation in healthy people are unclear. Illness associated with HHV-6 reactivation has been described primarily among immunocompromised recipients of solid organ and hematopoietic stem cell transplants. Among clinical findings associated with HHV-6 reactivation in these patients are fever, rash, hepatitis, bone marrow suppression, graft rejection, pneumonia, and encephalitis. A few cases of central nervous system symptoms have been reported in association with HHV-7 reactivation in immunocompromised hosts, but clinical findings generally have been reported less frequently with HHV-7 than with HHV-6 reactivation.

Etiology

HHV-6 and HHV-7 are lymphotropic agents that are closely related members of the Herpesviridae family, which, like all human herpesviruses, establish lifelong infection after initial exposure. HHV-6 strains have 2 distinct subgroups: variants A and B. Essentially all postnatally acquired primary infections in children are caused by variant B strains, except infections in some parts of Africa. Among congenital HHV-6 infections, however, as many as one-third may be caused by variant A.

Epidemiology

HHV-6 and HHV-7 cause ubiquitous infections in children worldwide. Humans are the only known natural host. Nearly all children acquire HHV-6 infection within the first 4 years of life, probably resulting from asymptomatic shedding of infectious virus in secretions of healthy family members or other close contacts. During the acute phase of primary infection, HHV-6 and HHV-7 can be isolated from peripheral blood mononuclear cells and from saliva of some children. Viral DNA subsequently can be detected throughout life by PCR assay in multiple body sites. Although HHV-6 and HHV-7 can be detected in blood mononuclear cells, salivary glands, lung, and skin, only HHV-6 frequently is found in brain and HHV-7 only in mammary glands. Virus-specific maternal antibody, which is present uniformly in the sera of infants at birth, provides transient partial protection. As the concentration of maternal antibody decreases during the first year of life, the rate of infection increases rapidly, peaking between 6 and 24 months of age. Infections occur throughout the year without a seasonal pattern. Secondary cases rarely are identified. Occasional outbreaks of roseola have been reported.

Congenital infection with HHV-6 occurs in approximately 1% of newborn infants as determined by the presence of HHV-6 DNA in cord blood. Most congenital infections appear to result from the germline passage of maternal or paternal chromosomally integrated HHV-6, a unique mechanism of transmission of human viral congenital infection. Transplacental HHV-6 infection also can occur from reinfection or reactivation of maternal HHV-6 infection or from reactivated maternal chromosomally integrated HHV-6. HHV-6 has not been identified in human milk.

HHV-7 infection usually occurs later in childhood compared with HHV-6. By adulthood, the seroprevalence of HHV-7 is approximately 85%. Infectious HHV-7 is present in more than 75% of saliva specimens obtained from healthy adults. Contact with infected respiratory tract secretions of healthy contacts is the probable mode of transmission of HHV-7 to young children. HHV-7 has been detected in human milk, peripheral blood mononuclear cells, cervical secretions, and other body sites. Congenital HHV-7 infection has not been demonstrated by the examination of large numbers of cord blood samples for HHV-7 DNA.

Incubation Period

HHV-6, mean of 9 to 10 days; HHV-7, unknown.

Diagnostic Tests

Multiple assays for detection of HHV-6 and HHV-7 have been developed, but few are available commercially, and many do not differentiate between new, past, and reactivated infection. Moreover, because laboratory diagnosis of HHV-6 or HHV-7 usually does not influence clinical management (infections among the severely immunocompromised can be an exception), these tests have limited utility in clinical practice. Diagnostic assays include serologic tests, isolation of the virus from tissue culture, and detection of viral DNA by qualitative and quantitative PCR and of RNA by reverse transcriptase PCR in blood, secretions, and tissues. Most of these assays are available only in research laboratories. Some serologic and DNA detection assays are available commercially.

Reference laboratories offer diagnostic testing for HHV-6 and HHV-7 infections by detection of viral DNA in blood and cerebrospinal fluid specimens. However, detection of HHV-6 DNA or HHV-7 DNA in peripheral blood mononuclear cells, other body fluids, and tissues generally does not differentiate between new infection and persistence of virus from past infection. DNA detection by PCR in plasma and sera has been used to diagnose acute primary infection, but these assays are not reliably sensitive in young children or specific in children with chromosomally integrated HHV-6 infection. Chromosomal integration of HHV-6 is indicated by consistently positive PCR tests for HHV-6 DNA in blood with high viral loads (≥ 1 copy of HHV-6 DNA per leukocyte) and is confirmed by detection of HHV-6 DNA in hair follicles.

Treatment

Supportive. Anecdotal reports suggest that use of ganciclovir or foscarnet may be beneficial for immunocompromised patients with serious HHV-6 disease, but resistance may occur.

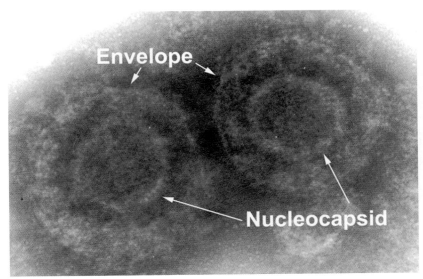

Image 66.1
Thin-section electron micrograph image of human herpesvirus 7, which causes roseola. Virions consist of a darkly staining core within the capsid that is surrounded by a proteinaceous tegument layer and enclosed within the viral envelope. Courtesy of Centers for Disease Control and Prevention.

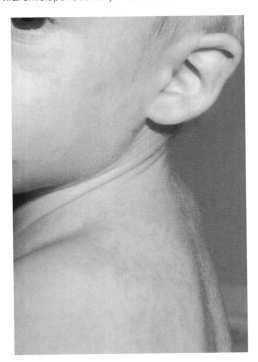

Image 66.2
A 13-month-old white male developed high fever that persisted for 4 days without recognized cause. The child appeared relatively well and the fever subsided, to be followed by a maculopapular rash that began on the trunk and spread to involve the face and extremities. The course was typical for roseola infantum. Courtesy of George Nankervis, MD.

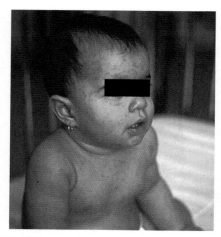

Image 66.3
A Hispanic female toddler with the exanthem of roseola following several days of high fever. Copyright Larry Frenkel, MD.

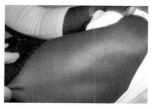

Image 66.4
A 3-year-old with 2 days of bounding fever to 103°F. Though febrile, he has still been active between fever spikes. He had a brief tonic-clonic seizure, but was not started on anticonvulsants because of his well appearance at the emergency department. He was diagnosed with a febrile seizure. The fever resolved, but the child was restricted from child care because of a fine rash all over. He was asymptomatic at the time his rash developed and was diagnosed with roseola. Despite reassurance, school admission was refused until the rash faded. Copyright Will Sorey, MD.

67

Human Herpesvirus 8

Clinical Manifestations

Human herpesvirus 8 (HHV-8) is the etiologic agent associated with Kaposi sarcoma (KS), primary effusion lymphoma, and multicentric Castleman disease (MCD). In regions with endemic disease, a primary infection syndrome in immunocompetent children has been described, which consists of fever and a maculopapular rash, often accompanied by upper respiratory tract signs. Primary infection among immunocompromised people and men who have sex with men tends to have more severe manifestations that include fever, rash, lymphadenopathy, splenomegaly, diarrhea, arthralgia, and KS. In parts of Africa, among children with and without HIV infection, KS is a frequent, aggressive malignancy. In the United States, KS rarely is observed among children. Most commonly, KS occurs among severely immunocompromised HIV patients in the United States. Among organ transplant recipients and other immunosuppressed patients, KS is an important cause of cancer-related deaths. Primary effusion lymphoma is rare among children. MCD has been described in adolescents, but the proportion of cases attributable to infection with HHV-8 is unknown.

Etiology

HHV-8 is a member of the family Herpesviridae, the gammaherpesvirus subfamily, and the *Rhadinovirus* genus.

Epidemiology

In regions with high endemicity, the epidemiology of HHV-8 closely reflects that observed for KS. In areas of Africa, the Amazon basin, Mediterranean, and Middle East, seroprevalence ranges from approximately 30% to 60%. Low rates of seroprevalence, generally less than 5%, have been reported in the United States, Northern and Central Europe, and most areas of Asia. Higher rates, however, occur in specific geographic regions, among adolescents and adults with or at high risk of acquiring HIV infection, injection drug users, and internationally adopted children coming from some Eastern European countries.

Acquisition of HHV-8 in areas with endemic infection frequently occurs before puberty, likely by oral inoculation of saliva of close contacts, especially secretions of mothers and siblings. Virus is shed frequently in saliva of infected people and becomes latent for life in peripheral blood mononuclear cells, primarily $CD^{19}+$ B lymphocytes, and lymphoid tissue. Sexual transmission appears to be the major route of infection among men who have sex with men. Transplantation of infected donor organs has been documented to result in HHV-8 infection. HHV-8 DNA has been detected in blood drawn at birth from infants born to HHV-8 seropositive mothers, suggesting vertical transmission is possible.

Incubation Period

Unknown.

Diagnostic Tests

Nucleic acid amplification testing and serologic assays for HHV-8 are available, and new assays with greater clinical usefulness are being developed. PCR tests may be used on peripheral blood and tissue biopsy specimens of patients with HHV-8–associated disease, such as KS. PCR detection of HHV-8 in peripheral blood specimens has been used in some patients to support the diagnosis of KS and to identify exacerbations of HHV-8–associated diseases, primarily MCD. However, HHV-8 DNA detection in the peripheral blood does not differentiate between latent and active replicating infection.

Currently available serologic assays measuring antibodies to HHV-8 include immunofluorescence assay (IFA), enzyme immunoassays, and Western blot assays using recombinant HHV-8 proteins. IFA is used most frequently. These serologic assays can detect both latent and lytic infection but are of limited use in the diagnosis and management of acute clinical disease.

Treatment

No antiviral treatment is approved for HHV-8 disease. HHV-8–associated malignancies can be treated with radiation and cancer chemotherapies.

68

HIV Infection

Clinical Manifestations

Human immunodeficiency virus (HIV) infection results in a wide array of clinical manifestations and varied natural history. HIV type 1 (HIV-1) is much more common in the United States than is HIV type 2 (HIV-2). Unless otherwise specified, this chapter addresses HIV-1 infection.

Acquired immunodeficiency syndrome (AIDS) is the name given to an advanced stage of HIV infection. The Centers for Disease Control and Prevention (CDC) uses a case definition that comprises AIDS-defining conditions for surveillance (Box 68.1). The CDC classifies all infected children younger than 13 years of age according to clinical stage of disease (Box 68.2) and immunologic status (Table 68.1). This pediatric classification system emphasizes the importance of the CD4+ T-lymphocyte count and percentage as critical immunologic parameters and as markers of prognosis. Data regarding plasma HIV-1 RNA concentration (viral load) are not included in this classification.

With timely diagnostic testing and appropriate treatment, clinical manifestations of HIV-1 infection and occurrence of AIDS-defining illnesses now are rare among children in the United States and other industrialized

Box 68.1
Case Definition of AIDS-Defining Conditions for Adults and Adolescents 13 Years of Age and Older[a]

- Candidiasis of bronchi, trachea, or lungs
- Candidiasis, esophageal
- Cervical cancer, invasive
- Coccidioidomycosis, disseminated or extrapulmonary
- Cryptococcosis, extrapulmonary
- Cryptosporidiosis, chronic intestinal (>1 mo duration)
- Cystoisosporiasis (isosporiasis), chronic intestinal (>1 mo duration)
- Cytomegalovirus disease (other than liver, spleen, or nodes)
- Cytomegalovirus retinitis (with loss of vision)
- Encephalopathy, HIV related
- Herpes simplex: chronic ulcer(s) (>1 mo duration) or bronchitis, pneumonitis, or esophagitis
- Histoplasmosis, disseminated or extrapulmonary
- Kaposi sarcoma
- Lymphoma, Burkitt (or equivalent term)
- Lymphoma, immunoblastic (or equivalent term)
- Lymphoma, primary or brain
- *Mycobacterium avium* complex or *Mycobacterium kansasii* infection, disseminated or extrapulmonary
- *Mycobacterium tuberculosis* infection, any site, pulmonary or extrapulmonary
- *Mycobacterium,* other species or unidentified species infection, disseminated or extrapulmonary
- *Pneumocystis jiroveci* pneumonia
- Pneumonia, recurrent
- Progressive multifocal leukoencephalopathy
- *Salmonella* septicemia, recurrent
- Toxoplasmosis of brain
- Wasting syndrome attributable to HIV
- CD4+ T-lymphocyte count <200/μL (0.20 x 10^9/L) or CD4+ T-lymphocyte percentage <15%

[a]Modified from Centers for Disease Control and Prevention. 1993 revised classification system for HIV infection and expanded surveillance case definition for AIDS among adolescents and adults. *MMWR Recomm Rep.* 1992;41(RR–17):1–19.

Box 68.2

Clinical Categories for Children Younger Than 13 Years With HIV Infection[a]

Category N: Not Symptomatic

Children who have no signs or symptoms considered to be the result of HIV infection or have only 1 of the conditions listed in Category A

Category A: Mildly Symptomatic

- Children with 2 or more of the conditions listed but none of the conditions listed in categories B and C
- Lymphadenopathy ($\geq$0.5 cm at >2 sites; bilateral at 1 site)
- Hepatomegaly
- Splenomegaly
- Dermatitis
- Parotitis
- Recurrent or persistent upper respiratory tract infection, sinusitis, or otitis media

Category B: Moderately Symptomatic

- Children who have symptomatic conditions other than those listed for category A or C that are attributed to HIV infection
- Anemia (hemoglobin <8 g/dL [<80 g/L]), neutropenia (white blood cell count <1,000/μL [<1.0 x 10^9/L]), and/or thrombocytopenia (platelet count <100 x 10^3/μL [<100 x 10^9/L]) persisting for $\geq$30 days
- Bacterial meningitis, pneumonia, or sepsis (single episode)
- Candidiasis, oropharyngeal (thrush), persisting (>2 mo) in children >6 mo
- Cardiomyopathy
- Cytomegalovirus infection, with onset before 1 mo of age
- Diarrhea, recurrent or chronic
- Hepatitis
- Herpes simplex virus (HSV) stomatitis, recurrent (>2 episodes within 1 year)
- HSV bronchitis, pneumonitis, or esophagitis with onset before 1 mo of age
- Herpes zoster (shingles) involving at least 2 distinct episodes or >1 dermatome
- Leiomyosarcoma
- Lymphoid interstitial pneumonia or pulmonary lymphoid hyperplasia complex
- Nephropathy
- Nocardiosis
- Persistent fever (lasting >1 mo)
- Toxoplasmosis, onset before 1 mo of age
- Varicella, disseminated (complicated chickenpox)

Box 68.2

Clinical Categories for Children Younger Than 13 Years With HIV Infection[a], continued

Category C: Severely Symptomatic

- Serious bacterial infections, multiple or recurrent (ie, any combination of at least 2 culture-confirmed infections within a 2-y period), of the following types: septicemia, pneumonia, meningitis, bone or joint infection, or abscess of an internal organ or body cavity (excluding otitis media, superficial skin or mucosal abscesses, and indwelling catheter-related infections)

- Candidiasis, esophageal or pulmonary (bronchi, trachea, lungs)

- Coccidioidomycosis, disseminated (at site other than or in addition to lungs or cervical or hilar lymph nodes)

- Cryptococcosis, extrapulmonary

- Cryptosporidiosis or cystoisosporiasis with diarrhea persisting >1 mo

- Cytomegalovirus disease with onset of symptoms after 1 mo of age (at a site other than liver, spleen, or lymph nodes)

- Encephalopathy (at least 1 of the following progressive findings present for at least 2 mo in the absence of a concurrent illness other than HIV infection that could explain the findings): (1) failure to attain or loss of developmental milestones or loss of intellectual ability, verified by standard developmental scale or neuropsychologic tests; (2) impaired brain growth or acquired microcephaly demonstrated by head circumference measurements or brain atrophy demonstrated by computed tomography or magnetic resonance imaging (serial imaging required for children <2 y; (3) acquired symmetric motor deficit manifested by ≥2 of the following: paresis, pathologic reflexes, ataxia, or gait disturbance

- HSV infection causing a mucocutaneous ulcer that persists for >1 mo or bronchitis, pneumonitis, or esophagitis for any duration affecting a child >1 mo

- Histoplasmosis, disseminated (at a site other than or in addition to lungs or cervical or hilar lymph nodes)

- Kaposi sarcoma

- Lymphoma, primary, in brain

- Lymphoma, small, noncleaved cell (Burkitt), or immunoblastic; or large-cell lymphoma of B-lymphocyte or unknown immunologic phenotype

- *Mycobacterium tuberculosis*, disseminated or extrapulmonary

- *Mycobacterium*, other species or unidentified species infection, disseminated (at a site other than or in addition to lungs, skin, or cervical or hilar lymph nodes)

- *Pneumocystis jiroveci* pneumonia

- Progressive multifocal leukoencephalopathy

- *Salmonella* (nontyphoid) septicemia, recurrent

- Toxoplasmosis of the brain with onset at after 1 mo of age

- Wasting syndrome in the absence of a concurrent illness other than HIV infection that could explain the following findings: (1) persistent weight loss >10% of baseline; (2) downward crossing of at least 2 of the following percentile lines on the weight-for-age chart (eg, 95th, 75th, 50th, 5th, 5th) in a child ≥1 y; OR (3) <5th percentile on weight-for-height chart on 2 consecutive measurements, ≥30 days apart; PLUS (1) chronic diarrhea (ie, at least 2 loose stools per day for >30 days); OR (2) documented fever (for >30 days, intermittent or constant)

[a] Modified from Centers for Disease Control and Prevention. 1994 revised classification system for human immunodeficiency virus infection in children less than 13 years of age. Official authorized addenda: human immunodeficiency virus infection codes and official guidelines for coding and reporting ICD-9-CM. *MMWR Recomm Rep.* 1994;43(RR-12);1-19.

Table 68.1
Pediatric HIV Classification for Children Younger Than 13 Years[a]

Immunologic Definitions	Immunologic Categories Age-Specific CD4+ T-Lymphocyte Count and Percentage of Total Lymphocytes[b]						Clinical Classifications[c]			
	<12 mo		1–5 y		6–12 y		N: No Signs or Symptoms	A: Mild Signs and Symptoms	B: Moderate Signs and Symptoms[d]	C: Severe Signs and Symptoms[d]
	µL	%	µL	%	µL	%				
1: No evidence of suppression	≥1,500	≥25	≥1,000	≥25	≥500	≥25	N1	A1	B1	C1
2: Evidence of moderate suppression	750–1,499	15–24	500–999	15–24	200–499	15–24	N2	A2	B2	C2
3: Severe suppression	<750	<15	<500	<15	<200	<15	N3	A3	B3	C3

[a]Modified from Centers for Disease Control and Prevention. 1994 revised classification system for human immunodeficiency virus infection in children less than 13 years of age. Official authorized addenda: human immunodeficiency virus infection codes and official guidelines for coding and reporting ICD-9-CM. *MMWR Recomm Rep.* 1994;43(RR-12):1–19.

[b]To convert values in µL to Système International units (x 10^9/L), multiply by 0.001.

[c]Children whose HIV infection status is not confirmed are classified by using this grid with a letter E (for perinatally exposed) placed before the appropriate classification code (eg, EN2).

[d]Lymphoid interstitial pneumonitis in category B or any condition in category C is reportable to state and local health departments as AIDS (AIDS-defining conditions).

countries. Early manifestations of pediatric HIV infection include unexplained fevers, generalized lymphadenopathy, hepatomegaly, splenomegaly, failure to thrive, persistent or recurrent oral and diaper candidiasis, recurrent diarrhea, parotitis, hepatitis, central nervous system (CNS) disease (eg, hyperreflexia, hypertonia, floppiness, developmental delay), lymphoid interstitial pneumonia, recurrent invasive bacterial infections, and other opportunistic infections (OIs) (eg, viral and fungal).

In the era of highly active antiretroviral therapy (HAART), there has been a substantial decrease in frequency of all OIs. The frequency of different OIs in the pre-HAART era varied by age, pathogen, previous infection history, and immunologic status. In the pre-HAART era, the most common OIs observed among children in the United States were infections caused by invasive encapsulated bacteria, *Pneumocystis jiroveci* (previously known as *Pneumocystis carinii)*, varicella-zoster virus, cytomegalovirus (CMV), *Herpes simplex* virus, *Mycobacterium avium* complex (MAC), and *Candida* species. Less commonly observed opportunistic pathogens included Epstein-Barr virus (EBV), *Mycobacterium tuberculosis, Cryptosporidium* species, *Cystoisospora* (formerly *Isospora*) species, other enteric pathogens, *Aspergillus* species, and *Toxoplasma gondii.*

Immune reconstitution inflammatory syndrome (IRIS) is a paradoxical clinical deterioration often seen in severely immunosuppressed people that occurs shortly after the initiation of HAART. Local symptoms develop secondary to an inflammatory response as cell-mediated immunity is restored. Underlying infection with mycobacteria (including *Mycobacterium tuberculosis),* herpesviruses, and fungi (including *Cryptococcal* species) predisposes to IRIS.

Malignant neoplasms in children with HIV-1 infection are relatively uncommon, but leiomyosarcomas and non-Hodgkin B-cell lymphomas of the Burkitt type (including some that occur in the CNS) occur more commonly in children with HIV infection than in immunocompetent children. Kaposi sarcoma is rare in children in the United States but has been documented in HIV-infected children

who have emigrated from sub-Saharan African countries. The incidence of malignant neoplasms in HIV-infected children has decreased during the HAART era.

Prognosis for survival is poor for untreated children who acquired HIV infection through mother-to-child transmission and who have high viral loads (ie, >100,000 copies/mL) and severe suppression of CD4+ T-lymphocyte counts (Table 68.1). In these children, AIDS-defining conditions developing during the first 6 months of life, including *P jiroveci* pneumonia (PCP), progressive neurologic disease, and severe wasting, are predictors of a poor outcome. When HAART regimens are begun early, prognosis and survival rates improve dramatically. Although deaths attributable to OIs have declined, non–AIDS-defining infections and multiorgan failure remain major causes of death. In the United States, mortality in HIV-infected children has declined from 7.2/100 person years in 1993 to 0.8/100 person years in 2006. The HIV mortality rate is approximately 30 times higher than for the general US pediatric population.

Etiology

As noted above, 2 types of HIV cause disease in humans: HIV-1 and HIV-2. These viruses are cytopathic lentiviruses belonging to the family Retroviridae, and they are related closely to the simian immunodeficiency viruses, agents in African green monkeys and sooty mangabeys. Three distinct genetic groups of HIV-1 exist worldwide: M (major), O (outlier), and N (new). Group M viruses are the most prevalent worldwide and comprise 8 genetic subtypes, or clades, known as A through H. The envelope glycoprotein interacts with the CD4 receptor and with 1 of 2 major coreceptors (CCR5 or CXCR4) on the host cell membrane. HIV-1 is an RNA virus that requires the activity of a viral enzyme, reverse transcriptase, to convert the viral RNA to DNA. A double-stranded DNA copy of the viral genome then can incorporate into the host cell genome, where it persists as a provirus.

HIV-2, the second AIDS-causing virus, predominantly is found in West Africa, with the highest rates of infection in Guinea-Bissau. The prevalence of HIV-2 in the United States is extremely low. HIV-2 is thought to have a milder disease course with a longer time to development of AIDS than HIV-1. Nonnucleoside reverse transcriptase inhibitors (NNRTIs) are not effective against HIV-2, whereas nucleoside reverse transcriptase inhibitors (NRTIs) and protease inhibitors have varying efficacy against HIV-2.

Epidemiology

Humans are the only known reservoir for HIV-1 and HIV-2. Latent virus persists in peripheral blood mononuclear cells and in cells of the brain, bone marrow, and genital tract even when plasma viral load is undetectable. Only blood, semen, cervicovaginal secretions, and human milk have been implicated epidemiologically in transmission of infection.

Established modes of HIV transmission include: (1) sexual contact (vaginal, anal, or orogenital); (2) percutaneous blood exposure (from contaminated needles or other sharp instruments); (3) mucous membrane exposure to contaminated blood or other body fluids; (4) mother-to-child transmission during pregnancy, around the time of labor and delivery, and postnatally through breastfeeding; and (5) transfusion with contaminated blood products. Cases of probable HIV transmission from HIV-infected caregiver to their infants through feeding blood-tinged premasticated food have been reported in the United States. As a result of highly effective screening methods, blood, blood components, and clotting factor virtually have been eliminated as a cause of HIV transmission in the United States since 1985. In the United States, transmission of HIV has not been documented with usual household contact. Transmission has been documented after contact of nonintact skin with blood-containing body fluids. Moreover, transmission of HIV has not been documented in schools or child care settings in the United States.

Pediatric AIDS cases account for fewer than 1% of all reported cases of AIDS in the United States. Since the mid 1990s, the number of reported pediatric AIDS cases decreased significantly, primarily because of interruption of mother-to-child transmission of HIV. The decrease in rate of mother-to-child transmission of HIV in the United States was attribut-

able to development and implementation of antenatal HIV testing programs and of interventions to prevent transmission: antiretroviral (ARV) prophylaxis during the antepartum, intrapartum, and postnatal periods; cesarean delivery before labor and before rupture of membranes; and complete avoidance of breastfeeding. Combination ARV regimens during pregnancy have been associated with lower rates of mother-to-child transmission than has zidovudine alone. Currently in the United States, most HIV-infected pregnant women receive 3-drug combination ARV regimens either for treatment of their own HIV infection or, if criteria for treatment are not yet met, for prevention of mother-to-child transmission of HIV (in which case the drugs are stopped after delivery). The CDC estimates that each year, 215 to 370 infants with HIV infection are born in the United States.

The risk of infection for an infant born to an HIV-seropositive mother who did not receive interventions to prevent transmission is estimated to range from 12% to 40% and is thought to average between 21% and 25% in the United States. Most mother-to-child transmission is intrapartum, with smaller proportions of transmission occurring in utero and postnatally through breastfeeding. Various risk factors for mother-to-child transmission of HIV have been identified and can be categorized as follows: (1) the amount of virus to which the child is exposed (especially the maternal viral load; a higher maternal viral load is associated with a lower maternal CD4+ T-lymphocyte count and with more advanced maternal clinical disease); (2) the duration of such exposure (eg, duration of ruptured membranes or of breastfeeding, vaginal vs cesarean delivery before labor and before rupture of membranes); and (3) factors that facilitate the transfer of virus from mother to child (eg, maternal breast pathologic lesions, infant oral candidiasis). In addition to these factors, characteristics of the virus and the child's susceptibility to infection are important. Of note, although maternal viral load is a critical determinant affecting the likelihood of mother-to-child transmission of HIV, transmissions have been observed across the entire range of maternal viral loads. The risk of mother-to-child transmission increases with each hour increase in the duration of rupture of membranes, and the duration of ruptured membranes should be considered when evaluating the need for special obstetric interventions. Cesarean delivery performed before onset of labor and before rupture of membranes has been shown to reduce mother-to-child intrapartum transmission. Current US guidelines recommend cesarean delivery before onset of labor and before rupture of membranes for HIV-infected women with a viral load greater than 1,000 copies/mL (irrespective of use of ARVs during pregnancy) and for women with unknown viral load near the time of delivery.

Postnatal transmission to neonates and young infants occurs mainly through breastfeeding. Worldwide, an estimated one-third to one-half of cases of mother-to-child transmission of HIV occurs as a result of breastfeeding. HIV genomes have been detected in cell-associated and cell-free fractions of human milk. In the United States, HIV-infected mothers are advised not to breastfeed, because safe alternatives to human milk are available readily. Because human milk cell-associated HIV can be detected even in women receiving antiretroviral therapy (ART), replacement (formula) feeding continues to be recommended for US mothers receiving ART. In resource-limited locations, women whose HIV infection status is unknown are encouraged to breastfeed their infants exclusively for the first 6 months of life, because the morbidity associated with formula feeding is unacceptably high. In addition, these women should be offered HIV testing. For HIV-infected mothers, 2010 World Health Organization guidelines recommend that exclusive breastfeeding be provided for the first 6 months of life. The introduction of complementary foods should occur after 6 months of life, and breastfeeding should continue through 12 months of life. Breastfeeding should be replaced only when a nutritionally adequate and safe diet can be maintained without human milk. In areas where ARVs are available, infants should receive daily nevirapine prophylaxis until 1 week after human milk consumption stops, or mothers should receive ARV prophylaxis (consisting of an ART regimen) for the first

6 months of their infants' lives. For infants known to be HIV-infected, mothers are encouraged to breastfeed exclusively for the first 6 months of life, and after the introduction of complementary foods, they should continue to breastfeed up to 2 years of age, as per recommendations for the general population.

Although the rate of acquisition of HIV infection among infants has decreased significantly in the United States, the rate of acquisition of HIV during adolescence and young adulthood continues to increase. HIV infection in adolescents occurs disproportionately among youth of minority race or ethnicity. Transmission of HIV among adolescents is attributable primarily to sexual exposure and secondarily to illicit intravenous drug use. Young men who have sex with men particularly are at high risk of acquiring HIV infection. Infection among young women primarily is acquired heterosexually. In 2006, 38% of new HIV infections in males 13 through 29 years of age were in men who have sex with men. From 2005 to 2008, respectively, the absolute number of newly diagnosed HIV infections in the United States decreased from 35,526 to 34,038, but the proportion of all new HIV infections contributed by this age group increased from 14% to 18%. In 2007, in 37 states and 5 dependent areas with confidential named-based HIV infection reporting, 4% of people living with HIV infection were people 13 through 24 years of age.

The ratio of male to female adolescents and young adults with a diagnosis of HIV infection increases with age at diagnosis. In 2007, 31% of people 13 through 19 years of age diagnosed with HIV infection were female, compared with 23% of young adults 20 through 24 years of age and 26% of adults 25 years of age and older. Most HIV-infected adolescents and young adults are asymptomatic and, without testing, remain unaware of their underlying serostatus.

Incubation Period

Approximately 12 to 18 months of age for untreated infants who acquired HIV infection through mother-to-child transmission, but some HIV-infected infants become ill in the first few months of life and others remain relatively asymptomatic for more than 5 to 11 years.

Diagnostic Tests

Laboratory diagnosis of HIV-1 infection during infancy is based on detection of the virus or viral nucleic acid (Table 68.2). Because infants born to HIV-infected mothers acquire maternal antibodies passively, antibody assays are not informative for diagnosis of infection in children younger than 18 months unless assay results are negative. However, in children 18 months of age and older, HIV antibody assays can be used for diagnosis.

In the United States, the preferred test for diagnosis of HIV infection in infants is the HIV DNA PCR assay. The DNA PCR assay can detect 1 to 10 DNA copies of proviral DNA in peripheral blood mononuclear cells. Approximately 30% to 40% of HIV-infected infants will have a positive HIV DNA PCR assay result in samples obtained before 48 hours of age. A positive result by 48 hours of age suggests in utero transmission. Approximately 93% of infected infants have detectable HIV DNA by 2 weeks of age, and approximately 95% of HIV-infected infants have a positive HIV DNA PCR assay result by 1 month of age. A single HIV DNA PCR assay has a sensitivity of 95% and a specificity of 97% for samples collected from infected children 1 to 36 months of age.

HIV isolation by culture is less sensitive, less available, and more expensive than the DNA PCR assay. Definitive results may take up to 28 days. This test no longer is recommended for routine diagnosis.

Detection of the antigen (including immune complex dissociated) is less sensitive than the HIV DNA PCR assay or culture. False-positive test results occur in samples obtained from infants younger than 1 month. This test generally should not be used, although newer assays have been reported to have sensitivities similar to HIV DNA PCR assays.

Plasma HIV RNA assays also have been used to diagnose HIV infection. However, a false-negative test result may occur in neonates receiving ARVs as prophylaxis. Although use of ART can reduce plasma viral loads to undetectable levels, results of DNA PCR assay, which detects cell-associated integrated HIV DNA, remain positive even among people with undetectable viral loads.

In the absence of therapy, plasma viral loads among infants who acquired HIV infection through mother-to-child transmission increase rapidly to very high levels (from several hundred thousand to more than 1 million copies/mL) after birth, decreasing only slowly to a

Table 68.2
Laboratory Diagnosis of HIV Infection

Test	Comment
HIV DNA PCR	Preferred test to diagnose HIV-1 subtype B infection in infants and children younger than 18 months of age; highly sensitive and specific by 2 weeks of age and available; performed on peripheral blood mononuclear cells. False-negative results can occur in non-B subtype HIV-1 infections.
HIV p24 Ag	Less sensitive, false-positive results during first month of life, variable results; not recommended.
ICD p24 Ag	Negative test result does not rule out infection; not recommended.
HIV culture	Expensive, not easily available, requires up to 4 weeks to do test; not recommended.
HIV RNA PCR	Preferred test to identify non-B subtype HIV-1 infections. Similar sensitivity and specificity to HIV DNA PCR in infants and children younger than 18 months of age, but DNA PCR is generally preferred due to greater clinical experience with that assay.

Abbreviations: Ag, antigen; HIV, human immunodeficiency virus; ICD, immune complex dissociated; PCR, polymerase chain reaction.

"set point" by approximately 2 years of age. This contrasts to infection in adults, in whom a viral load "set point" occurs approximately 6 months after acquisition of infection. An HIV RNA assay with only low-level viral copy number in an HIV-exposed infant may yield a false-positive result, reinforcing the importance of repeating any positive assay result to confirm the diagnosis of HIV infection in infancy. Like HIV DNA PCR assays, the sensitivity of HIV RNA assays for diagnosing infections in the first week of life is low (25%–40%), because transmission usually occurs around the time of delivery. The RNA assays approved by the US Food and Drug Administration provide quantitative results used to quantify virus as a predictor of disease progression rather than for routine diagnosis of HIV infection in infants. RNA assays are useful in monitoring changes in viral load during the course of antiretroviral therapy.

Diagnostic testing with HIV DNA or RNA assays is recommended at 14 to 21 days of age, and if results are negative, repeated at 1 to 2 months of age and again at 4 to 6 months of age. An infant is considered infected if 2 separate samples test positive by DNA or RNA PCR.

Viral diagnostic testing in the first few days of life (eg, <48 hours of age) is recommended by some experts to allow for early identification of infants with presumed in utero infection. If testing is performed at birth, umbilical cord blood should not be used because of possible contamination with maternal blood. Obtaining the sample as early as 14 days of age may facilitate decisions about initiating ARV therapy. If found to be infected, infants would be transitioned from neonatal ARV prophylaxis to ARV treatment. In nonbreastfed children younger than 18 months with negative HIV virologic test results, *presumptive* exclusion of HIV infection is based on

- Two negative HIV DNA or RNA virologic test results, from separate specimens, both of which were obtained at 2 weeks of age or older and one of which was obtained at 4 weeks of age or older **OR**
- One negative HIV DNA or RNA virologic test result from a specimen obtained at 8 weeks of age or older **OR**

- One negative HIV antibody test result obtained at 6 months of age or older **AND**
- No other laboratory or clinical evidence of HIV infection (ie, no subsequent positive results from virologic tests if tests were performed and no AIDS-defining condition for which there is no other underlying condition of immunosuppression)

In non-breastfed children younger than 18 months with negative HIV virologic test results, *definitive* exclusion of HIV is based on

- At least 2 negative HIV DNA or RNA virologic test results, from separate specimens, both of which were obtained at 1 month of age or older and one of which was obtained at 4 months of age or older
- At least 2 negative HIV antibody test results from separate specimens obtained at 6 months of age or older
- No other laboratory or clinical evidence of HIV infection (ie, no subsequent positive results from virologic tests if tests were performed and no AIDS-defining condition for which there is no other underlying condition of immunosuppression)

In children with 2 negative HIV DNA PCR test results, many clinicians will confirm the absence of antibody (ie, loss of passively acquired natural antibody) to HIV on testing at 12 through 18 months of age ("seroreversion"). A non-breastfed infant with 2 antibody-negative blood samples drawn at least 1 month apart and that were both obtained after 6 months of age is considered HIV uninfected.

Enzyme immunoassays (EIAs) are used widely as the initial test for serum HIV antibody. These tests are highly sensitive and specific. Repeated EIA testing of initially reactive specimens is common practice and is followed by Western blot analysis to confirm the presence of antibody specific to HIV. A positive HIV antibody test result (EIA followed by Western blot analysis) in a child 18 months of age or older almost always indicates infection, although passively acquired maternal antibody rarely can persist beyond 18 months of age. An HIV antibody test can be performed on samples of blood or oral fluid. Rapid tests for HIV antibodies have been licensed for use in the United States; these tests are used widely throughout the world, particularly to screen mothers of undocumented serostatus in maternity settings. As with standard EIA tests, confirmatory testing is required for a positive rapid test. Results from rapid testing are available within 20 minutes; however, confirmatory Western blot analysis results may take 1 to 2 weeks in some settings.

Infants who acquire HIV infection through mother-to-child transmission commonly have high viral set points with progressive cellular immune dysfunction and immunosuppression resulting from a decrease in the total number of circulating CD4+ T lymphocytes. Sometimes, T-lymphocyte counts do not decrease until late in the course of infection. Changes in cell populations frequently result in a decrease in the normal CD4+ to CD8+ T-lymphocyte ratio of 1.0 or greater. This nonspecific finding, although characteristic of HIV-1 infection, also occurs with other acute viral infections, including infections caused by CMV and EBV. The risk of OIs correlates with the CD4+ T-lymphocyte percentage and count. The normal values for peripheral CD4+ T-lymphocyte counts are age related, and the lower limits of normal are provided in Table 68.1.

Adolescents and HIV Testing. Routine screening be offered to all adolescents at least once by 16 through 18 years of age in health care settings is recommended when the prevalence of HIV in the patient population is more than 0.1%. In areas of lower community prevalence, routine HIV testing is encouraged for all sexually active adolescents and adolescents with other risk factors for HIV infection.

Consent for Diagnostic Testing. The CDC recommends that diagnostic HIV testing and opt-out HIV screening be part of routine clinical care in all health care settings for patients 13 through 64 years of age, thus preserving the patient's option to decline HIV testing and allowing a provider-patient relationship conducive to optimal clinical and preventive care. However, laws concerning consent and confidentiality for HIV care differ among states. Public health statutes and legal precedents allow for evaluation and treatment of minors for sexually transmitted infections without parental knowledge or consent, but not every

state has explicitly defined HIV infection as a condition for which testing or treatment may proceed without parental consent. Providing information regarding HIV infection, diagnostic testing, transmission, and implications of infection is an essential component of the anticipatory guidance provided to all adolescents as part of primary care.

Treatment

Because HIV treatment options and recommendations change with time and vary with occurrence of ARV drug resistance and adverse event profile, consultation with an expert in pediatric HIV infection is recommended in the care of HIV-infected infants, children, and adolescents. Current treatment recommendations for HIV-infected children are available online (**http://aidsinfo.nih.gov**). Whenever possible, enrollment of HIV-infected children in clinical trials should be encouraged. Information about trials for adolescents and children can be obtained by contacting the AIDS Clinical Trials Information Service.

ARV therapy is indicated for most HIV-infected children. The principal objectives of therapy are to suppress viral replication maximally, restore and preserve immune function, reduce HIV-associated morbidity and mortality, minimize drug toxicity, maintain normal growth and development, and improve quality of life. Initiation of ARV therapy depends on age of the child and on a combination of virologic, immunologic, and clinical criteria. Data from both observational studies and clinical trials indicate that very early initiation of therapy reduces morbidity and mortality compared with starting treatment when clinically symptomatic or immune suppressed. Effective administration of early therapy will maintain the viral load at low or undetectable concentrations and will reduce viral mutation and evolution.

Initiation of ARV therapy is recommended as follows. (1) HIV-infected infants should receive ARV therapy irrespective of clinical symptoms, immune status, or viral load. (2) Children from 1 to younger than 5 years should receive ARV therapy if they have AIDS or significant HIV-related symptoms, regardless of CD4+

T-lymphocyte counts or plasma viral load values; if they have a CD4+ T-lymphocyte percentage less than 25%, regardless of symptoms or viral load; or if they are asymptomatic or mildly symptomatic and they have a CD4+ T-lymphocyte percentage 25% or greater and a viral load of 100,000 copies/mL or greater. (3) Children 5 years or older should receive ARV therapy if they have AIDS or significant HIV-related symptoms), if they have a CD4+ T-lymphocyte count of 500 cells/mm³ or less, or if they are asymptomatic or mildly symptomatic and they have a CD4+ T-lymphocyte count greater than 500 cells/mm³ and a viral load of 100,000 copies/mL or greater. Starting ARV therapy should be considered for HIV-infected children from 1 to younger than 5 years who are asymptomatic or have mild symptoms and have a CD4+ T-lymphocyte percentage of 25% or greater and a viral load less than 100,000 copies/mL. Initiation of ARV therapy also should be considered for HIV-infected children 5 years or older who are asymptomatic or have mild symptoms and have a CD4+ T-lymphocyte count greater than 500 cells/mm³ and a viral load less than 100,000 copies/mL. The child and the child's primary caregiver must be able to adhere to the prescribed regimen.

Initiation of treatment of adolescents generally follows guidelines for adults, for whom initiation of treatment strongly is recommended: If an AIDS-defining illness is present or if the CD4+ T-lymphocyte count is less than 350 cells/mm³; if the CD4+ T-lymphocyte count is 350 to 500 cells/mm³; or regardless of CD4+ T-lymphocyte count in patients with HIV-associated nephropathy or with hepatitis B virus infection when treatment of hepatitis B virus is recommended. ARV treatment should be considered for patients with CD4+ T-lymphocyte counts greater than 500 cells/mm³. Dosages of ARVs should be prescribed according to Tanner staging of puberty, and not only on the basis of age; adolescents in early puberty (Tanner stages I and II) should be prescribed doses based on pediatric schedules, and adolescents in late puberty (Tanner stage V) should be prescribed doses based on adult schedules. In general, combination ARV therapy with at least 3 drugs is recommended for all HIV-infected individuals requiring ARV therapy. Drug regimens most often include 2 NRTIs plus either a protease inhibitor or an NNRTI (http://aidsinfo.nih.gov).

Immune globulin intravenous therapy has been used in combination with ARV therapy for HIV-infected children with hypogammaglobulinemia (IgG <400 mg/dL [4.0 g/L]) and could be considered for HIV-infected children who have recurrent, serious bacterial infections, such as bacteremia, meningitis, or pneumonia. Trimethoprim-sulfamethoxazole prophylaxis may provide comparable protection. Typically, neither form of prophylaxis is necessary for patients receiving effective ARV therapy.

Early prophylaxis, diagnosis, and aggressive treatment of OIs can prolong survival. This particularly is true for PCP, which accounts for approximately one-third of pediatric AIDS diagnoses overall and may occur early in the first year of life. Because mortality rates are high, chemoprophylaxis should be given to all HIV-exposed infants with indeterminate HIV infection status starting at 4 to 6 weeks of age. If PCP prophylaxis is started at 4 to 6 weeks of age in an HIV-exposed infant with indeterminate HIV infection status, prophylaxis can be stopped if the child subsequently meets criteria for presumptive or definitive lack of HIV infection. Prophylaxis is not recommended for infants who meet criteria for presumptive or definitive HIV uninfected status. Thus, for infants with negative HIV diagnostic test results at 2 and 4 weeks of age (and no positive tests or clinical symptoms and who are, therefore, presumptively not infected with HIV), PCP prophylaxis would not need to be initiated. All infants with HIV infection should receive PCP prophylaxis through 1 year of age regardless of immune status. The need for PCP prophylaxis for HIV-infected children 1 year of age and older is determined by the degree of immunosuppression, as determined by CD4+ T-lymphocyte counts.

Guidelines for prevention and treatment of OIs in children, adolescents, and adults provide indications for administration of drugs for infection with MAC, CMV, T gondii, and other organisms. Successful suppression of HIV replication in the blood to undetectable levels by ART has resulted in relatively normal CD4+ and CD8+ T-lymphocyte counts, leading to a dramatic decrease in the occurrence of most OIs. Limited data on the safety of discontinuing prophylaxis in HIV-infected children receiving ART are available. Prophylaxis should not be discontinued in HIV-infected infants. For older children, many experts consider discontinuing PCP prophylaxis for those who have received at least 6 months of ART on the basis of CD4+ T-lymphocyte count (1) for children 1 through 5 years of age: CD4+ T-lymphocyte percentage of at least 15% or CD4+ T-lymphocyte absolute count of at least 500 cells/µL for more than 3 consecutive months and (2) for children 6 years of age or older: CD4+ T-lymphocyte percentage of at least 15% or the CD4+ T-lymphocyte absolute count of at least 200 cells/µL for more than 3 consecutive months. Subsequently, the CD4+ T-lymphocyte absolute count or percentage should be reevaluated at least every 3 months. Prophylaxis should be reinstituted if the original criteria for prophylaxis are reached again.

Immunization Recommendations. All recommended childhood immunizations should be given to HIV-exposed infants. If HIV infection is confirmed, then guidelines for the HIV-infected child should be followed. Children with HIV infection should be immunized as soon as is age appropriate with inactivated vaccines. Trivalent inactivated influenza vaccine should be given annually according to the most current recommendations. Additionally, live-virus vaccines (measles-mumps-rubella [MMR] and varicella) can be given to asymptomatic HIV-infected children and adolescents with appropriate CD4+ T-lymphocyte percent-

ages (ie, >15% in children 1 through 5 years of age). Measles-mumps-rubella-varicella vaccine should not be administered to HIV-infected infants because of lack of safety data in this population. Rotavirus vaccine can be given to HIV-exposed and HIV-infected infants irrespective of CD4+ T-lymphocyte count. HIV-infected children should all receive a dose of 23-valent polysaccharide pneumococcal vaccine after 24 months of age, with a minimal interval of 8 weeks since the last conjugate pneumococcal vaccine. The suggested schedule for administration of these vaccines is provided in the recommended childhood and adolescent immunization schedule. The immunologic response to these vaccines in HIV-infected infants and children may be less robust and less persistent than in immunocompetent infants and children.

Children Who Are HIV Uninfected Residing in the Household of an HIV-Infected Person. Members of households in which an adult or child has HIV infection can receive MMR vaccine, because these vaccine viruses are not transmitted person to person. To decrease the risk of transmission of influenza to patients with symptomatic HIV infection, all household members 6 months of age or older should receive yearly influenza immunization. Immunization with varicella vaccine of siblings and susceptible adult caregivers of patients with HIV infection is encouraged to prevent acquisition of wild-type varicella-zoster virus infection, which can cause severe disease in immunocompromised hosts. Transmission of varicella vaccine virus from an immunocompetent host to a household contact is uncommon.

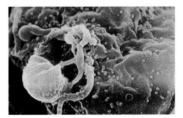

Image 68.1
Scanning electron micrograph of HIV-1 budding from cultured lymphocyte. Courtesy of Centers for Disease Control and Prevention/C. Goldsmith, P. Feorino, E.L. Palmer, W.R. McManus.

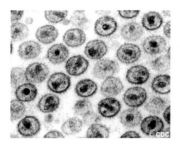

Image 68.2
HIV-1. Transmission electron micrograph. Cone-shaped cores are sectioned in various orientations. Viral genomic RNA is located in the electron-dense wide end of the core. Courtesy of Centers for Disease Control and Prevention/Dr Edwin P. Ewing, Jr.

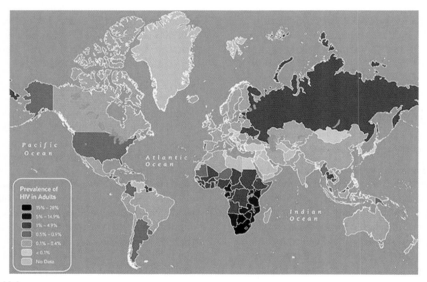

Image 68.3
HIV prevalence in adults, 2009. Courtesy of Centers for Disease Control and Prevention.

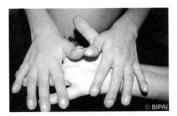

Image 68.4

Digital clubbing in a child with HIV infection and lymphoid interstitial pneumonitis/pulmonary lymphoid hyperplasia (LIP/PLH). Marked lymphadenopathy, hepatosplenomegaly, and salivary gland enlargement also are observed in many children with LIP/PLH. The clinical course of LIP/PLH is variable. Exacerbation of respiratory distress and hypoxemia can occur in association with intercurrent viral respiratory illnesses. Spontaneous clinical remission sometimes is observed. Copyright Baylor International Pediatric AIDS Initiative/Mark Kline, MD, FAAP.

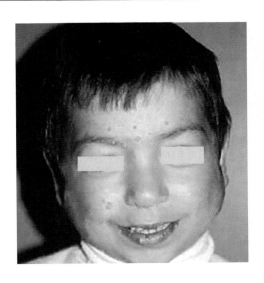

Image 68.5

Bilateral parotid gland enlargement in an HIV-infected male child with lymphoid interstitial pneumonitis/pulmonary lymphoid hyperplasia. Note the presence of multiple lesions of molluscum contagiosum, which are commonly seen in patients with HIV, particularly those with a low CD4 lymphocyte count. (See also **Molluscum Contagiosum.**) Copyright Baylor International Pediatric AIDS Initiative/Mark Kline, MD, FAAP.

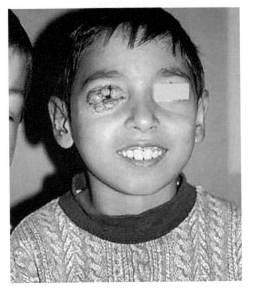

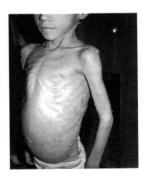

Image 68.6

Severe molluscum contagiosum in a boy with HIV infection. Some HIV-infected children develop molluscum contagiosum lesions that are unusually large or widespread. They are often seated more deeply in the epidermis. (See also **Molluscum Contagiosum.**) Copyright Baylor International Pediatric AIDS Initiative/Mark Kline, MD, FAAP.

Image 68.7

Norwegian (crusted) scabies in a boy with HIV infection. Generalized scaling and hyperkeratotic, crusted plaques are present. (See also **Scabies.**) Copyright Baylor International Pediatric AIDS Initiative/Mark Kline, MD, FAAP.

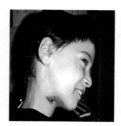

Image 68.8
An 8-year-old boy with HIV and tuberculous lymphadenitis (scrofula). Copious amounts of pus spontaneously drained from this lesion. In an immunocompromised child, other causes of lymphadenitis include infections with gram-positive bacteria, atypical mycobacterium, and *Bartonella henselae* (cat-scratch disease); malignant neoplasms such as lymphoma; masses such as branchial cleft cysts or cystic hygromas masquerading as lymph nodes; and adenitis due to HIV itself. (See also **Diseases Caused by Nontuberculous Mycobacteria.**) Copyright Baylor International Pediatric AIDS Initiative/ Mark Kline, MD, FAAP.

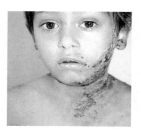

Image 68.9
Herpes zoster (shingles) in a boy with HIV infection. Such cases can be complicated by chronicity or dissemination. (See also **Varicella-Zoster Infections.**) Copyright Baylor International Pediatric AIDS Initiative/Mark Kline, MD, FAAP.

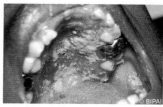

Image 68.11
Pseudomembranous candidiasis in a person with HIV infection. (See also **Candidiasis.**) Copyright Baylor International Pediatric AIDS Initiative/Mark Kline, MD, FAAP.

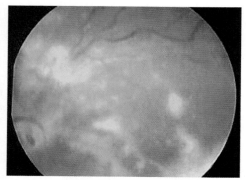

Image 68.10
Funduscopic examination of a 16-year-old female with HIV infection and cytomegalovirus retinitis. There are extensive areas of hemorrhage, with white retinal exudates. Children with cytomegalovirus retinitis usually present with painless visual impairment. (See also **Cytomegalovirus Infections.**) Copyright Baylor International Pediatric AIDS Initiative/Mark Kline, MD, FAAP.

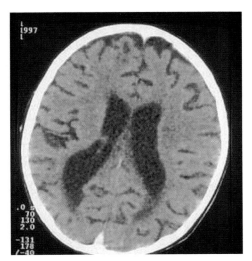

Image 68.12

Computed tomography scan of the brain of an 8-year-old boy with HIV infection and generalized brain atrophy. Cerebral atrophy is observed commonly among children with HIV-associated encephalopathy, but it also may be observed among children who are normal neurologically and developmentally. Copyright Baylor International Pediatric AIDS Initiative/Mark Kline, MD, FAAP.

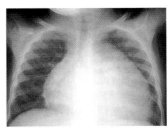

Image 68.13

Chest radiograph showing cardiomegaly in a 5-year-old girl with HIV infection, cardiomyopathy, and congestive heart failure. Many HIV-infected children with congestive heart failure respond well to medical management. Copyright Baylor International Pediatric AIDS Initiative/Mark Kline, MD, FAAP.

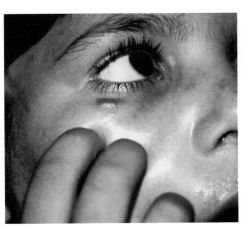

Image 68.14

A 7-year-old girl with HIV infection and a Kaposi sarcoma lesion. This tumor is rarely diagnosed among US children, with the occasional exceptions of children of Haitian descent with vertical HIV infection or older adolescents. Kaposi sarcoma is observed more commonly among HIV-infected children in some other geographic locales, including parts of Africa (eg, Zambia, Uganda) and Romania. Kaposi sarcoma has been linked to infection with a novel herpesvirus, now known as human herpesvirus 8 or Kaposi sarcoma–associated virus. Copyright Baylor International Pediatric AIDS Initiative/Mark Kline, MD, FAAP.

69

Influenza

Clinical Manifestations

Influenza typically begins with sudden onset of fever, often accompanied by chills or rigors, headache, malaise, diffuse myalgia, and non-productive cough. Subsequently, respiratory tract signs, including sore throat, nasal congestion, rhinitis, and cough, become more prominent. Conjunctival injection, abdominal pain, nausea, vomiting, and diarrhea less commonly are associated with influenza illness. In some children, influenza can manifest as an upper respiratory tract infection or as a febrile illness with few respiratory tract symptoms. Influenza is an important cause of otitis media. Acute myositis characterized by calf tenderness and refusal to walk has been described. In infants, influenza can produce a sepsis-like picture and occasionally can cause croup, bronchiolitis, or pneumonia. Although the large majority of children with influenza recover fully after 7 days, previously healthy children can have severe symptoms and complications. In the 2010–2011 influenza season, approximately 50% of all children hospitalized with influenza had no known underlying conditions. Neurologic complications associated with influenza range from febrile seizures to severe encephalopathy and encephalitis with status epilepticus, with resulting neurologic sequelae or death. Reye syndrome has been associated with influenza infection. Children with influenza or suspected influenza should not be given aspirin. Death from influenza-associated myocarditis has been reported. Invasive secondary infections or coinfections with group A streptococcus, *Staphylococcus aureus* (including methicillin-resistant *S aureus*), *Streptococcus pneumoniae*, or other bacterial pathogens can result in severe disease and death.

Etiology

Influenza viruses are orthomyxoviruses of 3 genera or types (A, B, and C). Epidemic disease is caused by influenza virus types A and B, and both influenza A and B virus antigens are included in influenza vaccines. Type C influenza viruses cause sporadic mild influenza-like illness in children, and antigens are not included in influenza vaccines. Influenza A viruses are subclassified into subtypes by 2 surface antigens, hemagglutinin (HA) and neuraminidase (NA). Examples of these include H1N1, H1N2, and H3N2 viruses. Specific antibodies to these various antigens, especially to HA, are important determinants of immunity. Minor variation within the same influenza B type or influenza A subtypes is called *antigenic drift*. Antigenic drift occurs continuously and results in new strains of influenza A and B viruses, leading to seasonal epidemics. *Antigenic shifts* are major changes in influenza A viruses that result in new subtypes that contain a new HA alone or with a new NA. Antigenic shift occurs only with influenza A viruses and can lead to pandemics if the new strain can infect humans and be transmitted efficiently from person to person in a sustained manner in the setting of little or no preexisting immunity.

From April 2009 to August 2010, the World Health Organization declared such a pandemic caused by influenza A (H1N1) virus. There now have been 4 influenza pandemics caused by antigenic shift in the 20th and 21st centuries. The 2009 pandemic was associated with 2 waves of substantial activity, occurring in the spring and fall of 2009 and extending well into winter 2010. During this time, more than 99% of virus isolates characterized were the 2009 pandemic influenza A (H1N1) virus. Humans, including children, occasionally are infected with influenza A viruses of swine or avian origin. Human infections with swine viruses have manifested as typical influenza-like illness, and confirmation of infection caused by an influenza virus of swine origin has been discovered retrospectively during routine typing of human influenza isolates. Rare but severe infections with influenza A subtype H5N1 viruses have been identified since 1997 in Asia, Africa, Europe, and the Middle East, areas where these viruses are present in domestic or wild birds. Other influenza subtypes of avian origin, including H7, also are identified occasionally in humans.

Epidemiology

Influenza is spread from person to person, primarily by respiratory tract droplets created by coughing or sneezing. Contact with respiratory tract droplet–contaminated surfaces is another possible mode of transmission. During community outbreaks of influenza, the highest incidence occurs among school-aged children. Secondary spread to adults and other children within a family is common. Incidence and disease severity depend, in part, on immunity developed as a result of previous experience (by natural disease) or recent influenza immunization with the circulating strain or a related strain. Antigenic drift in the circulating strain(s) is associated with seasonal epidemics. In temperate climates, seasonal epidemics usually occur during winter months. Peak influenza activity in the United States can occur anytime from November to May but most commonly occurs in January and February. Community outbreaks can last 4 to 8 weeks or longer. Circulation of 2 or 3 influenza virus strains in a community can be associated with a prolonged influenza season of 3 months or more and bimodal peaks in activity. Influenza is highly contagious, especially among semi-enclosed institutionalized populations and other ongoing, closed-group gatherings, such as school classrooms. Patients may become infectious during the 24 hours before onset of symptoms. Viral shedding in nasal secretions usually peaks during the first 3 days of illness and ceases within 7 days but can be prolonged in young children and immunodeficient patients. Viral shedding is correlated directly with degree of fever.

Incidence in healthy children generally is 10% to 40% each year, but illness rates as low as 3% also have been reported. Tens of thousands of children visit clinics and emergency departments because of influenza illness each season. Influenza and its complications have been reported to result in a 10% to 30% increase in the number of courses of antimicrobial agents prescribed to children during the influenza season. Although bacterial coinfections with a variety of pathogens have been reported, medical care encounters for children with influenza are an important cause of inappropriate antimicrobial use.

Hospitalization rates among children younger than 2 years are similar to hospitalization rates among people 65 years of age and older. Rates vary among studies (190–480 per 100,000 population) because of differences in methodology and severity of influenza seasons. However, children younger than 24 months consistently are at a substantially higher risk of hospitalization than older children. Antecedent influenza infection sometimes is associated with development of pneumococcal or staphylococcal pneumonia. Methicillin-resistant staphylococcal community-onset pneumonia, with a rapid clinical progression and a high fatality rate, has been reported in previously healthy children and adults with concomitant influenza infection. Rates of hospitalization and morbidity attributable to complications, such as pneumonia, are even greater in children with high-risk conditions, including hemoglobinopathies, bronchopulmonary dysplasia, asthma, cystic fibrosis, malignancy, diabetes mellitus, chronic renal disease, and congenital heart disease. Influenza virus infection in neonates also has been associated with considerable morbidity, including a sepsis-like syndrome, apnea, and lower respiratory tract disease.

Fatal outcomes, including sudden death, have been reported in both chronically ill and previously healthy children. Since influenza-related pediatric deaths became nationally notifiable in 2004, the number of deaths among children reported annually ranged from 46 to 153, until the 2009–2010 season, when the number increased to 279. During the entire influenza A (H1N1) pandemic period lasting from April 2009 to August 2010, a total of 344 laboratory-confirmed, influenza-associated pediatric deaths were reported. The 2010–2011 influenza season had at least 114 laboratory-confirmed, influenza-associated pediatric deaths. Most pediatric deaths are attributable to influenza A, and approximately 50% of children who died did not have a high-risk condition.

Incubation Period

2 days (range 1–4 days).

Diagnostic Tests

Specimens for viral culture or immunofluorescent or rapid diagnostic tests should be obtained, if possible, during the first 72 hours of illness, because the quantity of virus shed decreases rapidly as illness progresses beyond that point. Specimens of nasopharyngeal secretions obtained by swab, aspirate, or wash should be placed in appropriate transport media for culture. After inoculation into eggs or cell culture, influenza virus usually can be isolated within 2 to 6 days. Rapid diagnostic tests for identification of influenza A and B antigens in respiratory tract specimens are available commercially, although their reported sensitivity (44%–97%) and specificity (76%–100%) compared with viral culture are variable and differ by test and specimen type. Additionally, many rapid diagnostic antigen tests cannot distinguish between influenza subtypes, a feature that can be critical during seasons with strains that differ in antiviral susceptibility and/or relative virulence. Direct fluorescent antibody and indirect immunofluorescent antibody staining for detection of influenza A and B antigens in nasopharyngeal or nasal specimens are available at most hospital-based laboratories and can yield results in 3 to 4 hours. Results of immunofluorescent and rapid diagnostic tests should be interpreted in the context of clinical findings and local community influenza activity. Careful clinical judgment must be exercised, because the prevalence of circulating influenza viruses influences the positive and negative predictive values of these influenza screening tests. False-positive results are more likely to occur during periods of low influenza activity; false-negative results are more likely to occur during periods of peak influenza activity. Serologic diagnosis can be established retrospectively by a fourfold or greater increase in antibody titer in serum specimens obtained during the acute and convalescent stages of illness, as determined by hemagglutination inhibition testing, complement fixation testing, neutralization testing, or enzyme immunoassay; however, serologic testing rarely is useful in patient management, because 2 serum samples collected 10 to 14 days apart are required. Reverse transcriptase PCR (RT-PCR) testing of respiratory tract specimens is available at some institutions. Both RT-PCR and viral culture tests offer potential for high sensitivity as well as specificity and are recommended as the tests of choice.

Treatment

Influenza A viruses, including 2 subtypes (H1N1 and H3N2), and influenza B viruses circulate worldwide, but the prevalence of each can vary among communities and within a single community over the course of an influenza season. In the United States, 2 classes of antiviral medications currently are available for treatment or prophylaxis of influenza infections: neuraminidase inhibitors (oseltamivir and zanamivir) and adamantanes (amantadine and rimantadine).

Since 2005, all H3N2 strains in the United States have been resistant to adamantanes. Influenza B viruses intrinsically are resistant to adamantanes. Since January 2006, neuraminidase inhibitors (oseltamivir, zanamivir) have been the only recommended influenza antiviral drugs because of this widespread resistance to the adamantanes and the activity of neuraminidase inhibitors against influenza A and B viruses. Resistance to oseltamivir was documented for 1.3% of all tested 2010–2011 influenza viral samples. These resistance patterns among circulating influenza A virus strains simplify antiviral treatment, as 2009 influenza A (H1N1), influenza A (H3N2), and influenza B all were susceptible to neuraminidase inhibitors and resistant to adamantanes. Each year, options for treatment or chemoprophylaxis of influenza in the United States will depend on influenza strain resistance patterns.

Therapy for influenza virus infection should be offered to any child with presumed influenza or severe, complicated, or progressive illness, regardless of influenza-immunization status and for influenza infection of any severity in children with a condition that places them at increased risk. Children with severe influenza should be evaluated carefully for possible coinfection with bacterial pathogens (eg, S aureus) that might require antimicrobial therapy.

Table 69.1
Antiviral Drugs for Influenza[a]

Drug (Trade Name)	Virus	Administration	Treatment Indications	Prophylaxis Indications	Adverse Effects
Oseltamivir (Tamiflu)	A and B	Oral	≥1 y of age	≥1 y of age	Nausea, vomiting
Zanamivir (Relenza)	A and B	Inhalation	≥7 y of age	≥5 y of age	Bronchospasm
Amantadine[c] (Symmetrel)	A	Oral	≥1 y of age	≥1 y of age	Central nervous system, anxiety, gastrointestinal
Rimantadine[b] (Flumadine)	A	Oral	≥13 y of age	≥1 y of age	Central nervous system, anxiety, gastrointestinal

[a]For current recommendations about treatment and chemoprophylaxis of influenza, see **www.cdc.gov/flu/professionals/antivirals/index. htm** or **www.aapredbook.org/flu.**
[b]High levels of resistance to amantadine and rimantadine persist, and these drugs should not be used unless resistance patterns change significantly. Antiviral susceptibilities of viral strains are reported weekly at **www.cdc.gov/flu/weekly/fluactivity.htm.**

If antiviral therapy is prescribed, treatment should be started as soon after illness onset as possible and should not be delayed while waiting for a definitive influenza test result, because benefit is greatest when treatment is initiated within 48 hours of onset of symptoms. Treatment should be discontinued approximately 24 to 48 hours after symptoms resolve. The duration of treatment studied was 5 days for both the neuraminidase inhibitors (oseltamivir and zanamivir) and the adamantanes (amantadine and rimantadine). Only zanamivir, which is administered by inhalation, does not require adjustment for people with severe renal insufficiency.

Control of fever with acetaminophen or other appropriate antipyretic agents may be important in young children, because fever and other symptoms of influenza could exacerbate underlying chronic conditions. Children and adolescents with influenza should not receive aspirin or any salicylate-containing products because of the potential risk of developing Reye syndrome.

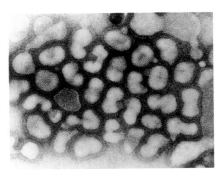

Image 69.1
Transmission electron micrograph of influenza A virus, late passage. Courtesy of Centers for Disease Control and Prevention/Dr Erskine Palmer.

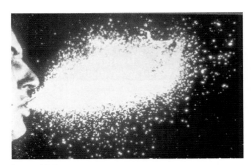

Image 69.2
Influenza, like many viral infections, is spread by droplet transmission or direct contact with items recently contaminated by infected naso-pharyngeal secretions. Courtesy of Centers for Disease Control and Prevention.

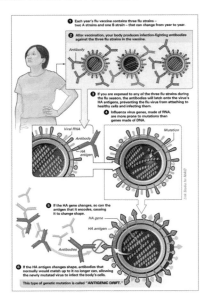

Image 69.3
Antigenic drift. Each year's flu vaccine contains 3 flu strains—2 A strains and 1 B strain—that can change from year to year. After vaccination, your body produces infection-fighting antibodies against the 3 flu strains in the vaccine. If you are exposed to any of the 3 flu strains during the flu season, the antibodies will latch onto the virus's hemagglutinin (HA) antigens, preventing the flu virus from attaching to healthy cells and infecting them. Influenza virus genes, made of RNA, are more prone to mutations than genes made of DNA. If the HA gene changes, so can the antigen that it encodes, causing it to change shape. If the HA antigen changes shape, antibodies that normally would match up to it no longer can, allowing the newly mutated virus to infect the body's cells. Courtesy of National Institute of Allergy and Infectious Diseases.

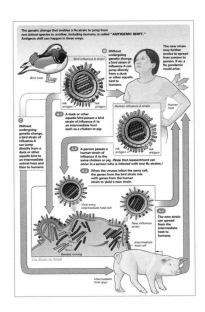

Image 69.4

Antigenic shift. The genetic change that enables a flu strain to jump from one animal species to another, including humans, is called antigenic shift. Antigenic shift can happen in 3 ways. *Antigenic shift 1:* A duck or other aquatic bird passes a bird strain of influenza A to an intermediate host, such as a chicken or pig. A person passes a human strain of influenza A to the same chicken or pig. When the viruses infect the same cell, genes from the bird strain mix with genes from the human strain to yield a new strain. The new strain can spread from the intermediate host to humans. *Antigenic shift 2:* Without undergoing genetic change, a bird strain of influenza A can jump directly from a duck or other aquatic bird to humans. *Antigenic shift 3:* Without undergoing genetic change, a bird strain of influenza A can jump directly from a duck or other aquatic bird to an intermediate animal host and then to humans. The new strain may further evolve to spread from person to person. If so, a flu pandemic could arise. Courtesy of National Institute of Allergy and Infectious Diseases.

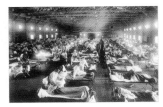

Image 69.5

Emergency hospital during 1918 influenza epidemic, Camp Funston, KS. Source: National Museum of Health and Medicine, Armed Forces Institute of Pathology, Washington, DC, Image NCP 1603. Courtesy of Immunization Action Coalition.

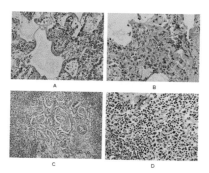

Image 69.6

Pathologic findings from a patient with confirmed influenza A (H5N1) infection (hematoxylin-eosin stain, magnification x40). Panel A shows hyaline membrane formation lining the alveolar spaces of the lung and vascular congestion with a few infiltrating lymphocytes in the interstitial areas. Reactive fibroblasts are also present. Panel B is an area of lung with proliferating reactive fibroblasts within the interstitial areas. Few lymphocytes are seen, and no viral intranuclear inclusions are visible. Panel C shows fibrinous exudates filling the alveolar spaces, with organizing formation and few hyaline membranes. The surrounding alveolar spaces contain hemorrhage. Panel D is from a section of spleen, showing numerous atypical lymphoid cells scattered around the white pulp. No viral intranuclear inclusions are seen. Courtesy of Centers for Disease Control and Prevention.

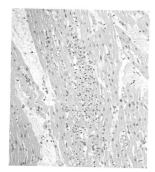

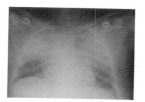

Image 69.8

Influenza pneumonia in a 12-year-old male with respiratory failure. Copyright Benjamin Estrada, MD.

Image 69.7

Focal myocarditis seen in the previous patient with influenza B infection. Note myocardial necrosis associated with areas of mostly mononuclear inflammation. Courtesy of Centers for Disease Control and Prevention.

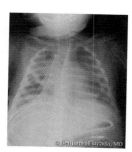

Image 69.10

Influenza A with *Staphylococcus aureus* superinfection in a 6-year-old. Note the presence of bilateral pneumatoceles. Copyright Benjamin Estrada, MD.

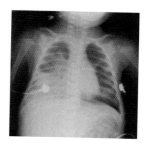

Image 69.9

Influenza A with *Staphylococcus aureus* pneumonia with empyema in a preschool-aged child. Copyright Benjamin Estrada, MD.

70

Isosporiasis (now designated as Cystoisosporiasis)

Clinical Manifestations

Watery diarrhea is the most common symptom and can be profuse and protracted, even in immunocompetent people. Manifestations are similar to those caused by other enteric protozoa (eg, *Cryptosporidium* and *Cyclospora* species) and can include abdominal pain, cramping, anorexia, nausea, vomiting, weight loss, and low-grade fever. Eosinophilia also can occur. The proportion of infected people who are asymptomatic is unknown. Severity of infection ranges from self-limiting in immunocompetent hosts to debilitating and life-threatening in immunocompromised patients, particularly people infected with HIV. Infections of the biliary system also have been reported.

Etiology

Cystoisospora belli (formerly *Isospora belli*) is a coccidian protozoan; oocysts (rather than cysts) are passed in stools.

Epidemiology

Infection occurs predominantly in tropical and subtropical regions of the world and can cause traveler's diarrhea. Infection results from ingestion of sporulated oocysts (eg, in contaminated food and water). Humans are the only known host for *C belli* and shed non-infective oocysts in feces. These oocysts must mature (sporulate) outside the host in the environment to become infective. Under favorable conditions, sporulation can be completed in 1 to 2 days and perhaps more quickly. Oocysts probably are resistant to most disinfectants and can remain viable for prolonged periods in a cool, moist environment.

Incubation Period

Uncertain; range 7 to 12 days in reported cases.

Diagnostic Tests

Identification of oocysts in feces or in duodenal aspirates or finding developmental stages of the parasite in biopsy specimens (eg, of the small intestine) is diagnostic. Oocysts in stool are elongate and ellipsoidal (length, 25–30 μm). Oocysts can be shed in low numbers, even by people with profuse diarrhea. This constraint underscores the utility of repeated stool examinations, sensitive recovery methods (eg, concentration methods), and detection methods that highlight the organism (eg, oocysts stain bright red with modified acid-fast techniques and autofluoresce when viewed by ultraviolet fluorescent microscopy). PCR is an emerging and promising tool for diagnosis.

Treatment

Trimethoprim-sulfamethoxazole, typically for 7 to 10 days, is the drug of choice. Immunocompromised patients may need higher doses and longer duration of therapy. Pyrimethamine (plus leucovorin, to prevent myelosuppression) is an alternative treatment for people who cannot tolerate trimethoprim-sulfamethoxazole. Ciprofloxacin is less effective than trimethoprim-sulfamethoxazole. Nitazoxanide also has been reported to be effective. Maintenance therapy to prevent recurrent disease may be indicated for people infected with HIV.

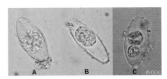

Image 70.1

Oocysts of *Cystoisospora belli* (iodine stain). The oocysts are large (25–30 µm) and have a typical ellipsoidal shape. When excreted, they are imma-ture and contain 1 sporoblast (A, B). The oocyst matures after excretion: the single sporoblast divides into 2 sporoblasts (C), which develop cyst walls, becoming sporocysts, which eventually contain 4 sporozoites each. Courtesy of Centers for Disease Control and Prevention.

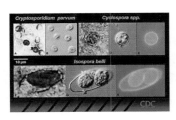

Image 70.2

Oocysts of *Cystoisospora belli* also can be stained with acid-fast stain and visualized by epifluorescence on wet mounts, as illustrated. Three coccidian parasites that most commonly infect humans, seen in acid-fast stained smears (A, C, F), bright-field differential interference contrast (B, D, G), and epifluorescence (C, E, H; *Cryptosporidium parvum* oocysts do not auto-fluoresce). Courtesy of Centers for Disease Control and Prevention.

71

Kawasaki Disease

Clinical Manifestations

Kawasaki disease is a febrile, exanthematous, multisystem vasculitis recognized on all continents. If untreated, approximately 20% of children can develop coronary artery abnormalities, including aneurysms. Approximately 80% of cases of Kawasaki disease occur in children younger than 5 years. The illness is characterized by fever and the following clinical features: (1) bilateral bulbar conjunctival injection with limbic sparing and without exudate; (2) erythematous mouth and pharynx, strawberry tongue, and red, cracked lips; (3) a polymorphous, generalized, erythematous rash that can be morbilliform, maculopapular, or scarlatiniform or can resemble erythema multiforme; (4) changes in the peripheral extremities consisting of induration of the hands and feet with erythematous palms and soles, often with later periungual desquamation; and (5) acute, nonsuppurative, usually unilateral, cervical lymphadenopathy with at least one node 1.5 cm in diameter. For diagnosis of classic Kawasaki disease, patients should have fever for at least 5 days (or fever until the date of treatment if given before the fifth day of illness) and at least 4 of the above 5 features without alternative explanation for the findings. The epidemiologic case definition also allows diagnosis of incomplete Kawasaki disease when a child has fewer than 4 principal clinical criteria in the presence of fever and coronary artery abnormalities. Irritability, abdominal pain, diarrhea, and vomiting commonly are associated features. Other findings include urethritis with sterile pyuria (70% of cases), mild anterior uveitis (25%–50%), mild hepatic enzyme elevation (50%), arthritis or arthralgia (10%–20%), meningismus with cerebrospinal fluid pleocytosis (25%), pericardial effusion of at least 1 mm (<5%), gallbladder hydrops (<10%), and myocarditis manifested by congestive heart failure (<5%). A persistent resting tachycardia and the presence of an S3 gallop often are appreciated. Fine desquamation in the groin area can occur in the acute phase of disease. Inflammation or ulceration can be observed at the inoculation scar of previous bacille Calmette-Guérin immuniza-

tion. Rarely, Kawasaki disease can present with what appears to be septic shock with need for intensive care; these children often have significant thrombocytopenia at admission. Group A streptococcal or *Staphylococcus aureus* toxic shock syndrome should be excluded in such cases.

Incomplete Kawasaki disease can be diagnosed in febrile patients when fever plus fewer than 4 of the characteristic features are present. Patients with fewer than 4 of the characteristic features and who have additional findings not listed above (eg, purulent conjunctivitis) should not be considered to have incomplete Kawasaki disease. The proportion of children with Kawasaki disease with incomplete manifestations is higher among patients younger than 12 months. Infants with Kawasaki disease also have a higher risk of developing coronary artery aneurysms than do older children, making diagnosis and timely treatment especially important in this age group. Laboratory findings in incomplete cases are similar to findings in classic cases. Therefore, although laboratory findings in Kawasaki disease are nonspecific, they may prove useful in increasing or decreasing the likelihood of incomplete Kawasaki disease. If coronary artery ectasia or dilatation is evident, diagnosis can be made with certainty. A normal early echocardiographic study is typical and does not exclude the diagnosis but can be useful in evaluation of patients with suspected incomplete Kawasaki disease. Incomplete Kawasaki disease should be considered in any child with unexplained fever for 5 days or longer in association with 2 or more of the principal features of this illness and supportive laboratory data (eg, erythrocyte sedimentation rate [ESR] ≥40 mm/hour or C-reactive protein [CRP] concentration ≥3.0 mg/dL). Image 71.1 is the American Heart Association algorithm for diagnosis and treatment of suspected incomplete Kawasaki disease.

The average duration of fever in untreated Kawasaki disease is 10 days; however, fever can last 2 weeks or longer. After fever resolves, patients can remain anorectic and/or irritable for 2 to 3 weeks. During this phase, desquamation of the groin, fingers, and toes and fine desquamation of other skin may occur. Recurrent disease occurring months to years later develops in approximately 2% of patients.

Coronary artery abnormalities can be demonstrated with 2-dimensional echocardiography in approximately 20% of patients who are not treated within 10 days of onset of fever. Increased risk of developing coronary artery aneurysms is associated with male sex; age younger than 12 months or older than 8 years; Asian or Hispanic ethnicity, high baseline neutrophil (>30,000 cells/mm³) and band count; low hemoglobin concentration (<10 g/dL); hypoalbuminemia, hyponatremia, or thrombocytopenia at presentation; fever persisting 48 hours or occurring after immune globulin intravenous (IGIV) administration; and persistence of elevated ESR or CRP for more than 30 days, or recurrent elevations. Aneurysms of the coronary arteries have been demonstrated by echocardiography as early as 5 to 7 days after onset of illness but more typically occur between 1 and 4 weeks after onset of illness; their initial appearance later than 6 weeks is uncommon. Giant coronary artery aneurysms (diameter ≥8 mm) likely are associated with long-term complications. Aneurysms occurring in other medium-sized arteries (eg, iliac, femoral, renal, and axillary vessels) are uncommon and generally do not occur in the absence of significant coronary abnormalities. In addition to coronary artery disease, carditis can involve the pericardium, myocardium, or endocardium, and mitral or aortic regurgitation or both can develop. Carditis generally resolves when fever resolves.

In children with mild coronary artery dilation or ectasia, coronary artery dimensions often return to baseline within 6 to 8 weeks after onset of disease. Approximately 50% of coronary aneurysms (fewer giant aneurysms) regress to normal luminal size within 1 to 2 years, although this process can be accompanied by development of coronary stenosis. In addition, regression of aneurysm(s) may result in a poorly compliant, fibrotic vessel wall.

The current case-fatality rate in the United States and Japan is less than 0.2%. The principal cause of death is myocardial infarction resulting from coronary artery occlusion attributable to thrombosis or progressive stenosis. Rarely, a large coronary artery aneurysm may rupture. The relative risk of mortality is highest within 6 weeks of onset of symptoms, but myocardial infarction and sudden death can occur months to years after the acute episode.

Etiology

The cause is unknown. Epidemiologic and clinical features suggest an infectious cause or trigger.

Epidemiology

Peak age of occurrence in the United States is between 18 and 24 months. Fifty percent of patients are younger than 2 years, and 80% are younger than 5 years. In children younger than 6 months, the diagnosis often is delayed, because the clinical complex of Kawasaki disease is incomplete. The male-to-female ratio is approximately 1.5:1. In the United States, 4,000 to 5,500 cases are estimated to occur each year. Kawasaki disease first was described in Japan, where a pattern of endemic occurrence with superimposed epidemic outbreaks was recognized. A similar pattern of disease occurrence with occasional sharply defined community-wide epidemics has been recognized in North America and Hawaii. Clusters generally occur during winter and spring. No evidence indicates person-to-person or common-source spread, although the incidence is slightly higher in siblings of children with the disease.

Incubation Period

Unknown.

Diagnostic Tests

No specific diagnostic test is available. The diagnosis is established by fulfillment of the clinical criteria and clinical or laboratory exclusion of other similar illnesses, such as staphylococcal or streptococcal toxin-mediated disease; drug reactions (eg, Stevens-Johnson syndrome); measles, adenovirus, parvovirus B19, or enterovirus infections; rickettsial exanthems; leptospirosis; systemic onset juvenile idiopathic arthritis; and reactive arthritis. A greatly increased ESR and serum CRP concentration during the first 2 weeks of illness and an increased platelet count (>450,000/mm³) on days 10 to 21 of illness almost are universal laboratory features. ESR and platelet count usually return to normal within 6 to 8 weeks; CRP concentration returns to normal much sooner.

Treatment

Management during the acute phase is directed at decreasing inflammation of the myocardium and coronary artery wall and providing supportive care. Therapy should be initiated when the diagnosis is established or strongly suspected, optimally within the first 10 days of illness. Once the acute phase has passed, therapy is directed at prevention of coronary artery thrombosis. Specific recommendations for therapy include the following measures.

IGIV. Therapy with high-dose IGIV and aspirin initiated within 10 days of the onset of fever substantially decreases progression to coronary artery dilatation and aneurysms, compared with treatment with aspirin alone, and results in more rapid resolution of fever and other clinical and laboratory indicators of acute inflammation. Therapy with IGIV should be initiated as soon as possible. However, therapy with IGIV and aspirin should be provided for patients diagnosed after day 10 who have manifestations of continuing inflammation (eg, fever or elevated ESR or CRP concentration) or of evolving coronary artery disease. Despite prompt treatment with IGIV and aspirin, 2% to 4% of patients develop coronary artery abnormalities.

Dose. A dose of 2 g/kg as a single dose, given over 10 to 12 hours, has been proven to reduce the risk of coronary artery aneurysm from 17% to 4%.

Retreatment. Many patients have fever in the 24 hours after completing the IGIV infusion. Persistent or recrudescent fever that is present 48 hours after the end of the IGIV infusion is used to define IGIV-resistant cases. Up to 15% of Kawasaki patients can be IGIV resistant. In these situations, the diagnosis of Kawasaki disease should be reevaluated. If Kawasaki disease still is considered to be most likely, re-treatment with IGIV and continued high-dose aspirin therapy generally is given. For the limited number of patients who are refractory to at least 2 doses of IGIV, infliximab or intravenous methylprednisolone may be administered. Lack of data on use of these modalities precludes definitive recommendations.

Aspirin. Aspirin is used for anti-inflammatory and antithrombotic actions, although aspirin alone does not decrease risk of coronary artery abnormalities. The optimal dose or duration of aspirin treatment is unknown. Aspirin is administered in doses of 80 to 100 mg/kg per day in 4 divided doses once the diagnosis is made. Children with acute Kawasaki disease have decreased aspirin absorption and increased clearance and rarely achieve therapeutic serum concentrations. High-dose aspirin is discontinued on day 14 of illness or when the child has been afebrile for 72 hours; low-dose aspirin then is continued. If no coronary artery abnormalities have been detected by 6 to 8 weeks after onset of illness, low-dose aspirin is discontinued. Low-dose aspirin therapy should be continued indefinitely for people in whom coronary artery abnormalities are present. In general, ibuprofen should be avoided in children with coronary aneurysms taking aspirin for its antiplatelet effects, because ibuprofen antagonizes the platelet inhibition that is induced by aspirin. The child and household contacts should be given influenza vaccine at the time of diagnosis of Kawasaki disease according to seasonal recommendations.

Cardiac Care. An echocardiogram should be obtained at the time of diagnosis and repeated at 2 weeks and 6 to 8 weeks after diagnosis. Children at higher risk may require more frequent echocardiograms to guide the need for additional therapies. Children also should be assessed during this time for arrhythmias, congestive heart failure, and valvular regurgitation. The care of patients with significant cardiac abnormalities should involve a pediatric cardiologist experienced in management of patients with Kawasaki disease and in assessing echocardiographic studies of coronary arteries in children. Long-term management of Kawasaki disease should be based on the extent of coronary artery involvement.

Subsequent Immunization. Measles and varicella-containing vaccines should be deferred for 11 months after receipt of high-dose IGIV for treatment of Kawasaki disease. If the child's risk of exposure to measles or varicella is high, the child should be immunized and then reimmunized at least 11 months after administration of IGIV. The schedule for administration of inactivated childhood vaccines should not be interrupted.

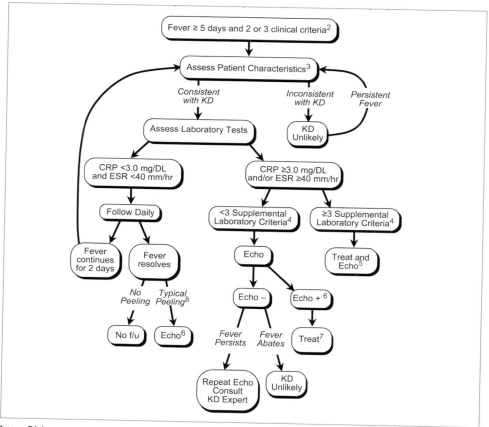

Image 71.1

Evaluation of suspected incomplete Kawasaki disease. (1) In the absence of gold standard for diagnosis, this algorithm cannot be evidence based but rather represents the informed opinion of the expert committee. Consultation with an expert should be sought any time assistance is needed. (2) Infants ≤6 months old on day ≥7 of fever without other explanation should undergo laboratory testing and, if evidence of systemic inflammation is found, an echocardiogram, even if the infants have no clinical criteria. (3) Patient characteristics suggesting Kawasaki disease are provided in text. Characteristics suggesting disease other than Kawasaki disease include exudative conjunctivitis, exudative pharyngitis, discrete intraoral lesions, bullous or vesicular rash, or generalized adenopathy. Consider alternative diagnoses. (4) Supplemental laboratory criteria include albumin ≤3.0 g/dL, anemia for age, elevation of alanine aminotransferase, platelets after 7 d ≥450,000/mm3, white blood cell count ≥15,000/mm3, and urine ≥10 white blood cells/high-power field. (5) Can treat before performing echocardiogram. (6) Echocardiogram is considered positive for purposes of this algorithm if any of 3 conditions are met: z score of LAD or RCA ≥2.5, coronary arteries meet Japanese Ministry of Health criteria for aneurysms, or ≥3 other suggestive features exist, including perivascular brightness, lack of tapering, decreased LV function, mitral regurgitation, pericardial effusion, or z scores in LAD or RCA of 2–2.5. (7) If the echocardiogram is positive, treatment should be given to children within 10 d of fever onset and those beyond day 10 with clinical and laboratory signs (CRP, ESR) of ongoing inflammation. (8) Typical peeling begins under nail bed of fingers and then toes. Reprinted from Newburger JW, Takahashi M, Gerber MA, et al. Diagnosis, treatment and long-term management of Kawasaki disease: a statement for health professionals from the Committee on Rheumatic Fever, Endocarditis and Kawasaki Disease, Council on Cardiovascular Disease in the Young, American Heart Association. *Pediatrics.* 2004;114(6):1708–1733.

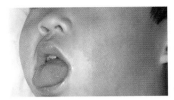

Image 71.2
A child with Kawasaki disease with striking facial rash and erythema of the oral mucous membrane.

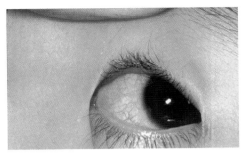

Image 71.3
A child with Kawasaki disease with conjunctivitis. Note the absence of conjunctival discharge.

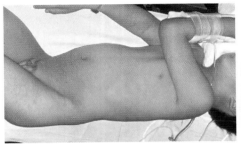

Image 71.4
Characteristic distribution of erythroderma of Kawasaki disease. The rash is accentuated in the perineal area in approximately two-thirds of patients.

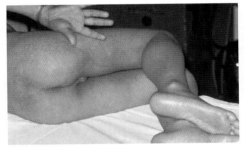

Image 71.5
Generalized erythema and early perianal and palmar desquamation. This is the same patient as in Image 71.4.

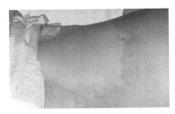

Image 71.6
Characteristic desquamation of the skin over the abdomen in a patient with Kawasaki disease. This is the same patient as in images 71.4 and 71.5.

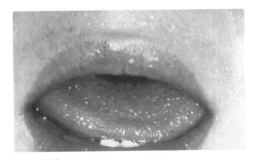

Image 71.7
Erythematous lips and injection of the oropharyngeal membranes in a patient with Kawasaki disease. Scarlet fever, toxic shock syndrome, staphylococcal scalded skin syndrome, and measles may be confused with this disease.

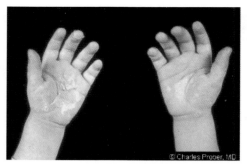

Image 71.8
A child with the characteristic desquamation of the hands in a later stage of Kawasaki disease. Copyright Charles Prober, MD.

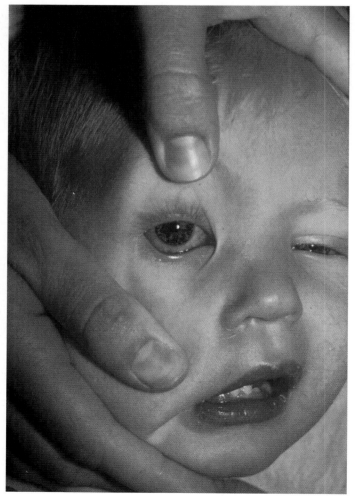

Image 71.9
This 1-year-old white child presented with fever, generalized erythroderma, and conjunctivitis compatible with Kawasaki disease. Courtesy of George Nankervis, MD.

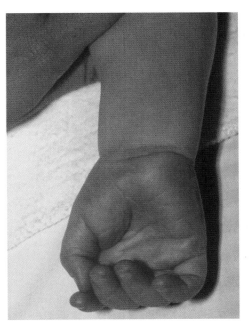

Image 71.10
Erythroderma of the palm of the hand of the child in Image 71.9 with Kawasaki disease. Courtesy of George Nankervis, MD.

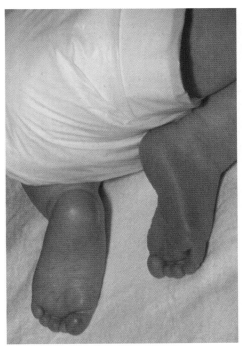

Image 71.11
Erythroderma of the plantar foot surface of the child in images 71.9 and 71.10 with Kawasaki disease. Courtesy of George Nankervis, MD.

72

Legionella pneumophila Infections

Clinical Manifestations

Legionellosis is associated with 2 clinically and epidemiologically distinct illnesses: Legionnaires disease and Pontiac fever. **Legionnaires disease** varies in severity from mild to severe pneumonia characterized by fever, cough, and progressive respiratory distress. Legionnaires disease can be associated with chills, myalgia, gastrointestinal tract, central nervous system, and renal manifestations. Respiratory failure and death can occur. **Pontiac fever** is a milder febrile illness without pneumonia that occurs in epidemics and is characterized by an abrupt onset and a self-limited, influenza-like illness.

Etiology

Legionella species are fastidious aerobic bacilli that stain gram negative after recovery on buffered charcoal yeast extract media. At least 20 different species have been implicated in human disease, but the most common species causing infections in the United States is *Legionella pneumophila*, with most isolates belonging to serogroup 1.

Epidemiology

Legionnaires disease is acquired through inhalation of aerosolized water contaminated with *L pneumophila*. Person-to-person transmission has not been demonstrated. More than 80% of cases are sporadic; the sources of infection can be related to exposure to *L pneumophila*–contaminated water in the home, workplace, or hospitals or other medical facilities or to aerosol-producing devices in public places. Outbreaks have been ascribed to common-source exposure to contaminated cooling towers, evaporative condensers, potable water systems, whirlpool spas, humidifiers, and respiratory therapy equipment. Outbreaks have occurred in hospitals, hotels, and other large buildings as well as on cruise ships. Health care–associated infections can occur and often are related to contamination of the hot water supply. Legionnaires disease occurs most commonly in people who are elderly, are immunocompromised, or have underlying lung disease.

Infection in children is rare and usually is asymptomatic or mild and unrecognized. Severe disease has occurred in children with malignant neoplasms, severe combined immunodeficiency, chronic granulomatous disease, organ transplantation, end-stage renal disease, underlying pulmonary disease, and immunosuppression; in children receiving systemic corticosteroids; and as a health care–associated infection in newborn infants.

Incubation Period

Legionnaires disease, 2 to 10 days; Pontiac fever, 1 to 2 days.

Diagnostic Tests

Recovery of *Legionella* from respiratory tract secretions, lung tissue, pleural fluid, or other normally sterile fluid specimens by using charcoal-based media provides definitive evidence of infection, but the sensitivity of culture is laboratory dependent. Detection of *Legionella* antigen in urine by commercially available immunoassays is highly specific. Such tests are sensitive for *L pneumophila* serogroup 1, but these tests rarely detect antigen in patients infected with other *L pneumophila* serogroups or other *Legionella* species. Genus-specific PCR-based assays have been developed that detect *Legionella* DNA in respiratory secretions as well as in blood and urine of some patients with pneumonia. For serologic diagnosis, a fourfold increase in titer of antibodies to *L pneumophila* serogroup 1, measured by indirect immunofluorescent antibody (IFA) assay, confirms a recent infection. Convalescent serum samples should be obtained 3 to 4 weeks after onset of symptoms; however, a titer increase can be delayed for 8 to 12 weeks. The positive predictive value of a single titer of 1:256 or greater is low and does not provide definitive evidence of infection. Antibodies to several gram-negative organisms, including *Pseudomonas* species, *Bacteroides fragilis,* and *Campylobacter jejuni,* can cause false-positive IFA test results.

Treatment

Intravenous azithromycin has replaced intravenous erythromycin as the drug of choice. Once the condition of a patient is improving, oral therapy can be substituted. Levofloxacin (or another fluoroquinolone) is the drug of choice for immunocompromised patients, because fluoroquinolone antimicrobial agents are bactericidal and are more effective than macrolides in vitro and in animal models of infection. Fluoroquinolones are not approved for this indication in children younger than 18 years. Doxycycline and trimethoprim-

sulfamethoxazole are alternative drugs. Doxycycline should not be used for pregnant women or for children younger than 8 years. Duration of therapy is 5 to 10 days for azithromycin, 14 to 21 days for other drugs, and longer for patients who are immunocompromised or who have severe disease.

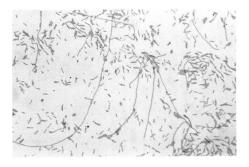

Image 72.1

This Gram-stained micrograph reveals chains and solitary gram-negative *Legionella pneumophila* bacteria found within a sample taken from a victim of the 1976 Legionnaires disease outbreak in Philadelphia. Legionnaires disease is the more severe form of legionellosis and is characterized by pneumonia, commencing 2 to 10 days after exposure. Pontiac fever is an acute-onset, flu-like, non-pneumonic illness, occurring within 1 to 2 days of exposure. Courtesy of Centers for Disease Control and Prevention.

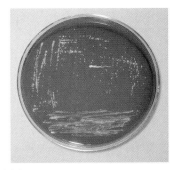

Image 72.2

Charcoal-yeast extract agar plate culture of *Legionella pneumophila*. Courtesy of Centers for Disease Control and Prevention/Dr Jim Feeley.

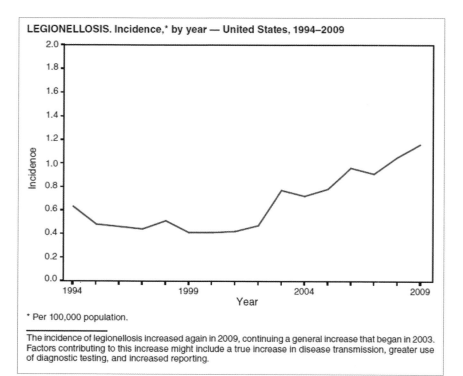

LEGIONELLOSIS. Incidence,* by year — United States, 1994–2009

* Per 100,000 population.

The incidence of legionellosis increased again in 2009, continuing a general increase that began in 2003. Factors contributing to this increase might include a true increase in disease transmission, greater use of diagnostic testing, and increased reporting.

Image 72.3
Legionellosis. Incidence by year—United States, 1994–2009. Courtesy of *Morbidity and Mortality Weekly Report.*

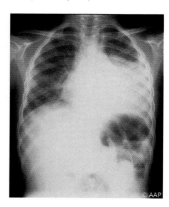

Image 72.4
An adult with pneumonia due to *Legionella pneumophila. Legionella* infections are rare in otherwise healthy children. Though nosocomial infections and hospital outbreaks are reported, this infection is not transmitted from person to person.

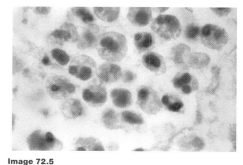

Image 72.5
This hematoxylin-eosin stained micrograph of lung tissue biopsied from a patient with Legionnaires disease revealed the presence of an intraalveolar exudate consisting of macrophages, and polymorphonuclear leucocytes. The *Legionella pneumophila* bacteria are not stained in this preparation (magnification x500). Courtesy of Centers for Disease Control and Prevention.

73

Leishmaniasis

Clinical Manifestations

The 3 major clinical syndromes are as follows:
- *Cutaneous Leishmaniasis.* After inoculation by the bite of an infected female phlebotomine sandfly, parasites proliferate locally in mononuclear phagocytes, leading to an erythematous papule, which typically slowly enlarges to become a nodule and then a shallow painless ulcerative lesion with raised borders. Ulcerative lesions can become dry and crusted or can develop a moist granulating base with an overlying exudate. Lesions can persist as nodules or papules and may be single or multiple. Lesions commonly are located on exposed areas of the body (eg, face and extremities) and can be accompanied by satellite lesions, which appear as sporotrichoid-like nodules, and regional adenopathy. Clinical manifestations of Old World and New World (American) cutaneous leishmaniasis are similar. Spontaneous resolution of lesions can take weeks to years and usually results in a flat atrophic (cigarette paper) scar. Cutaneous leishmaniasis attributable to the *Viannia* subspecies seldom heals without treatment.
- *Mucosal Leishmaniasis (Espundia).* Hematogenous mucocutaneous leishmaniasis (**espundia**) primarily is associated with the *Viannia* subspecies. Mucosal involvement can occur by extension of facial lesions attributable to other species. Mucosal infection is primarily found in the New World. It may become evident clinically from months to years after the cutaneous lesions heal; sometimes mucosal and cutaneous lesions are noted simultaneously. Parasites may disseminate to the naso-oropharyngeal mucosa. Granulomatous inflammation may cause hypertrophy of the nose and lips. In some patients, granulomatous ulceration and necrosis follow, leading to facial disfigurement, secondary infection, and mucosal perforation, which may occur months to years after the initial cutaneous lesion heals.

- *Visceral Leishmaniasis (Kala-azar).* After cutaneous inoculation of parasites by the sandfly vector, organisms spread throughout the mononuclear macrophage system to the spleen, liver, and bone marrow. The resulting clinical illness typically manifests as fever, anorexia, weight loss, splenomegaly, hepatomegaly, anemia, leukopenia, thrombocytopenia sometimes associated with hemorrhage, hypoalbuminemia, and hypergammaglobulinemia. Peripheral lymphadenopathy is commonly seen in Sudan and East Africa. Kala-azar ("black sickness") refers to hyperpigmentation of skin seen in late-stage disease in patients in the Indian subcontinent. Secondary gram-negative enteric infections and tuberculosis may occur as a result of suppression of the cell-mediated immune response. Untreated fully manifested visceral infection is nearly always fatal. At the other end of the spectrum are patients who are minimally symptomatic but harbor viable parasites lifelong. Reactivation of latent visceral infection can occur in patients who become immunocompromised, including people with concurrent HIV infection and recipients of stem cell or solid organ transplants.

Etiology

In the human host, *Leishmania* species are obligate intracellular parasites of mononuclear phagocytes. Cutaneous leishmaniasis typically is caused by Old World species (*Leishmania tropica, Leishmania major,* and *Leishmania aethiopica*) and by New World species (*Leishmania mexicana, Leishmania amazonensis, Leishmania braziliensis, Leishmania panamensis, Leishmania guyanensis,* and *Leishmania peruviana*). Mucosal leishmaniasis typically is caused by *Leishmania (V) braziliensis, L (V) panamensis,* and *L (V) guyanensis.* Visceral leishmaniasis is caused by *Leishmania donovani* and *Leishmania infantum (Leishmania chagasi* is synonymous). *L donovani* and *L infantum* can cause cutaneous leishmaniasis. However, people with typical cutaneous leishmaniasis caused by these organisms rarely develop visceral leishmaniasis.

Epidemiology

Leishmaniasis typically is a zoonosis with a variety of mammalian reservoir hosts, including canines and rodents. However, the only proven reservoir of *L donovani* in the Indian subcontinent consists of infected humans, and transmission has a large anthroponotic component in East Africa as well. Transmission primarily is vector-borne through the bite of infected female phlebotomine sandflies. Congenital and parenteral transmission also have been reported. Leishmaniasis is endemic in 88 countries, from northern Argentina to southern Texas (not including Uruguay or Chile), in southern Europe, China and Central Asia, the Indian subcontinent, the Middle East, and Africa (particularly East and North Africa, with sporadic cases elsewhere) but not in Australia or Oceania. Overall, visceral leishmaniasis is found in focal areas of approximately 65 countries. Most (>90%) of the world's cases of visceral leishmaniasis occur in the Indian subcontinent (India, Bangladesh, and Nepal), Sudan, and Brazil. The estimated annual number of new cases of cutaneous leishmaniasis is approximately 1.5 million; more than 90% of these occur in Afghanistan, Algeria, Iran, Iraq, Saudi Arabia, and Syria (Old World) and in Brazil and Peru (New World). Approximately 90% of cases of mucosal leishmaniasis occur in 3 countries: Bolivia, Brazil, and Peru. Geographic distribution of cases evaluated in the developed world reflects travel and immigration patterns. The number of cases has increased as a result of increased travel to areas with endemic infection; for example, with ecotourism activities in Central and South America and military activities in Iraq and Afghanistan, the number of imported cases within North America has increased.

Incubation Period

For the different forms of leishmaniasis, incubation periods range from several days to several years but usually are in the range of several weeks to 6 months. In cutaneous leishmaniasis, primary skin lesions typically appear several weeks after parasite inoculation. In visceral infection, the incubation period typically ranges from 2 to 6 months.

Diagnostic Tests

Definitive diagnosis is made by demonstration of the presence of the parasite. A common way of identifying the parasite is by microscopic identification of intracellular leishmanial organisms (amastigotes) on Wright- or Giemsa-stained smears or histologic sections of infected tissues. In cutaneous disease, tissue can be obtained by a 3-mm punch biopsy, by lesion scrapings, or by needle aspiration of the raised non-necrotic edge of the lesion. In visceral leishmaniasis, the organisms can be identified in the spleen and, less commonly, in bone marrow and the liver. The sensitivity is highest for splenic aspiration (approximately 95%), but so is the risk of hemorrhage or bowel perforation. In East Africa in patients with lymphadenopathy, the organisms also can be identified in lymph nodes. Buffy-coat preparations have been positive in some patients, and organisms occasionally may be observed in blood smears or cultured from buffy-coat preparations in HIV-infected patients. Isolation of parasites (promastigotes) by culture of appropriate tissue specimens in specialized media may take days to several weeks but should be attempted when possible. Knowledge of the infecting species may affect prognosis and influence treatment decisions.

The diagnosis of some forms of leishmaniasis can be aided by performance of serologic testing, which is available at the Centers for Disease Control and Prevention (CDC). Serologic test results usually are positive in cases of visceral and mucosal leishmaniasis if the patient is immunocompetent but often are negative in cutaneous leishmaniasis. False-positive results may occur in patients with other infectious diseases, especially American trypanosomiasis.

Treatment

The decision whether to treat leishmaniasis should be made on an individual basis, with the assistance of infectious disease experts or consultation from the CDC Division of Parasitic Diseases and Malaria. Treatment always is indicated for patients with mucosal or visceral leishmaniasis. Liposomal amphotericin B is the only treatment approved by the US Food and Drug Administration for visceral leishmaniasis and is the most efficacious and least toxic of the antileishmanial drugs available in the United States. Paromomycin intramuscular injection is approved for the treatment of visceral leishmaniasis in several countries. Treatment of cutaneous leishmaniasis should be considered, especially if skin lesions are or could become disfiguring or disabling (eg, facial lesions or lesions near joints), are persistent, or are known to be or might be caused by leishmanial species that can disseminate to the naso-oropharyngeal

mucosa. Local wound care and treatment of bacterial superinfection also must be considered in cutaneous leishmaniasis. Miltefosine, the first oral agent for treatment of leishmaniasis, is not licensed or available in the United States. Miltefosine has demonstrated degrees of efficacy in visceral leishmaniasis and in New and Old World cutaneous lesions but is contraindicated in pregnancy. Meglumine antimoniate by injection is supported by the World Health Organization for treatment of leishmaniasis but is not available in the United States.

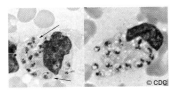

Image 73.1

Leishmania tropica amastigotes from a skin touch preparation. (A) A still intact macrophage is practically filled with amastigotes, several of which have a clearly visible nucleus and a kinetoplast (arrows). (B) Amastigotes are being freed from a rupturing macrophage. The patient has a history of travel to Egypt, Africa, and the Middle East. Culture in Novy-MacNeal-Nicolle medium followed by isoenzyme analysis identified the species as *L tropica* minor. Courtesy of Centers for Disease Control and Prevention.

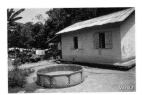

Image 73.3

Homes built in newly cleared forest areas (here, outside Rio de Janeiro) expose settlers to the sandflies that transmit leishmaniasis. Courtesy of World Health Organization.

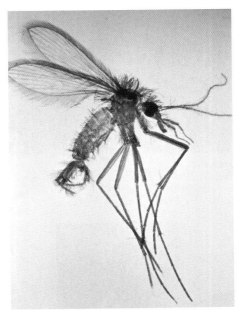

Image 73.2

This image depicts a mounted male *Phlebotomus* sp fly, which due to its resemblance may be mistaken for a mosquito. *Phlebotomus* spp sandflies are bloodsucking insects that are very small and sometimes act as the vectors for various diseases, such as leishmaniasis and bartonellosis (also known as Carrión disease). Courtesy of Centers for Disease Control and Prevention/ Donated by the World Health Organization.

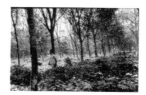

Image 73.4
Natural uncut forests are transmission sites for leishmaniasis. People who collect rubber or clear such areas for agriculture are prone to infection. Courtesy of World Health Organization/TDR/ Lainson, Wellcome Trust.

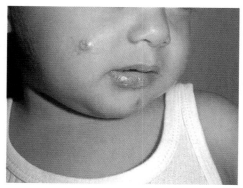

Image 73.5
Cutaneous leishmaniasis, as in this boy from India, seldom disseminates in immunocompetent persons. Multiple organisms usually can be found on biopsy of the border of a lesion.

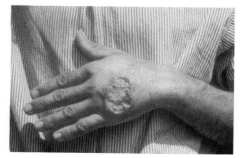

Image 73.6
Skin ulcer due to leishmaniasis, hand of Central American adult. Courtesy of Centers for Disease Control and Prevention/Dr D.S. Martin.

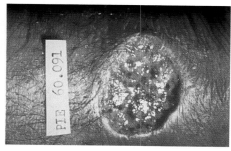

Image 73.7
Crater lesion of leishmaniasis, skin. Courtesy of Centers for Disease Control and Prevention.

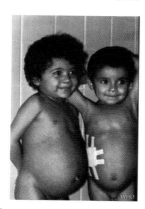

Image 73.8
Two young boys suffering visceral leishmaniasis, with distended abdomens due to hepatospleno-megaly. Courtesy of World Health Organization/ TDR/Marsden, Wellcome Trust.

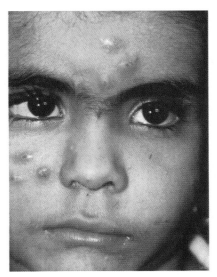

Image 73.9
A young girl with cutaneous leishmaniasis with multiple cutaneous lesions.
Courtesy of World Health Organization.

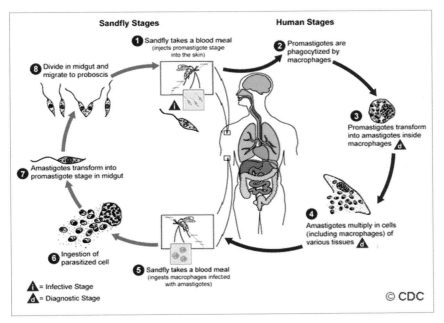

Image 73.10
Leishmaniasis is transmitted by the bite of female phlebotomine sandflies. The sandflies inject the infective stage, promastigotes, during blood meals (1). Promastigotes that reach the puncture wound are phagocytized by macrophages (2) and transform into amastigotes (3). Amastigotes multiply in infected cells and affect different tissues, depending in part on the *Leishmania* species (4). This originates the clinical manifestations of leishmaniasis. Sandflies become infected during blood meals on an infected host when they ingest macrophages infected with amastigotes (5, 6). In the sandfly's midgut, the parasites differentiate into promastigotes (7), which multiply and migrate to the proboscis (8). Courtesy of Centers for Disease Control and Prevention/Alexander J. da Silva, PhD/Blaine Mathison.

74

Leprosy

Clinical Manifestations

Leprosy (Hansen disease) is a curable infection involving skin, peripheral nerves, mucosa of the upper respiratory tract, and testes. The clinical forms of leprosy reflect the cellular immune response to *Mycobacterium leprae* and the organism's unique tropism for peripheral nerves. In the United States, the Redley-Jopling scale is used and has 5 classifications that correlate with histologic findings: (1) polar tuberculoid, (2) borderline tuberculoid, (3) borderline, (4) borderline lepromatous, and (5) polar lepromatous.

The cell-mediated immunity of most patients and their clinical presentation occur between the 2 extremes of tuberculoid and lepromatous forms. Leprosy lesions usually do not itch or hurt; they lack sensation to heat, touch, and pain. The classic presentation of the "leonine facies" and loss of lateral eyebrows (madarosis) occurs in patients with end-stage lepromatous leprosy. A simplified scheme introduced by the World Health Organization, for situations in which there is no doctor, classifies leprosy involving 1 patch of skin as (1) paucibacillary single lesion; (2) paucibacillary (2–5 lesions; usually tuberculous leprosy); and (3) multibacillary (>5 lesions, usually lepromatous leprosy).

Serious consequences of leprosy occur from immune reactions and nerve involvement with resulting anesthesia, which can lead to repeated unrecognized trauma, ulcerations, fractures, and bone resorption. Injuries can have a significant effect on quality of life, because leprosy is a leading cause of permanent physical disability among communicable diseases worldwide. Eye involvement can occur, and patients should be examined by an ophthalmologist. A diagnosis of leprosy should be considered in any patient with hypoesthetic or anesthetic skin rash.

Leprosy Reactions: Acute clinical exacerbations reflect abrupt changes in immunologic balance, especially common during initial years of treatment, but can occur in the absence of therapy. Two major types are seen. Type 1 (reversal reaction) is predominantly observed in borderline tuberculoid and borderline lepromatous leprosy and is the result of a sudden increase in effective cell-mediated immunity. Acute tenderness and swelling at the site of cutaneous and neural lesions with development of new lesions are major manifestations. Ulcerations can occur. Fever and systemic toxicity are uncommon. Type 2 (erythema nodosum leprosum) occurs in borderline and lepromatous forms as a systemic inflammatory response. Tender, red dermal papules or nodules resembling erythema nodosum along with high fever, migrating polyarthralgia, painful swelling of lymph nodes and spleen, iridocyclitis and, rarely, nephritis can occur.

Etiology

Leprosy is caused by *M leprae,* an obligate intracellular, acid-fast bacillus that has variable staining by Gram stain. *M leprae* is the only bacterium known to infect nerves.

Epidemiology

Leprosy primarily is a disease of poverty. Approximately 5% of people genetically are susceptible to infection with *M leprae*; several genes now have been identified that are associated with susceptibility to *M leprae*. Accordingly, spouses of leprosy patients are not likely to develop leprosy, but biological parents, children, and siblings who are household contacts of untreated patients with leprosy are at increased risk. The major source of infectious material probably is nasal secretions from patients with untreated infection. Little shedding of *M leprae* from involved intact skin occurs. People with HIV infection do not appear to be at increased risk of becoming infected with *M leprae*. There currently are approximately 6,500 leprosy cases in the United States; approximately 3,300 require active medical management. As of early 2009, the World Health Organization new case detection rate for the United States was less than 0.1 per 100,000 population. Most cases of leprosy reported were in native-born US citizens from Texas and Louisiana and among immigrants in California, Florida, New York, and Massachusetts. More than 65% of the world's leprosy patients reside in South and Southeast Asia—most of these patients are in India. High endemicity remains in some areas of Angola, Brazil, Central African Republic, Democratic Republic of Congo, India, Madagascar, Mozambique, Nepal, Republic of the Marshall Islands, the Federated States of Micronesia, and the United Republic of Tanzania.

The infectivity of lepromatous patients ceases within 24 hours of the first administration of multidrug therapy, the standard antimicrobial treatment for leprosy.

Incubation Period

Range, 1 to many years, usually 3 to 5 years. Tuberculoid is shorter than lepromatous form. Symptoms can take up to 20 years to develop.

Diagnostic Tests

Histopathologic examination of skin biopsy by an experienced pathologist is the best method of establishing the diagnosis and is the basis for classification of leprosy. These specimens can be sent to National Hansen's Disease (Leprosy) Programs (NHDP) (800/642-2477; **www.hrsa.gov/hansens**) in formalin or embedded in paraffin. Acid-fast bacilli can be found in slit-smears or biopsy specimens of skin lesions but rarely from patients with tuberculoid and indeterminate forms of disease. Organisms have not been cultured successfully in vitro. A PCR test for *M leprae* is available on a limited basis after consultation with the NHDP

Treatment

Therapy for patients with leprosy should be undertaken in consultation with an expert in leprosy. The NHDP provides medications for leprosy at no charge as well as consultation on clinical and pathologic issues and information about local Hansen disease clinics.

Leprosy is curable. The primary goal of therapy is prevention of permanent nerve damage, which can be accomplished by early diagnosis and treatment. Combination antimicrobial multidrug therapy (MDT) to minimize development of antimicrobial-resistant organisms is

necessary. Adults are treated with dapsone, rifampin, and clofazimine. Resistance to all 3 drugs has been documented but is rare in the United States.

Treatment Regimens Recommended by the NHDP

Multibacillary leprosy (6 patches or more)
1. Dapsone for 24 months **and**
2. Rifampin for 24 months **and**
3. Clofazimine for 24 months (Clarithromycin can be used in place of clofazimine for children.)

Paucibacillary leprosy (1–5 patches)
1. Dapsone for 12 months **and**
2. Rifampin for 12 months

Before beginning antimicrobial therapy, patients should be tested for glucose-6-phosphate dehydrogenase deficiency, have baseline complete blood cell counts and liver function test results documented, and be evaluated for any evidence of tuberculosis infection, especially if the patient is infected with HIV. This consideration is important to avoid monotherapy of active tuberculosis with rifampin while treating active leprosy.

Adverse reactions of MDT commonly include darkening of skin caused by daily clofazimine therapy. This will resolve within several months of completing therapy.

All patients with leprosy should be educated about signs and symptoms of neuritis and cautioned to report signs and symptoms of neuritis immediately so that corticosteroid therapy can be instituted. Patients should receive counseling because of the social and psychological effects of this disease.

Relapse of disease after completing MDT is rare (0.01%–0.14%); the presentation of new skin patches usually is attributable to a late type 1 reaction. Self-examination is critical for any patient with loss of sensitivity in the foot. When it does occur, relapse usually is attributable to reactivation of drug-susceptible organisms. People with relapses of disease require another course of MDT.

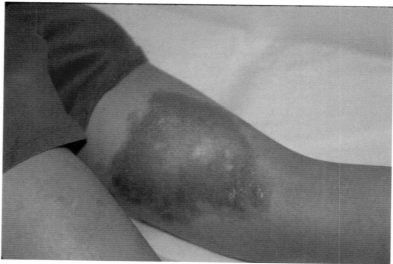

Image 74.1
Hansen disease. A young Vietnamese boy who spent 2 years in a refugee camp in the Philippines presented with the nodular violaceous skin lesion shown. The results of a biopsy of the lesion showed acid-fast organisms surrounding blood vessels. A diagnosis of lepromatous leprosy was made and the child was treated with a multidrug regimen. Copyright Barbara Jantausch, MD, FAAP.

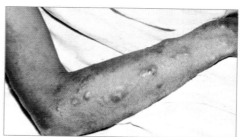

Image 74.3
An adult male with lepromatous leprosy. Courtesy of Hugh Moffet, MD.

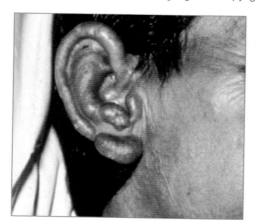

Image 74.2
Lepromatous leprosy in an Asian man. Newly diagnosed cases are considered contagious until treatment is established and should be reported to local and state public health departments. Courtesy of Hugh Moffet, MD.

75

Leptospirosis

Clinical Manifestations

Leptospirosis is an acute febrile disease with varied manifestations characterized by vasculitis. The severity of disease ranges from asymptomatic or subclinical to self-limited systemic illness (approximately 90% of patients) to life-threatening illness with jaundice, renal failure, and hemorrhagic pneumonitis. Clinical presentation typically is biphasic, with an acute septicemia phase usually lasting 1 week, followed by a second immune-mediated phase. Regardless of its severity, the acute phase is characterized by nonspecific symptoms, including fever, chills, headache, nausea, vomiting, and a transient rash. The most distinct clinical findings are conjunctival suffusion without purulent discharge (30%–99% of cases) and myalgias of the calf and lumbar regions (40%–100% of cases). In some patients, the 2 phases are separated by a short-lived abatement of fever (3–4 days). Findings commonly associated with the immune-mediated phase include fever, aseptic meningitis, conjunctival suffusion, uveitis, muscle tenderness, adenopathy, and purpuric rash. Approximately 10% of patients have severe illness, including jaundice and renal dysfunction (Weil syndrome), hemorrhagic pneumonitis, cardiac arrhythmias, or circulatory collapse associated with a case-fatality rate of 5% to 15%. The overall duration of symptoms for both phases of disease varies from less than 1 week to several months. Asymptomatic or subclinical infection with seroconversion is frequent, especially in settings of endemic infection.

Etiology

Leptospirosis is caused by pathogenic spirochetes of the genus *Leptospira*. Leptospires previously were classified into 2 species, which then were subdivided into more than 200 antigenically defined serovars, grouped into serogroups on the basis of serologic relatedness. Currently, the molecular classification divides the genus into 20 named pathogenic and nonpathogenic genomospecies as determined by DNA-DNA hybridization.

Epidemiology

The reservoirs for *Leptospira* species include a wide range of wild and domestic animals that may shed organisms asymptomatically for years. *Leptospira* organisms excreted in animal urine, amniotic fluid, or placental tissue may remain viable in moist soil or water for weeks to months in warm climates. Humans usually become infected via entry of leptospires through contact of mucosal surfaces or abraded skin with contaminated soil, water, or animal tissues. Infection may be acquired through direct contact with infected animals or their tissues or through contact with infective urine or fluids from carrier animals or urine-contaminated soil or water. People who are predisposed by occupation include abattoir and sewer workers, miners, veterinarians, farmers, and military personnel. Recreational exposures and clusters of disease have been associated with wading, swimming (especially being submerged in or swallowing water), or boating in contaminated water, particularly during flooding or following heavy rainfall. Person-to-person transmission is rare.

Incubation Period

5 to 14 days; range, 2 to 30 days.

Diagnostic Tests

Leptospira organisms can be isolated from blood or cerebrospinal fluid specimens during the early septicemic phase (first 7–10 days) of illness and subsequently from urine specimens. However, isolation of the organism may be difficult, requiring special media and techniques and incubation for up to 16 weeks. In addition, the sensitivity of culture for diagnosis is low. For these reasons, serum specimens always should be obtained to facilitate diagnosis. Antibodies can develop as early as 5 to 7 days after onset of illness, and can be measured by commercially available immunoassays; however, increases in antibody titer may not be detected until more than 10 days after onset, especially if antimicrobial therapy is initiated. Antibody increases can be transient, delayed, or absent in some patients. Microscopic agglutination, the confirmatory serologic test, is performed only in reference laboratories and requires seroconversion demonstrated between acute and convalescent specimens obtained at least 10 days apart. Immunohistochemical techniques can detect leptospiral antigens in infected tissues. PCR assays for detection of *Leptospira* organisms have been developed but are available only in research laboratories.

Treatment

Intravenous penicillin is the drug of choice for patients with severe infection requiring hospitalization and is effective as late as 7 days into the course of illness. Penicillin G decreases the duration of systemic symptoms and persistence of associated laboratory abnormalities and may prevent development of leptospiruria. As with other spirochetal infections, a Jarisch-Herxheimer reaction (an acute febrile reaction accompanied by headache, myalgia, and an aggravated clinical picture lasting less than 24 hours) can develop after initiation of penicillin therapy. Parenteral cefotaxime, doxycycline, and ceftriaxone have been demonstrated in randomized clinical trials to be equal in efficacy to penicillin G for treatment of severe leptospirosis. Severe cases also require appropriate supportive care, including fluid and electrolyte replacement, and often dialysis. For patients with mild disease, oral doxycycline has been shown to shorten the course of illness and decrease occurrence of leptospiruria. Doxycycline should not be used in pregnant women or children younger than 8 years unless no other treatment options are available. Azithromycin has been demonstrated in a clinical trial to be as effective as doxycycline and can be used as an alternative to doxycycline in patients for whom doxycycline is contraindicated.

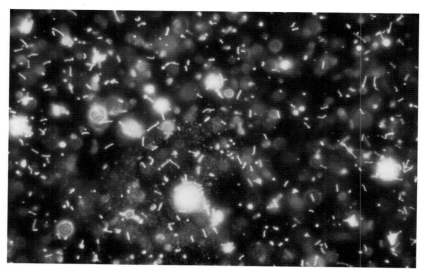

Image 75.1
Photomicrograph of leptospiral microscopic agglutination test with live antigen (dark field microscopy technique). Leptospirosis is a common global zoonotic disease of humans and several warm-blooded animals, especially in subtropic regions of the world, caused by the spirochete bacteria *Leptospira*. Courtesy of Centers for Disease Control and Prevention/Mrs M. Gatton.

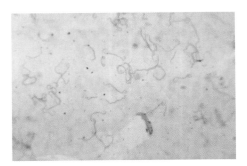

Image 75.2

A photomicrograph of a liver smear, using a silver staining technique, taken from a patient with a fatal case of leptospirosis. Humans become infected by swallowing water contaminated by infected animals or through skin contact, especially with mucosal surfaces, such as the eyes or nose, or with broken skin. The disease is not known to be spread from person to person. Courtesy of Centers for Disease Control and Prevention/Dr Martin Hicklin.

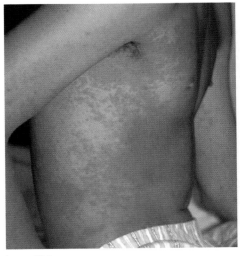

Image 75.3

Leptospirosis rash in an adolescent male that shows the generalized vasculitis caused by this infection.

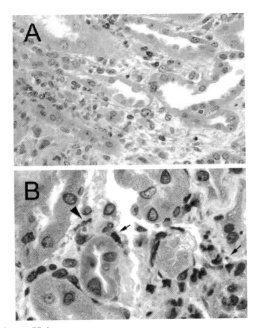

Image 75.4

(A) Renal biopsy shows inflammatory cell infiltrate in the interstitium and focal denudation of tubular epithelial cells (hematoxylin-eosin, original magnification x100). (B) Immunostaining of fragmented leptospire (arrowhead) and granular form of bacterial antigens (arrows) (original magnification x158). Courtesy of Meites E, Jay MT, Deresinski S, et al. Reemerging leptospirosis, California. *Emerg Infect Dis*. 2004;10(3):406–412.

76

Listeria monocytogenes Infections
(Listeriosis)

Clinical Manifestations

Listeriosis is a relatively uncommon but severe invasive infection caused by *Listeria monocytogenes*. Listeriosis transmission predominantly is foodborne and occurs most frequently among pregnant women and their fetuses or newborn infants, people of advanced age, and immunocompromised patients. In pregnant women, infections can be asymptomatic or associated with an influenza-like illness with fever, malaise, headache, gastrointestinal tract symptoms, and back pain. Approximately 65% of pregnant women with *Listeria* infection experience a prodromal illness before the diagnosis of listeriosis in their newborn infant. Amnionitis during labor, brown staining of amniotic fluid, or asymptomatic perinatal infection can occur. Fetal infection results from transplacental transmission following maternal bacteremia, although some infections can occur through ascending spread from vaginal colonization. Pregnancy-associated infections can result in spontaneous abortion, fetal death, preterm delivery, and neonatal illness or death. Neonatal illnesses have early-onset and late-onset syndromes similar to those of group B streptococcal infections. Preterm birth, pneumonia, and septicemia are common in early-onset disease. An erythematous rash with small, pale papules characterized histologically by granulomas, termed granulomatosis infantisepticum, can occur in severe newborn infection. Late-onset infections occur after the first week of life and usually result in meningitis. Late-onset neonatal infection can result from acquisition of the organism during passage through the birth canal or from environmental sources, followed by hematogenous invasion of the organism from the intestine. Clinical features characteristic of invasive listeriosis outside the neonatal period or pregnancy are septicemia and meningitis with or without parenchymal brain involvement in (1) immunocompromised patients, including people with organ transplantation, AIDS, hematologic malignancies, or immunosuppression attributable to corticosteroids; (2) people older than 50 years; or (3) patients for whom reports from the laboratory indicate "diphtheroids" on Gram stain or culture from normally sterile sources. *L monocytogenes* also can cause rhombencephalitis (brain stem encephalitis), brain abscess, and endocarditis. Outbreaks of febrile gastroenteritis caused by food contaminated with *L monocytogenes* have been reported.

Etiology

L monocytogenes is a facultative anaerobic, non-spore–forming, motile, gram-positive bacillus that multiplies intracellularly.

Epidemiology

L monocytogenes causes an estimated 2,500 cases of invasive disease and 500 deaths annually in the United States. The saprophytic organism is distributed widely in the environment and is an important cause of zoonoses, especially in ruminants. Foodborne transmission causes outbreaks and sporadic infections. Incriminated foods include unpasteurized milk, dairy products, and soft cheeses, including Mexican-style cheese; prepared ready-to-eat deli foods, such as hot dogs, cold cut meats, deli salads, hummus, and pâté; undercooked poultry; precooked seafood and smoked or cured fish; melons and fruit salads; and unwashed raw vegetables. In 2011, a large outbreak of listeriosis occurred in the United States associated with contaminated cantaloupe. The incidence of listeriosis has decreased substantially since 1989, when US regulatory agencies began enforcing rigorous screening guidelines for *L monocytogenes* in ready-to-eat foods. The prevalence of stool carriage of *L monocytogenes* among healthy, asymptomatic adults is estimated to be 1% to 5%.

Incubation Period

Range, 1 day to more than 3 weeks.

Diagnostic Tests

The organism can be recovered on trypticase soy agar containing 5% sheep, horse, or rabbit blood from cultures of blood, cerebrospinal fluid, meconium, gastric washings, placental or fetal tissue specimens, amniotic fluid, and other infected tissue specimens, including joint, pleural, or pericardial fluid. *L monocytogenes* can be mistaken for a contaminant because of its morphologic similarity to diphtheroids and non-pathogenic streptococci.

Treatment

Initial therapy with intravenous ampicillin and an aminoglycoside, usually gentamicin, is recommended for severe infections, including meningitis and encephalitis, endocarditis, and infections in neonates and immunocompromised people. This combination is more effective than ampicillin alone in vitro and in animal models of *L monocytogenes* infection. In immunocompetent patients with mild infections, ampicillin alone can be given. For people with serious penicillin allergy, some experts recommend skin testing and desensitization. For patients who fail to respond to therapy or those with a history of anaphylaxis, wheezing, or angioedema, trimethoprim-sulfamethoxazole can be considered. Treatment failures with vancomycin have been reported. Cephalosporins are not active against *L monocytogenes*.

Box 76.1
Dietary Recommendations for People at Higher Risk of Listeriosis[a]

1. Foods to avoid include
   - Raw or unpasteurized milk, including goat milk
   - Soft cheeses (eg, feta, goat, Brie, Camembert, Gorgonzola, blue-veined, and Mexican-style queso fresco cheese)
   - Dairy products that contain unpasteurized milk
   - Foods from delicatessen counters (eg, prepared salads, meats, cheeses) that have not been heated/reheated adequately
   - Refrigerated pâtés, other meat spreads, and refrigerated, smoked seafood that have not been heated/reheated adequately
2. Ways to reduce risk include
   - Cook leftover or ready-to-eat foods (eg, hot dogs) until steaming hot before eating (165°F).
   - Wash raw vegetables.
   - Wash hands, knives, utensils, and cutting boards after exposure to uncooked or ready-to-eat foods.
   - Prevent contamination from fluids of uncooked meats, hot dogs, and packaging onto other foods or food preparation surfaces by keeping them separate from vegetables, uncooked foods, and ready-to-eat foods.
   - Use a refrigerator thermometer to set the refrigerator temperature to 40°F or lower and the freezer temperature to 0°F or lower.
   - Clean up all spills in the refrigerator immediately, especially juices from hot dog packages, raw meat, or poultry.
   - Clean the inside walls and shelves of your refrigerator with hot water and liquid soap, then rinse.
   - Divide leftovers into shallow containers; cover with airtight lids or enclose in plastic wraps or aluminum foil; use leftovers within 3 to 4 days.
   - Use precooked or ready-to-eat food as soon as possible; hot dogs should be eaten within 1 week once the package is opened and within 2 weeks if the package is unopened; deli meat should be eaten within 3 to 5 days once the package is opened and 2 weeks if the package is unopened.

[a]Pregnant women, older adults, and people who are immunocompromised by illness or therapy are at higher risk of invasive listeriosis.

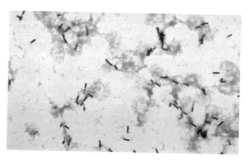

Image 76.1

Cerebrospinal fluid showing characteristic gram-positive rods (Gram stain). Listeriosis is a severe but relatively uncommon infection. Listeriosis occurs most frequently among pregnant women and their fetuses or newborn infants, people of advanced age, or immunocompromised people. Copyright Martha Lepow, MD.

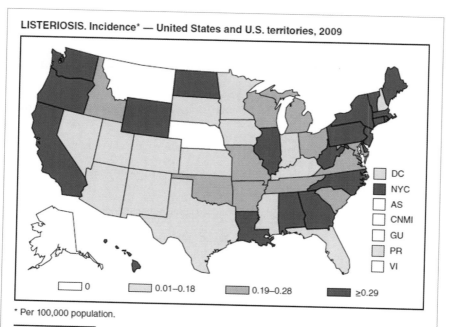

LISTERIOSIS. Incidence* — United States and U.S. territories, 2009

DC
NYC
AS
CNMI
GU
PR
VI

0　　0.01–0.18　　0.19–0.28　　≥0.29

* Per 100,000 population.

Listeriosis is primarily foodborne and occurs most frequently among older adults or persons who are pregnant or immunocompromised. Although the infection is relatively uncommon, listeriosis is a leading cause of death attributable to foodborne illness in the United States. Recent outbreaks have been linked to Mexican-style cheese.

Image 76.2

Listeriosis. Incidence—United States and US territories, 2009. Courtesy of *Morbidity and Mortality Weekly Report.*

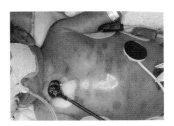

Image 76.3

Skin lesions present at birth in a neonate with congenital pneumonia. *Listeria monocytogenes* was isolated from blood and skin lesion cultures.

77

Lyme Disease

(Lyme Borreliosis, *Borrelia burgdorferi* Infection)

Clinical Manifestations

Clinical manifestations of Lyme disease are divided into 3 stages: early localized, early disseminated, and late disease. Early localized disease is characterized by a distinctive rash, erythema migrans, at the site of a recent tick bite. Erythema migrans is the most common manifestation of Lyme disease in children. Only a small proportion is diagnosed at the stage of early disseminated or late Lyme disease; most of these children do not have a history of erythema migrans. Erythema migrans begins as a red macule or papule that usually expands over days to weeks to form a large, annular, erythematous lesion that typically increases in size to 5 cm or more in diameter, sometimes with partial central clearing. The lesion usually but not always is painless and not pruritic. Localized erythema migrans can vary greatly in size and shape, can have vesicular or necrotic areas in its center, and can be confused with cellulitis. Fever, malaise, headache, mild neck stiffness, myalgia, and arthralgia often accompany the rash of early localized disease.

Approximately 20% of children with Lyme disease come to medical attention with early disseminated disease, most commonly multiple erythema migrans. This rash usually occurs several weeks after an infective tick bite and consists of secondary annular, erythematous lesions similar to but usually smaller than the primary lesion. These lesions reflect spirochetemia with cutaneous dissemination. Other manifestations of early disseminated illness occurring with or without rash are palsies of the cranial nerves (especially cranial nerve VII), ophthalmic conditions (optic neuritis, episcleritis, keratitis, uveitis, conjunctivitis), and lymphocytic meningitis. Systemic symptoms, such as fever, arthralgia, myalgia, headache, and fatigue, also are common during the early disseminated stage. Lymphocytic meningitis can occur and frequently has a more subacute onset than viral meningitis. Carditis, which usually manifests as various degrees of heart block, occurs rarely in children. Occasionally, people with early Lyme disease have concurrent human granulocytic anaplasmosis or babesiosis, transmitted by the same tick, which may contribute to symptomatology.

Late disease is characterized most commonly by arthritis that usually is pauciarticular and affects large joints, particularly knees. Arthritis can occur without a history of earlier stages of illness (including erythema migrans). Peripheral neuropathy and central nervous system manifestations also can occur rarely during late disease. Children who are treated with antimicrobial agents in the early stage of disease almost never develop late disease.

Because congenital infection occurs with other spirochetal infections, there has been concern that an infected pregnant woman could transmit *Borrelia burgdorferi* to her fetus. No causal relationship between maternal Lyme disease and abnormalities of pregnancy or congenital disease caused by *B burgdorferi* has been documented. There is no evidence that Lyme disease can be transmitted via human milk.

Etiology

In the United States, Lyme disease is caused by the spirochete *B burgdorferi* sensu stricto. In Eurasia, *B burgdorferi*, *Borrelia afzelii*, and *Borrelia garinii* cause borreliosis.

Epidemiology

Lyme disease occurs primarily in 3 distinct geographic regions of the United States. Most cases occur in southern New England and in the eastern mid-Atlantic states. The disease also occurs, but with lower frequency, in the upper Midwest, especially Wisconsin and Minnesota, and less commonly on the West Coast, especially northern California. The occurrence of cases in the United States correlates with the distribution and frequency of infected tick vectors—*Ixodes scapularis* in the east and Midwest and *Ixodes pacificus* in the west. In Southern states, *Ixodes* feed on reptiles rather than small mammals (as in the northeast). Reptile blood is bacteriostatic for *B burgdorferi*, which explains why the disease is not endemic in the south. Reported cases from states without known enzootic risks may have been acquired in states with endemic infection or may be misdiagnoses resulting from false-positive serologic test results. In addition, a rash similar to erythema migrans known as "southern tick-associated rash illness" or STARI has been reported in south central states without endemic *B burgdorferi* infection; however, the etiology of this condition remains unknown. Most cases of early Lyme disease occur between April and October; more than 50% of cases occur during June and July. People of all ages can be affected, but incidence in the United States is highest among children 5 through 9 years of age and adults 55 through 59 years of age.

Incubation Period

From bite to appearance of erythema migrans, 1 to 32 days with a median of 11 days. Endemic Lyme disease transmitted by ixodid ticks occurs in Canada, Europe, states of the former Soviet Union, China, and Japan. The primary tick vector in Europe is *Ixodes ricinus* and the primary tick vector in Asia is *Ixodes persulcatus*. Clinical manifestations of infection vary somewhat from manifestations seen in the United States, probably because of different genomospecies of *Borrelia*.

Diagnostic Tests

During the early stages of Lyme disease, the diagnosis is best made clinically by recognizing the characteristic rash, a singular lesion of erythema migrans, because antibodies against *B burgdorferi* are not detectable in most people within the first few weeks after infection. During the first 4 weeks of infection, serodiagnostic tests are insensitive and generally are not recommended. Diagnosis in patients with early disseminated disease who have multiple lesions of erythema migrans also is made clinically. Diagnosis of early disseminated disease without rash or late Lyme disease should be made on the basis of clinical findings and serologic test results. Some patients who are treated with antimicrobial agents for early Lyme disease never develop antibodies against *B burgdorferi*; they are cured and are not at risk of late disease. Most patients with early disseminated disease and virtually all patients with late disease have antibodies against *B burgdorferi*. Once such antibodies develop, they persist for many years and perhaps for life. Consequently, tests for antibodies should not be repeated or used to assess the success of treatment.

A 2-step approach is recommended for serologic diagnosis of *B burgdorferi*. First, a quantitative screening test for serum antibodies should be performed using a sensitive enzyme immunoassay (EIA) or immunofluorescent antibody assay (IFA). Serum specimens that yield positive or equivocal results then should be tested by a standardized Western immunoblot for presence of antibodies to *B burgdorferi*; serum specimens that yield negative results by EIA or IFA should not be tested further by immunoblot testing. Immunoblot testing should not be performed if the EIA result is negative or instead of or before an EIA; the specificity of immunoblot testing diminishes if this test is performed alone. When testing to confirm early disseminated disease without rash, immunoglobulin (Ig) G and IgM immunoblot assays should be performed. To confirm late disease, only an IgG immunoblot assay should be performed, because false-positive results may occur with the IgM immunoblot. In people with symptoms lasting longer than 1 month, a positive IgM test result alone (ie, with a negative IgG result) is likely to represent a false-positive result and should not be the basis on which to diagnose Lyme disease. A positive result of an IgG immunoblot test requires detection of antibody ("bands") to 5 or more of the following: 18, 23/24, 28, 30, 39, 41, 45, 60, 66, and 93 kDa polypeptides. A positive test result of IgM immunoblot requires detection of antibody to at least 2 of the 23/24, 39, and 41 kDa polypeptides. Two-step testing is needed, because EIA and IFA may yield false-positive results because of the presence of antibodies directed against spirochetes in normal oral flora that cross-react with antigens of *B burgdorferi* or because of cross-reactive antibodies in patients with other spirochetal infections (eg, syphilis, leptospirosis, relapsing fever), certain viral infections (eg, varicella, Epstein-Barr virus), or certain autoimmune diseases (eg, systemic lupus erythematosus).

The widespread practice of ordering serologic tests for patients with nonspecific symptoms, such as fatigue or arthralgia, who have a low probability of having Lyme disease or because of parental pressure, is discouraged. Almost all positive serologic test results in these patients are false-positive results. In areas with endemic infection, subclinical infection and seroconversion also can occur, and the patient's symptoms merely are coincidental. Patients with acute Lyme disease almost always have objective signs of infection (eg, erythema migrans, facial nerve palsy, arthritis). Nonspecific symptoms commonly accompany these specific signs but almost never are the only evidence of Lyme disease.

Treatment

Consensus practice guidelines for assessment, treatment, and prevention of Lyme disease have been published and the recommendations for children are summarized in Table 77.1. Except for doxycycline, the treatment for pregnant women is the same as for children. Anti-microbial therapy for nonspecific symptoms or for asymptomatic seropositivity is discouraged. Use of alternative diagnostic approaches or therapies without adequate validation studies and publication in peer-reviewed scientific literature also are discouraged.

The Jarisch-Herxheimer reaction (an acute febrile reaction accompanied by headache, myalgia, and an aggravated clinical picture lasting <24 hours) can occur when therapy is initiated. Nonsteroidal anti-inflammatory agents may be beneficial, and the antimicrobial agent should be continued.

Table 77.1
Recommended Treatment of Lyme Disease in Children

Disease Category	Drug(s) and Dose[a]
Early Localized Disease[a]	
8 y of age or older	Doxycycline 14–21 days[b]
Younger than 8 y of age or unable to tolerate doxycycline	Amoxicillin for 14–21 days **OR** Cefuroxime, for 14–21 days
Early Disseminated and Late Disease	
Multiple erythema migrans	Same oral regimen as for early localized disease, but for 21 days
Isolated facial palsy	Same oral regimen as for early localized disease, but for 14–21 days[c,d]
Arthritis	Same oral regimen as for early localized disease, but for 28 days
Persistent or recurrent arthritis[e]	Ceftriaxone sodium once a day for 14–28 days Alternatives Penicillin IV for 14–28 days **OR** Cefotaxime 14–28 days **OR** Same oral regimen as for early disease (re-treatment) but for 28 days
Atrioventricular heart block or carditis	Oral regimen as for early disease if asymptomatic[f] but for 14–21 days Ceftriaxone or penicillin IV for symptomatic: see persistent or recurrent arthritis for dosing, but for 14–21 days
Meningitis	Ceftriaxone[g] or cefotaxime with alternative of penicillin[g]: for 14 days (range, 10–28 days) **OR** Doxycycline for 14 days (range, 10–28 days)[b]
Encephalitis or other late neurologic disease[h]	Ceftriaxone[g] or alternatives of penicillin[g] or cefotaxime[g]: see persistent or recurrent arthritis for dosing, duration also for 14–28 days

Abbreviation: IV, intravenously.
[a] For patients who are allergic to penicillin, cefuroxime and erythromycin are alternative drugs.
[b] Tetracyclines are contraindicated in pregnancy and in children younger than 8 years.
[c] Corticosteroids should not be given.
[d] Treatment has no effect on the resolution of facial nerve palsy; its purpose is to prevent late disease.
[e] Arthritis is not considered persistent or recurrent unless objective evidence of synovitis exists at least 2 months after treatment is initiated. Some experts administer a second course of an oral agent before using an IV-administered antimicrobial agent.
[f] Symptoms for heart block or carditis includes syncope, dyspnea, or chest pain.
[g] Ceftriaxone and penicillin should be administered IV for treatment of meningitis or encephalitis.
[h] Other late neurologic manifestations include peripheral neuropathy or encephalopathy.

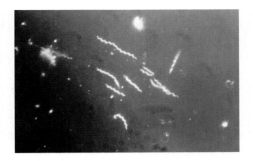

Image 77.1

Using darkfield microscopy technique, this photomicrograph reveals the presence of spirochetes, or corkscrew-shaped bacteria known as *Borrelia burgdorferi,* which is the pathogen responsible for causing Lyme disease (magnification x400). *B burgdorferi* are helical-shaped bacteria, and are about 10 to 25 μm long. These bacteria are transmitted to humans by the bite of an infected deer tick. Courtesy of Centers for Disease Control and Prevention.

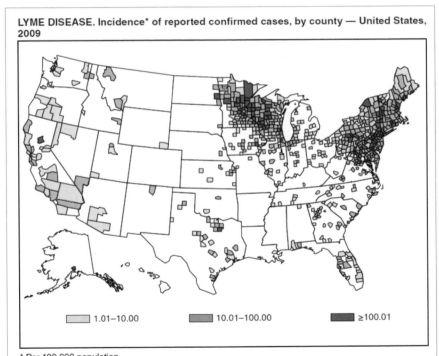

LYME DISEASE. Incidence* of reported confirmed cases, by county — United States, 2009

1.01–10.00	10.01–100.00	≥100.01

* Per 100,000 population.

Approximately 90% of confirmed Lyme disease cases are reported from states in the northeastern and upper midwestern United States. A rash that can be confused with early Lyme disease sometimes occurs following bites of the lone star tick (*Amblyomma americanum*). These ticks, which do not transmit the Lyme disease bacterium, are common human-biting ticks in southern and southeastern United States.

Image 77.2

Number of reported US Lyme disease cases by county, 2009. Courtesy of *Morbidity and Mortality Weekly Report.*

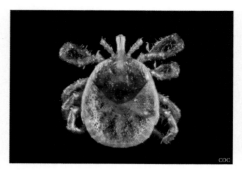

Image 77.3

This photograph depicts a dorsal view of an immature, or nymphal, Lone Star tick, *Amblyomma americanum.* Nymphal ticks are much smaller than adult ticks, and people might not notice a nymph until it has been feeding for a few days. Nymphs are, therefore, more likely than adult ticks to transmit diseases to people. Courtesy of Centers for Disease Control and Prevention/James Gathany.

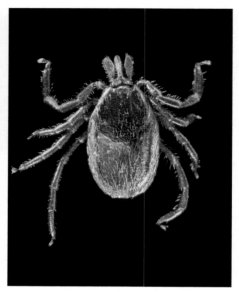

Image 77.4

This photograph depicts a dorsal view of an adult female western blacklegged tick, *Ixodes pacificus,* which has been shown to transmit *Borrelia burgdorferi,* the agent of Lyme disease, and *Anaplasma phagocytophilum,* the agent of human granulocytic anaplasmosis, which was previously known as human granulocytic ehrlichiosis, in the western United States. The small scutum does not cover its entire abdomen, thereby allowing the abdomen to expand many times when this tick ingests its blood meal, and which identifies this specimen as a female. The 4 pairs of jointed legs places these ticks in the phylum Arthropoda and the class Arachnida. Courtesy of Centers for Disease Control and Prevention/James Gathany.

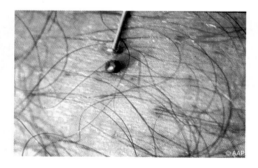

Image 77.5

Despite engorgement, the deer tick is still small and its size approximates the head of a small nail. The ticks that transmit *Rickettsia rickettsii,* usually the dog or Lone Star ticks, are larger, particularly when engorged.

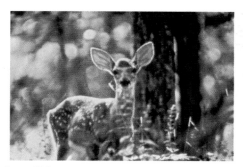

Image 77.6

This photograph of a whitetail deer, *Odocoileus virginianus,* was taken during a Lyme disease field investigation in 1993. Whitetail deer are investigated during outbreaks of Lyme disease because they serve as hosts to the ticks that carry *Borrelia burgdorferi,* the bacteria responsible for Lyme disease. Courtesy of Centers for Disease Control and Prevention.

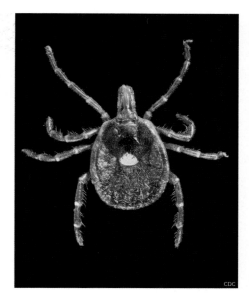

Image 77.7

This photograph depicts a dorsal view of a female Lone Star tick, *Amblyomma americanum.* Note the characteristic "lone star" marking located centrally on its dorsal surface, at the distal tip of its scutum. Courtesy of Centers for Disease Control and Prevention/James Gathany.

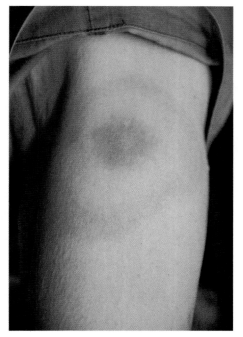

Image 77.8

This photograph depicts the pathognomonic erythematous rash (erythema migrans) in the pattern of a bull's-eye, which developed at the site of a tick bite on this Maryland woman's posterior right upper arm. The expanding rash reflects migration of the spirochetes after introduction of the organism during the tick bite. Courtesy of Centers for Disease Control and Prevention/James Gathany.

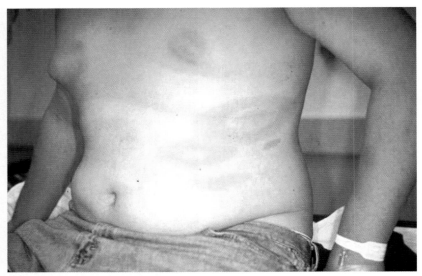

Image 77.9
A 14-year-old boy with multiple annular skin lesions and worsening headache associated with photophobia. Results from a lumbar puncture revealed a cerebrospinal fluid pleocytosis and aseptic meningitis. The characteristic erythema migrans skin lesions helped to determine the diagnosis of Lyme disease. The patient was treated with intravenous ceftriaxone. Copyright Barbara Jantausch, MD, FAAP.

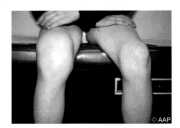

Image 77.10
Borrelia burgdorferi synovitis with marked swelling and only mild tenderness. Arthritis occurs usually within 1 to 2 months following the appearance of erythema migrans, and the knees are the most commonly affected joints.

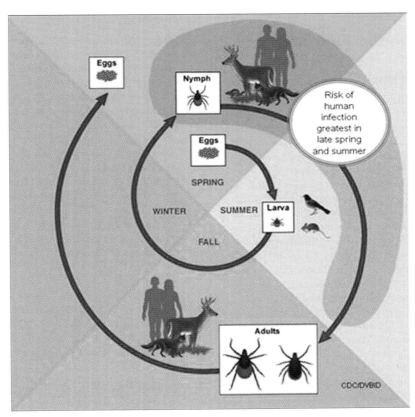

Image 77.11

Life cycle of blacklegged ticks. Blacklegged ticks live for 2 years and have 3 feeding stages: larvae, nymph, and adult. Tick eggs are laid in the spring and hatch as larvae in the summer. Larvae feed on mice, birds, and other small animals in the summer and early fall. When a young tick feeds on an infected animal, the tick takes bacteria into its body along with the blood meal, and it remains infected for the rest of its life. After this initial feeding, the larvae become inactive as they grow into nymphs. The following spring, nymphs seek blood meals in order to fuel their growth into adults. When the tick feeds again, it can transmit the bacterium to its new host. Usually the new host is another small rodent, but sometimes the new host is a human. Most cases of human illness occur in the late spring and summer when the tiny nymphs are most active and human outdoor activity is greatest. Adult ticks feed on large animals, and sometimes on humans. In the spring, adult female ticks lay their eggs on the ground, completing the life cycle. Although adult ticks often feed on deer, these animals do not become infected. Deer are nevertheless important in transporting ticks and maintaining tick populations. Courtesy of Centers for Disease Control and Prevention.

78

Lymphatic Filariasis
(Bancroftian, Malayan, and Timorian)

Clinical Manifestations

Lymphatic filariasis is caused by infection with adult worms, *Wuchereria bancrofti, Brugia malayi,* or *Brugia timori.* Adult worms cause lymphatic dilatation and dysfunction, which results in abnormal lymph flow and may eventually predispose an infected person to lymphedema in the legs, scrotal area, and arms. Recurrent secondary bacterial infections hasten progression of lymphedema to its advanced stage, known as elephantiasis. Although the initial infection usually occurs in young children living in areas with endemic infection, chronic manifestations of infection, such as hydrocele and lymphedema, can occur in people younger than 20 years. Most filarial infections remain asymptomatic but cause subclinical lymphatic dilatation and dysfunction. Lymphadenopathy, most frequently of the inguinal, crural, and axillary lymph nodes, is the most clinical sign of lymphatic filariasis in children. Death of the adult worm triggers an acute inflammatory response, which progresses distally (retrograde) along the affected lymphatic vessel, usually in the limbs. If present, systemic symptoms, such as headache or fever, generally are mild. In postpubertal males, adult *W bancrofti* organisms are found most commonly in the intrascrotal lymphatic vessels; thus, inflammation resulting from adult worm death may present as funiculitis (inflammation of the spermatic cord), epididymitis, or orchitis. A tender granulomatous nodule may be palpable at the site of the dead adult worms. Chyluria can occur as a manifestation of bancroftian filariasis. Tropical pulmonary eosinophilia, characterized by cough, fever, marked eosinophilia, and high serum immunoglobulin E concentrations, is an uncommon manifestation of lymphatic filariasis.

Etiology

Filariasis is caused by 3 filarial nematodes: *W bancrofti, B malayi,* and *B timori.*

Epidemiology

The parasite is transmitted by the bite of infected species of various genera of mosquitoes, including *Culex, Aedes, Anopheles,* and *Mansonia. W bancrofti,* the most prevalent cause of lymphatic filariasis, is found in Haiti, the Dominican Republic, Guyana, northeast Brazil, sub-Saharan and North Africa, and Asia, extending from India through the Indonesian archipelago to the western Pacific islands. Humans are the only definitive host for the parasite. *B malayi* is found mostly in Southeast Asia and parts of India. *B timori* is restricted to certain islands at the eastern end of the Indonesian archipelago. Live adult worms release microfilariae into the bloodstream, and because adult worms live an average of 5 to 8 years and reinfection is common, microfilariae infective for mosquitoes may remain in the patient's blood for decades; individual microfilaria have a lifespan up to 1.5 years. The adult worm is not transmissible from person to person or by blood transfusion, but microfilariae can be transmitted by transfusion.

Incubation Period

From acquisition to appearance of microfilariae in blood, 3 to 12 months, depending on the species of parasite.

Diagnostic Tests

Microfilariae generally can be detected microscopically on blood smears obtained at night (10 pm–4 am), although variations in the periodicity of microfilaremia have been described depending on the parasite and the geographic location of the host. Adult worms or microfilariae can be identified in tissue specimens obtained at biopsy. Serologic enzyme immunoassays are available, but interpretation of results is affected by cross-reactions of filarial antibodies with antibodies against other helminths. Assays for circulating parasite antigen of *W bancrofti* are available commercially but are not licensed by the US Food and Drug Administration. Ultrasonography can be used to visualize adult worms. Lymphatic filariasis often must be diagnosed clinically, because in patients with lymphedema, microfilariae no longer may be present.

Treatment

The main goal of treatment of an infected person is to kill the adult worm. Diethylcarbamazine citrate (DEC), which is both microfilaricidal and active against the adult worm, is the drug of choice for lymphatic filariasis. Once lymphedema is established (the late phase of chronic disease), the disease is not affected by chemotherapy. Ivermectin is effective against the microfilariae of *W bancrofti* but has no effect on the adult parasite. In some studies, combination therapy with single-dose DEC-albendazole or ivermectin-albendazole has been shown to be more effective than any one drug alone in suppressing microfilaremia.

Complex decongestive physiotherapy may be effective for treating lymphedema. Chyluria originating in the bladder responds to fulguration; chyluria originating in the kidney usually cannot be corrected. Prompt identification and treatment of bacterial superinfections, particularly streptococcal and staphylococcal infections, and careful treatment of intertriginous and ungual fungal infections are important aspects of therapy for lymphedema.

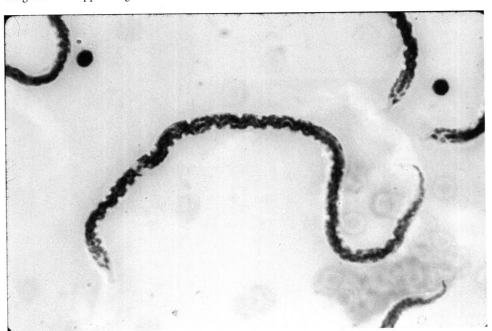

Image 78.1
Giemsa stain of thick blood smear filiariasis.

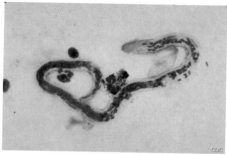

Image 78.2

This photomicrograph shows the inner body and cephalic space of a *Brugia malayi* microfilaria in a thick blood smear. *B malayi,* a nematode that can inhabit the lymphatics and subcutaneous tissues in humans, is one of the causative agents for lymphatic filariasis. The vectors for this parasite are mosquito species from the genera *Mansonia* and *Aedes.* Courtesy of Centers for Disease Control and Prevention/Mae Melvin, MD.

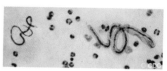

Image 78.3

Microfilariae of *Loa loa* (right) and *Mansonella perstans* (left) in a patient in Cameroon (thick blood smear; hematoxylin stain). *L loa* is sheathed, with a relatively dense nuclear column; its tail tapers and is frequently coiled, and nuclei extend to the end of the tail. *M perstans* is smaller, has no sheath, and has a blunt tail with nuclei extending to the end of the tail. Courtesy of Centers for Disease Control and Prevention.

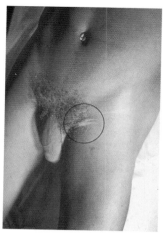

Image 78.5

Inguinal lymph nodes enlarged due to filariasis. Courtesy of Centers for Disease Control and Prevention.

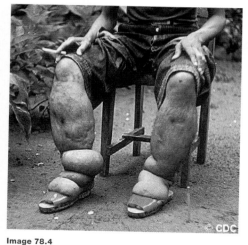

Image 78.4

Elephantiasis of both legs due to filariasis. Luzon, Philippines. Courtesy of Centers for Disease Control and Prevention.

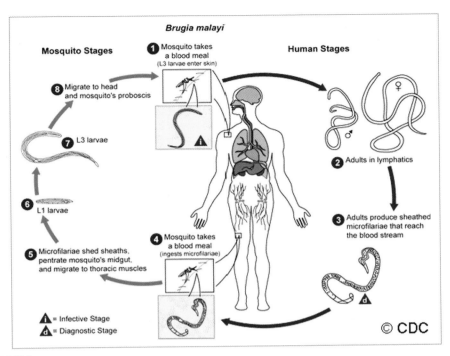

Image 78.6
The typical vector for *Brugia malayi* filariasis are mosquito species from the genera *Mansonia* and *Aedes*. During a blood meal, an infected mosquito introduces third-stage filarial larvae onto the skin of the human host, where they penetrate into the bite wound (1). They develop into adults that commonly reside in the lymphatics (2). The adult worms resemble those of *Wuchereria bancrofti* but are smaller. Female worms measure 43 to 55 mm in length by 130 to 170 μm in width, and males measure 13 to 23 mm in length by 70 to 80 μm in width. Adults produce microfilariae, measuring 177 to 230 μm in length and 5 to 7 μm in width, that are sheathed and have nocturnal periodicity. The microfilariae migrate into lymph and enter the bloodstream, reaching the peripheral blood (3). A mosquito ingests the microfilariae during a blood meal (1).

After ingestion, the microfilariae lose their sheaths and work their way through the wall of the proventriculus and cardiac portion of the midgut to reach the thoracic muscles (5). There the microfilariae develop into first-stage larvae (6) and subsequently into third-stage larvae (7). The third-stage larvae migrate through the hemocoel to the mosquito's proboscis (8) and can infect another human when the mosquito takes a blood meal (1). Courtesy of Centers for Disease Control and Prevention.

79

Lymphocytic Choriomeningitis

Clinical Manifestations

Child and adult infections are asymptomatic in approximately one-third of cases. Symptomatic infection can result in a mild to severe influenza-like illness, including fever, malaise, myalgia, retro-orbital headache, photophobia, anorexia, and nausea. Initial symptoms can last up to 1 week. A biphasic febrile course is common; after a few days without symptoms, the second phase occurs in up to half of symptomatic patients, consisting of neurologic manifestations that vary from aseptic meningitis to severe encephalitis. Transmission of lymphocytic choriomeningitis (LCM) virus through organ transplantation can result in fatal disseminated infection with multiple organ failure. In the past, LCM virus has caused up to 10% to 15% of all cases of aseptic meningitis, and it was a common cause of aseptic meningitis during winter months. Arthralgia or arthritis, respiratory tract symptoms, orchitis, and leukopenia develop occasionally. Recovery without sequelae is the usual outcome. LCM virus infection should be suspected in presence of (1) aseptic meningitis or encephalitis during the fall-winter season; (2) febrile illness, followed by brief remission, followed by onset of neurologic illness; and (3) cerebrospinal fluid (CSF) findings of lymphocytosis and hypoglycorrhachia.

Infection during pregnancy has been associated with spontaneous abortion. Congenital infection may cause severe abnormalities, including hydrocephalus, chorioretinitis, intracranial calcifications, microcephaly, and mental retardation. Congenital LCM etiology should be envisaged when a congenital infection syndrome is suspected. Patients with immune abnormalities may experience severe or fatal illness, as observed in patients receiving organs from LCM virus-infected donors.

Etiology

LCM virus is an arenavirus.

Epidemiology

LCM is a chronic infection of common house mice, which often are infected asymptomatically, but chronically shed virus in urine and other excretions. Pet hamsters, laboratory mice, guinea pigs, and colonized golden hamsters can have chronic infection and can be sources of human infection. Humans are infected by aerosol or by ingestion of dust or food contaminated with the virus from the urine, feces, blood, or nasopharyngeal secretions of infected rodents. The disease is observed more frequently in young adults. Human-to-human transmission has occurred during pregnancy from infected mothers to their fetus and through solid organ transplantation from an undiagnosed, acutely LCM virus-infected organ donor. Several such clusters of cases have been described following transplantation, and 1 case was traced to a pet hamster purchased by the donor. A number of laboratory-acquired LCM virus infections have occurred, both through contaminated tissue culture stocks and infected laboratory animals.

Incubation Period

Usually 6 to 13 days; occasionally 3 weeks.

Diagnostic Tests

In patients with central nervous system disease, mononuclear pleocytosis often exceeding 1,000 cells/µL is present in CSF. Hypoglycorrhachia can occur. LCM virus usually can be isolated from CSF obtained during the acute phase of illness and, in severe disseminated infections, also from blood, urine, and nasopharyngeal secretion specimens. Reverse transcriptase PCR assays can be used for CSF. Serum specimens from the acute and convalescent phases of illness can be tested for increases in antibody titers by enzyme immunoassays. Demonstration of virus-specific immunoglobulin M antibodies in serum or CSF specimens is useful. In congenital infections, diagnosis usually is suspected at the sequela phase, and diagnosis usually is made by serologic testing. Diagnosis can be made retrospectively by immunohistochemistry assay of tissues obtained from necropsy.

Treatment

Supportive.

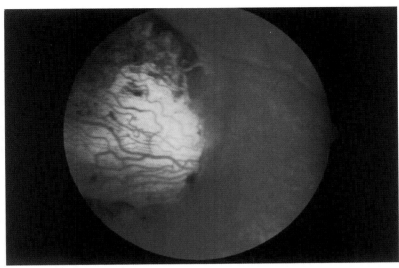

Image 79.1

Fundus photograph of a 9-month-old girl with congenital lymphocytic choriomeningitis virus infection. Extensive chorioretinal scarring is visible. Hydrocephalus and periventricular calcification were visible on computed tomography scan and magnetic resonance imaging. Copyright Leslie L. Barton, MD, FAAP.

80

Malaria

Clinical Manifestations

The classic symptoms of malaria are high fever with chills, rigor, sweats, and headache, which may be paroxysmal. If appropriate treatment is not administered, fever and paroxysms can occur in a cyclic pattern. Depending on the infecting species, fever classically appears every other or every third day. Other manifestations can include nausea, vomiting, diarrhea, cough, tachypnea, arthralgia, myalgia, and abdominal and back pain. Anemia and thrombocytopenia are common, and pallor and jaundice caused by hemolysis can occur. Hepatosplenomegaly may be present. More severe disease occurs in people without previous exposure, young children, and people who are pregnant or immunocompromised.

Infection with *Plasmodium falciparum,* 1 of the 5 *Plasmodium* species that infect humans, potentially is fatal and most commonly manifests as a febrile nonspecific illness without localizing signs. Severe disease (most commonly caused by *P falciparum*) can manifest as one of the following clinical syndromes, each of which are medical emergencies and fatal unless treated:

- **Cerebral malaria,** which can have variable neurologic manifestations, including generalized seizures, signs of increased intracranial pressure, confusion, and progression to stupor, coma, and death
- **Hypoglycemia,** which can occur with metabolic acidosis and hypotension associated with hyperparasitemia or be associated with quinine treatment
- **Renal failure** caused by acute tubular necrosis (rare in children <8 years)
- **Respiratory failure and metabolic acidosis,** without pulmonary edema
- **Severe anemia** attributable to high parasitemia, sequestration and hemolysis associated with hypersplenism
- **Vascular collapse and shock** associated with hypothermia and adrenal insufficiency (People with asplenia who become infected can be at increased risk of more severe illness and death.)

Syndromes primarily associated with *Plasmodium vivax* and *Plasmodium ovale* infection is as follows:

- **Anemia** attributable to acute parasitemia
- **Hypersplenism** with danger of late splenic rupture
- **Relapse,** for as long as 3 to 5 years after the primary infection, attributable to latent hepatic stages (hypnozoites)

Syndromes associated with *Plasmodium malariae* infection include

- **Chronic asymptomatic parasitemia** for as long as several years after the last exposure
- **Nephrotic syndrome** from deposition of immune complexes in the kidney

Plasmodium knowlesi is a primate malaria parasite that also can infect humans. *P knowlesi* malaria has been misdiagnosed commonly as the more benign *P malariae* malaria. Disease can be characterized by very rapid replication of the organism and hyperparasitemia resulting in severe disease. Severe disease in patients with *P knowlesi* infection should be treated aggressively, because hepatorenal failure and subsequent death have been reported.

Congenital malaria secondary to perinatal transmission rarely can occur. Most congenital cases have been caused by *P vivax* and *P falciparum*; *P malariae* and *P ovale* account for fewer than 20% of such cases. Manifestations can resemble those of neonatal sepsis, including fever and nonspecific symptoms of poor appetite, irritability, and lethargy.

Etiology

The genus *Plasmodium* includes species of intraerythrocytic parasites that infect a wide range of mammals, birds, and reptiles. The 5 species that frequently infect humans are *P falciparum, P vivax, P ovali, P malariae,* and *P knowlesi.* Coinfection with multiple species increasingly is recognized as PCR technology is applied to the diagnosis of malaria.

Epidemiology

Malaria is endemic throughout the tropical areas of the world and is acquired from the bite of the female nocturnal-feeding *Anopheles* genus of mosquito. Half of the world's population lives in areas where transmission occurs. Worldwide, 243 million cases and 863,000 reported deaths occur each year. Most deaths occur in young children. Infection by the malaria parasite poses substantial risks to pregnant women and their fetuses and may result in spontaneous abortion and stillbirth. Malaria also contributes significantly to low birth weight in countries with endemic infection. The risk of malaria is highest, but variable, for travelers to sub-Saharan Africa, Papua New Guinea, the Solomon Islands, and Vanuatu; the risk is intermediate on the Indian subcontinent and is low in most of Southeast Asia and Latin America. The potential for malaria transmission is ongoing in areas where malaria previously was eliminated if infected people return and the mosquito vector is still present. These conditions have resulted in recent cases in travelers to areas such as Jamaica, the Dominican Republic, and the Bahamas. Health care professionals should check an up-to-date source (**wwwn.cdc.gov/travel**) to determine malaria endemicity when providing pretravel malaria advice or evaluating a febrile returned traveler. Transmission is possible in more temperate climates, including areas of the United States where anopheline mosquitoes are present. Nearly all of the approximately 1,400 annual reported cases in the United States result from infection acquired abroad. Rarely, mosquitoes in airplanes flying from areas with endemic malaria have been the source of cases in people working or residing near international airports. Local transmission also occurs rarely in the United States.

P vivax and *P falciparum* are the most common species worldwide. *P vivax* malaria is prevalent on the Indian subcontinent and in Central America. *P falciparum* malaria is prevalent in Africa, Papua New Guinea, and on the island of Hispaniola (Haiti and the Dominican Republic). *P vivax* and *P falciparum* species are the most common malaria species in southern and Southeast Asia, Oceania, and South America. *P malariae*, although much less common, has a wide distribution. *P ovale* malaria occurs most often in West Africa but has been reported in other areas.

Relapses can occur in *P vivax* and *P ovale* malaria because of a persistent hepatic (hypnozoite) stage of infection. Recrudescence of *P falciparum* and *P malariae* infection occurs when a persistent low-concentration parasitemia causes recurrence of symptoms of the disease or when drug resistance prevents elimination of the parasite. In areas of Africa and Asia with hyperendemic infection, reinfection in people with partial immunity results in a high prevalence of asymptomatic parasitemia.

The spread of chloroquine-resistant *P falciparum* strains throughout the world is of increasing concern. In addition, resistance to other antimalarial drugs also is occurring in many areas where the drugs are used widely. *P falciparum* resistance to sulfadoxine-pyrimethamine is common throughout Africa, mefloquine resistance has been documented in Burma (Myanmar), Laos, Thailand, Cambodia, China, and Vietnam and emerging resistance to artemisinins has been observed at the Cambodia-Thailand border. Chloroquine-resistant *P vivax* has been reported in Indonesia, Papua New Guinea, the Solomon Islands, Myanmar, India, and Guyana. Malaria symptoms can develop as soon as 7 days after exposure in an area with endemic malaria to as late as several months after departure. More than 80% of cases diagnosed in the United States occur in people who have onset of symptoms after their return to the United States.

Diagnostic Tests

Definitive diagnosis relies on identification of the parasite microscopically on stained blood films. Both thick and thin blood films should be examined. The thick film allows for concentration of the blood to find parasites that may be present in small numbers, whereas the thin film is most useful for species identification and determination of the degree of parasitemia (the percentage of erythrocytes harboring parasites). If initial blood smears test negative for *Plasmodium* species but malaria remains a possibility, the smear should be repeated every 12 to 24 hours during a 72-hour period.

Confirmation and identification of the species of malaria parasites on the blood smear is important in guiding therapy. Serologic testing generally is not helpful, except in epidemiologic surveys. PCR assay is available in reference laboratories and some state health departments. DNA probes and malarial ribosomal RNA testing may provide rapid and accurate diagnosis in the future but currently are used in experimental studies only. A new US Food and Drug Administration–approved test for antigen detection is available in the United States. It is the only antigen-detection kit available. However, an evaluation by the World Health Organization found that this product had poor sensitivity for detecting low-density *P vivax* infections. Rapid diagnostic testing is recommended to be conducted in parallel with routine microscopy to provide further information needed for patient treatment, such as the percentage of erythrocytes harboring parasites. Also, information about the sensitivity of rapid diagnostic tests for the 2 less common species of malaria, *P ovale* and *P malariae,* is limited. More information about rapid diagnostic testing for malaria is available at **www.cdc.gov/malaria/diagnosis_treatment/index.html.**

Treatment

The choice of malaria chemotherapy is based on the infecting species, possible drug resistance, and severity of disease. Severe malaria is defined as any one or more of the following: parasitemia greater than 5% of red blood cells, signs of central nervous system or other end-organ involvement, shock, acidosis, and/or hypoglycemia. Patients with severe malaria require intensive care and parenteral treatment until the parasite density decreases to less than 1% and they are able to tolerate oral therapy. Exchange transfusion may be warranted when parasitemia exceeds 10% or if there is evidence of complications (eg, cerebral malaria or renal failure) at lower parasite densities. For patients with severe malaria in the United States who do not tolerate or cannot easily access quinidine, intravenous artesunate has become available through a Centers for Disease Control and Prevention investigational new drug protocol. For patients with *P falciparum* malaria, sequential blood smears to determine percentage of erythrocytes harboring parasites can be useful in monitoring treatment.

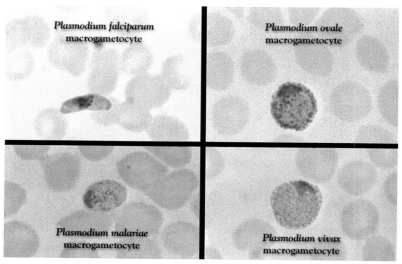

Image 80.1

This Giemsa-stained slide reveals a *Plasmodium falciparum, Plasmodium ovale, Plasmodium malariae,* and *Plasmodium vivax* gametocyte. The male (microgametocytes) and female (macrogametocytes) are ingested by an *Anopheles* mosquito during its blood meal. Known as the sporogonic cycle, while in the mosquito's stomach, the microgametes penetrate the macrogametes generating zygotes. Courtesy of Centers for Disease Control and Prevention/Steven Glenn, Laboratory and Consultation Division.

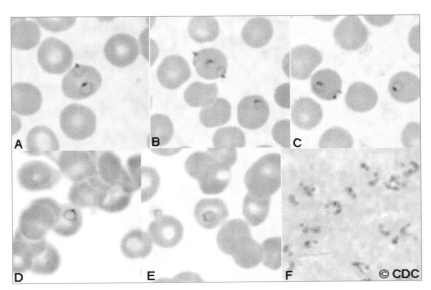

Image 80.2

Plasmodium falciparum: ring stage smears from patients. *P falciparum* rings have delicate cytoplasm and 1 or 2 small chromatin dots. Red blood cells (RBCs) that are infected are not enlarged; multiple infection of RBCs is more common in *P falciparum* than in other species. Occasional appliqué forms (rings appearing on the periphery of the RBC) can be present. (A–C) Multiply infected RBCs with appliqué forms in thin blood smears. (D) Signet ring form. (E) Double chromatin dot. (F) A thick blood smear showing many ring forms of *P falciparum.* Courtesy of Centers for Disease Control and Prevention.

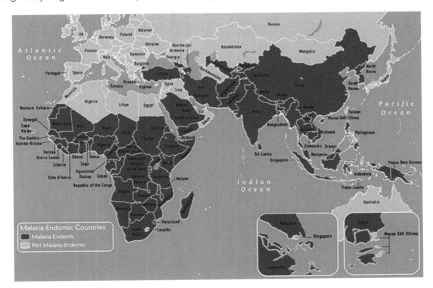

Image 80.3

Malaria-endemic countries in the eastern hemisphere. Courtesy of Centers for Disease Control and Prevention.

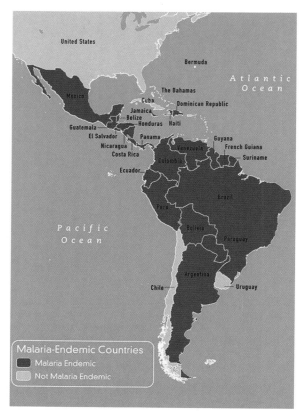

Image 80.4
Malaria-endemic countries in the western hemisphere. Courtesy of Centers for Disease Control and Prevention.

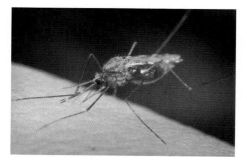

Image 80.5
This photograph depicts an *Anopheles funestus* mosquito partaking in a blood meal from its human host. Note the blood passing through the proboscis, which has penetrated the skin and entered a miniscule cutaneous blood vessel. The *A funestus* mosquito, which along with *Anopheles gambiae,* is 1 of the 2 most important malaria vectors in Africa, where more than 80% of the world's malarial disease and deaths occurs. Courtesy of Centers for Disease Control and Prevention/James Gathany.

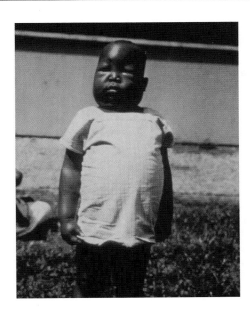

Image 80.6

The edema exhibited by this African child was brought on by nephrosis associated with malaria. Infection with one type of malaria, *Plasmodium falciparum,* if not promptly treated, may cause kidney failure. Swelling of the abdomen, eyes, feet, and hands are some of the symptoms of nephrosis brought on by the damaged kidneys. Courtesy of Centers for Disease Control and Prevention/ Dr Myron Schultz.

81

Measles

Clinical Manifestations

Measles is an acute viral disease characterized by fever, cough, coryza, conjunctivitis, an erythematous maculopapular rash, and a pathognomonic enanthema (Koplik spots). Complications including otitis media, bronchopneumonia, laryngotracheobronchitis (croup), and diarrhea occur commonly in young children. Acute encephalitis, which often results in permanent brain damage, occurs in approximately 1 of every 1,000 cases. In the post measles elimination era, death, predominantly resulting from respiratory and neurologic complications, has occurred in 1 to 3 of every 1,000 cases reported in the United States. Case-fatality rates are increased in children younger than 5 years and immunocompromised children, including children with leukemia, HIV infection, and severe malnutrition. Sometimes the characteristic rash does not develop in immunocompromised patients.

Subacute sclerosing panencephalitis (SSPE) is a rare degenerative central nervous system disease characterized by behavioral and intellectual deterioration and seizures that occurs 7 to 10 years after wild-type measles virus infection. Widespread measles immunization has led to the virtual disappearance of SSPE in the United States.

Etiology

Measles virus is an enveloped RNA virus with 1 serotype, classified as a member of the genus Morbillivirus in the Paramyxoviridae family.

Epidemiology

The only natural hosts of measles virus are humans. Measles is transmitted by direct contact with infectious droplets or, less commonly, by airborne spread. Measles is one of the most highly communicable of all infectious diseases. In temperate areas, the peak incidence of infection usually occurs during late winter and spring. In the prevaccine era, most cases of measles in the United States occurred in preschool- and young school-aged children, and few people remained susceptible

by 20 years of age. The childhood and adolescent immunization program in the United States has resulted in a greater than 99% decrease in the reported incidence of measles and interruption of endemic disease transmission since measles vaccine first was licensed in 1963.

From 1989 to 1991, the incidence of measles in the United States increased because of low immunization rates in preschool-aged children, especially in urban areas. Following improved coverage in preschool-aged children and implementation of a routine second dose of measles-mumps-rubella vaccine for children, the incidence of measles declined to extremely low levels (<1 case per 1 million population). In 2000, an independent panel of internationally recognized experts reviewed available data and unanimously agreed that measles no longer was endemic (continuous, year-round transmission) in the United States. In the post elimination era, from 2001 through 2010, the incidence of measles in the United States has been low (37–140 cases reported per year), consistent with an absence of endemic transmission. Cases of measles continue to occur, however, as a result of importation of the virus from other countries. Cases are considered international importations if the rash onset occurs within 21 days after entering the United States. During 2011, 222 cases of measles were reported to the Centers for Disease Control and Prevention (CDC) from 30 states—the highest number of reported measles cases since 1996. Seventy-two of the cases were direct importations from 22 countries, and 17 outbreaks (≥3 cases) occurred. Most (approximately 85%) of the cases were people who were unimmunized or had unknown immunization status, including 27 cases in infants younger than 12 months, some of whom had traveled abroad.

Vaccine failure occurs in as many as 5% of people who have received a single dose of vaccine at 12 months of age or older. Although waning immunity after immunization may be a factor in some cases, most cases of measles in previously immunized children seem to occur in people in whom response to the vaccine was inadequate (ie, primary vaccine failures). This was the main reason a 2-dose vaccine schedule was recommended routinely for children and high-risk adults.

Patients are contagious from 4 days before the rash to 4 days after appearance of the rash. Immunocompromised patients who may have prolonged excretion of the virus in respiratory tract secretions can be contagious for the duration of the illness. Patients with SSPE are not contagious.

Incubation Period

8 to 12 days from exposure to onset; in family studies, average is 14 days (range, 7–21).

Diagnostic Tests

Measles virus infection can be diagnosed by a positive serologic test result for measles immunoglobulin (Ig) M antibody, a significant increase in measles IgG antibody concentration in paired acute and convalescent serum specimens by any standard serologic assay, or isolation of measles virus or identification of measles RNA (by reverse transcriptase PCR assay) from clinical specimens, such as urine, blood, or throat or nasopharyngeal secretions. State public health laboratories or the CDC Measles Laboratory will process these viral specimens. The simplest method of establishing the diagnosis of measles is testing for IgM antibody on a single serum specimen obtained during the first encounter with a person suspected of having disease. The sensitivity of measles IgM assays varies by timing of specimen collection and immunization status of the case. The IgM level may be diminished during the first 72 hours after rash onset. If the result is negative for measles IgM and the patient has a generalized rash lasting more than 72 hours, a second serum specimen should be obtained, and the measles IgM test should be repeated. A negative IgM test should not be used to exclude the diagnosis in immunized people. People with febrile rash illness who are seronegative for measles IgM should be tested for rubella using the same specimens. Genotyping of viral isolates allows determination of patterns of importation and transmission, and genome sequencing can be used to differentiate between wild-type and vaccine virus infection in those who have been immunized recently. Measles now is on the list of nationally notifiable diseases that should be reported to the CDC within 24 hours.

Treatment

No specific antiviral therapy is available. Vitamin A treatment of children with measles in developing countries has been associated with decreased morbidity and mortality rates. Low serum concentrations of vitamin A also have been found in children in the United States, and children with more severe measles illness have lower vitamin A concentrations. The World Health Organization currently recommends vitamin A for all children with acute measles, regardless of their country of residence. Vitamin A for treatment of measles is administered once daily for 2 days. Parenteral and oral formulations of vitamin A are available in the United States.

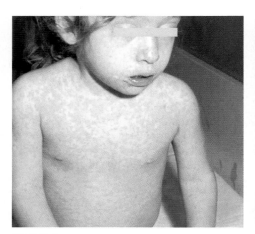

Image 81.1
Child with rubeola who has the characteristic rash and irritable, ill appearance.

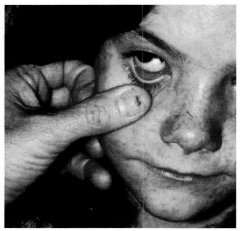

Image 81.2
Measles (rubeola) rash and conjunctivitis. Conjunctivitis results in clear tearing. Photophobia is common.

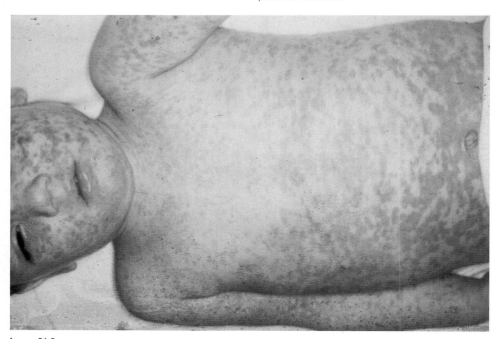

Image 81.3
The near confluent exanthem of measles (rubeola) in a 2-year-old white male. Courtesy of Paul Wehrle, MD.

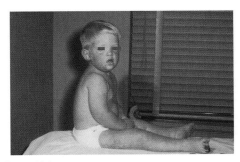

Image 81.4
This child with measles is displaying the characteristic red blotchy pattern on his face and body during the third day of the rash. Courtesy of Centers for Disease Control and Prevention.

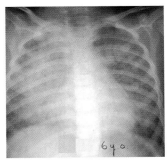

Image 81.6
Measles (rubeola) pneumonia in a 6-year-old child with acute lymphoblastic leukemia. The child died of respiratory failure.

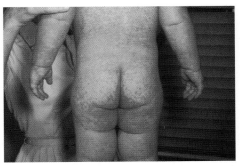

Image 81.5
This child with measles is showing the characteristic red blotchy rash on his buttocks and back during the third day of the rash. Measles is an acute, highly communicable viral disease with prodromal fever, conjunctivitis, coryza, cough, and Koplik spots on the buccal mucosa. A red, blotchy rash appears around day 3 of the illness, first on the face and then becoming generalized. Courtesy of Centers for Disease Control and Prevention.

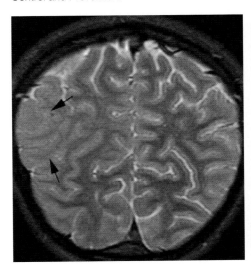

Image 81.7
This coronal T2-weighted magnetic resonance image shows swelling and hyperintensity of the right parietal occipital cortex (arrows) in a patient with measles encephalitis.

82

Meningococcal Infections

Clinical Manifestations

Invasive infection usually results in meningo-coccemia, meningitis, or both. Onset can be insidious and nonspecific but typically is abrupt, with fever, chills, malaise, myalgia, limb pain, prostration, and a rash that initially can be macular, maculopapular, petechial, or purpuric. The maculopapular and petechial rash are indistinguishable from the rash caused by some viral infections. Purpura can occur in severe sepsis caused by other bacterial patho-gens. In fulminant cases, purpura, limb isch-emia, coagulopathy, pulmonary edema, shock, coma, and death can ensue in hours despite appropriate therapy. Signs and symptoms of meningococcal meningitis are indistinguish-able from those associated with acute menin-gitis caused by other meningeal pathogens (eg, *Streptococcus pneumoniae*). In severe and fatal cases of meningococcal meningitis, raised intracranial pressure is a predominant presenting feature. The overall case-fatality rate for meningococcal disease is 10% and is higher in adolescents and lower in infants. Death is associated with coma, hypotension, leukopenia, thrombocytopenia, and absence of meningitis. Less common manifestations of meningococcal infection include conjunctivi-tis, pneumonia, febrile occult bacteremia, sep-tic arthritis, and chronic meningococcemia. Invasive infections can be complicated by arthritis, myocarditis, pericarditis, and endo-phthalmitis. A self-limiting postinfectious inflammatory syndrome (immune complex mediated) occurs in less than 10% of cases 4 or more days after onset of meningococcal infec-tion and most commonly presents as fever and arthritis or vasculitis. Iritis, scleritis, conjunc-tivitis, pericarditis, and polyserositis are less common manifestations of postinfectious inflammatory syndrome.

Sequelae associated with meningococcal disease occur in 11% to 19% of survivors and include hearing loss, neurologic disability, digit or limb amputations, and skin scarring.

Etiology

Neisseria meningitidis is a gram-negative diplococcus with at least 13 serogroups based on capsule type.

Epidemiology

Strains belonging to groups A, B, C, Y, and W-135 are implicated most commonly in inva-sive disease worldwide. Serogroup A has been associated frequently with epidemics outside the United States, primarily in sub-Saharan Africa. An increase in cases of serogroup W-135 meningococcal disease has been associated with the Hajj pilgrimage in Saudi Arabia. Since 2002, serogroup W-135 meningococcal disease has been reported in sub-Saharan African countries during epidemic seasons. Prolonged outbreaks of serogroup B meningococcal dis-ease have occurred in New Zealand, France, and Oregon. Serogroup X causes a substantial number of cases of meningococcal disease in parts of Africa but is rare on other continents.

The incidence of meningococcal disease var-ies over time and by age and location. During the past 60 years, the annual incidence of meningococcal disease in the United States has varied from 0.5 to 1.5 cases per 100,000 population. Incidence cycles have occurred over multiple years. Since the early 2000s, annual incidence rates have decreased and are sustained. The reasons for this decrease, which preceded introduction of meningococcal polysaccharide-protein conjugate vaccine into the immunization schedule, are not known but may be related to immunity of the population to circulating meningococcal strains and to the changes in behavioral risk factors (eg, smoking).

Distribution of meningococcal serogroups in the United States has shifted in the past 2 decades. Serogroups B, C, and Y each account for approximately 30% of reported cases, but serogroup distribution varies by age, location, and time. Approximately three-quarters of cases among adolescents and young adults are caused by serogroups C, Y, or W-135 and poten-tially are preventable with available vaccines. In infants, 50% to 60% of cases are caused by serogroup B and are not preventable with vac-cines available in the United States.

Since introduction in the United States of *Haemophilus influenzae* type b and pneumococcal polysaccharide-protein conjugate vaccines for infants, *N meningitidis* has become the leading cause of bacterial meningitis in children and remains an important cause of septicemia. Disease most often occurs in children 2 years of age or younger; the peak incidence occurs in children younger than 1 year of age. Another peak occurs in adolescents and young adults 16 through 21 years of age. Historically, freshman college students who lived in dormitories and military recruits in boot camp had a higher rate of disease compared with people who are the same age and who are not living in such accommodations. Close contacts of patients with meningococcal disease are at increased risk of becoming infected. Patients with persistent complement component deficiencies (eg, C5–C9, properdin, or factor H or factor D deficiencies) or anatomic or functional asplenia are at increased risk of invasive and recurrent meningococcal disease. Patients are considered capable of transmitting the organism for up to 24 hours after initiation of effective antimicrobial treatment. Asymptomatic colonization of the upper respiratory tract provides the source from which the organism is spread. Transmission occurs from person-to-person through droplets from the respiratory tract and requires close contact.

Outbreaks occur in communities and institutions, including child care centers, schools, colleges, and military recruit camps. However, most cases of meningococcal disease are endemic, with fewer than 5% associated with outbreaks. The attack rate for household contacts is 500 to 800 times the rate for the general population. Serologic typing, multilocus sequence typing, multilocus enzyme electrophoresis, and pulsed-field gel electrophoresis of enzyme-restricted DNA fragments can be useful epidemiologic tools during a suspected outbreak to detect concordance among invasive strains.

Incubation Period

1 to 10 days, usually less than 4 days.

Diagnostic Tests

Cultures of blood and cerebrospinal fluid (CSF) are indicated for patients with suspected invasive meningococcal disease. Cultures of a petechial or purpuric lesion scraping, synovial fluid, and other usually sterile body fluid specimens yield the organism in some patients. A Gram stain of a petechial or purpuric scraping, CSF, and buffy coat smear of blood can be helpful. Because *N meningitidis* can be a component of the nasopharyngeal flora, isolation of *N meningitidis* from this site is not helpful diagnostically. Bacterial antigen detection in CSF supports the diagnosis of a probable case if the clinical illness is consistent with meningococcal disease. A serogroup-specific PCR test to detect *N meningitidis* from clinical specimens is used routinely in the United Kingdom and some European countries, where up to 56% of cases are confirmed by PCR testing alone. This test particularly is useful in patients who receive antimicrobial therapy before cultures are obtained. In the United States, PCR-based assays are available in some research and public health laboratories.

Case definitions for invasive meningococcal disease are given in Box 82.1.

Treatment

The priority in management of meningococcal disease is treatment of shock in meningococcemia and of raised intracranial pressure in severe cases of meningitis. Empiric therapy for suspected meningococcal disease should include an extended-spectrum cephalosporin, such as cefotaxime or ceftriaxone. Once the microbiologic diagnosis is established, definitive treatment with penicillin G (300,000 U/kg/day; maximum, 12 million U/day, divided every 4–6 hours), ampicillin, or an extended-spectrum cephalosporin (cefotaxime or ceftriaxone), is recommended. Some experts recommend susceptibility testing before switching to penicillin. However, susceptibility testing is not standardized, and clinical significance of intermediate susceptibility is unknown. Resistance of *N meningitidis* to penicillin is rare in the United States. Ceftriaxone clears nasopharyngeal carriage effectively

Box 82.1
Surveillance Case Definitions for Invasive Meningococcal Disease

Confirmed

A clinically compatible case and isolation of *Neisseria meningitidis* from a usually sterile site, for example
- Blood
- Cerebrospinal fluid
- Synovial fluid
- Pleural fluid
- Pericardial fluid
- Isolation from skin scraping of petechial or purpuric lesions

Probable

A clinically compatible case with either a positive result of antigen test or immunohistochemistry of formalin-fixed tissue or a positive PCR test of blood or cerebrospinal fluid without a positive sterile site culture

Suspect
- A clinically compatible case and gram-negative diplococci in any sterile fluid, such as cerebrospinal fluid, synovial fluid, or scraping from a petechial or purpuric lesion
- Clinical purpura fulminans without a positive blood culture

after 1 dose and allows outpatient management for completion of therapy when appropriate. For patients with a serious penicillin allergy characterized by anaphylaxis, chloramphenicol is recommended, if available. If chloramphenicol is not available, meropenem can be used, although the rate of cross-reactivity in penicillin-allergic adults is 2% to 3%. For travelers from areas where penicillin resistance has been reported, cefotaxime, ceftriaxone, or chloramphenicol is recommended. Five to 7 days of

antimicrobial therapy is adequate. In meningococcemia presenting with shock, early and rapid fluid resuscitation and early use of inotropic and ventilatory support may reduce mortality. In view of the lack of evidence in pediatric populations, adjuvant therapies are not recommended. The postinfectious inflammatory syndromes associated with meningococcal disease often respond to nonsteroidal anti-inflammatory drugs.

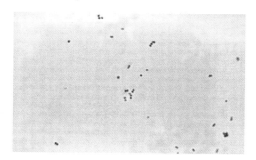

Image 82.1

This micrograph depicts the presence of aerobic gram-negative *Neisseria meningitidis* diplococcal bacteria (magnification ×1,150). Meningococcal disease is an infection caused by a bacterium called *N meningitidis* or meningococcus. Courtesy of Centers for Disease Control and Prevention/ Dr Brodsky.

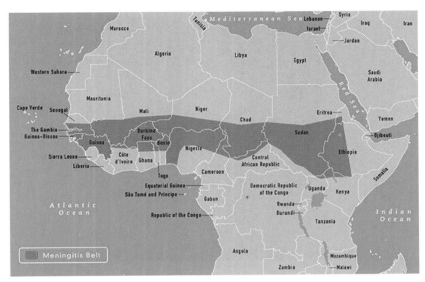

Image 82.2
Areas with frequent epidemics of meningococcal meningitis. Courtesy of Centers for Disease Control and Prevention.

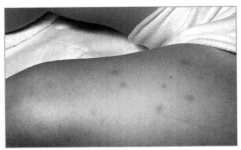

Image 82.3
Papular skin lesions of early meningococcemia.

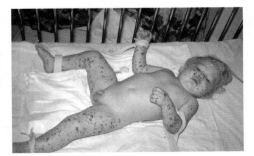

Image 82.4
Young boy with meningococcemia that demonstrates striking involvement of the extremities with sparing of the trunk. Copyright Martin G. Myers, MD.

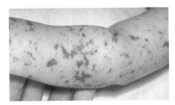

Image 82.5
The arm of the boy shown in Image 82.4, which demonstrates striking extremity involvement and characteristic angular lesions. Copyright Martin G. Myers, MD.

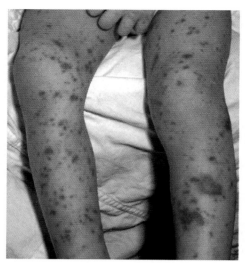

Image 82.6
Meningococcemia lesions of the lower extremities.

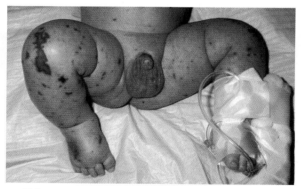

Image 82.7
Meningococcemia in an infant male. Courtesy of Ed Fajardo, MD.

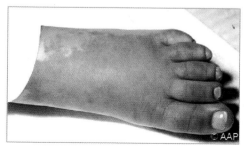

Image 82.8
Marked purpura of the left foot.

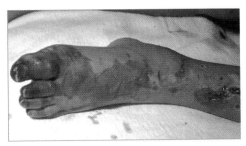

Image 82.9
Patient shown in Image 82.8 with gangrene of the toes.

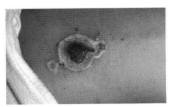

Image 82.10
Patient shown in images 82.8 and 82.9 with cutaneous necrosis.

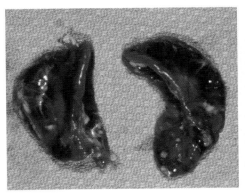

Image 82.11
Adrenal hemorrhage in a patient with gram-negative sepsis, a major complication of meningococcal disease with increased mortality. Courtesy of Dimitris P. Agamanolis, MD.

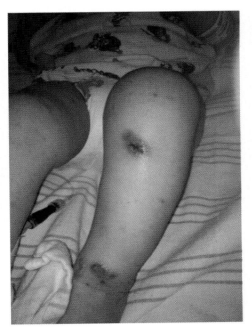

Image 82.12
A 6-month-old infant with meningococcemia and meningitis who responded well to supportive and antibiotic therapy. However, on day 4 of treatment he developed a low-grade fever, irritability especially when moving his lower extremities, and a few purpuric lesions became elevated and fluid filled, typical of the postinfectious complication, vasculitis. All symptoms resolved with use of a nonsteroidal anti-inflammatory agent. Courtesy of Carol J. Baker, MD.

83

Human Metapneumovirus

Clinical Manifestations

Since discovery in 2001, human metapneumovirus (HMPV) has been shown to cause acute respiratory tract illness in patients of all ages. HMPV is one of the leading causes of bronchiolitis in infants and also causes pneumonia, asthma exacerbations, croup, and upper respiratory tract infections with concomitant acute otitis media in children as well as acute exacerbations of chronic obstructive pulmonary disease in adults. Otherwise healthy young children infected with HMPV usually have mild or moderate symptoms, but occasionally young children have severe disease requiring hospitalization. HMPV infection in the immunosuppressed also can result in severe disease, and fatalities from HMPV infection have been reported in hematopoietic stem cell or lung transplant recipients. Preterm birth and underlying cardiopulmonary disease likely are risk factors, but the degree of risk associated with these conditions is not defined fully.

Recurrent infection occurs throughout life and, in healthy people, usually is mild or asymptomatic.

Etiology

HMPV is an enveloped single-stranded negative-sense RNA virus of the family Paramyxoviridae. Four major genotypes of virus have been identified, and these viruses are classified into 2 major antigenic subgroups (designated A and B), which usually cocirculate each year.

Epidemiology

Humans are the only source of infection. Transmission studies have not been reported, but transmission is likely to occur by direct or close contact with contaminated secretions. Health care–associated infections have been reported. HMPV infections usually occur in annual epidemics during late winter and early spring in temperate climates. Serologic studies suggest that all children are infected at least once by 5 years of age. The population incidence of HMPV hospitalizations is thought to be generally lower than respiratory syncytial virus (RSV), but comparable to influenza and parainfluenza 3 in children younger than 5 years. The HMPV season in a community generally coincides with or overlaps the latter half of the RSV season. During this overlapping period, bronchiolitis has been caused by either or both viruses. Sporadic infection may occur throughout the year. In otherwise healthy infants, the duration of viral shedding is 1 to 2 weeks. Prolonged shedding (weeks to months) has been reported in severely immunocompromised hosts.

Incubation Period

Estimated at 3 to 5 days.

Diagnostic Tests

Rapid diagnostic immunofluorescent assays based on HMPV antigen detection by monoclonal antibodies are available commercially. The reported sensitivity of these assays varies from 65% to 90%. HMPV-specific molecular diagnostic tests using reverse transcriptase PCR amplification of viral genes (both conventional and real time) have been developed. Some of these assays (including multiplex PCR assays for multiple respiratory tract viruses) are available commercially and increasingly are being used. Serologic testing of acute and convalescent serum specimens is used in research settings only.

Treatment

Treatment is supportive and includes hydration, careful clinical assessment of respiratory status, including measurement of oxygen saturation, use of supplemental oxygen and, if necessary, mechanical ventilation. The rate of bacterial lung infection or bacteremia associated with HMPV infection is unknown, but is suspected to be low. Thus antimicrobial agents are not indicated in treatment of infants hospitalized with uncomplicated HMPV bronchiolitis or pneumonia unless evidence exists for the presence of a secondary bacterial infection.

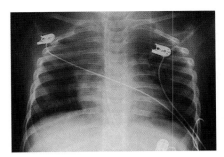

Image 83.1

Human metapneumovirus bronchiolitis in a 12-month-old male. Copyright Benjamin Estrada, MD.

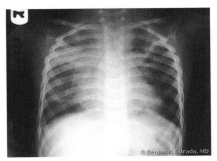

Image 83.2

Bilateral human metapneumovirus pneumonia in a 3-year-old male. Copyright Benjamin Estrada, MD.

84

Microsporidia Infections
(Microsporidiosis)

Clinical Manifestations

Patients with intestinal infection have watery, nonbloody diarrhea, generally without fever. Abdominal cramping also can occur. Data suggest that asymptomatic infection is more common than originally suspected. Symptomatic intestinal infection is most common in immunocompromised people, especially people who are infected with HIV with low CD4+ lymphocyte counts, in whom infection often results in chronic diarrhea. The clinical course can be complicated by malnutrition and progressive weight loss. Chronic infection in immunocompetent people is rare. Other clinical syndromes that can occur in HIV-infected and immunocompromised patients include keratoconjunctivitis, sinusitis, myositis, nephritis, hepatitis, cholangitis, peritonitis, prostatitis, cystitis, disseminated disease, and wasting syndrome.

Etiology

Microsporidia are obligate intracellular, spore-forming organisms. They have been reclassified from protozoa to fungi. Multiple genera, including *Encephalitozoon, Enterocytozoon, Nosema, Pleistophora, Trachipleistophora, Brachiola, Vittaforma,* and *Microsporidium,* have been implicated in human infection, as have unclassified species. *Enterocytozoon bieneusi* and *Encephalitozoon (Septata) intestinalis* are causes of chronic diarrhea in HIV-infected people.

Epidemiology

Most microsporidian infections are transmitted by oral ingestion of spores. Microsporidium spores commonly are found in surface water, and human strains have been identified in municipal water supplies and ground water. Several studies indicate that waterborne transmission occurs. Person-to-person spread by the fecal-oral route also occurs. Spores also have been detected in other body fluids, but their role in transmission is unknown.

Incubation Period

Unknown.

Diagnostic Tests

Infection with gastrointestinal *Microsporidia* species can be documented by identification of organisms in biopsy specimens from the small intestine. *Microsporidia* species spores also can be detected in formalin-fixed stool specimens or duodenal aspirates stained with a chromotrope-based stain (a modification of the trichrome stain) and examined by an experienced microscopist. Gram, acid-fast, periodic acid-Schiff, and Giemsa stains also can be used to detect organisms in tissue sections. Organisms often are not noticed, because they are small (1–4 μm), stain poorly, and evoke minimal inflammatory response. Use of stool concentration techniques does not seem to improve the ability to detect *E bieneusi* spores. PCR assay also can be used for diagnosis. Identification for classification purposes and diagnostic confirmation of species requires electron microscopy or molecular techniques.

Treatment

Restoration of immune function is critical in control of any microsporidian infection. For some patients, albendazole, fumagillin, metronidazole, atovaquone, and nitazoxanide have been reported to decrease diarrhea but without eradication of the organism. Albendazole is the drug of choice for infections caused by *E intestinalis* but is ineffective against *E bieneusi* infections, which may respond to fumagillin. However, fumagillin is associated with significant toxicity, and recurrence of diarrhea is common after therapy is discontinued. In HIV-infected patients, antiretroviral therapy, which is associated with improvement in the CD4+ T-lymphocyte cell count, can modify the course of disease favorably. None of these therapies have been studied in children with *Microspordia* infection.

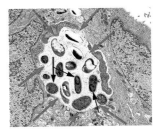

Image 84.1
Transmission electron micrograph showing developing forms of *Encephalitozoon intestinalis* inside a parasitophorous vacuole (red arrows) with mature spores (black arrows). Microsporidiosis, parasite. Courtesy of Centers for Disease Control and Prevention.

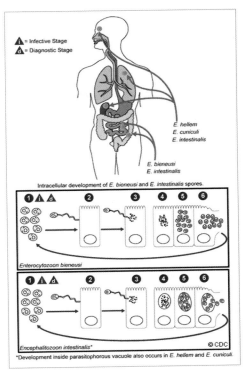

Image 84.2
Life cycle. The infective form of microsporidia is the resistant spore and it can survive for a long time in the environment (1). The spore extrudes its polar tubule and infects the host cell (2). The spore injects the infective sporoplasm into the eukaryotic host cell through the polar tubule (3). Inside the cell, the sporoplasm undergoes extensive multiplication either by merogony (binary fission) (4) or schizogony (multiple fission). This development can occur either in direct contact with the host cell cytoplasm (eg, *Enterocytozoon bieneusi*) or inside a vacuole termed parasitophorous vacuole (eg, *Encephalitozoon intestinalis*). Either free in the cytoplasm or inside a parasitophorous vacuole, microsporidia develop by sporogony to mature spores (5). During sporogony, a thick wall is formed around the spore that provides resistance to adverse environmental conditions. When the spores increase in number and completely fill the host cell cytoplasm, the cell membrane is disrupted and releases the spores to the surroundings (6). These free mature spores can infect new cells, thus continuing the cycle. Courtesy of Centers for Disease Control and Prevention.

85

Molluscum Contagiosum

Clinical Manifestations

Molluscum contagiosum is a benign viral infection of the skin with no systemic manifestations. It usually is characterized by 1 to 20 discrete, 2- to 5-mm–diameter, flesh-colored to translucent, dome-shaped papules, some with central umbilication. Lesions commonly occur on the trunk, face, and extremities but rarely are generalized. Molluscum contagiosum is a self-limited infection that usually resolves spontaneously in 6 to 12 months but may take as long as 4 years to disappear completely. An eczematous reaction encircles lesions in approximately 10% of patients. People with eczema, immunocompromising conditions, and HIV infection tend to have more widespread and prolonged eruptions.

Etiology

The cause is a poxvirus, which is the sole member of the genus *Molluscipoxvirus*. DNA subtypes can be differentiated, but subtype is not significant in pathogenesis.

Epidemiology

Humans are the only known source of the virus, which is spread by direct contact, including sexual contact, or by fomites. Vertical transmission has been suggested in case reports of neonatal molluscum contagiosum infection. Lesions can be disseminated by autoinoculation. Infectivity generally is low, but occasional outbreaks have been reported, including outbreaks in child care centers. The period of communicability is unknown.

Incubation Period

2 to 7 weeks, but can be as long as 6 months.

Diagnostic Tests

The diagnosis usually is made clinically from the characteristic appearance of the lesions. Wright or Giemsa staining of cells expressed from the central core of a lesion reveals characteristic intracytoplasmic inclusions. Electron microscopic examination of these cells identifies typical poxvirus particles. Nucleic acid testing via PCR is available at certain reference centers. Adolescents and young adults with genital molluscum contagiosum should have screening tests for other sexually transmitted infections.

Treatment

There is no consensus on management of molluscum contagiosum in children and adolescents. Genital lesions should be treated to prevent spread to sexual contacts. Treatment of nongenital lesions is mainly for cosmetic reasons. Lesions in healthy people typically are self-limited, and treatment is not necessary. However, therapy may be warranted to (1) alleviate discomfort, including itching; (2) reduce autoinoculation; (3) limit transmission of the virus to close contacts; (4) reduce cosmetic concerns; and (5) prevent secondary infection. Physical destruction of the lesions is the most rapid and effective means of curing molluscum contagiosum lesions. Modalities available for physical destruction include curettage, cryotherapy with liquid nitrogen, electrodesiccation, and chemical agents designed to initiate a local inflammatory response (podophyllin, tretinoin, cantharidin, 25%–50% trichloroacetic acid, liquefied phenol, silver nitrate, tincture of iodine, or potassium hydroxide). These options require a trained physician and can result in postprocedural pain, irritation, and scarring. Imiquimod cream is a local immunomodulatory agent that has been reported as a potentially effective topical treatment in several small clinical trials. Cidofovir is a cytosine nucleotide analogue with in vitro activity against molluscum contagiosum; successful intravenous treatment of immunocompromised adults with severe lesions has been reported. However, use of cidofovir should be reserved for severe cases because of potential carcinogenicity and known toxicities (nephrotoxicity, neutropenia) associated with systemic administration of cidofovir. Successful treatment using topical cidofovir, in a combination vehicle, has been reported in both adult and pediatric cases, most of which were immunocompromised. Genital lesions in children usually are not acquired by sexual transmission and do not necessarily denote sexual abuse, as other modes of direct contact with the virus, including autoinoculation, may result in genital disease.

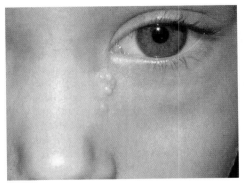

Image 85.1
Molluscum contagiosum lesions adjacent to nasal bridge. Copyright Edward Marcuse.

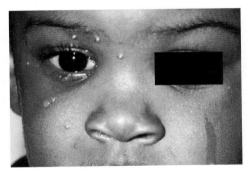

Image 85.2
Molluscum contagiosum is characterized by one or more translucent or white papules. Intracytoplasmic inclusions may be seen with Wright or Giemsa staining of material expressed from the core of a lesion.

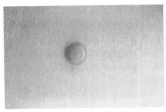

Image 85.3
A molluscum contagiosum lesion with characteristic umbilication.

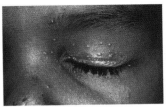

Image 85.4
Pearly papules on the forehead and eyelid in a child with molluscum contagiosum lesions, which commonly occur on the face.

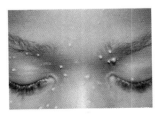

Image 85.5
This 10-year-old girl has had multiple small bumps on the face for the past month. These started as a solitary papule on her eyebrow, but spread over several weeks. They have developed a small pointed core and are an embarrassment to the child. School pictures are pending. The family demands treatment. There is a family history of keloids. The family was counseled on the limited treatment options due to the potential for permanent scarring and keloid formation. Consultation with a dermatologist was arranged at the parents' request. Copyright Will Sorey, MD.

86

Mumps

Clinical Manifestations

Mumps is a systemic disease characterized by swelling of one or more of the salivary glands, usually the parotid glands. Approximately one-third of infections do not cause clinically apparent salivary gland swelling and can be asymptomatic (subclinical) or manifest primarily as a respiratory tract infection. More than 50% of people with mumps have cerebrospinal fluid pleocytosis, but fewer than 10% have symptoms of viral meningitis. Orchitis is a commonly reported complication after puberty, but sterility rarely occurs. Rare complications include arthritis, thyroiditis, mastitis, glomerulonephritis, myocarditis, endocardial fibroelastosis, thrombocytopenia, cerebellar ataxia, transverse myelitis, encephalitis, pancreatitis, oophoritis, and permanent hearing impairment. In the absence of an immunization program, mumps typically occurs during childhood. Infection among adults is more likely to result in complications. An association between maternal mumps infection during the first trimester of pregnancy and an increase in the rate of spontaneous abortion or intrauterine fetal death has been reported in some studies but not in others. Although mumps virus can cross the placenta, no evidence exists that this results in congenital malformation.

Etiology

Mumps is an RNA virus in the Paramyxoviridae family. Other infectious causes of parotitis include Epstein-Barr virus, cytomegalovirus, parainfluenza virus types 1 and 3, influenza A virus, enteroviruses, lymphocytic choriomeningitis virus, HIV, nontuberculous *Mycobacterium* and, less often, gram-positive and gram-negative bacteria.

Epidemiology

Mumps occurs worldwide, and humans are the only known natural hosts. The virus is spread by contact with infectious respiratory tract secretions and saliva. Mumps virus is the only known cause of epidemic parotitis. Historically, the peak incidence of mumps was between January and May and among children younger than 10 years. Mumps vaccine was licensed in the United States in 1967 and recommended for routine childhood immunization in 1977. After implementation of the 1-dose mumps vaccine recommendation, the incidence of mumps in the United States declined from an incidence of 50 to 251 per 100,000 in the prevaccine era to 2 per 100,000 in 1988. After implementation of the 2-dose measles-mumps-rubella vaccine recommendation in 1989 for measles control, mumps further declined to extremely low levels, with an incidence of 0.1/100,000 by 1999. From 2000 to 2005, seasonality no longer was evident, and there were fewer than 300 reported cases per year (incidence of 0.1/100,000), representing a greater than 99% reduction in disease incidence since the prevaccine era. In early 2006, a large-scale mumps outbreak occurred in the Midwestern United States, with 6,584 reported cases (incidence of 2.2/100,000). Most of the cases occurred among people 18 through 24 years of age, many of whom were college students who had received 2 doses of mumps vaccine. Another outbreak in 2009–2010 affected more than 3,500 people, primarily members of traditional observant communities in New York and New Jersey. Because 2 doses of mumps-containing vaccine are not 100% effective, in settings of high immunization coverage such as the United States, most mumps cases likely will occur in people who have received 2 doses. The period of maximum communicability is considered to be several days before and after parotitis onset. Virus has been isolated from saliva from 7 days before through 8 days after onset of swelling.

Incubation Period

16 to 18 days, but occasionally 12 to 25 days after exposure.

Diagnostic Tests

Despite the outbreaks in 2006 and 2009–2010, mumps is an uncommon infection in the United States, and parotitis has many etiologies. People with parotitis without other apparent cause should undergo diagnostic testing to confirm mumps virus as the cause or to diagnose other etiologies. Mumps can be confirmed by isolation of mumps virus or detection of mumps virus nucleic acid by reverse transcriptase PCR (RT-PCR) in specimens from buccal swabs (Stenson duct exudates), throat washings, saliva, or spinal fluid; by detection of mumps-specific immunoglobulin (Ig) M antibody; or by a significant increase between acute and convalescent titers in serum mumps IgG antibody titer determined by semiquantitative serologic assay. With the availability of RT-PCR assays, culture rarely is performed anymore.

Confirming the diagnosis of mumps in highly immunized populations is challenging, because the IgM response can be absent or

short lived; acute IgG titers already can be high, and mumps virus might be present in clinical specimens only during the first few days after illness onset. Emphasis should be placed on obtaining clinical specimens within 1 to 3 days after onset of symptoms (usually parotitis). In immunized cases, a negative IgM result does not rule out the diagnosis.

Treatment

Supportive.

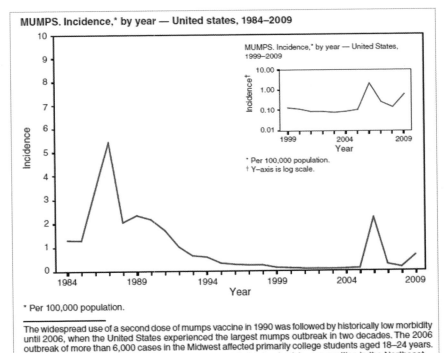

MUMPS. Incidence,* by year — United states, 1984–2009

MUMPS. Incidence,* by year — United States, 1999–2009

* Per 100,000 population.
† Y–axis is log scale.

* Per 100,000 population.

The widespread use of a second dose of mumps vaccine in 1990 was followed by historically low morbidity until 2006, when the United States experienced the largest mumps outbreak in two decades. The 2006 outbreak of more than 6,000 cases in the Midwest affected primarily college students aged 18–24 years. A second large outbreak began in 2009 and affected Orthodox Jewish communities in the Northeast.

Image 86.1
Mumps. Incidence per year—United States, 1984–2009. Courtesy of *Morbidity and Mortality Weekly Report*.

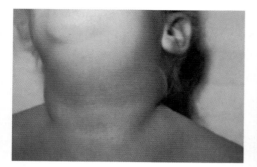

Image 86.2

This is a photograph of a patient with bilateral swelling in the submaxillary regions due to mumps. Prior to vaccine licensure in 1967, 100,000 to 200,000 mumps cases are estimated to have occurred in the United States each year. Courtesy of Centers for Disease Control and Prevention/Dr Heinz F. Eichenwald.

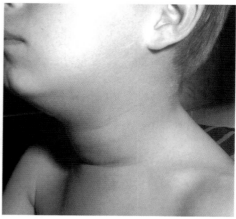

Image 86.3

Mumps parotitis with cervical and presternal edema and erythema that resolved spontaneously.

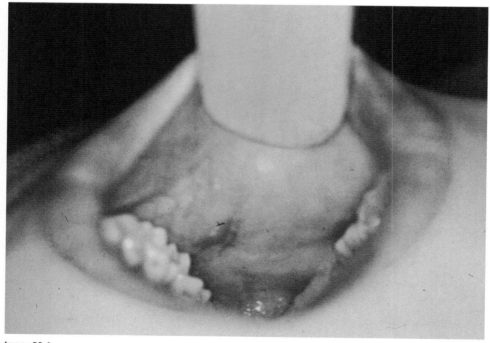

Image 86.4

Swelling and erythema of the Stensen duct in the above 10-year-old white male with mumps parotitis. Courtesy of Paul Wehrle, MD.

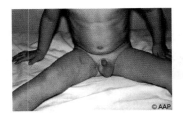

Image 86.5

Mumps orchitis in a 6-year-old boy. This complication is unusual in prepubertal boys. The highest risk for orchitis is in males between 15 and 29 years of age.

87

Mycoplasma pneumoniae and Other Mycoplasma Species Infections

Clinical Manifestations

Mycoplasma pneumoniae is a frequent cause of upper and lower respiratory tract infections in children, including pharyngitis, acute bronchitis, and pneumonia. Acute otitis media is uncommon. Bullous myringitis, once considered pathognomonic for mycoplasma, now is known to occur with other pathogens as well. Coryza, sinusitis, and croup are rare. Symptoms are variable and can include cough, malaise, fever and, occasionally, headache. Acute bronchitis and upper respiratory tract illness caused by M pneumoniae generally are mild and self-limited. Approximately 10% of infected school-aged children will develop pneumonia with cough and widespread rales by physical examination within days after onset of constitutional symptoms. Cough often initially is nonproductive but later can become productive. Cough can persist for 3 to 4 weeks and can be accompanied by wheezing. Approximately 10% of children with M pneumoniae infection will exhibit a rash, which most often is maculopapular. Radiographic abnormalities are variable. Bilateral diffuse infiltrates or focal abnormalities, such as consolidation, effusion, or hilar adenopathy, can occur.

Unusual manifestations include nervous system disease (eg, aseptic meningitis, encephalitis, acute disseminated encephalomyelitis, cerebellar ataxia, transverse myelitis, peripheral neuropathy) as well as myocarditis, pericarditis, polymorphous mucocutaneous eruptions (including classic and atypical Stevens-Johnson syndrome) hemolytic anemia, and arthritis. In patients with sickle cell disease, Down syndrome, immunodeficiencies, and chronic cardiorespiratory disease, severe pneumonia with pleural effusion may develop. Acute chest syndrome and pneumonia have been associated with M pneumoniae in patients with sickle cell disease. It also has been associated with exacerbations of asthma.

Several other Mycoplasma species colonize mucosal surfaces of humans and can produce disease in children. Mycoplasma hominis infection has been reported in neonates (especially at scalp electrode monitor site) and children (both immunocompetent and immunocompromised). Intra-abdominal abscesses, septic arthritis, endocarditis, pneumonia, meningoencephalitis, brain abscess, and surgical wound infections all have been reported. The diagnosis should be considered in children with a bacterial culture-negative purulent infection.

Etiology

Mycoplasmas, including M pneumoniae, are pleomorphic bacteria that lack a cell wall. Mycoplasmas cannot be detected using light microscopy.

Epidemiology

Mycoplasmas are ubiquitous in animals and plants, but M pneumoniae causes disease only in humans. M pneumoniae is transmissible by respiratory droplets during close contact with a symptomatic person. Outbreaks have been described in hospitals, military bases, colleges, and summer camps. Occasionally M pneumoniae causes ventilator-associated pneumonia. M pneumoniae is a leading cause of pneumonia in school-aged children and young adults and less frequently causes pneumonia in children younger than 5 years. Infections occur throughout the world, in any season, and in all geographic settings. In family studies, approximately 30% of household contacts develop pneumonia. Asymptomatic carriage after infection may occur for weeks to months. Immunity after infection is not long lasting.

Incubation Period

2 to 3 weeks; range, 1 to 4 weeks.

Diagnostic Tests

When Gram stain of colonies is performed, no bacteria are noted. M pneumoniae can be grown but most clinical facilities lack the capacity to perform this culture. Isolation takes up to 21 days. PCR tests for M pneumoniae increasingly are available and have been used as diagnostic tests at many medical centers.

Where available, PCR has replaced other tests, because PCR enables more rapid diagnosis in acutely ill patients. Identification of *M pneumoniae* by PCR or in culture from a patient with compatible clinical manifestations suggests causation. PCR testing is available commercially; sensitivity and specificity are between 80% and 100%. Performance characteristics of individual institutions' non–US Food and Drug Administration–approved PCR tests, using different primer sequences and targeting different genes, is not generalizable. Attributing a nonclassic clinical disorder to *Mycoplasma* on the basis of PCR test or culture results is problematic, because *M pneumoniae* can colonize the respiratory tract for several weeks after acute infection, even after appropriate antimicrobial therapy.

Immunofluorescent tests and enzyme immunoassays that detect *M pneumoniae*–specific immunoglobulin (Ig) M and IgG antibodies in sera are available commercially. IgM antibodies generally are not detectable within the first 7 days after onset of symptoms. Although the presence of IgM antibodies can indicate recent *M pneumoniae* infection, false-positive test results occur often. Conversely, IgM antibodies may not be elevated in older children and adults who have had recurrent *M pneumoniae* infection. Serologic diagnosis is best made by demonstrating a fourfold or greater increase in antibody titer between acute and convalescent serum specimens. IgM antibody titer peaks at approximately 3 to 6 weeks and persists for 2 to

3 months after infection. False-positive IgM test results occur frequently, particularly when results are near the threshold for positivity. False-negative results also occur frequently with single specimen testing, with sensitivity ranging from 50% to 60%.

The diagnosis of mycoplasma-associated central nervous system disease (acute or postinfectious) is controversial because of the lack of a reliable cerebrospinal fluid test for *Mycoplasma*. No single test has adequate sensitivity or specificity to establish this diagnosis.

Treatment

Observational data indicate that children with pneumonia attributable to *M pneumoniae* have shorter duration of symptoms and fewer relapses when treated with an antimicrobial agent active against *M pneumoniae*. There is no evidence that treatment of upper respiratory tract or nonrespiratory tract disease with antimicrobial agents alters the course of illness. Because mycoplasmas lack a cell wall, they inherently are resistant to beta-lactam agents. Macrolides, including erythromycin, azithromycin, and clarithromycin, are the preferred antimicrobial agents for treatment of pneumonia in children younger than 8 years. Tetracycline and doxycycline also are effective and may be used for children 8 years of age and older. Fluoroquinolones are effective but are not recommended as first-line agents for children.

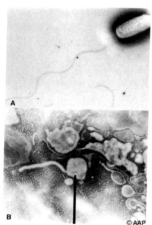

Image 87.1

(A) Typical structure of a common gram-negative bacterium (*Pseudomonas aeruginosa*) and its flagellum, as seen on electron microscopy. (B) Pleomorphic structure of *Mycoplasma pneumoniae,* as seen on electron microscopy. The bacterium is indicated by the black pointer. Mycoplasmas, including *M pneumoniae,* lack a cell wall.

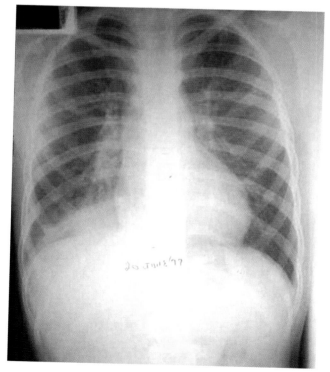

Image 87.2

A preadolescent boy with bilateral perihilar infiltration and right lower lobe pneumonia and pleural effusion due to *Mycoplasma pneumoniae.* Courtesy of Edgar O. Ledbetter, MD, FAAP.

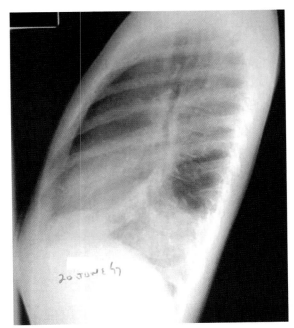

Image 87.3
Right lateral radiograph of the patient in Image 87.2 with pneumonia and pleural effusion. Pleural effusions associated with *Mycoplasma pneumoniae* infections generally resolve spontaneously without drainage. Courtesy of Edgar O. Ledbetter, MD, FAAP.

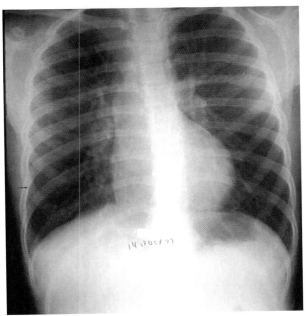

Image 87.4
Preadolescent boy with bilateral perihilar infiltrates caused by *Mycoplasma pneumoniae*.

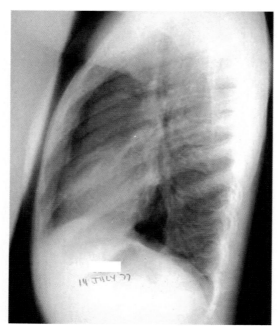

Image 87.5
Lateral radiograph of the patient in Image 87.4 with pneumonia caused by *Mycoplasma pneumoniae.*

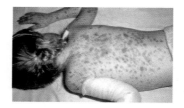

Image 87.6
Erythema multiforme rash (Stevens-Johnson syndrome) associated with *Mycoplasma pneumoniae* infection in a preadolescent girl. Copyright Charles Prober, MD.

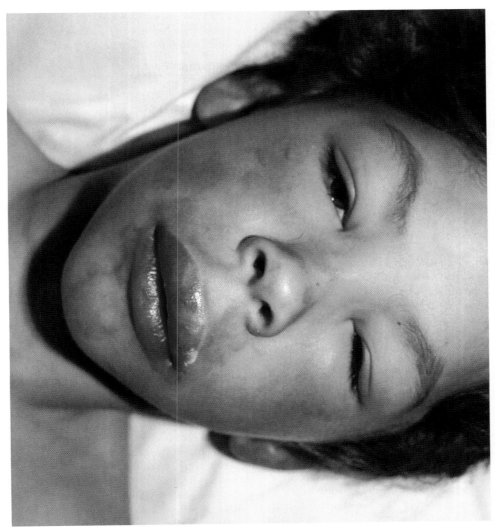

Image 87.7
Erythema multforme associated with mycoplasma infection. This 10-year-old boy presented with fever and macular lesions on the face, chest, arms, and back, as well as facial swelling. He had a 4-day period of increasing cough and low-grade fever prior to the onset of the skin lesions and facial swelling. Chest x-ray revealed mild increased infiltrates in the right lung. Cold agglutinins were markedly elevated and he had a greater than four-fold rise in complement fixation antibody to *Mycoplasma pneumoniae.* Courtesy of Neal Halsey, MD.

88

Nocardiosis

Clinical Manifestations

Immunocompetent children typically develop cutaneous or lymphocutaneous disease with pustular or ulcerative lesions that remain localized after soil contamination of a skin injury. Invasive disease occurs most commonly in immunocompromised patients, particularly people with chronic granulomatous disease, organ transplantation, HIV infection, or disease requiring long-term systemic corticosteroid therapy. In these children, infection characteristically begins in the lungs, and illness can be acute, subacute, or chronic. Pulmonary disease commonly manifests as rounded nodular infiltrates that can undergo cavitation. Hematogenous spread can occur from the lungs to the brain (single or multiple abscesses), in skin (pustules, pyoderma, abscesses, mycetoma), or occasionally in other organs. Some experts recommend neuroimaging in patients with pulmonary disease attributable to the frequency of concurrent central nervous system (CNS) disease, which initially can be asymptomatic. Nocardia organisms can be recovered from patients with cystic fibrosis, but their role as a lung pathogen in these patients is not clear.

Etiology

Nocardia species are aerobic actinomycetes, a large and diverse group of gram-positive bacteria, which include Actinomyces israelii (the cause of actinomycosis), Rhodococcus equi, and Tropheryma whipplei (formerly Tropheryma whippelii) (Whipple disease). Pulmonary or disseminated disease most commonly is caused by the Nocardia asteroides complex. Primary cutaneous disease most commonly is caused by Nocardia brasiliensis. Nocardia pseudobrasiliensis is associated with pulmonary, CNS, or systemic nocardiosis.

Epidemiology

Found worldwide, Nocardia species are ubiquitous environmental saprophytes living in soil, organic matter, and water. Lungs are the portals of entry for pulmonary or disseminated disease. Direct skin inoculation occurs, often as the result of contact with contaminated soil after trauma. Person-to-person and animal-to-human transmission does not occur.

Incubation Period

Unknown.

Diagnostic Tests

Isolation of Nocardia organisms from body fluid, abscess material, or tissue specimens provides a definitive diagnosis. Stained smears of sputum, body fluids, or pus demonstrating beaded, branched, weakly gram-positive, variably acid-fast rods suggest the diagnosis. Brown and Brenn and methenamine silver stains are recommended to demonstrate microorganisms in tissue specimens. Nocardia organisms are slow growing but grow readily on blood and chocolate agar in 3 to 5 days. Cultures from normally sterile sites should be maintained for 3 weeks in an appropriate liquid medium. Serologic tests for Nocardia species are not useful.

Treatment

Trimethoprim-sulfamethoxazole or a sulfonamide alone (eg, sulfisoxazole or sulfamethoxazole) has been the drug of choice for mild infections. Sulfonamides that are less urine soluble, such as sulfadiazine, should be avoided. For patients with immunocompromised or severe disease, use of combination therapy is recommended for the first 4 to 12 weeks. Suggested combinations include amikacin plus ceftriaxone or amikacin plus meropenem or imipenem. Immunocompetent patients with primary lymphocutaneous disease usually respond after 6 to 12 weeks of therapy. Drainage of abscesses is beneficial. Immunocompromised patients and patients with serious disease should be treated for 6 to 12 months and for at least 3 months after apparent cure because of the tendency for relapse. Patients with HIV infection may need even longer therapy, and low-dose maintenance therapy should be continued for life.

If infection does not respond to trimethoprim-sulfamethoxazole, other agents, such as clarithromycin (Nocardia nova), amoxicillin-clavulanate (N brasiliensis and N abscessus), or meropenem may be beneficial. Drug susceptibility testing is recommended by the Clinical and Laboratory Standards Institute for isolates from patients with invasive disease and patients who are unable to tolerate a sulfonamide or who fail sulfonamide therapy.

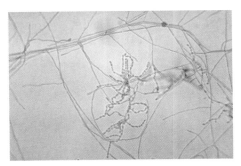

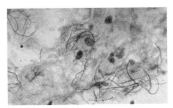

Image 88.2
Nocardia asteroides colony (tissue acid-fast stain).

Image 88.1
This gram-positive aerobic *Nocardia asteroides* slide culture reveals chains of aerial mycelia. The filamentous structure of these bacteria tend toward a branching pattern terminating in a rod- or coccoid-shaped morphologic appearance. Courtesy of Centers for Disease Control and Prevention/Dr Lucille K. Georg.

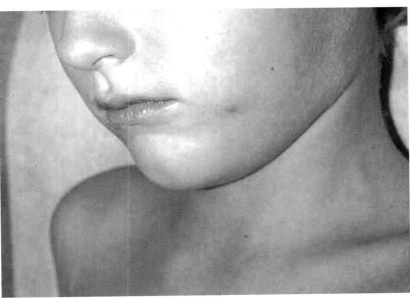

Image 88.3
Cutaneous *Nocardia asteroides* lesion in a 10-year-old male with no evidence of disseminated disease. Courtesy of Edgar O. Ledbetter, MD, FAAP.

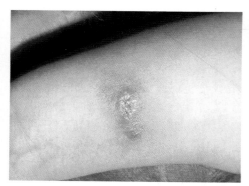

Image 88.4
Cutaneous nocardiosis of forearm in an immuno-competent preschool-aged male.

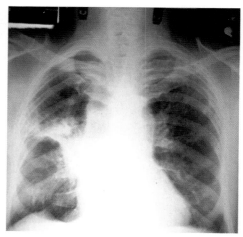

Image 88.5
Nocardia pneumonia, bilateral, in an immuno-compromised child. Invasive nocardiosis is unusual in immunocompetent children.

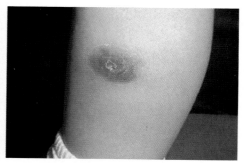

Image 88.6
Cutaneous nocardiosis of the lower leg of immu-nocompetent preschool-aged female.

89

Onchocerciasis
(River Blindness, Filariasis)

Clinical Manifestations

The disease involves skin, subcutaneous tissues, lymphatic vessels, and eyes. Subcutaneous, nontender nodules that can be up to several centimeters in diameter containing adult worms develop 6 to 12 months after initial infection. In patients in Africa, nodules tend to be found on the lower torso, pelvis, and lower extremities, whereas in patients in Central and South America, the nodules more often are located on the upper body (the head and trunk) but can occur on the extremities. After the worms mature, microfilariae are produced that migrate to the dermis and can cause a papular dermatitis. Pruritus often is highly intense, resulting in patient-inflicted excoriations over the affected areas. After a period of years, skin can become lichenified and hypo- or hyperpigmented. Microfilariae can invade ocular structures, leading to inflammation of the cornea, iris, ciliary body, retina, choroid, and optic nerve. Loss of visual acuity and blindness can result if the disease is untreated.

Etiology

Onchocerca volvulus is a filarial nematode.

Epidemiology

O volvulus has no significant animal reservoir. Microfilariae in human skin infect *Simulium* species flies (black flies) when they take a blood meal and then in 10 to 14 days develop into infectious larvae that are transmitted with subsequent bites. Black flies breed in fast-flowing streams and rivers (hence, the colloquial name of the disease, "river blindness"). The disease occurs primarily in equatorial Africa, but small foci are found in southern Mexico, Guatemala, northern South America, and Yemen. Prevalence is greatest among people who live near vector breeding sites. The infection is not transmissible by person-to-person contact or by blood transfusion.

Incubation Period

6 to 18 months from inoculation to microfilariae in skin but can be as long as 3 years.

Diagnostic Tests

Direct examination of a 1- to 2-mg shaving or biopsy specimen of the epidermis and upper dermis (usually taken from the posterior iliac crest area) can reveal microfilariae. Microfilariae are not found in blood. Adult worms may be demonstrated in excised nodules that have been sectioned and stained. A slit-lamp examination of the anterior chamber of an involved eye can reveal motile microfilariae or "snowflake" corneal lesions. Eosinophilia is common. Specific serologic tests and PCR techniques for detection of microfilariae in skin are available only in research laboratories.

Treatment

Ivermectin, a microfilaricidal agent, is the drug of choice for treatment of onchocerciasis. Treatment decreases dermatitis and the risk of developing severe ocular disease but does not kill adult worms (which can live for more than a decade) and, thus, is not curative. One single oral dose of ivermectin should be given every 6 to 12 months until asymptomatic. Adverse reactions to treatment are caused by death of microfilariae and can include rash, edema, fever, myalgia and, rarely, asthma exacerbation and hypotension. Such reactions are more common in people with higher skin loads of microfilaria and decrease with repeated treatment in the absence of reexposure. Treatment of patients with high levels of circulating *Loa loa* microfilariaemia with ivermectin sometimes can result in fatal encephalopathy. A 6-week course of doxycycline also is being used to kill adult worms through depletion of the endosymbiotic rickettsia-like bacteria, which appear to be required for survival of *O volvulus*. This approach may provide adjunctive therapy for children 8 years of age or older and nonpregnant adults. This treatment should be initiated several days after treatment with ivermectin.

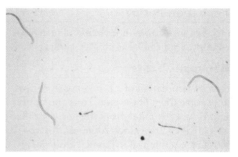

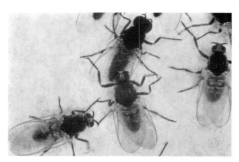

Image 89.1

This is a glycerine mount photomicrograph of the microfilarial pathogen *Onchocerca volvulus* in its larval form. Courtesy of Centers for Disease Control and Prevention/Ladene Newton.

Image 89.2

These are *Simulium* sp of flies, or "black flies," a vector of the disease onchocerciasis, or "river blindness." Courtesy of World Health Organization.

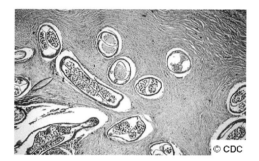

Image 89.3

Histopathologic features of *Onchocerca* nodule in onchocerciasis. Courtesy of Centers for Disease Control and Prevention/Dr Mae Melvin.

90

Human Papillomaviruses

Clinical Manifestations

Most human papillomavirus (HPV) infections are inapparent clinically. However, HPVs can cause benign epithelial proliferation (warts) of the skin and mucous membranes and are associated with cervical, anogenital, and oropharyngeal dysplasias and cancers. Cutaneous nongenital warts include common skin warts, plantar warts, flat warts, thread-like (filiform) warts, and epidermodysplasia verruciformis. Warts also occur on the mucous membranes, including the anogenital, oral, nasal, and conjunctival areas and the respiratory tract, where respiratory papillomatosis occurs.

Common **skin warts** are dome-shaped with conical projections that give the surface a rough appearance. They usually are painless and multiple, occurring commonly on the hands and around or under the nails. When small dermal vessels become thrombosed, black dots appear in the warts. Plantar warts on the foot may be painful and are characterized by marked hyperkeratosis, sometimes with black dots.

Flat warts ("juvenile warts") commonly are found on the face and extremities of children and adolescents. They usually are small, multiple, and flat topped; seldom exhibit papillomatosis; and rarely cause pain. Filiform warts occur on the face and neck. Cutaneous warts are benign.

Anogenital warts, also called **condylomata acuminata,** are skin-colored warts with a cauliflower-like surface that range in size from a few millimeters to several centimeters. In males, these warts may be found on the penis, scrotum, or anal and perianal area. In females, these lesions may occur on the vulva or perianal areas and less commonly in the vagina or on the cervix. Anogenital warts often are multiple and attract attention because of their appearance. Warts usually are painless, although they may cause itching, burning, local pain, or bleeding.

Persistent anogenital HPV infection may be associated with clinically apparent dysplastic lesions, particularly in the female genital tract (cervix and vagina). Abnormal cells associated with these lesions often are detected during Papanicolaou (Pap) testing of the cervix and are classified morphologically as representing low- or high-grade squamous intraepithelial lesions (L-SIL or H-SIL, respectively). On biopsy, these precursor lesions are classified as low-grade cervical intraepithelial neoplasia (CIN 1) or high-grade cervical intraepithelial neoplasia (CIN 2 or 3). Similar dysplastic lesions can develop at other genital and anal mucosal sites. Over 1 to 2 decades, persistent HPV infection with high-risk HPV types can undergo neoplastic progression and lead to invasive cancers of the cervix, vagina, vulva, penis, anus, or oropharynx.

Juvenile recurrent respiratory papillomatosis is a rare condition characterized by recurring papillomas in the larynx or other areas of the upper respiratory tract. This condition is diagnosed most commonly in children between 2 and 5 years of age and manifests as a voice change, stridor, or abnormal cry. Respiratory papillomas can cause respiratory tract obstruction in young children. Adult onset also has been described.

Epidermodysplasia verruciformis (EV) is a rare, inherited disorder believed to be a consequence of a deficiency of cell-mediated immunity resulting in an abnormal susceptibility to certain HPV types and manifesting as chronic cutaneous HPV infection and frequent development of skin cancer. Lesions may resemble flat warts but often are similar to tinea versicolor, covering the torso and upper extremities. Most appear during the first decade of life, but malignant transformation, which occurs in 30% to 60% of affected people, usually is delayed until adulthood. EV-like HPV disease also can occur in people with HIV infection.

Etiology

HPVs are members of the *Papillomaviridae* family and are DNA viruses. More than 100 types have been identified. These viruses are grouped into cutaneous and mucosal types on the basis of their tendency to infect particular types of epithelium. Most often, HPV types found in nongenital warts will be cutaneous types, and those in respiratory papillomatosis, anogenital warts, dysplasias, or cancers will be mucosal types. More than 40 HPV types can infect the genital tract. More than 14 high-risk types are recognized, with types 16 and 18 most frequently being associated with cervical cancer and type 16 most frequently being associated with other anogenital cancers and oropharyngeal cancers. Types 6 and 11 frequently are associated with condylomata acuminata, recurrent respiratory papillomatosis, and conjunctival papillomas.

Epidemiology

Papillomaviruses are distributed widely among mammals and are species-specific. Cutaneous warts occur commonly among school-aged children; the prevalence rate is as high as 50%. HPV infections are transmitted from person to person by close contact. Nongenital warts are acquired through contact with HPV and minor trauma to the skin. An increase in the incidence of plantar warts has been associated with swimming in public pools. The intense and often widespread appearance of cutaneous warts in patients with compromised cellular immunity (particularly patients who have undergone transplantation and people with HIV infection) suggests that alterations in immunity predispose to reactivation of latent intraepithelial infection.

Anogenital HPV infection is the most common sexually transmitted infection in the United States. Most infections are subclinical and clear spontaneously within 2 years. Persistent infection with high-risk types of HPV is associated with development of cervical cancer, with more than 12,000 new cases and 4,000 deaths attributed to HPV annually in the United States, as well as with vulvar, vaginal, penile, and anal cancers and a significant percentage of oropharyngeal cancers. The risk of development of

dysplastic cancer precursor lesions is greater in people with HIV infection and people with cellular immune deficiencies.

Respiratory papillomatosis is believed to be acquired by aspiration of infectious secretions during passage through an infected birth canal. When anogenital warts are identified in a child who is beyond infancy but is prepubertal, sexual abuse must be considered.

Incubation Period

Estimated range, 3 months to several years. Chronic persistent infection, usually occurring more than 10 years after infection, is associated with the rare sequelae, malignant anogenital and pharyngeal neoplasias.

Diagnostic Tests

Most cutaneous and anogenital warts are diagnosed clinically. Respiratory papillomatosis is diagnosed using endoscopy and biopsy. Cervical dysplasias are detected via (1) cytologic examination of exfoliated cells in a Pap test, either by conventional or liquid-based cytologic methods, or (2) histologic examination of cervical tissue biopsy. Cervical biopsy can show HPV-associated lesions, such as warts, dysplasias, and carcinomas. Although characteristic cytologic and histologic changes may suggest the presence of HPV, diagnosing infection requires a molecular test.

Although HPV can be propagated under special laboratory conditions, HPV cannot be isolated from patient samples; therefore, a definitive diagnosis of HPV infection is based on detection of viral nucleic acid (DNA or RNA) or capsid protein. Three tests that detect high-risk types of HPV DNA in exfoliated cells obtained from the cervix are available for clinical use (Digene HC2 High-Risk HPV DNA test [Qiagen Inc, Valencia, CA], Cervista HPV HR test [Hologic, Bedford, MA], and cobas HPV test [Roche Molecular Diagnostics]). The tests detect any of 13 to 14 high-risk HPV types known to be associated with cervical cancer, and the result is reported as negative or positive. Two tests detect type-specific infection, the Cervista HPV 16/18 and the cobas test, which in addition to reporting presence of any of 14 HPV types also reports detection of HPV

16 and/or 18. These tests are recommended by some organizations for use in combination with Pap testing in women 30 years of age or older and for triage of women 20 years of age or older in specific circumstances to help determine whether further assessments, such as colposcopy, are necessary. However, these tests are not recommended for routine use in adolescents. Serologic testing does not inform clinical decisions and is not indicated.

Treatment

Treatment of HPV infection is directed toward eliminating lesions that result from infection rather than HPV. Treatment of anogenital warts may differ from treatment of cutaneous nongenital warts, so treatment options for these warts should be discussed with a health care professional. Spontaneous regression of genital warts occurs within months in some cases. The optimal treatment for genital warts that do not resolve spontaneously has not been identified. Most nongenital warts eventually regress spontaneously but can persist for months or years. Most methods of treatment use chemical or physical destruction of the infected epithelium, including application of salicylic acid products, cryotherapy with liquid nitrogen, or laser or surgical removal of warts. Daily treatment with tretinoin has been useful for widespread flat warts in children. Care must be taken to avoid a deleterious cosmetic result with therapy. Pharmacologic treatments for refractory warts, including cimetidine, have been used with varied success.

Treatments are characterized as patient applied or administered by health care professionals and include ablational/excisional treatments, antiproliferative methods, and immune-modulating therapy. Although most forms of therapy are successful for initial removal of warts, treatment does not eradicate HPV infection from the surrounding tissue. Recurrences are common and may be attributable to reactivation rather than reinfection. Patients should be followed up during and after treatment for genital warts, because many treatments can result in local symptoms or adverse effects.

Cervical Cancer Screening. HPV infection of the cervix is common in sexually active adolescents and can be associated with epithelial dysplasia, which commonly are low-grade lesions. However, most HPV infections eventually clear, and cervical cancer is rare in adolescence. The American College of Obstetricians and Gynecologists and other professional organizations recommend that Pap testing be initiated at 21 years of age for all otherwise healthy women, regardless of their sexual history. This approach recognizes the importance of avoiding unnecessary treatment for cervical dysplasia, which can have substantial economic, emotional, and reproductive adverse effects, including higher risk of preterm birth. Female adolescents with a recent diagnosis of HIV infection should undergo cervical Pap test screening twice in the first year after diagnosis and annually thereafter. Sexually active female adolescents who have had an organ transplant or are receiving long-term corticosteroid therapy also should undergo similar cervical Pap test screening. If cytologic screening has been initiated before 21 years of age, patients with abnormal Pap test results should be cared for by a physician who is knowledgeable in the management of cervical dysplasia.

Respiratory papillomatosis is difficult to treat and is best managed by an otolaryngologist. Local recurrence is common, and repeated surgical procedures for removal often are necessary. Extension or dissemination of respiratory papillomas from the larynx into the trachea, bronchi, or lung parenchyma can result in increased morbidity and mortality; rarely, carcinoma can occur. Intralesional interferon, indole-3-carbinole, photodynamic therapy, and intralesional cidofovir have been used as investigational treatments and may be of benefit for patients with frequent recurrences.

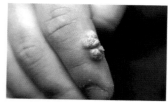

Image 90.1
Digitate human papillomavirus wart with finger-like projections on a child's index finger. Copyright Gary Williams, MD.

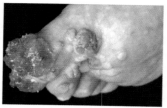

Image 90.2
Human papillomavirus warts on the foot of an immunocompromised 14-year-old male. Copyright Gary Williams, MD.

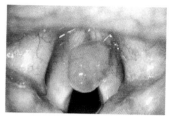

Image 90.3
Laryngeal papillomas may cause hoarseness. Though rare, they can occur in infants of mothers infected with human papillomavirus.

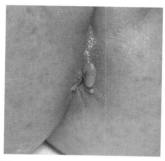

Image 90.4
A 13-month-old girl with condylomata acuminata around the anus from sexual abuse (sodomy). Copyright Martin G. Myers, MD.

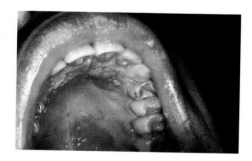

Image 90.5
This HIV-positive patient was exhibiting signs of a secondary condylomata acuminata infection (ie, venereal warts). This intraoral eruption of condylomata acuminata was caused by human papillomavirus (HPV). Though oral HPV is a rare occurrence, HIV reduces the body's immune response and, therefore, such secondary infections can manifest themselves. Courtesy of Centers for Disease Control and Prevention/Sol Silverman, Jr, DDS.

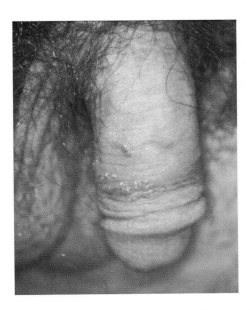

Image 90.6
This patient with condylomata acuminata presented with soft, wart-like growths on the penis; 12 hours post-podophyllin application. Condylomata acuminata refers to an epidermal manifestation caused by epidermotropic human papillomavirus. The most commonly affected areas are the penis, vulva, vagina, cervix, perineum, and perianal area. Courtesy of Centers for Disease Control and Prevention/ Susan Lindsley.

91

Paracoccidioidomycosis
(South American Blastomycosis)

Clinical Manifestations

Disease occurs primarily in adults, in whom the site of initial infection is the lungs. Clinical patterns are categorized as an acute-subacute form that predominates in childhood and a chronic form that is the typical clinical pattern in adults. In both forms, constitutional symptoms, such as fever, malaise, and weight loss, are common. In the acute-subacute form, the initial pulmonary infection usually is asymptomatic, and manifestations are related to dissemination of infection to the reticulo-endothelial system, resulting in enlarged lymph nodes and involvement of liver, spleen, and bone marrow. Involvement of bones, joints, skin, and mucous membranes is less common. Occasionally, enlarged lymph nodes coalesce and form abscesses or fistulas. The chronic form of the illness can be localized to the lungs or can disseminate. Oral, upper respiratory tract, and gastrointestinal tract granulomatous or ulcerative mucosal lesions are less common manifestations of disease in children than in adults. Infection can be latent for years before causing illness.

Etiology

Paracoccidioides brasiliensis is a thermally dimorphic fungus with yeast and mycelia phases.

Epidemiology

The infection occurs throughout Latin America. The natural reservoir is unknown, although soil is suspected. The mode of transmission is unknown; person-to-person transmission does not occur.

Incubation Period

Highly variable; range, 1 month to many years.

Diagnostic Tests

Round, multiple-budding cells with a distinguishing pilot's wheel appearance can be seen in 10% potassium hydroxide preparations of sputum, bronchoalveolar lavage specimens, scrapings from ulcers, and material from lesions or in tissue biopsy specimens. The organism can be cultured on most enriched media. A number of serologic tests are available; quantitative immunodiffusion is the preferred test. The antibody titer by immunodiffusion usually is 1:32 or greater in acute infection.

Treatment

Amphotericin B is preferred by many experts for initial treatment of severe paracoccidioidomycosis. An alternative is intravenous trimethoprim-sulfamethoxazole. Children treated initially by the intravenous route can transition to orally administered therapy after clinical improvement has been observed, usually after 3 to 6 weeks.

Oral therapy with itraconazole is the treatment of choice for less severe or localized infection and to complete treatment when amphotericin B is used initially. Prolonged therapy for 6 to 12 months is necessary to minimize the relapse rate. Children with severe disease can require a longer course. Voriconazole is as well tolerated and effective as itraconazole in adults, but data for its use in children with paracoccidioidomycosis are not available. Trimethoprim-sulfamethoxazole orally is an alternative, but treatment must be continued for 2 years or longer to lessen the risk of relapse.

Serial serologic testing by quantitative immunodiffusion is useful for monitoring the response to therapy. The expected response is a progressive decline in titers after 1 to 3 months of treatment with stabilization at a low titer.

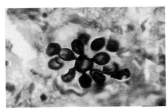

Image 91.1
Histopathologic features of paracoccidioidomycosis. Budding cell of *Paracoccidioides brasiliensis* (methenamine silver stain). Courtesy of
Centers for Disease Control and Prevention.

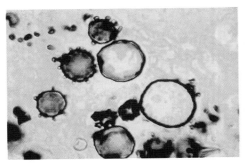

Image 91.2
Histopathologic features of paracoccidioidomycosis, liver. Minute buds on several cells of
Paracoccidioides brasiliensis (methenamine silver
stain). Courtesy of Centers for Disease Control
and Prevention/Dr Lucille K. Georg.

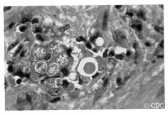

Image 91.3
Histopathologic features of paracoccidioidomy-
cosis from skin sample. Cells of *Paracoccidioides
brasiliensis* are visible. Courtesy of Centers for
Disease Control and Prevention/ Dr Lucille
K. George.

92

Paragonimiasis

Clinical Manifestations

There are 2 major forms of paragonimiasis: (1) disease attributable to *Paragonimus westermani, Paragonimus heterotremus, Paragonimus africanus,* and *Paragonimus uterobilateralis,* causing primary pulmonary disease with or without extrapulmonary manifestations and (2) disease attributable to other species of *Paragonimus,* most notably *Paragonimus skrjabini,* for which humans are accidental hosts and manifestations generally are extrapulmonary, resulting in a larva migrans syndrome. The disease has an insidious onset and a chronic course. Pulmonary disease is associated with chronic cough and dyspnea, but most infections probably are inapparent or result in mild symptoms. Heavy infestations cause paroxysms of coughing that often produce blood-tinged sputum that is brown because of the presence of *Paragonimus* species eggs. Hemoptysis can be severe. Pleural effusion, pneumothorax, bronchiectasis, and pulmonary fibrosis with clubbing can develop. Extrapulmonary manifestations also may involve liver, spleen, abdominal cavity, intestinal wall, intra-abdominal lymph nodes, skin, and central nervous system, with meningoencephalitis, seizures, and space-occupying tumors attributable to invasion of the brain by adult flukes, usually occurring within a year of pulmonary infection. Symptoms tend to subside after approximately 5 years but can persist for as many as 20 years.

Extrapulmonary paragonimiasis is associated with migratory allergic subcutaneous nodules containing juvenile worms. Pleural effusion is common, as is invasion of the brain.

Etiology

In Asia, classical paragonimiasis is caused by adult flukes and eggs of *P westermani* and *P heterotremus.* In Africa, adult flukes and eggs of *P africanus* and *P uterobilateralis* produce the disease. The adult flukes of *P westermani* are up to 12 mm long and 7 mm wide and occur throughout the Far East. A triploid parthenogenetic form of *P westermani,* which is larger, produces more eggs, and elicits greater disease, has been described in Japan, Korea, Taiwan, and parts of eastern China. *P heterotremus* occurs in Southeast Asia and adjacent parts of China. Extrapulmonary paragonimiasis is caused by larval stages of *P skrjabini* and *Paragonimus miyazakii.* The worms rarely mature. *P skrjabini* occurs in China, and *P miyazakii* occurs in Japan. *Paragonimus mexicanus* and *Paragonimus ecuadoriensis* occur in Mexico, Costa Rica, Ecuador, and Peru. *Paragonimus kellicotti,* a lung fluke of mink and opossums in the United States, also can cause a zoonotic infection in humans.

Epidemiology

Transmission occurs when raw or undercooked freshwater crabs or crayfish containing larvae (metacercariae) are ingested. The metacercariae excyst in the small intestine and penetrate the abdominal cavity, where they remain for a few days before migrating to the lungs. *P westermani* and *P heterotremus* mature within the lungs over 6 to 10 weeks, when they then begin egg production. Eggs escape from pulmonary capsules into the bronchi and exit from the human host in sputum or feces. Eggs hatch in freshwater within 3 weeks, giving rise to miracidia. Miracidia penetrate freshwater snails and emerge several weeks later as cercariae, which encyst within the muscles and viscera of freshwater crustaceans before maturing into infective metacercariae. Transmission also occurs when humans ingest raw pork, usually from wild pigs, containing the juvenile stages of *Paragonimus* species in Japan.

Humans are accidental ("dead-end") hosts for *P skrjabini* and *P miyazakii.* These flukes cannot mature in humans and, hence, do not produce eggs. *Paragonimus* species also infect a variety of other mammals, such as canids, mustelids, felids, and rodents, which can serve as animal reservoir hosts.

Incubation Period

Variable; egg production begins approximately 8 weeks after ingestion of *P westermani* metacercariae.

Diagnostic Tests

Microscopic examination of stool, sputum, pleural effusion, cerebrospinal fluid, and other tissue specimens may reveal eggs. A Western blot serologic antibody test based on *P westermani* antigen, available at the Centers for Disease Control and Prevention (CDC), is sensitive and specific; antibody levels detected by immunoblot decrease slowly after the infection is cured by treatment. Charcot-Leyden crystals and eosinophils in sputum are useful in diagnosis. Chest radiographs can appear normal or resemble radiographs from patients with tuberculosis. Misdiagnosis is likely unless paragonimiasis is suspected.

Treatment

Praziquantel in a 2-day course is the treatment of choice and is associated with high cure rates as demonstrated by disappearance of egg production and radiographic lesions in the lungs. The drug also is effective for some extrapulmonary manifestations. Bithionol, available from the CDC, is an alternative drug.

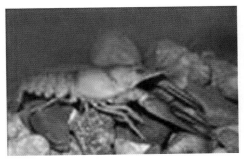

Image 92.2
Eating raw or undercooked crabs or crayfish can result in human paragonimiasis, a parasitic disease caused by *Paragonimus westermani* and *Paragonimus heterotremus*. Courtesy of Centers for Disease Control and Prevention.

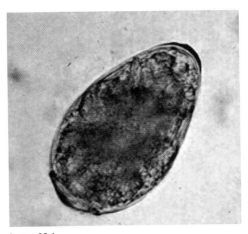

Image 92.1
Ovum of *Paragonimus westermani*. The average ovum size is 85 by 53 μm (range, 68–118 μm by 39–67 μm). They are yellow-brown and ovoid or elongate, with a thick shell, and often asymmetric with one end slightly flattened. At the large end, the operculum is clearly visible. The opposite (abopercular) end is thickened. The ova of *P westermani* are excreted unembryonated and may be found in the stool or sputum. Courtesy of Centers for Disease Control and Prevention.

Paragonimiasis (*Paragonimus westermani*)

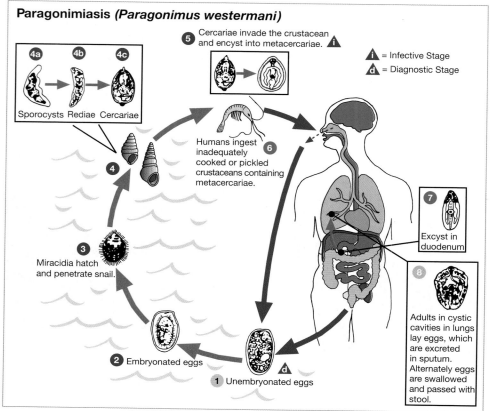

Image 92.3

Life cycle of *Paragonimus westermani*. The eggs are excreted unembryonated in the sputum, or alternately they are swallowed and passed with stool (1). In the external environment, the eggs become embryonated (2), and miracidia hatch and seek the first intermediate host, a snail, and penetrate its soft tissues (3). Miracidia develop in the snail (4): sporocysts (4a), rediae (4b), giving rise to many cercariae (4c), which emerge from the snail. The cercariae invade the second intermediate host (a crustacean), where they encyst and become metacercariae. This is the infective stage for the mammalian host (5). Human infection occurs by eating inadequately cooked or pickled crab or crayfish that harbor metacercariae (6). The metacercariae excyst in the duodenum (7), penetrate through the intestinal wall into the peritoneal cavity, through the abdominal wall and diaphragm into the lungs, where they encapsulate and develop into adults (8) (7.5–12 mm by 4–6 mm).

The worms can also reach other tissues (brain and striated muscles). However, completion of the life cycles is not achieved, because the eggs laid cannot exit these sites. Time from infection to oviposition is 65 to 90 days. Infections may persist for 20 years in humans. Animals such as pigs, dogs, and a variety of feline species can also harbor *P westermani*. Courtesy of Centers for Disease Control and Prevention/Alexander J. da Silva, PhD/Melanie Moser.

93

Parainfluenza Viral Infections

Clinical Manifestations

Parainfluenza viruses are the major cause of laryngotracheobronchitis (croup), but they also commonly cause upper respiratory tract infection, pneumonia, and/or bronchiolitis. Parainfluenza virus types 1 and 2 are the most common pathogens associated with croup, and parainfluenza virus type 3 most commonly is associated with bronchiolitis and pneumonia in infants and young children. Rarely, parotitis, aseptic meningitis, and encephalitis have been associated with type 3 infections. Parainfluenza virus infections can exacerbate symptoms of chronic lung disease and asthma in children and adults. Severe and persistent infections occur in immunodeficient children and are associated most commonly with type 3 virus. Infections with type 4 parainfluenza virus are not as well characterized, but studies using reverse transcriptase PCR (RT-PCR) assays suggest that they may be more common than previously appreciated. Parainfluenza infections do not confer complete protective immunity; thus, reinfections can occur with all serotypes and at any age, but reinfections usually cause a mild illness limited to the upper respiratory tract.

Etiology

Parainfluenza viruses are enveloped RNA viruses classified in the family Paramyxoviridae. Four antigenically distinct types—1, 2, 3, and 4 (with 2 subtypes, 4A and 4B)—have been identified.

Epidemiology

Parainfluenza viruses are transmitted from person to person by direct contact and exposure to contaminated nasopharyngeal secretions through respiratory tract droplets and fomites. Parainfluenza virus infections can be sporadic or associated with outbreaks of acute respiratory tract disease. Seasonal patterns of infection are distinct, predictable, and cyclic.

Different serotypes have distinct epidemiologic patterns. Type 1 virus tends to produce outbreaks of respiratory tract illness, usually croup, in the autumn of every other year. A major increase in the number of cases of croup in the autumn usually indicates a parainfluenza type 1 outbreak. Type 2 virus also can cause outbreaks of respiratory tract illness in the autumn, often in conjunction with type 1 outbreaks, but type 2 outbreaks tend to be less severe, irregular, and less common. Parainfluenza type 3 virus usually is prominent during spring and summer in temperate climates but often continues into autumn, especially in years when autumn outbreaks of parainfluenza virus types 1 or 2 are absent. Infections with type 4 parainfluenza virus are recognized less commonly and can be associated with mild to severe illnesses.

The age of primary infection varies with serotype. Primary infection with all types usually occurs by 5 years of age. Infection with type 3 virus more often occurs in infants and is a prominent cause of lower respiratory tract illnesses in this age group. By 12 months of age, 50% of infants have acquired type 3 parainfluenza infection. Infections between 1 and 5 years of age are more commonly associated with type 1 and, to a lesser extent, type 2 parainfluenza viruses. Age at acquisition of type 4 parainfluenza infection is not as well defined. Rates of parainfluenza virus hospitalizations for children younger than 5 years are estimated to be 1 per 1,000, with the highest rates in infants 0 to 5 months of age (3 per 1,000).

Immunocompetent children with primary parainfluenza infection can shed virus for up to 1 week before onset of clinical symptoms and for 1 to 3 weeks after symptoms have disappeared, depending on serotype. Severe lower respiratory tract disease with prolonged shedding of the virus can develop in immunodeficient people. In these patients, infection can spread beyond the respiratory tract to liver and lymph nodes.

Incubation Period

2 to 6 days.

Diagnostic Tests

Rapid antigen identification techniques, including immunofluorescent assays and enzyme immunoassays, can be used to detect the virus in nasopharyngeal secretions, but sensitivities of the tests vary. Virus may be isolated from nasopharyngeal secretions usually within 4 to 7 days of culture inoculation or earlier by using centrifugation of the specimen onto a monolayer of susceptible cells with subsequent staining for viral antigen (shell vial assay). Highly sensitive and specific RT-PCR assays are available for detection and differentiation of parainfluenza viruses, and they are becoming the standard diagnostic approach for these viruses. Serologic diagnosis, made retrospectively by a significant increase in antibody titer between serum specimens obtained during acute infection and convalescence, is less useful, because infection may not always be accompanied by a significant homotypic antibody response.

Treatment

Specific antiviral therapy is not available. Most infections are self-limited and require no treatment. Monitoring for hypoxia and hypercapnia in more severely affected children with lower respiratory tract disease can be helpful. Racemic epinephrine aerosol commonly is given to severely affected, hospitalized patients with laryngotracheobronchitis to decrease airway obstruction. Parenteral dexamethasone in high doses, oral dexamethasone, and nebulized corticosteroids have been demonstrated to lessen the severity and duration of respiratory and hospitalization in patients with moderate to severe laryngotracheobronchitis. Oral dexamethasone also is effective for outpatients with less severe croup. Management otherwise is supportive.

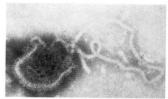

Image 93.1
Electron micrograph of parainfluenza virus.
Copyright Charles Prober, MD.

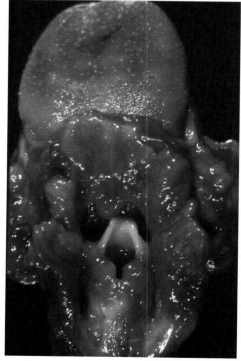

Image 93.2
Fatal croup. Edema, congestion, and inflammation of larynx and pharynx. Courtesy of Dimitris P. Agamanolis, MD.

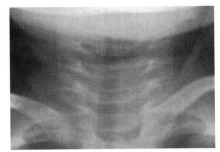

Image 93.3

Parainfluenza laryngotracheitis with the steeple sign in a 2-year-old. Copyright Benjamin Estrada, MD.

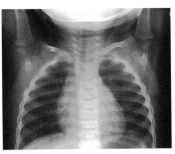

Image 93.4

Parainfluenza laryngotracheitis in a 2-year-old male. Copyright Benjamin Estrada, MD.

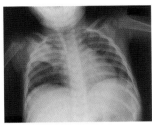

Image 93.5

Parainfluenza pneumonia in a 2-year-old male. Copyright Benjamin Estrada, MD.

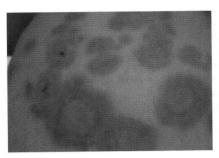

Image 93.6

Erythema multiforme minor in a 2-year-old male with parainfluenza. Copyright Benjamin Estrada, MD.

94

Parasitic Diseases

Many parasitic diseases traditionally have been considered exotic and, therefore, frequently are not included in differential diagnoses of patients in the United States, Canada, and Europe. Nevertheless, a number of these organisms are endemic in industrialized countries and, overall, parasites are among the most common causes of morbidity and mortality in various and diverse geographic locations worldwide. Outside the tropics and subtropics, parasitic diseases particularly are common among tourists returning to their own countries, immigrants from areas with highly endemic infection, and immunocompromised people. Some of these infections disproportionately affect impoverished populations, such as black and Hispanic people living in the United States, and aboriginal people living in

Alaska and the Canadian Arctic. Physicians and clinical laboratory personnel need to be aware of where these infections may be acquired, their clinical presentations, and methods of diagnosis and should advise people how to prevent infection.

Consultation and assistance in diagnosis and management of parasitic diseases are available from the Centers for Disease Control and Prevention; state health departments, and university departments or divisions of geographic medicine, tropical medicine, pediatric infectious diseases, international health, and public health.

Important human parasitic infections are discussed in individual chapters; the diseases are arranged alphabetically. The recommendations for administration of drugs given in the disease-specific chapters are similar.

Table 94.1

Parasitic Diseases Not Covered Elsewhere

Disease and/or Agent	Where Infection May Be Acquired	Definitive Host	Intermediate Host	Modes of Human Infection	Directly Communicable (Person to Person)	Diagnostic Laboratory Tests in Humans	Causative Form of Parasite	Manifestations in Humans
Angiostrongylus cantonensis (neurotropic disease)	Widespread in the tropics, particularly Pacific Islands, Southeast Asia, and Central and South America	Rats	Snails and slugs	Eating improperly cooked infected mollusks or food contaminated by mollusk secretions containing larvae	No	Eosinophils in CSF; rarely, identification of larvae in CSF or at autopsy; serologic test	Larval worms	Eosinophilia, meningo-encephalitis
Angiostrongylus costaricensis (gastrointestinal tract disease)	Central and South America	Rodents	Snails and slugs	Eating improperly poorly cooked infected mollusks or food contaminated by mollusk secretions containing larvae	No	Gel diffusion; identification of larvae and eggs in tissue	Larval worms	Abdominal pain, eosinophilia
Anisakiasis	Cosmopolitan, mainly Japan	Marine mammal	Certain saltwater fish, squid, and octopus	Eating uncooked infected fish	No	Identification of recovered larvae in granulomas or vomitus	Larval worms	Acute gastrointestinal tract disease
Clonorchis sinensis, Opisthorchis viverrini, Opisthorchis felineus (flukes)	East Asia, Eastern Europe, Russian Federation	Humans, cats, dogs, other mammals	Certain freshwater snails	Eating uncooked infected freshwater fish	No	Eggs in stool or duodenal fluid	Larvae and mature flukes	Abdominal pain; hepatobiliary disease

Table 94.1

Parasitic Diseases Not Covered Elsewhere, continued

Disease and/ or Agent	Where Infection May Be Acquired	Definitive Host	Intermediate Host	Modes of Human Infection	Directly Communicable (Person to Person)	Diagnostic Laboratory Tests in Humans	Causative Form of Parasite	Manifestations in Humans
Dracunculiasis (Dracunculus medinensis) (guinea worm)	Foci in Africa	Humans	Crustacea (copepods)	Drinking infested water	No	Identification of emerging or adult worm in subcutaneous tissues	Adult female worm	Emerging round-worm; inflamma-tory response; systemic and local blister or ulcer in skin
Fasciolopsiasis (Fasciolopsis buski)	East Asia	Humans, pigs, dogs	Certain fresh-water snails, plants	Eating uncooked infected plants	No	Eggs or worm in feces or duodenal fluid	Larvae and mature worms	Diarrhea, consti-pation, vomiting, anorexia, edema of face and legs, ascites
Intestinal capillariasis (Capillaria philippinensis)	Philippines, Thailand	Humans, fish-eating birds	Fish	Ingestion of uncooked infected fish	Uncertain	Eggs and parasite in feces	Larvae and mature worms	Protein-losing enteropathy, diarrhea, malab-sorption, asci-tes, emaciation

Abbreviation: CSF, cerebrospinal fluid.

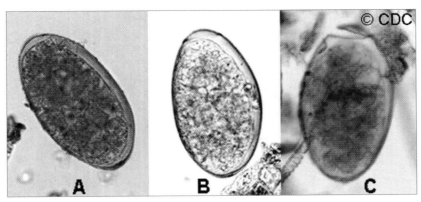

Image 94.1
Fasciola hepatica eggs. Wet mounts with iodine. The eggs are ellipsoidal. They have a small, barely distinct operculum (A, B, upper end of the eggs). The operculum can be opened (egg C), for example, when a slight pressure is applied to the coverslip. The eggs have a thin shell that is slightly thicker at the abopercular end. They are passed unembryonated. The size ranges from 120 to 150 μm by 63 to 90 μm. Fascioliasis is caused by the sheep liver fluke infecting the liver and biliary system. Courtesy of Centers for Disease Control and Prevention.

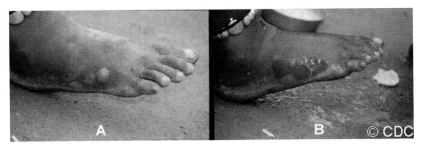

Image 94.2
Dracunculiasis. The female guinea worm *(Dracunculus medinensis)* induces a painful blister (A); after rupture of the blister, the worm emerges as a whitish filament (B) in the center of a painful ulcer, which is often secondarily infected. Courtesy of Centers for Disease Control and Prevention.

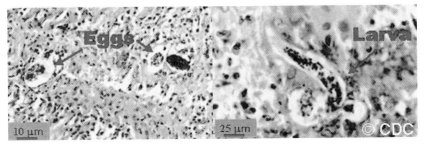

Image 94.3
Eggs and larva of *Angiostrongylus costaricensis*. In humans, eggs and larvae are not normally excreted, but remain sequestered in tissues. Both eggs and larvae (occasionally adult worms) of *A costaricensis* can be identified in biopsy or surgical specimens of intestinal tissue. The larvae need to be distinguished from larvae of *Strongyloides stercoralis;* however, the presence of granulomas containing thin-shelled eggs and/or larvae serve to distinguish *A costaricensis* infections. The larval infection can cause mesenteric arteritis and abdominal pain, occurring primarily in people in Central and South America. Courtesy of Centers for Disease Control and Prevention.

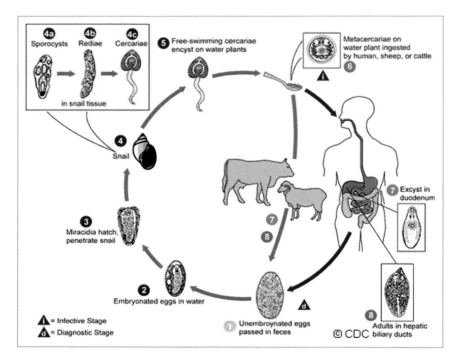

Image 94.4

Fasciola hepatica (life cycle). Immature eggs are discharged in the biliary ducts and in the stool (1). Eggs become embryonated in water (2) and release miracidia (3), which invade a suitable snail intermediate host (4), including many species of the genus *Lymnae*. In the snail the parasites develop (sporocysts [4a], rediae [4b], and cercariae [4c]). The cercariae are released from the snail (5) and encyst as metacercariae on aquatic vegetation or other surfaces. Mammals acquire the infection by eating vegetation containing metacercariae. Humans can become infected by ingesting metacercariae-containing freshwater plants, especially watercress (6). After ingestion, the metacercariae excyst in the duodenum (7) and migrate through the intestinal wall, the peritoneal cavity, and the liver parenchyma into the biliary ducts, where they develop into adults (8). In humans, maturation from metacercariae into adult flukes takes approximately 3 to 4 months. The adult flukes reside in the large biliary ducts of the mammalian host. *F hepatica* infect various animal species, mostly herbivores. Courtesy of Centers for Disease Control and Prevention.

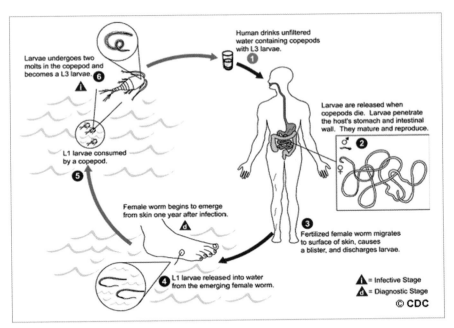

Image 94.5

Dracunculus medinensis. Humans become infected by drinking unfiltered water containing copepods (small crustaceans) that are infected with larvae of *D medinensis* (1). Following ingestion, the copepods die and release the larvae, which penetrate the host stomach and intestinal wall and enter the abdominal cavity and retroperitoneal space (2). After maturation into adults and copulation, the male worms die and the females (length, 70–120 cm) migrate in the subcutaneous tissues toward the skin surface (3). Approximately 1 year after infection, the female worm induces a blister on the skin, generally on the distal lower extremity, which ruptures. When this lesion comes into contact with water, a contact that the patient seeks to relieve the local discomfort, the female worm emerges and releases larvae (4). The larvae are ingested by a copepod (5) and after 2 weeks (and 2 molts) have developed into infective larvae (6). Ingestion of the copepods closes the cycle. Courtesy of Centers for Disease Control and Prevention/Alexander J. da Silva, PhD/Melanie Moser.

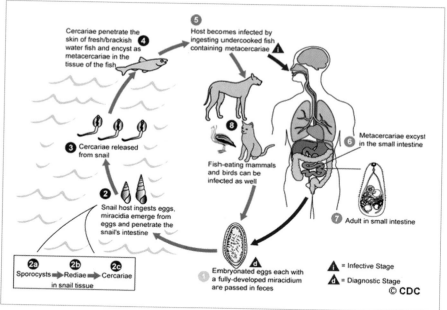

Image 94.6

Heterophyes heterophyes. Adults release embryonated eggs each with a fully developed miracidium, and eggs are passed in the host's feces (1). After ingestion by a suitable snail (first intermediate host), the eggs hatch and release miracidia, which penetrate the snail's intestine (2). Genera *Cerithidia* and *Pironella* are important snail hosts in Asia and the Middle East, respectively. The miracidia undergo several developmental stages in the snail (ie, sporocysts [2a], rediae [2b], and cercariae [2c]). Many cercariae are produced from each redia. The cercariae are released from the snail (3) and encyst as metacercariae in the tissues of a suitable fresh/brackish water fish (second intermediate host) (4). The definitive host becomes infected by ingesting undercooked or salted fish containing metacercariae (5). After ingestion, the metacercariae excyst, attach to the mucosa of the small intestine (6), and mature into adults (measuring 1.0–1.7 mm by 0.3–0.4 mm) (7). In addition to humans, various fish-eating mammals (eg, cats and dogs) and birds can be infected by *H heterophyes* (8). Geographic distribution: Egypt, the Middle East, and Far East. Courtesy of Centers for Disease Control and Prevention/ Alexander J. da Silva, PhD/Melanie Moser.

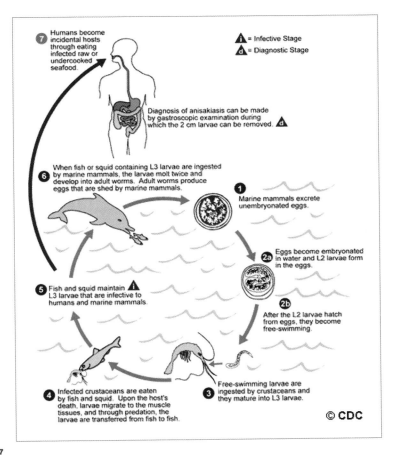

Image 94.7

Adult stages of *Anisakis simplex* or *Pseudoterranova decipiens* reside in the stomach of marine mammals, where they are embedded in the mucosa, in clusters. Unembryonated eggs produced by adult females are passed in the feces of marine mammals (1). The eggs become embryonated in water, and first-stage larvae are formed in the eggs. The larvae molt, becoming second-stage larvae (2a), and after the larvae hatch from the eggs, they become free-swimming (2b). Larvae released from the eggs are ingested by crustaceans (3). The ingested larvae develop into third-stage larvae that are infective to fish and squid (4). The larvae migrate from the intestine to the tissues in the peritoneal cavity and grow up to 3 cm in length. On the host's death, larvae migrate to the muscle tissues, and through predation, the larvae are transferred from fish to fish. Fish and squid maintain third-stage larvae that are infective to humans and marine mammals (5). When fish or squid containing third-stage larvae are ingested by marine mammals, the larvae molt twice and develop into adult worms. The adult females produce eggs that are shed by marine mammals (6). Humans become infected by eating raw or undercooked infected marine fish (7). After ingestion, the *Anisakis* larvae penetrate the gastric and intestinal mucosa, causing the symptoms of anisakiasis. Courtesy of Centers for Disease Control and Prevention/Alexander J. da Silva, PhD/Melanie Moser.

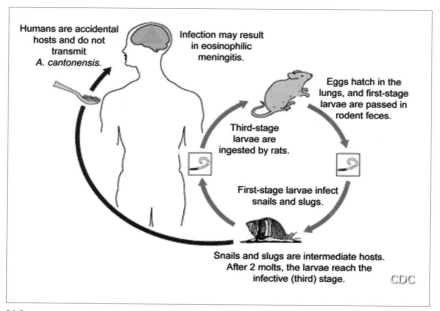

Image 94.8

Life cycle of *Angiostrongylus cantonensis.* Courtesy of Centers for Disease Control and Prevention.

95

Parvovirus B19
(Erythema Infectiosum, Fifth Disease)

Clinical Manifestations

Infection with parvovirus B19 is recognized most often as erythema infectiosum (EI), or fifth disease, which is characterized by a distinctive rash that may be preceded by mild systemic symptoms, including fever in 15% to 30% of patients. The facial rash can be intensely red with a "slapped cheek" appearance that often is accompanied by circumoral pallor. A symmetric, macular, lace-like, and often pruritic rash also occurs on the trunk, moving peripherally to involve the arms, buttocks, and thighs. The rash can fluctuate in intensity and recur with environmental changes, such as temperature and exposure to sunlight, for weeks to months. A brief, mild, nonspecific illness consisting of fever, malaise, myalgia, and headache often precedes the characteristic exanthem by approximately 7 to 10 days. Arthralgia and arthritis occur in fewer than 10% of infected children but commonly occur among adults, especially women. Knees are involved most commonly in children, but a symmetric polyarthropathy of knees, fingers, and other joints is common in adults.

Human parvovirus B19 also can cause an asymptomatic infection. Other manifestations (Table 95.1) include a mild respiratory tract illness with no rash, a rash atypical for EI that may be rubelliform or petechial, papulopurpuric gloves-and-socks syndrome (PPGSS; painful and pruritic papules, petechiae, and purpura of hands and feet, often with fever and an enanthem), polyarthropathy syndrome (arthralgia and arthritis in adults in the absence of other manifestations of EI), chronic erythroid hypoplasia with severe anemia in immunodeficient patients (eg, HIV-infected patients, patients receiving immune suppressive therapy), and transient aplastic crisis lasting 7 to 10 days in patients with hemolytic anemias (eg, sickle cell disease and autoimmune hemolytic anemia) and other conditions associated with low hemoglobin concentrations, including hemorrhage, severe anemia, and thalassemia. Patients with transient aplastic crisis can have a prodromal illness with fever, malaise, and myalgia, but rash usually is absent. The B19-associated red blood cell aplasia is related to caspase-10–mediated apoptosis of erythrocyte precursors. In addition, parvovirus B19 infection sometimes has been associated with decreases in numbers of platelets, lymphocytes, and neutrophils.

Parvovirus B19 infection occurring during pregnancy can cause fetal hydrops, intrauterine growth retardation, isolated pleural and pericardial effusions, and death, but parvovirus B19 is not a proven cause of congenital anomalies. The risk of fetal death is between 2% and 6% when infection occurs during pregnancy. The greatest risk appears to occur during the first half of pregnancy.

Etiology

Human parvovirus B19 is a small, nonenveloped, single-stranded DNA virus in the family Parvoviridae, genus *Erythrovirus*. Three major genetic variants of the virus have been described. Parvovirus B19 replicates in human erythrocyte precursors, which accounts for some of the clinical manifestations following infection.

Table 95.1
Clinical Manifestations of Human Parvovirus B19 Infection

Conditions	Usual Hosts
Erythema infectiosum (fifth disease)	Immunocompetent children
Polyarthropathy syndrome	Immunocompetent adults (more common in women)
Chronic anemia/pure red cell aplasia	Immunocompromised hosts
Transient aplastic crisis	People with hemolytic anemia (ie, sickle cell anemia)
Hydrops fetalis/congenital anemia	Fetus (first 20 weeks of pregnancy)

Epidemiology

Parvovirus B19 is distributed worldwide and is a common cause of infection in humans, who are the only known hosts. Modes of transmission include contact with respiratory tract secretions, percutaneous exposure to blood or blood products, and vertical transmission from mother to fetus. Since 2002, plasma derivatives have been screened using nucleic acid amplification tests to decrease the risk of parvovirus B19 transmission. Parvovirus B19 infections are ubiquitous, and cases of EI can occur sporadically or in outbreaks in elementary or junior high schools during late winter and early spring. Secondary spread among susceptible household members is common, with infection occurring in approximately 50% of susceptible contacts in some studies. The transmission rate in schools is less, but infection can be an occupational risk for school and child care personnel, with approximately 20% of susceptible contacts becoming infected. In young children, antibody seroprevalence generally is 5% to 10%. In most communities, approximately 50% of young adults and often more than 90% of elderly people are seropositive. The annual seroconversion rate in women of childbearing age has been reported to be approximately 1.5%. Timing of the presence of parvovirus B19 DNA in serum and respiratory tract secretions indicates that people with EI are most infectious before rash onset and are unlikely to be infectious after onset of the rash and/or joint symptoms. In contrast, patients with aplastic crises are contagious from before the onset of symptoms through at least the week after onset. Symptoms of the PPGSS occur in association with viremia and before development of antibody response, and affected patients should be considered infectious.

Incubation Period

Usually 4 to 14 days but can be as long as 21 days. Rash and joint symptoms occur 2 to 3 weeks after infection.

Diagnostic Tests

Parvovirus B19 cannot be propagated in standard cell culture. In the immunocompetent host, detection of serum parvovirus B19-specific immunoglobulin (Ig) M antibody is the preferred diagnostic test. A positive IgM test result indicates that infection probably occurred within the previous 2 to 4 months. On the basis of enzyme immunoassay results, antibody can be detected in 90% or more of patients at the time of the EI rash and by the third day of illness in patients with transient aplastic crisis. Serum IgG antibody appears by approximately day 7 of EI and persists for life; thus, presence of parvovirus B19 IgG is not necessarily indicative of acute infection. These assays are available through commercial laboratories. However, their sensitivity and specificity can vary, particularly for IgM antibody. The optimal method for detecting chronic infection in the immunocompromised patient is demonstration of virus by PCR assays, because parvovirus B19 antibody is present variably in persistent infection. Because parvovirus B19 DNA can be detected at low levels by PCR assay in serum for up to 9 months after the acute viremic phase, detection does not necessarily indicate acute infection. Parvovirus DNA has been detected by PCR in tissues (skin, heart, cerebellum), independent of disease.

Treatment

For most patients, only supportive care is indicated. Patients with aplastic crises can require red blood cell and platelet transfusions. For treatment of chronic infection in immunodeficient patients, immune globulin intravenous therapy often is effective and should be considered. Some cases of parvovirus B19 infection concurrent with hydrops fetalis have been treated successfully with intrauterine blood transfusions.

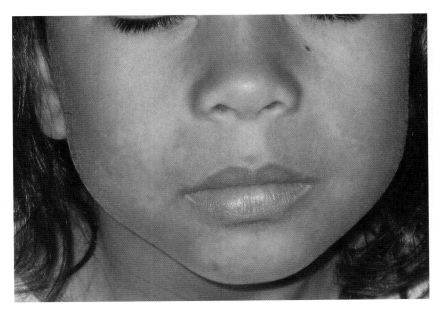

Image 95.1

This healthy 6-year-old girl developed an asymptomatic symmetric red papular eruption on her face, extremities, and trunk, which became confluent on her face 1 week earlier. Courtesy of H. Cody Meissner, MD, FAAP.

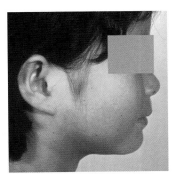

Image 95.2

Parvovirus B19 infection (erythema infectiosum, fifth disease) with typical facial erythema, commonly referred to as the "slapped cheek sign."

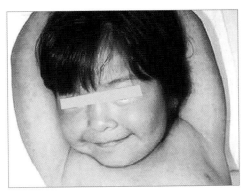

Image 95.3

Characteristic "slapped cheek" appearance of the face in a child who has fifth disease. The characteristic rash also is present on the arms.

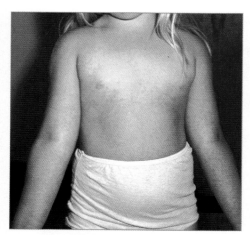

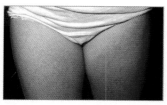

Image 95.5
Parvovirus B19 infection (erythema infectiosum, fifth disease). This is the same child as in Image 95.4.

Image 95.4
Parvovirus B19 infection (erythema infectiosum, fifth disease) in a 5-year-old girl.

96

Pasteurella Infections

Clinical Manifestations

The most common manifestation in children is cellulitis at the site of a scratch or bite of a cat, dog, or other animal. Cellulitis typically develops within 24 hours of the injury and includes swelling, erythema, tenderness, and serous or sanguinopurulent discharge at the site. Regional lymphadenopathy, chills, and fever can occur. Local complications, such as septic arthritis, osteomyelitis, and tenosynovitis, are common. Less common manifestations of infection include septicemia, meningitis, endocarditis, respiratory tract infections (eg, pneumonia, pulmonary abscesses, pleural empyema), appendicitis, hepatic abscess, peritonitis, urinary tract infection, and ocular infections (eg, conjunctivitis, corneal ulcer, endophthalmitis). People with liver disease or underlying host defense abnormalities are predisposed to bacteremia attributable to *Pasteurella multocida.*

Etiology

Species of the genus *Pasteurella* are nonmotile, facultative anaerobic, gram-negative coccobacilli that are primary pathogens in animals. The most common human pathogen is *P multocida.*

Epidemiology

Pasteurella species are found in the oral flora of 70% to 90% of cats, 25% to 50% of dogs, and many other animals. Transmission can occur from the bite or scratch of a cat or dog or, less commonly, from another animal. Respiratory tract spread from animals to humans also occurs. In a significant proportion of cases, no animal exposure can be identified. Human-to-human spread has been documented vertically from mother to neonate, horizontally from colonized humans, and by contaminated blood products.

Incubation Period

Usually less than 24 hours.

Diagnostic Tests

The isolation of *Pasteurella* species from skin lesion drainage or other sites of infection (eg, blood, joint fluid, cerebrospinal fluid, sputum, pleural fluid, or suppurative lymph nodes) is diagnostic. Although *Pasteurella* species resemble several other organisms morphologically and grow on many culture media at 37°C (98°F), laboratory differentiation is not difficult.

Treatment

The drug of choice is penicillin. Other effective oral agents include ampicillin, amoxicillin, cefuroxime, cefixime, cefpodoxime, doxycycline, and fluoroquinolones. For patients who are allergic to beta-lactam agents, azithromycin or trimethoprim-sulfamethoxazole is an alternative choice, but clinical experience with these agents is limited. Doxycycline is effective but should be avoided in children younger than 8 years whenever possible. For suspected polymicrobial infection, oral amoxicillin-clavulanate or, for severe infection, intravenous ampicillin-sulbactam, ticarcillin-clavulanate, or piperacillin-tazobactam can be given. Alternative agents for systemic infection include ceftriaxone or a carbapenem. Isolates usually are resistant to vancomycin, clindamycin, and erythromycin. Penicillin resistance is rare, but beta-lactamase–producing strains have been recovered, especially from adults with pulmonary disease. Wound drainage or debridement may be necessary.

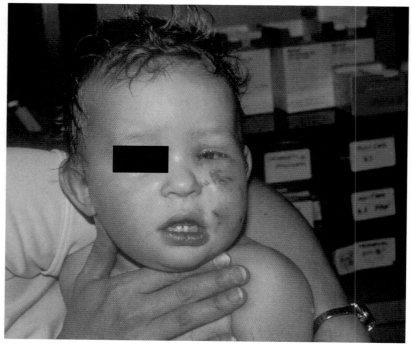

Image 96.1
Pasteurella multocida cellulitis secondary to multiple cat bites about the face of a 1-year-old child.
Courtesy of George Nankervis, MD.

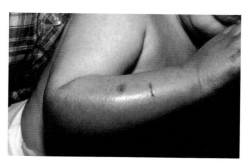

Image 96.2
Right forearm of 1-year-old boy bitten by a stray cat. The infant developed fever, redness, and swelling
10 hours after the bite. The child was taking amoxicillin for otitis media at the time of the bite. The
child responded to treatment with intravenous cefuroxime, although the fever persisted for 36 hours.
Pasturella multocida was cultured from purulent material obtained from the wound the day after
admission. Courtesy of Larry I. Corman, MD.

97

Pediculosis Capitis

(Head Lice)

Clinical Manifestations

Itching is the most common symptom of head lice infestation, but many children are asymptomatic. Adult lice or eggs (nits) are found on the hair and are most readily apparent behind the ears and near the nape of the neck. Excoriations and crusting caused by secondary bacterial infection can occur and often are associated with regional lymphadenopathy. Head lice usually deposit their eggs on a hair shaft 4 mm or less from the scalp. Because hair grows at a rate of approximately 1 cm per month, the duration of infestation can be estimated by the distance of the nit from the scalp.

Etiology

Pediculus humanus capitis is the head louse. Both nymphs and adult lice feed on human blood.

Epidemiology

In the United States, head lice infestation is most common in children attending child care and elementary school. Head lice infestation is not a sign of poor hygiene. All socioeconomic groups are affected. In the United States, infestations are less common in black children than in children of other ethnicities. Head lice infestation is not influenced by hair length or frequency of shampooing or brushing. Head lice are not a health hazard, because they are not responsible for spread of any disease. Head lice only are able to crawl; therefore, transmission occurs mainly by direct head-to-head contact with hair of infested people. Transmission by contact with personal belongings, such as combs, hair brushes, and hats, is uncommon. Away from the scalp, head lice survive less than 2 days at room temperature, and their eggs generally become nonviable within a week and cannot hatch at a lower ambient temperature than that near the scalp.

Incubation Period

From the laying of eggs to hatching of the first nymph, 8 to 9 days; range, 7 to 12 days but shorter in hot climates. Lice mature to adult stage approximately 9 to 12 days later. Adult females then may lay eggs (nits), but these will develop only if the female has mated.

Diagnostic Tests

Identification of eggs (nits), nymphs, and lice with the naked eye is possible; diagnosis can be confirmed by using a hand lens or microscope. Nymphal and adult lice shun light and move rapidly and conceal themselves. Wetting the hair with water, oil, or a conditioner and using a fine-tooth comb may improve the ability to diagnose infestation and shorten examination time. It is important to differentiate nits from dandruff, benign hair casts (a layer of follicular cells that may slide easily off the hair shaft), plugs of desquamated cells, external hair debris, and fungal infections of the hair. Because nits remain affixed to the hair firmly, even if dead or hatched, the mere presence of nits is not a sign of an active infestation.

Treatment

A number of effective pediculicidal agents are available to treat head lice infestation. Safety is a major concern with pediculicides, because the infestation itself presents minimal risk to the host. Pediculicides should be used only as directed and with care. Instructions on proper use of any product should be explained carefully. Therapy can be started with over-the-counter 1% permethrin or with a pyrethrin combined with piperonyl butoxide product, both of which have good safety profiles. However, resistance to these compounds has been documented in the United States. For treatment failures not attributable to improper use of an over-the-counter pediculicide, malathion, benzyl alcohol lotion, or spinosad suspension should be used. Lice resistant to all topical agents may be treated with ivermectin. No drug truly is ovicidal, but of the available topical agents, only malathion has ovicidal activity. Pediculicides usually require more than one application. Ideally, re-treatment should occur after the eggs that are present at the time of initial treatment have hatched but before any new eggs have been produced.

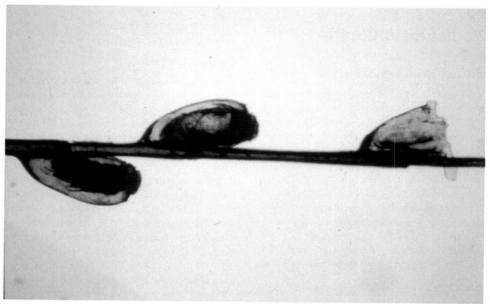

Image 97.1
Head lice. Nits on a hair shaft. Copyright James Brien, DO.

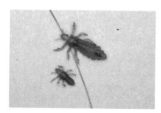

Image 97.2
Head louse, baby louse, and hair. Copyright Gary Williams, MD.

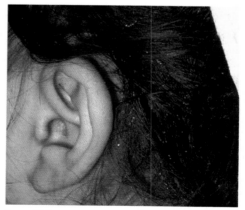

Image 97.3
Nits on the hair shafts. Copyright Ed Marcuse, MD.

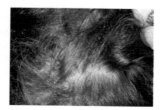

Image 97.4
An 8-year-old girl with an earache. This child complained of otalgia. During the course of oto-scopic evaluation, she was noted to have a very large number of nits in her hair as well as active lice. On questioning, she states she has had itching of the scalp. She was treated with topical permethrin with temporary resolution. Reinfestation occurred after sharing a riding helmet with a cousin. Copyright Will Sorey, MD.

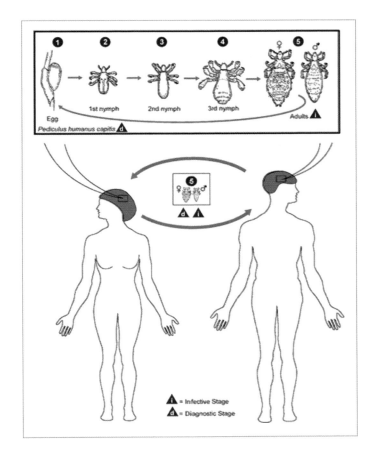

Image 97.5

The life cycle of the head louse has 3 stages: egg, nymph, and adult. **Eggs:** Nits are head lice eggs. They are hard to see and are often confused for dandruff or hair spray droplets. Nits are laid by the adult female and are cemented at the base of the hair shaft nearest the scalp (1). They are 0.8 by 0.3 mm, oval, and usually yellow to white. Nits take about 1 week to hatch (range, 6–9 days). Viable eggs are usually located within 6 mm of the scalp. **Nymphs:** The egg hatches to release a nymph (2). The nit shell then becomes a more visible dull yellow and remains attached to the hair shaft. The nymph looks like an adult head louse, but is about the size of a pinhead. Nymphs mature after 3 molts (3, 4) and become adults about 7 days after hatching. **Adults:** The adult louse is about the size of a sesame seed, has 6 legs (each with claws), and is tan to grayish-white (5). In persons with dark hair, the adult louse will appear darker. Females are usually larger than males and can lay up to 8 nits per day. Adult lice can live up to 30 days on a person's head. To live, adult lice need to feed on blood several times daily. Without blood meals, the louse will die within 1 to 2 days off the host. Courtesy of Centers for Disease Control and Prevention/Alexander J. da Silva, PhD/Melanie Moser.

98

Pediculosis Corporis
(Body Lice)

Clinical Manifestations

Intense itching, particularly at night, is common with body lice infestations. Bites manifest as small erythematous macules, papules, and excoriations primarily on the trunk. In heavily bitten areas, typically around the mid-section, the skin can become thickened and discolored. Secondary bacterial infection of the skin caused by scratching is common.

Etiology

Pediculus humanus corporis (or *humanus*) is the body louse. Nymphs and adult lice feed on human blood.

Epidemiology

Body lice generally are restricted to people living in crowded conditions without access to regular bathing or changes of clothing (refugees, victims of war or natural disasters, homeless people). Under these conditions, body lice can spread rapidly through direct contact or contact with contaminated clothing or bedding. Body lice live in clothes or bedding, lay their eggs on or near the seams of clothing, and move to the skin to feed. Body lice cannot survive away from a blood source

for longer than approximately 5 to 7 days at room temperature. In contrast with head lice, body lice are well-recognized vectors of disease (eg, epidemic typhus, trench fever, epidemic relapsing fever, and bacillary angiomatosis).

Incubation Period

From laying eggs to hatching of the first nymph, approximately 1 to 2 week. Lice mature and are capable of reproducing 9 to 19 days after hatching.

Diagnostic Tests

Identification of eggs, nymphs, and lice with the naked eye is possible; diagnosis can be confirmed by using a hand lens or microscope. Adult and nymphal body lice seldom are seen on the body, because they generally are sequestered in clothing.

Treatment

Treatment consists of improving hygiene and regular changes of clean clothes and bedding. Infested materials can be decontaminated by washing in hot water (at least 130°F), by machine drying at hot temperatures, by dry cleaning, or by pressing with a hot iron. Temperatures exceeding 53.5°C (128.3°F) for 5 minutes are lethal to lice and eggs. Pediculicides usually are not necessary if materials are laundered at least weekly.

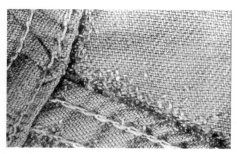

Image 98.1

This is a piece of clothing the seams of which contained lice eggs from the body louse *Pediculus humanus* var *corporis*. The most important factor in the control of body lice infestation is the ability to change and wash clothing. Courtesy of Centers for Disease Control and Prevention/Reed & Carnrick Pharmaceuticals.

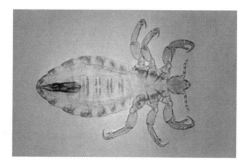

Image 98.2

This body louse, *Pediculus humanus corporis*, was photographed during a 1972 study of migrant labor camp disease vectors. Body lice, family Pediculidae, are parasitic insects that live on the body and in the clothing or bedding of infested humans. Infestation is common, and is found worldwide. Itching and rash are common with lice infestation. Courtesy of Centers for Disease Control and Prevention.

99

Pediculosis Pubis

(Pubic Lice, Crab Lice)

Clinical Manifestations

Pruritus of the anogenital area is a common symptom in pubic lice infestations ("crabs" or "pthiriasis"). The parasite most frequently is found in the pubic region, but infestation can involve the eyelashes, eyebrows, beard, axilla, perianal area and, rarely, the scalp. A characteristic sign of heavy pubic lice infestation is the presence of bluish or slate-colored macules (maculae ceruleae) on the chest, abdomen, or thighs.

Etiology

Phthirus pubis is the pubic or crab louse. Nymphs and adult lice feed on human blood.

Epidemiology

Pubic lice infestations are more prevalent in adults and usually are transmitted through sexual contact. Transmission by contaminated items, such as towels, is uncommon. Pubic lice on the eyelashes or eyebrows of children may be evidence of sexual abuse, although other modes of transmission are possible. Infested people should be examined for other sexually transmitted infections. Adult pubic lice can survive away from a host for up to 36 hours, and their eggs can remain viable for up to 10 days under suitable environmental conditions.

Incubation Period

From the laying of eggs to the hatching of the first nymph, approximately 6 to 10 days. Adult lice become capable of reproducing approximately 2 to 3 weeks after hatching.

Diagnostic Tests

Identification of eggs (nits), nymphs, and lice with the naked eye is possible; the diagnosis can be confirmed by using a hand lens or microscope.

Treatment

All areas of the body with coarse hair should be examined for evidence of pubic lice infestation. Lice and their eggs can be removed manually, or the hairs can be shaved to eliminate infestation immediately. Caution should be used when inspecting, removing, or treating lice on or near the eyelashes. Pediculicides used to treat other kinds of louse infestations are effective for treatment of pubic lice. Re-treatment is recommended as for head lice. Topical pediculicides should not be used for treatment of pubic lice infestation of eyelashes; rather an ophthalmic-grade petrolatum ointment should be applied to the eyelashes 2 to 4 times daily for 8 to 10 days.

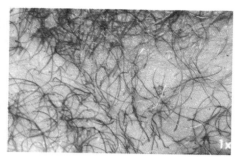

Image 99.1

This photograph reveals the presence of crab lice, *Phthirus pubis,* with reddish-brown crab feces. Pubic lice are generally found in the genital area on pubic hair, but may occasionally be found on other coarse body hair, such as leg hair, armpit hair, mustache, beard, eyebrows, and eyelashes. Courtesy of Centers for Disease Control and Prevention/Reed & Carnrick Pharmaceuticals.

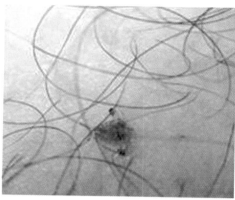

Image 99.2

Pediculosis, the infestation of humans by lice, has been documented for millennia. Three species of lice infest humans: *Pediculus humanus humanus,* the body louse; *Pediculus humanus capitis,* the head louse; and *Phthirus pubis,* the crab louse. The hallmark of louse infestation is pruritus at the site of bites. Lice are more active at night, frequently disrupting the sleep of the host, which is the derivation of the term "feeling lousy." Adult crab lice can survive without a blood meal for 36 hours. Unlike head lice, which may travel up to 23 cm/min, pubic lice are sluggish, traveling a maximum of 10 cm/day. Viable eggs on pubic hairs may hatch up to 10 days later. Crab louse infestation is localized most frequently to the pubic and perianal regions but may spread to the mustache, beard, axillae, eyelashes, or scalp hair. Infestation usually is acquired through sexual contact, and the finding of pubic lice in children (often limited to the eyelashes) should raise concern for possible sexual abuse. Courtesy of H. Cody Meissner, MD, FAAP.

100

Pertussis (Whooping Cough)

Clinical Manifestations

Pertussis begins with mild upper respiratory tract symptoms similar to the common cold (catarrhal stage) and progresses to cough and then usually to paroxysms of cough (paroxysmal stage), characterized by inspiratory whoop and commonly followed by vomiting. Fever is absent or minimal. Symptoms wane gradually over weeks to months (convalescent stage). Cough illness in immunized children and adults can range from typical to mild and unrecognized. The duration of classic pertussis is 6 to 10 weeks. Approximately half of adolescents with pertussis cough for 10 weeks or longer. Complications among adolescents and adults include syncope, sleep disturbance, incontinence, rib fractures, and pneumonia; among adults, complications increase with age. Pertussis is most severe when it occurs during the first 6 months of life, particularly in preterm and unimmunized infants. Disease in infants younger than 6 months can be atypical with a short catarrhal stage, gagging, gasping, bradycardia, or apnea as prominent early manifestations; absence of whoop; and prolonged convalescence. Sudden unexpected death can be caused by pertussis. Complications among infants include pneumonia (22%), seizures (2%), encephalopathy (<0.5%), hernia, subdural bleeding, conjunctival bleeding, and death. Case-fatality rates are approximately 1% in infants younger than 2 months and less than 0.5% in infants 2 through 11 months of age.

Etiology

Pertussis is caused by a fastidious, gram-negative, pleomorphic bacillus, *Bordetella pertussis*. Other causes of sporadic prolonged cough illness include *Bordetella parapertussis, Mycoplasma pneumoniae, Chlamydia trachomatis, Chlamydophila pneumoniae, Bordetella bronchiseptica*, and certain respiratory tract viruses, particularly adenoviruses and respiratory syncytial viruses.

Epidemiology

Humans are the only known hosts of *B pertussis*. Transmission occurs by close contact via aerosolized droplets. Cases occur year-round, typically with a late summer-autumn peak. Neither infection nor immunization provides lifelong immunity. Lack of natural boosting events and waning immunity since childhood immunization were responsible for the increase in cases of pertussis in people older than 10 years noted before use of the adolescent booster immunization. Additionally, waning maternal immunity and reduced transplacental antibody has led to an increase in pertussis in very young infants. More than 42,000 cases of pertussis were reported in the United States in 2012. As many as 80% of immunized household contacts of pertussis cases acquire infection, mainly because of waning immunity, with symptoms varying from asymptomatic infection to classic pertussis. Older siblings (including adolescents) and adults with mild or unrecognized atypical disease are important sources of pertussis for infants and young children. Infected people are most contagious during the catarrhal stage and the first 2 weeks after cough onset. Factors affecting the length of communicability include age, immunization status or previous infection, and appropriate antimicrobial therapy.

Incubation Period

7 to 10 days; range, 5 to 21 days.

Diagnostic Tests

Culture is considered the gold standard for laboratory diagnosis of pertussis. Although culture is 100% specific, *B pertussis* is a fastidious organism that requires careful specimen collection and transport. A nasopharyngeal specimen, obtained by aspiration or with Dacron (polyethylene terephthalate) or calcium alginate swab, must be placed into special transport media immediately and not allowed to dry while being transported promptly to the laboratory. Culture can be negative if taken from a previously immunized person, if antimicrobial therapy has been initiated, if more than 3 weeks has elapsed since cough onset, or if the specimen is not handled appropriately.

PCR assay increasingly is used for detection of *B pertussis* because of its improved sensitivity and more rapid turnaround time. PCR requires collection of an adequate nasopharyngeal specimen using a Dacron swab or nasopharyngeal wash or aspirate. Calcium alginate swabs are inhibitory to PCR and should not be used. PCR for pertussis lacks sensitivity in previously immunized people but still may be more sensitive than culture. Unacceptably high rates of false-positive results are reported from some laboratories, and a pseudo-outbreak linked to contaminated specimens also has been reported. Multiple DNA target sequences are required to distinguish between *Bordetella* species. Direct fluorescent antibody testing no longer is recommended.

Commercial serologic tests for pertussis infection can be helpful for diagnosis, especially later in illness. Cutoff points for diagnostic values of immunoglobulin (Ig) G antibody to pertussis toxin (PT) have not been established, and IgA and IgM assays lack adequate sensitivity and specificity. In the absence of recent immunization, an elevated serum IgG antibody to PT after 2 weeks of onset of cough is suggestive of recent *B pertussis* infection. An increasing concentration or a single IgG anti-PT value of approximately 94 EU/mL or greater (using standard reference sera as a comparator) can be used for diagnosis.

An increased white blood cell count attributable to absolute lymphocytosis is suggestive of pertussis in infants and young children but often is absent in adolescents and adults with pertussis and can be only mildly abnormal in young infants at the time of presentation.

Treatment

Antimicrobial agents administered during the catarrhal stage may ameliorate the disease. After the cough is established, antimicrobial agents have no discernible effect on the course of illness but are recommended to limit spread of organisms to others. Azithromycin, erythromycin, or clarithromycin are appropriate first-line agents for treatment and prophylaxis. Resistance of *B pertussis* to macrolide antimicrobial agents has been reported rarely. Penicillins and first- and second-generation cephalosporins are not effective against *B pertussis*.

Antimicrobial agents for infants younger than 6 months require special consideration. An association between orally administered erythromycin and infantile hypertrophic pyloric stenosis (IHPS) has been reported in infants younger than 1 month. Until additional information is available, azithromycin is the drug of choice for treatment or prophylaxis of pertussis in infants younger than 1 month, in whom the risk of developing severe pertussis and life-threatening complications outweighs the potential risk of IHPS with azithromycin.

Trimethoprim-sulfamethoxazole is an alternative for patients older than 2 months who cannot tolerate macrolides. However, studies evaluating trimethoprim-sulfamethoxazole as treatment for pertussis are limited.

Young infants are at increased risk of respiratory failure attributable to apnea or secondary bacterial pneumonia and are at risk of cardiopulmonary failure from pulmonary hypertension. Hospitalized young infants with pertussis should be managed in a setting/facility where these complications can be recognized and managed emergently.

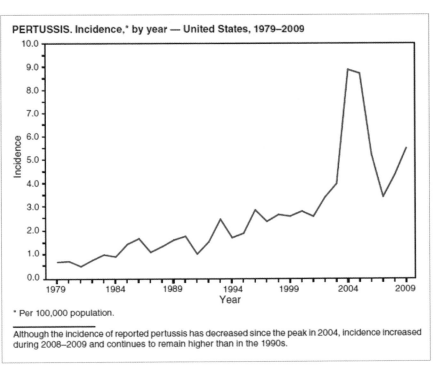

PERTUSSIS. Incidence,* by year — United States, 1979–2009

*Per 100,000 population.

Although the incidence of reported pertussis has decreased since the peak in 2004, incidence increased during 2008–2009 and continues to remain higher than in the 1990s.

Image 100.1
Pertussis. Incidence per year—United States, 1979–2009. Courtesy of *Morbidity and Mortality Weekly Report.*

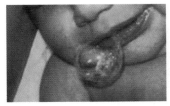

Image 100.2
Thick bronchopulmonary secretions of pertussis in an infant. Copyright Charles Prober, MD.

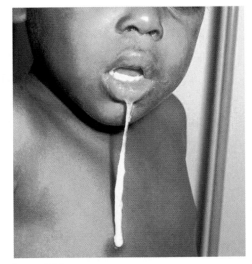

Image 100.3
A preschool-aged male with pertussis. Thick respiratory secretions were produced by a paroxysmal coughing spell. Courtesy of Edgar O. Ledbetter, MD, FAAP.

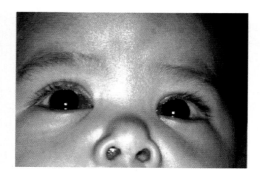

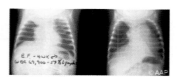

Image 100.5

A 4-week-old neonate with pertussis pneumonia with pulmonary air trapping and progressive atelectasis confirmed at autopsy. The neonate acquired the infection from the mother shortly after birth. Segmented and lobar atelectasis are not uncommon complications of pertussis.

Image 100.4

Bilateral subconjunctival hemorrhages and thick nasal mucus in an infant with pertussis.

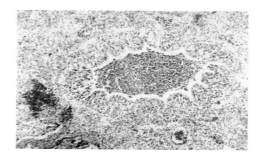

Image 100.6

Bronchiolar plugging in the neonate in Image 100.5 who died of pertussis pneumonia. Infants and children often acquire pertussis from an infected adult or sibling contact.

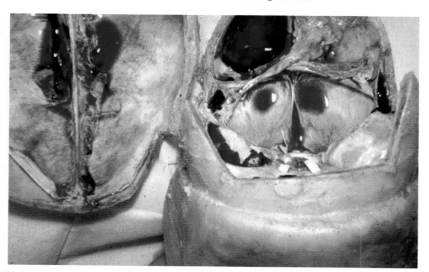

Image 100.7

Subdural bleeding secondary to whooping cough in the same patient as in Image 100.5. In the pre-vaccine era, pertussis resulted in as many as 8,000 deaths annually in the United States, with most deaths occurring in the first 6 months of life.

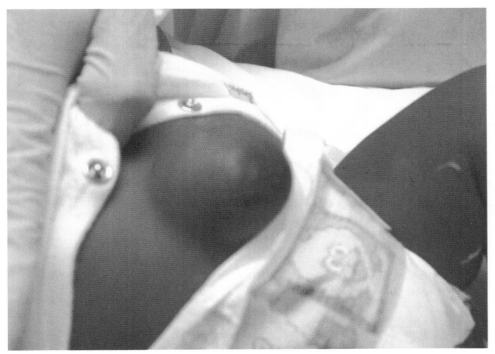

Image 100.8
Umbilical hernia more prominent as a result of persistent pertussis cough in a 4-month-old male.
Copyright Benjamin Estrada, MD.

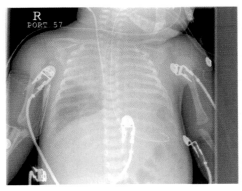

Image 100.9
Pertussis pneumonia in a 2-month-old infant 2 days after hospital admission. His mother had been coughing since shortly after delivery. Courtesy of Carol J. Baker, MD.

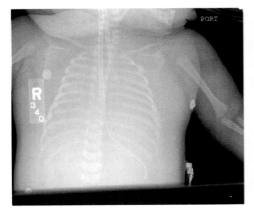

Image 100.10
The infant in Image 100.9 who required mechanical ventilation because of respiratory failure. Courtesy of Carol J. Baker, MD.

101

Pinworm Infection

(Enterobius vermicularis)

Clinical Manifestations

Although some people are asymptomatic, pinworm infection (enterobiasis) can cause pruritus ani and, rarely, pruritus vulvae. Bacterial superinfections can result from scratching and excoriation of the area. Pinworms have been found in the lumen of the appendix, but most evidence indicates that they do not cause acute appendicitis. Many clinical findings, such as grinding of teeth at night, weight loss, and enuresis, have been attributed to pinworm infections, but proof of a causal relationship has not been established. Urethritis, vaginitis, salpingitis, or pelvic peritonitis may occur from aberrant migration of an adult worm from the perineum.

Etiology

Enterobius vermicularis is a nematode or roundworm.

Epidemiology

Enterobiasis occurs worldwide and commonly clusters within families. Prevalence rates are higher in preschool- and school-aged children, in primary caregivers of infected children, and in institutionalized people; up to 50% of these populations may be infected.

Egg transmission occurs by the fecal-oral route either directly or indirectly via contaminated hands or fomites such as shared toys, bedding, clothing, toilet seats, and baths. Female pinworms usually die after depositing up to 10,000 fertilized eggs within 24 hours on the perianal skin. Reinfection occurs either by autoinfection or by infection following ingestion of eggs from another person. A person remains infectious as long as female nematodes are discharging eggs on perianal skin. Eggs remain infective in an indoor environment usually for 2 to 3 weeks. Humans are the only known natural hosts; dogs and cats do not harbor *E vermicularis*.

Incubation Period

From ingestion of an egg until an adult gravid female migrates to the perianal region, 1 to 2 months or longer.

Diagnostic Tests

Diagnosis is made when adult worms are visualized in the perianal region, which is best examined 2 to 3 hours after the child is asleep. No egg shedding occurs inside the intestinal lumen; thus, very few ova are present in stool, so examination of stool specimens for ova and parasites is not recommended. Alternatively, diagnosis is made by touching the perianal skin with transparent (not translucent) adhesive tape to collect any eggs that may be present; the tape is then applied to a glass slide and examined under a low-power microscopic lens. Specimens should be obtained on 3 consecutive mornings when the patient first awakens, before washing. Eosinophilia is unusual and should not be attributed to pinworm infection.

Treatment

Because pinworms largely are innocuous, the risk versus benefit of treatments should be weighed. Drugs of choice for treatment are mebendazole, pyrantel pamoate, and albendazole, all of which are given in a single dose and repeated in 2 weeks. Pyrantel pamoate is available without prescription. Reinfection with pinworms occurs easily; prevention should be discussed when treatment is given. Infected people should bathe in the morning; bathing removes a large proportion of eggs. Frequently changing the infected person's underclothes, bedclothes, and bed sheets may decrease the egg contamination of the local environment and risk of reinfection. Specific personal hygiene measures (eg, exercising hand hygiene before eating or preparing food, keeping fingernails short, avoiding scratching of the perianal region, and avoiding nail biting) may decrease risk of autoinfection and continued transmission. All household members should be treated as a group in situations in which multiple or repeated symptomatic infections occur.

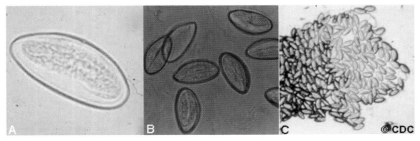

Image 101.1

(A, B) Enterobius egg(s). (C) Enterobius eggs on cellulose tape prep. Courtesy of Centers for Disease Control and Prevention.

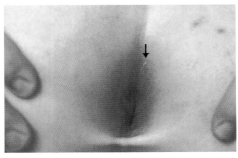

Image 101.2

Adult pinworm *(Enterobius vermicularis)* in the perianal area of a 14-year-old boy. Perianal inspection 2 to 3 hours after the child goes to sleep may reveal pinworms that have migrated outside of the intestinal tract. Copyright Gary Williams, MD.

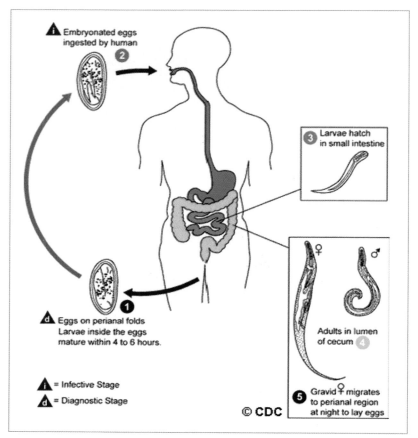

Eggs on perianal folds
Larvae inside the eggs
mature within 4 to 6 hours.

= Infective Stage
= Diagnostic Stage

Larvae hatch
in small intestine

Adults in lumen
of cecum

Gravid ♀ migrates
to perianal region
at night to lay eggs

© CDC

Image 101.3

Eggs are deposited on perianal folds (1). Self-infection occurs by transferring infective eggs to the mouth with hands that have scratched the perianal area (2). Person-to-person transmission can also occur through handling of contaminated clothes or bed linens. Enterobiasis may also be acquired through surfaces in the environment that are contaminated with pinworm eggs (eg, curtains, carpeting). Some small number of eggs may become airborne and inhaled. These could be swallowed and follow the same development as ingested eggs. Following ingestion of infective eggs, the larvae hatch in the small intestine (3) and the adults establish themselves in the colon (4). The time interval from ingestion of infective eggs to oviposition by the adult females is about 1 month. The life span of the adults is about 2 months. Gravid females migrate nocturnally outside the anus and oviposit while crawling on the skin of the perianal area (5). The larvae contained inside the eggs develop (the eggs become infective) in 4 to 6 hours under optimal conditions (1). Retroinfection, or the migration of newly hatched larvae from the anal skin back into the rectum, may occur but the frequency with which this happens is unknown. Courtesy of Centers for Disease Control and Prevention.

102

Pityriasis Versicolor

(Tinea Versicolor)

Clinical Manifestations

Pityriasis versicolor (formerly tinea versicolor) is a common superficial yeast infection of the skin characterized by multiple scaling, oval, and patchy macular lesions usually distributed over upper portions of the trunk, proximal areas of the arms, and neck. Facial involvement particularly is common in children. Lesions can be hypopigmented or hyperpigmented (fawn colored or brown), and both types of lesions can coexist in the same person. Lesions fail to tan during the summer and during the winter are relatively darker, hence the term *versicolor*. Common conditions confused with this disorder include pityriasis alba, postinflammatory hypopigmentation, vitiligo, melasma, seborrheic dermatitis, pityriasis rosea, pityriasis lichenoides, and dermatologic manifestations of secondary syphilis.

Etiology

The cause of pityriasis versicolor is *Malassezia* species, a group of lipid-dependent yeasts that exist on healthy skin in yeast phase and cause clinical lesions only when substantial growth of hyphae occurs. Moist heat and lipid-containing sebaceous secretions encourage rapid overgrowth.

Epidemiology

Pityriasis versicolor occurs worldwide but is more prevalent in tropical and subtropical areas. Although primarily a disorder of adolescents and young adults, pityriasis versicolor also may occur in prepubertal children and infants. *Malassezia* species commonly colonize the skin in the first year of life and usually are harmless commensals. *Malassezia* infection can be associated with bloodstream infections, especially in neonates receiving total parenteral nutrition with lipids.

Incubation Period

Unknown.

Diagnosis

Clinical appearance usually is diagnostic. Involved areas are fluorescent-yellow under Wood light examination. Skin scrapings examined microscopically in a potassium hydroxide wet mount preparation or stained with methylene blue or May-Grünwald-Giemsa stain disclose the pathognomonic clusters of yeast cells and hyphae ("spaghetti and meatball" appearance). Growth of this yeast in culture requires a source of long-chain fatty acids, which can be provided by overlaying Sabouraud dextrose agar medium with sterile olive oil.

Treatment

Topical treatment with selenium sulfide as 2.5% lotion or 1% shampoo has been the traditional treatment of choice. The lotion should be applied in a thin layer covering the body surface from the face to the knees for 10 minutes daily for 7 days. Off-label, monthly applications for 3 months may help prevent recurrences. Other US Food and Drug Administration–approved topical treatments for tinea versicolor include ciclopirox and oxiconazole. Because *Malassezia* species are part of normal flora, relapses are common. Multiple topical treatments may be necessary.

Oral antifungal therapy has advantages over topical therapy, including ease of administration and shorter duration of treatment, but oral therapy is more expensive and associated with a greater risk of adverse reactions. A single dose of fluconazole or a 5-day course of itraconazole has been effective in adults. Exercise to increase sweating and skin concentrations of medication may enhance the effectiveness of systemic therapy.

Patients should be advised that repigmentation may not occur for several months after successful treatment.

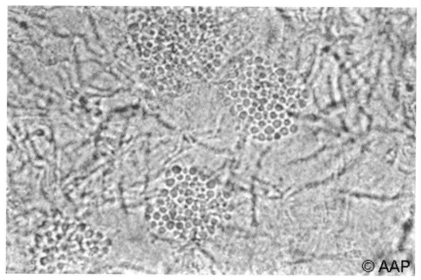

Image 102.1
The spores and pseudohyphae of *Malassezia furfur* (a yeast that can cause pityriasis versicolor) resemble "spaghetti and meatballs" on a potassium hydroxide slide.

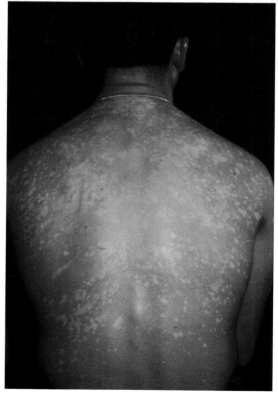

Image 102.2
Tinea versicolor. Copyright James Brien, DO.

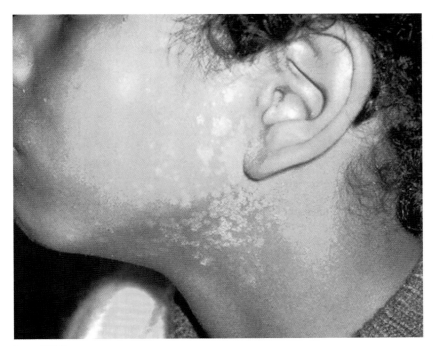

Image 102.3
Pityriasis versicolor. Copyright Edward Marcuse, MD.

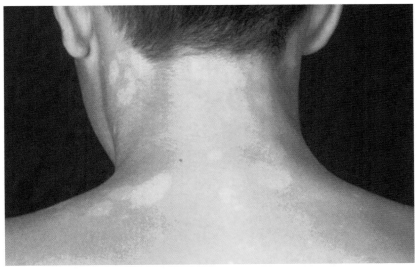

Image 102.4
Pityriasis versicolor in a 14-year-old boy. Copyright Gary Williams, MD.

103

Plague

Clinical Manifestations

Naturally acquired plague most commonly manifests in the **bubonic form**, with acute onset of fever and painful swollen regional lymph nodes (buboes). Buboes develop most commonly in the inguinal region but also occur in axillary or cervical areas. Less commonly, plague manifests in the **septicemic form** (hypotension, acute respiratory distress, purpuric skin lesions, intravascular coagulopathy, organ failure) or as **pneumonic plague** (cough, fever, dyspnea, and hemoptysis) and **rarely as** meningeal, pharyngeal, ocular, or gastrointestinal plague. Abrupt onset of fever, chills, headache, and malaise are characteristic in all cases. Occasionally, patients have symptoms of mild lymphadenitis or prominent gastrointestinal tract symptoms, which may obscure the correct diagnosis. When left untreated, plague often will progress to overwhelming sepsis with renal failure, acute respiratory distress syndrome, hemodynamic instability, diffuse intravascular coagulation, necrosis of distal extremities, and death. Plague has been referred to as the Black Death.

Etiology

Plague is caused by *Yersinia pestis,* a pleomorphic, bipolar-staining, gram-negative coccobacillus.

Epidemiology

Plague is a zoonotic infection primarily maintained in rodents and their fleas. Humans are incidental hosts who develop bubonic or primary septicemic manifestations typically through the bite of infected fleas carried by rodent or rarely other animals or through direct contact with contaminated tissues. Secondary pneumonic plague arises from hematogenous seeding of the lungs with *Y pestis* in patients with untreated bubonic or septicemic plague. Primary pneumonic plague is acquired by inhalation of respiratory tract droplets from a human or animal with pneumonic plague. Only the pneumonic form has been shown to be transmitted person-to-person, and the last known case of person-to-person transmission in the United States occurred in 1924. Rarely, humans can develop primary pneumonic plague following exposure to domestic cats with respiratory tract plague infections. Plague occurs worldwide with enzootic foci in parts of Asia, Africa, and the Americas. Most human plague cases are reported from rural, underdeveloped areas and mainly occur as isolated cases or in focal clusters. Since 2000, more than 95% of the approximately 22,000 cases reported to the World Health Organization have been from countries in sub-Saharan Africa. In the United States, plague is endemic in western states, with most (approximately 85%) of the 37 cases reported from 2006 through 2010 being from New Mexico, Colorado, Arizona, and California. Cases of peripatetic plague have been identified in states without endemic plague, such as Connecticut (2008) and New York (2002).

Incubation Period

2 to 8 days for bubonic plague; 1 to 6 days for primary pneumonic plague.

Diagnostic Tests

Diagnosis of plague usually is confirmed by culture of *Y pestis* from blood, bubo aspirate, sputum, or another clinical specimen. The organism has a bipolar (safety-pin) appearance when viewed with Wayson or Gram stains. A positive fluorescent antibody test result for the presence of *Y pestis* in direct smears or cultures of blood, bubo aspirate, sputum, or another clinical specimen provides presumptive evidence of *Y pestis* infection. A single positive serologic test result by passive hemagglutination assay or enzyme immunoassay in an unimmunized patient who previously has not had plague also provides presumptive evidence of infection. Seroconversion, defined as a fourfold difference in antibody titer between 2 serum specimens obtained at least 2 weeks apart, also confirms the diagnosis of plague. PCR assay and immunohistochemical staining for rapid diagnosis of *Y pestis* are available in some reference or public health laboratories. In regions with endemic plague with limited laboratory capacity, a rapid dipstick (immunostrip) test, which uses monoclonal antibodies to detect F1 antigen, can be used to test a bubo aspirate or sputum specimen for case confirmation, per World Health Organization recommendations.

Treatment

For children, gentamicin or streptomycin administered intramuscularly or intravenously appear to be equally effective. Tetracycline, doxycycline, chloramphenicol, trimethoprim-sulfamethoxazole, and ciprofloxacin are alternative drugs. Fluoroquinolone or chloramphenicol is appropriate treatment for plague meningitis. Fluoroquinolones also have been found to be effective in treating plague in animal and in vitro studies but are not approved by the US Food and Drug Administration for this indication. Drainage of abscessed buboes may be necessary; drainage material is infectious until effective antimicrobial therapy has been administered.

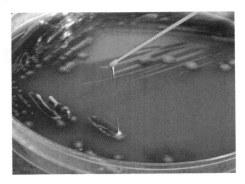

Image 103.1
This photograph depicts the colonial morphology displayed by gram-negative *Yersinia pestis* bacteria, which were grown on a medium of sheep blood agar for a 48-hour period at a temperature of 37°C. There is a tenacious nature of these colonies when touched by an inoculation loop, and their tendency to form "stringy," sticky strands. Morphologic characteristics after 48 hours of *Y pestis* colonial growth include an average colonial diameter of 1.0 to 2.0 mm and an opaque coloration that ranges from gray-white to yellowish. If permitted to continue growing, *Y pestis* colonies take on what is referred to as a "fried egg" appearance, which becomes more prominent as the colonies age. Older colonies also display what is termed a "hammered copper" texture to their surfaces. Courtesy of Centers for Disease Control and Prevention/Pete Seidel.

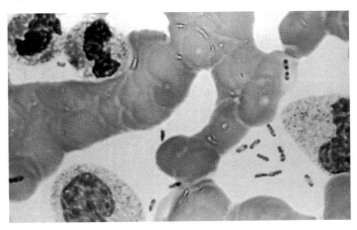

Image 103.2
Dark-stained bipolar ends of *Yersinia pestis* can clearly be seen in this Wright stain of blood from a plague victim. The actual cause of the disease is the plague bacillus *Y pestis*. It is a nonmotile, non-spore–forming, gram-negative, non-lactose fermenting, bipolar, ovoid, safety-pin–shaped bacterium. Courtesy of Centers for Disease Control and Prevention.

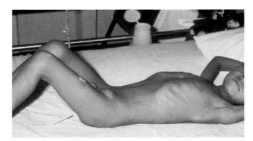

Image 103.3
Inguinal plague buboes in an 8-year-old boy. If left untreated, bubonic plague often becomes septicemic, with meningitis occurring in 6% of cases.

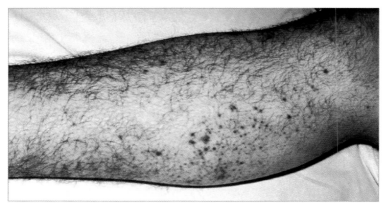

Image 103.4
Small hemorrhages on the skin of a plague victim. Capillary fragility is one of the manifestations of a plague infection, evident here on the leg of an infected patient. Courtesy of Centers for Disease Control and Prevention.

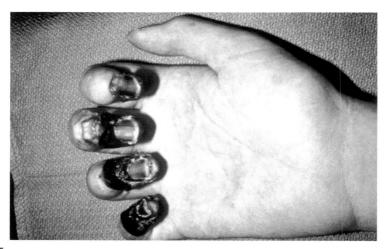

Image 103.5
Right hand of a plague patient displaying acral gangrene. Gangrene is one of the manifestations of plague and is the origin of the term "black death" given to plague throughout the ages. Disseminated intravascular coagulation is not uncommon in septicemic plague. Courtesy of Centers for Disease Control and Prevention.

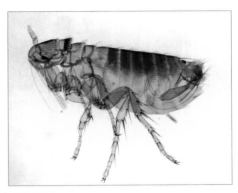

Image 103.6

This photograph depicts an adult male *Oropsylla montana* flea, formerly known as *Diamanus montana.* This flea is a common ectoparasite of the rock squirrel, *Citellus variegatus,* and in the western United States, is an important vector for the bacterium *Yersinia pestis,* the pathogen responsible for causing plague. Courtesy of Centers for Disease Control and Prevention/ John Montenieri.

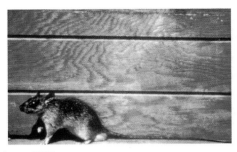

Image 103.7

This image shows the roof rat or black rat, *Rattus rattus,* a carrier of the plague bacterium *Yersinia pestis.* The roof rat can be differentiated from the Norway rat by its smaller size, and its body is generally 6 to 8 inches (16–20 cm) in length with a 7- to 10-inch (19–25 cm) tail. It is a climber and nests largely in buildings and trees. Courtesy of Centers for Disease Control and Prevention.

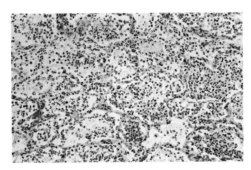

Image 103.8

This photomicrograph depicts the histopathologic changes in lung tissue in a case of fatal human plague pneumonia (hematoxylin-eosin stain, magnification x160). Note the presence of many polymorphonuclear leukocytes, capillary engorgement, and intra-alveolar debris, all indicative of an acute infection. Courtesy of Centers for Disease Control and Prevention/Dr Marshal Fox.

104

Pneumococcal Infections

Clinical Manifestations

Streptococcus pneumoniae is a common cause of invasive bacterial infections in children, including febrile bacteremia. Pneumococci also are a common cause of acute otitis media, sinusitis, community-acquired pneumonia, pleural empyema, and conjunctivitis. *S pneumoniae* can cause meningitis, but this is infrequent since the introduction of the pneumococcal conjugate vaccine in 2000. Pneumococci occasionally cause mastoiditis, periorbital cellulitis, endocarditis, osteomyelitis, pericarditis, peritonitis, pyogenic arthritis, soft tissue infection, overwhelming septicemia in patients with splenic dysfunction, and neonatal septicemia. Hemolytic uremic syndrome can accompany complicated invasive disease (eg, pneumonia with pleural empyema).

Etiology

S pneumoniae organisms (pneumococci) are lancet-shaped, gram-positive catalase-negative diplococci. More than 90 pneumococcal serotypes have been identified on the basis of unique polysaccharide capsules.

Epidemiology

Pneumococci are ubiquitous, with many people having transient colonization of the upper respiratory tract. In children, nasopharyngeal carriage rates range from 21% in industrialized countries to more than 90% in resource-limited countries. Transmission is from person to person by respiratory droplet contact. The period of communicability is unknown and may be as long as the organism is present in respiratory tract secretions but probably is less than 24 hours after effective antimicrobial therapy is begun. Among young children who acquire a new pneumococcal serotype in the nasopharynx, illness (eg, otitis media) occurs in approximately 15%, usually within a few days of acquisition. Viral upper respiratory tract infections, including influenza, can predispose to pneumococcal infection and transmission. Pneumococcal infections are most prevalent during winter months. Rates of infection are highest in infants; young children; elderly people; and black, Alaska Native, and some American Indian populations. The incidence and severity of infections are increased in people with congenital or acquired humoral immunodeficiency, HIV infection, absent or deficient splenic function (eg, sickle cell disease, congenital or surgical asplenia), or abnormal innate immune responses. Children with cochlear implants have high rates of pneumococcal meningitis, as do children with congenital or acquired cerebrospinal fluid (CSF) leaks. Other categories of children at presumed high risk or at moderate risk of developing invasive pneumococcal disease are outlined in Table 104.1. Since introduction of the 7-valent conjugate vaccine, racial disparities have diminished.

The 7-valent pneumococcal conjugate vaccine (PCV7) (containing serotypes 4, 6B, 9V, 14, 18C, 19F, and 23F) was introduced into the routine infant immunization platform in 2000. From 1998 to 2007, the incidence of vaccine-type invasive pneumococcal infections decreased by 99%, and the incidence of all invasive pneumococcal disease (IPD) decreased by 76% in children younger than 5 years. In adults 65 years of age and older, IPD caused by PCV7 serotypes decreased 92% compared with baseline and all serotype invasive disease by 37%. The reduction in cases in these latter groups indicates the significant indirect benefits of PCV7 immunization by interruption of transmission of pneumococci from children to adults. However, new serotypes emerged, in particular type 19A, and in 2010, 13-valent pneumococcal conjugate vaccine (PCV13) (containing types 1, 3, 5, 6A, 7F, and 19A in addition to the 7 PCV7 components) replaced PCV7.

Incubation Period

Varies by type of infection, but can be as short as 1 to 3 days.

Diagnostic Tests

Recovery of *S pneumoniae* from a suppurative focus or from blood confirms the diagnosis. The finding of lancet-shaped gram-positive organisms and white blood cells in expectorated sputum or pleural exudate suggests pneumococcal pneumonia in older children and adults. Recovery of pneumococci by culture of an upper respiratory tract swab specimen is

Table 104.1

Underlying Medical Conditions That Are Indications for Pneumococcal Immunization Among Children, by Risk Group[a]

Risk Group	Condition
Immunocompetent children	Chronic heart disease[b] Chronic lung disease[c] Diabetes mellitus Cerebrospinal fluid leaks Cochlear implant
Children with functional or anatomic asplenia	Sickle cell disease and other hemoglobinopathies Chronic or acquired asplenia, or splenic dysfunction
Children with immunocompromising conditions	HIV infection Chronic renal failure and nephrotic syndrome Disease associated with treatment with immuno-suppressive drugs or radiation therapy, including malignant neoplasms, leukemias, lymphomas, and Hodgkin disease; or solid organ transplantation Congenital immunodeficiency[d]

[a] Centers for Disease Control and Prevention. Licensure of a 13-valent pneumococcal conjugate vaccine (PCV13) and recommendations for use among children. Advisory Committee on Immunization Practices (ACIP). *Morb Mortal Wkly Rep.* 2010;59(9):258–261.
[b] Particularly cyanotic congenital heart disease and cardiac failure.
[c] Including asthma if treated with prolonged high-dose oral corticosteroids.
[d] Includes B-(humoral) or T-lymphocyte deficiency; complement deficiencies, particularly C_1, C_2, C_3 and C_4 deficiency; and phagocytic disorders (excluding chronic granulomatous disease).

not sufficient to assign an etiologic diagnosis of pneumococcal disease involving the middle ear, lower respiratory tract, or sinus. Real-time PCR using *lyt*A is investigational but may be specific and significantly more sensitive than culture of pleural fluid, CSF, and blood, particularly in patients who have received recent antimicrobial therapy.

Susceptibility Testing. All *S pneumoniae* isolates from normally sterile body fluids (eg, CSF, blood, middle ear fluid, pleural or joint fluid) should be tested for antimicrobial susceptibility to determine the minimum inhibitory concentration (MIC) of penicillin and cefotaxime or ceftriaxone. CSF isolates also should be tested for susceptibility to vancomycin and meropenem. *Nonsusceptible* includes both *intermediate* and *resistant* isolates. Breakpoints vary depending on whether an isolate is from a nonmeningeal or meningeal source. Accordingly, current definitions by the Clinical and Laboratory Standards Institute (CLSI) for susceptibility and nonsusceptibility are provided in Table 104.2 for non-meningeal and meningeal isolates.

For patients with meningitis caused by an organism that is nonsusceptible to penicillin, susceptibility testing of rifampin also should be performed.

Quantitative MIC testing using reliable methods, such as broth microdilution or antimicrobial gradient strips, should be performed on isolates from children with invasive infections. When quantitative testing methods are not available or for isolates from noninvasive infections, the qualitative screening test using a 1-μg oxacillin disk on an agar plate reliably identifies all penicillin-*susceptible* pneumococci using meningitis breakpoints (ie, disk-zone diameter of 20 mm or greater). Organisms with an oxacillin disk-zone size of less than 20 mm potentially are nonsusceptible for treatment of meningitis and require quantitative susceptibility testing. The oxacillin disk test is used as a screening test for resistance to beta-lactam drugs (ie, penicillins and cephalosporins).

Treatment

S pneumoniae strains that are nonsusceptible to penicillin G, cefotaxime, ceftriaxone, and other antimicrobial agents using meningitis

Table 104.2

Clinical and Laboratory Standards Institute Definitions of In Vitro Susceptibility and Nonsusceptibility of Nonmeningeal and Meningeal Pneumococcal Isolates[a,b]

Drug and Isolate Location	Susceptible, µg/mL	Nonsusceptible, µg/mL	
		Intermediate	Resistant
Penicillin (oral)[c]	≤0.06	0.12–1.0	≥2.0
Penicillin (intravenous)[d]			
Nonmeningeal	≤2.0	4.0	≥8.0
Meningeal	≤0.06	None	≥0.12
Cefotaxime **OR** ceftriaxone			
Nonmeningeal	≤1.0	2.0	≥4.0
Meningeal	≤0.5	1.0	≥2.0

[a] Clinical and Laboratory Standards Institute. *Performance Standards for Antimicrobial Susceptibility Testing: 18th Informational Supplement.* CLSI Publication No. M100-S21. Wayne, PA: Clinical and Laboratory Standards Institute; 2011.
[b] Centers for Disease Control and Prevention. Effects of new penicillin susceptibility breakpoints for *Streptococcus pneumoniae*—United States, 2006–2007. *MMWR Morb Mortal Wkly Rep.* 2008;57(50):1353–1355.
[c] Without meningitis.
[d] Treated with intravenous penicillin.

breakpoints have been identified throughout the United States and worldwide but are uncommon using nonmeningeal breakpoints.

Recommendations for treatment of pneumococcal infections are as follows.

***Bacterial Meningitis Possibly or Proven to Be Caused by* S pneumoniae.** Combination therapy with vancomycin and cefotaxime or ceftriaxone should be administered initially to all children 1 month of age or older with definite or probable bacterial meningitis because of the increased prevalence of *S pneumoniae* resistant to penicillin, cefotaxime, and ceftriaxone.

For children with serious hypersensitivity reactions to beta-lactam antimicrobial agents (ie, penicillins and cephalosporins), the combination of vancomycin and rifampin should be considered. Vancomycin should not be given alone, because bactericidal concentrations in CSF are difficult to sustain, and clinical experience to support use of vancomycin as monotherapy is minimal. Rifampin also should not be given as monotherapy, because resistance can develop during therapy. Meropenem also can be given as an alternative drug.

Once results of susceptibility testing are available, therapy should be modified according to the guidelines in Table 104.3. Vancomycin should be discontinued and penicillin should be continued if the organism is susceptible to

penicillin; if the isolate is penicillin nonsusceptible, cefotaxime or ceftriaxone should be continued. Vancomycin should be continued only if the organism is nonsusceptible to penicillin and to cefotaxime or ceftriaxone.

Dexamethasone. For infants and children 6 weeks of age and older, adjunctive therapy with dexamethasone may be considered after weighing the potential benefits and possible risks. If used, dexamethasone should be given before or concurrently with the first dose of antimicrobial agents.

Nonmeningeal Invasive Pneumococcal Infections Requiring Hospitalization. For nonmeningeal invasive infections in previously healthy children who are not critically ill, antimicrobial agents currently used to treat infections with *S pneumoniae* and other potential pathogens should be initiated at the usually recommended dosages (Table 104.4).

For critically ill infants and children with invasive infections potentially attributable to *S pneumoniae,* vancomycin in addition to usual antimicrobial therapy (eg, cefotaxime or ceftriaxone or others) can be considered for strains that possibly are nonsusceptible to penicillin, cefotaxime, or ceftriaxone. Such patients include those with myopericarditis or severe multilobar pneumonia with hypoxia or hypotension. If vancomycin is administered, it

Table 104.3
Antimicrobial Therapy for Infants and Children With Meningitis Caused by *Streptococcus pneumoniae* on the Basis of Susceptibility Test Results

Susceptibility Test Results	Antimicrobial Management[a]
Susceptible to penicillin	**Discontinue vancomycin** **AND** Begin penicillin (and discontinue cephalosporin) **OR** Continue cefotaxime or ceftriaxone alone[b]
Nonsusceptible to penicillin (*intermediate* or *resistant*) **AND** *Susceptible* to cefotaxime and ceftriaxone	**Discontinue vancomycin** **AND** Continue cefotaxime or ceftriaxone
Nonsusceptible to penicillin (*intermediate* or *resistant*) **AND** *Nonsusceptible* to cefotaxime and ceftriaxone (*intermediate* or *resistant*) **AND** *Susceptible* to rifampin	Continue vancomycin and high-dose cefotaxime or ceftriaxone **AND** Rifampin may be added in selected circumstances (see text)

[a] Some experts recommend the maximum dosages. Initial therapy for nonallergic children older than 1 month should be vancomycin and cefotaxime or ceftriaxone. See Bacterial Meningitis Possibly or Proven to Be Caused by *S pneumoniae*, p 000.
[b] Some physicians may choose this alternative for convenience and cost savings, but only in treatment of meningitis.

Table 104.4
Dosages of Intravenous Antimicrobial Agents for Invasive Pneumococcal Infections in Infants and Children[a]

Antimicrobial Agent	Meningitis		Nonmeningeal Infections	
	Dose/kg per Day	Dose Interval	Dose/kg per Day	Dose Interval
Penicillin G	250,000–400,000 U[b]	4–6 h	250,000–400,000 U[b]	4–6 h
Cefotaxime	225–300 mg	8 h	75–100 mg	8 h
Ceftriaxone	100 mg	12–24 h	50–75 mg	12–24 h
Vancomycin	60 mg	6 h	40–45 mg	6–8 h
Rifampin[c]	20 mg	12 h	Not indicated	...
Chloramphenicol[d]	75–100 mg	6 h	75–100 mg	6 h
Clindamycin	Not indicated	...	25–40 mg	6–8 h
Meropenem[e]	120 mg	8 h	60 mg	8 h

[a] Doses are for children 1 month of age or older.
[b] Because 1 U = 0.6 µg/mL, this range is equal to 150 to 240 mg/kg per day.
[c] Indications for use are not defined completely.
[d] Drug should be considered only for patients with life-threatening allergic response after administration of beta-lactam antimicrobial agents.
[e] Drug is approved for pediatric patients 3 months of age and older.

should be discontinued as soon as antimicrobial susceptibility test results demonstrate effective alternative agents.

If the organism has in vitro resistance to penicillin, cefotaxime, and ceftriaxone by CLSI standards, therapy should be modified on the basis of clinical response, susceptibility to other antimicrobial agents, and results of follow-up cultures of blood and other infected body fluids. Consultation with an infectious disease specialist should be considered.

For children with severe hypersensitivity to beta-lactam antimicrobial agents (ie, penicillins and cephalosporins), consultation with an infectious disease specialist should be considered.

Nonmeningeal Invasive Pneumococcal Infections in the Immunocompromised Host. The preceding recommendations for management of possible pneumococcal infections requiring hospitalization also apply to immunocompromised children. Vancomycin should be discontinued as soon as antimicrobial susceptibility test results indicate that effective alternative antimicrobial agents are available.

Acute Otitis Media. According to clinical practice guidelines of the American Academy of Pediatrics and the American Academy of Family Physicians on acute otitis media (AOM), high-dose amoxicillin is recommended, except in select cases in which the option of observation without antimicrobial therapy is warranted. Patients who fail to respond to initial management should be reassessed at 48 to 72 hours to confirm the diagnosis of AOM and exclude other causes of illness. If the patient has failed initial antibacterial therapy, a change in antibacterial agent is indicated. Suitable alternative agents should be active against penicillin-nonsusceptible pneumococci as well as beta-lactamase–producing *Haemophilus influenzae* and *Moraxella catarrhalis*. Such agents include high-dose oral amoxicillin-clavulanate; oral cefdinir, cefpodoxime, or cefuroxime; or intramuscular ceftriaxone in a 3-day course.

Myringotomy or tympanocentesis should be considered for children failing to respond to second-line therapy and for severe cases to obtain cultures to guide therapy. For multidrug–resistant strains of *S pneumoniae,* use of clindamycin, rifampin, or other agents should be considered in consultation with an expert on infectious diseases.

Sinusitis. Antimicrobial agents effective for treatment of AOM also are likely to be effective for acute sinusitis and are recommended.

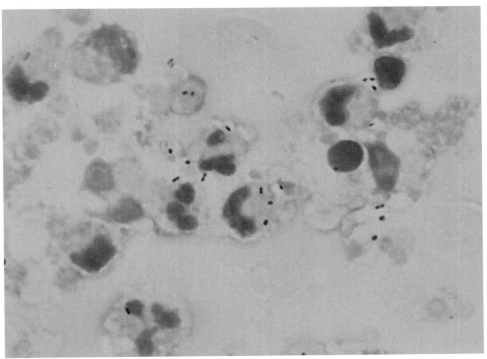

Image 104.1
Streptococcus pneumoniae (pneumococcus) in a Gram stain of cerebrospinal fluid. Courtesy of H. Cody Meissner, MD, FAAP.

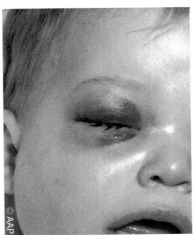

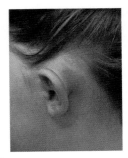

Image 104.3
Streptococcus pneumoniae mastoiditis in a 7-year-old female. Copyright Benjamin Estrada, MD.

Image 104.2
Periorbital cellulitis with purulent exudate from which *Streptococcus pneumoniae* and *Haemophilus influenzae* type b were grown on culture. *S pneumoniae* was isolated on blood culture. The cerebrospinal fluid culture was negative.

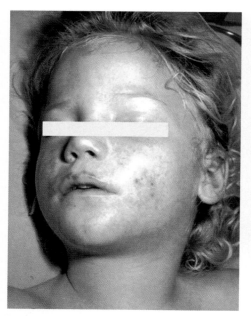

Image 104.4
Streptococcus pneumoniae sepsis with purpura fulminans in a child who had undergone splenectomy for refractory idiopathic thrombocytopenic purpura.

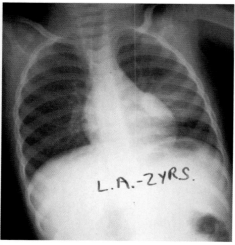

Image 104.5
Segmental (nodular) pneumonia due to *Streptococcus pneumoniae.*

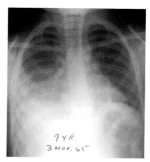

Image 104.6
Pneumococcal pneumonia with pleural effusion on the right. Courtesy of Edgar O. Ledbetter, MD, FAAP.

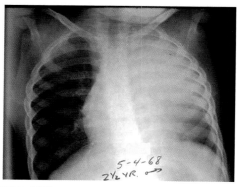

Image 104.7
A 2½-year-old boy with lobar pneumonia and empyema. Blood and empyema cultures were positive for *Streptococcus pneumoniae.* Courtesy of Edgar O. Ledbetter, MD, FAAP.

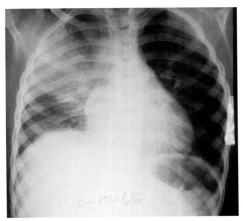

Image 104.8
Pneumonia with right subpleural empyema due to
Streptococcus pneumoniae in a child with sickle
cell disease.

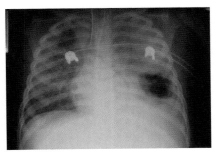

Image 104.10
Streptococcus pneumoniae pneumonia with
pneumatocele formation in the left lung. Copyright Benjamin Estrada, MD.

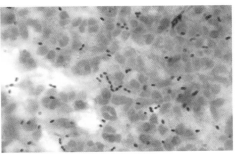

Image 104.9
Streptococcus pneumoniae in pleural exudate
(Gram stain).

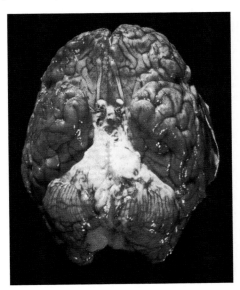

Image 104.11
A ventral view of the brain depicting purulent
exudate from fatal *Streptococcus pneumoniae*
meningitis. Courtesy of Centers for Disease
Control and Prevention.

105

Pneumocystis jiroveci Infections

Clinical Manifestations

Infants and children develop a characteristic syndrome of subacute diffuse pneumonitis with dyspnea, tachypnea, oxygen desaturation, nonproductive cough, and fever. However, intensity of these signs and symptoms can vary, and in some immunocompromised children and adults, onset can be acute and fulminant. Chest radiographs often show bilateral diffuse interstitial or alveolar disease; rarely, lobar, miliary, cavitary, and nodular lesions or even no lesions are seen. Most children with *Pneumocystis* pneumonia are hypoxic with low arterial oxygen pressure. The mortality rate in immunocompromised patients ranges from 5% to 40% in patients treated and approaches 100% without therapy.

Etiology

Nomenclature for *Pneumocystis* species has evolved. Originally considered a protozoan, *Pneumocystis* now is classified as a fungus on the basis of DNA sequence analysis. Because of this, human *Pneumocystis* now is called *Pneumocystis jiroveci*, reflecting the fact that *Pneumocystis carinii* only infects rats. *P carinii* or *P carinii f* sp *hominis* sometimes still are used to refer to human *Pneumocystis*. *P jiroveci* is an atypical fungus, with several morphologic and biologic similarities to protozoa, including susceptibility to a number of antiprotozoal agents but resistance to most antifungal agents. In addition, the organism exists as 2 distinct morphologic forms: the 5- to 7-μm–diameter cysts, which contain up to 8 intracystic bodies, and the smaller, 1- to 5-μm–diameter trophozoite or trophic form.

Epidemiology

Pneumocystis species are ubiquitous in mammals worldwide, particularly rodents, and have a tropism for growth on respiratory tract epithelium. *Pneumocystis* isolates recovered from mice, rats, and ferrets differ genetically from each other and from human *P jiroveci*.

Infections are species-specific, and cross-species infections are not known to occur. Asymptomatic human infection occurs early in life, with more than 85% of healthy children acquiring antibody by 20 months of age. In resource-limited countries and in times of famine, *P jiroveci* pneumonia (PCP) can occur in epidemics, primarily affecting malnourished infants and children. Epidemics also have occurred among preterm infants. In industrialized countries, PCP occurs almost entirely in immunocompromised people with deficient cell-mediated immunity, particularly people with HIV infection, recipients of immunosuppressive therapy after organ transplantation or treatment for malignant neoplasm, and children with congenital immunodeficiency syndromes. Although decreasing in frequency because of effective prophylaxis and antiretroviral therapy, PCP remains one of the most common serious opportunistic infections in infants and children with perinatally acquired HIV infection. Although onset of disease can occur at any age, including rare instances during the first month of life, PCP most commonly occurs in HIV-infected children in the first year of life, with peak incidence at 3 through 6 months of age. The mode of transmission is unknown. Animal studies have demonstrated animal-to-animal transmission by the airborne route; evidence suggests airborne transmission among humans. Evidence also exists for vertical transmission. Although reactivation of latent infection with immunosuppression has been proposed as an explanation for disease after the first 2 years of life, animal models of PCP do not support the existence of latency. Studies of patients with AIDS with more than one episode of PCP suggest reinfection rather than relapse. In patients with cancer, the disease can occur during remission or relapse. The period of communicability is unknown.

Incubation Period

Unknown, but possibly a median of 53 days from exposure to clinical infection.

Diagnostic Tests

A definitive diagnosis of PCP is made by visualization of organisms in lung tissue or respiratory tract secretion specimens. The most sensitive and specific diagnostic procedures involve specimen collection from open lung biopsy and, in older children, transbronchial biopsy. However, bronchoscopy with bronchoalveolar lavage, induction of sputum in older children and adolescents, and intubation with deep endotracheal aspiration are less invasive, can be diagnostic, and are sensitive in patients with HIV infection who have a large number of *Pneumocystis* organisms. Extracystic trophozoite forms are identified with Giemsa stain, modified Wright-Giemsa stain, and fluorescein-conjugated monoclonal antibody stain. The sensitivity of all microscopy-based methods depends on the skill of the laboratory technician. PCR assays for detecting *P jiroveci* infection have been shown to be sensitive even with noninvasive isolates, such as oral wash or expectorated sputum, but are not yet available commercially.

Treatment

The drug of choice is intravenous trimethoprim-sulfamethoxazole (TMP-SMX), usually administered intravenously. Oral therapy should be reserved for patients with mild disease who do not have malabsorption or diarrhea or for patients with a favorable clinical response to initial intravenous therapy. Duration of therapy is 21 days. The rate of adverse reactions to TMP-SMX (eg, rash, neutropenia, anemia, thrombocytopenia, renal toxicity, hepatitis, nausea, vomiting, and diarrhea) is higher in HIV-infected children than in non–HIV-infected patients. It is not necessary to discontinue therapy for most mild adverse reactions. At least half of the patients with more severe reactions (excluding anaphylaxis) requiring interruption of therapy subsequently will tolerate TMP-SMX if rechallenged after the reaction resolves.

Intravenously administered pentamidine is an alternative drug for children and adults who cannot tolerate TMP-SMX or who have severe disease and have not responded to TMP-SMX after 5 to 7 days of therapy. The therapeutic efficacy of intravenous pentamidine in adults with PCP is similar to that of TMP-SMX. Pentamidine is associated with a high incidence of adverse reactions, including pancreatitis, diabetes mellitus, renal toxicity, electrolyte abnormalities, hypoglycemia, hyperglycemia, hypotension, cardiac arrhythmias, fever, and neutropenia. Atovaquone is approved for oral treatment of mild to moderate PCP in adults who are intolerant of TMP-SMX. Experience with use of atovaquone in children is limited. Adverse reactions to atovaquone are limited to rash, nausea, and diarrhea.

Corticosteroids appear to be beneficial in treatment of HIV-infected adults with moderate to severe PCP (as defined by an arterial oxygen pressure of <70 mm Hg in room air or an arterial-alveolar gradient >35 mm Hg). Studies have shown that use of corticosteroids can lead to reduced acute respiratory failure, decreased need for ventilation, and reduced mortality in children with PCP. Although no controlled studies of the use of corticosteroids in young children have been performed, most experts would recommend corticosteroids as part of therapy for children with moderate to severe PCP disease.

Chemoprophylaxis is highly effective in preventing PCP among some high-risk groups. Prophylaxis against a first episode of PCP is indicated for many patients with significant immunosuppression, including people with HIV and people with primary or acquired cell-mediated immunodeficiency.

Prophylaxis for PCP is recommended for children who have received hematopoietic stem cell transplants or solid organ transplants; children with hematologic malignancies (eg, leukemia or lymphoma) and some non-hematologic malignancies; children with severe cell-mediated immunodeficiency, including children who received adrenocorticotropic hormone for treatment of infantile spasm; and children who otherwise are immunosuppressed and who have had a previous episode of PCP. In general, for this diverse group of immunocompromised hosts, the risk of PCP increases with duration and intensity of chemotherapy, other immunosuppressive therapies, and neutropenia as well as with coinfection with immunosuppresive viruses (eg, cytomegalovirus) and rates of PCP for similar patients in a given locale. Consequently, the recommended duration of PCP prophylaxis will vary depending on individual circumstances.

The recommended drug regimen for PCP prophylaxis for all immunocompromised patients is TMP-SMX administered orally on 3 consecutive days each week. Alternatively, TMP-SMX can be administered daily, 7 days a week. For patients who cannot tolerate TMP-SMX, alternative choices include oral atovaquone or dapsone. Atovaquone is effective and safe but expensive. Dapsone is effective and inexpensive but associated with more serious adverse effects than atovaquone. Aerosolized pentamidine is recommended for children who cannot tolerate TMP-SMX, atovaquone, or dapsone and are old enough to use a Respirgard II nebulizer.

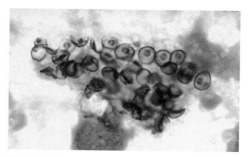

Image 105.1

Cysts of *P jiroveci* in a smear from bronchoalveolar lavage (Gomori methenamine silver stain). Courtesy of Russell Byrnes.

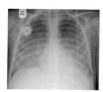

Image 105.2

Pneumocystis jiroveci (formerly *Pneumocystis carinii*) pneumonia. This pathogen is an important cause of pulmonary infections in immunocompromised patients. Characteristic signs and symptoms include dyspnea at rest, tachypnea, nonproductive cough, fever, and hypoxia with an increased oxygen requirement. The intensity of the signs and symptoms can vary, and onset may be acute and fulminant. Chest radiographs frequently demonstrate diffuse bilateral interstitial or alveolar disease. This is a chest radiograph from a 5-year-old boy demonstrating bilateral perihilar infiltrates due to *P jiroveci*. Courtesy of Beverly P. Wood, MD, FAAP, MSEd, PhD.

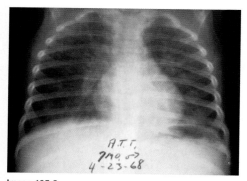

Image 105.3

Pneumocystis jiroveci pneumonia with hyperaeration in an infant with congenital agammaglobulinemia.

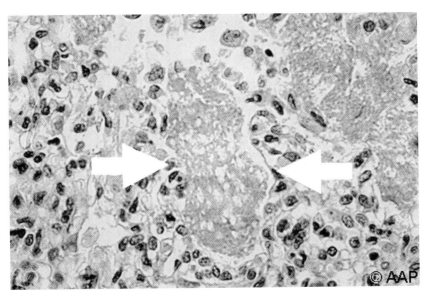

Image 105.4

Foamy intra-alveolar exudate in lung biopsy specimen from a patient with *Pneumocystis jiroveci* pneumonia (hematoxylin-eosin stain).

106

Poliovirus Infections

Clinical Manifestations

Approximately 72% of poliovirus infections in susceptible children are asymptomatic. Nonspecific illness with low-grade fever and sore throat (minor illness) occurs in 24% of people who become infected. Aseptic meningitis, sometimes with paresthesias, occurs in 1% to 5% of patients a few days after the minor illness has resolved. Rapid onset of asymmetric acute flaccid paralysis with areflexia of the involved limb occurs in fewer than 1% of infections, and residual paralytic disease involving the motor neurons (paralytic poliomyelitis), occurs in approximately two-thirds of people with acute motor neuron disease. Cranial nerve involvement (bulbar poliomyelitis) often showing a tripod sign and paralysis of respiratory tract muscles, can occur. Findings in cerebrospinal fluid (CSF) are characteristic of viral meningitis with mild pleocytosis and lymphocytic predominance.

Adults who contracted paralytic poliomyelitis during childhood can develop the noninfectious postpolio syndrome 15 to 40 years later. Postpolio syndrome is characterized by slow and irreversible exacerbation of weakness most likely occurring in those muscle groups involved during the original infection. Muscle and joint pain also are common manifestations. The prevalence and incidence of postpolio syndrome is unclear. Studies estimate the range of postpolio syndrome in poliomyelitis survivors is from 25% to 40%.

Etiology

Polioviruses are group C RNA enteroviruses and consist of serotypes 1, 2, and 3.

Epidemiology

Poliovirus infections occur only in humans. Spread is by the fecal-oral and respiratory routes. Infection is more common in infants and young children and occurs at an earlier age among children living in poor hygienic conditions. In temperate climates, poliovirus infections are most common during summer and autumn; in the tropics, the seasonal pattern is less pronounced.

The last reported case of poliomyelitis attributable to indigenously acquired, wild-type poliovirus in the United States occurred in 1979 during an outbreak among unimmunized people that resulted in 10 paralytic cases. The only identified imported case of paralytic poliomyelitis since 1986 occurred in 1993 in a child transported to the United States for medical care. Since 1986, all other cases acquired in the United States have been vaccine-associated paralytic poliomyelitis (VAPP) occurring in vaccine recipients or their contacts and attributable to oral poliovirus (OPV) vaccine. From 1980 to 1997, the average annual number of cases of VAPP reported in the United States was 8. Fewer VAPP cases were reported in 1998 and 1999, after a shift in United States immunization policy from use of OPV to a sequential inactivated poliovirus (IPV) vaccine beginning in 1997. Implementation of an all-IPV vaccine schedule in 2000 essentially ended the occurrence of VAPP cases in the United States. In 2005, however, a healthy, unimmunized young adult from the United States acquired VAPP abroad during a study program in Central America, most likely from an infant grandchild of the host family who recently had been immunized with OPV. In 2005, a type 1 vaccine-derived poliovirus was identified in the stool of an asymptomatic, unimmunized, immunodeficient child in Minnesota. Subsequently, poliovirus infections in 7 other unimmunized children (35% of all children tested) within the index patient's community were documented. None of the infected children had paralysis. Phylogenetic analysis suggested that the vaccine-derived poliovirus circulated in the community for approximately 2 months before the infant's infection was detected and that the initiating OPV dose had been given (likely in another country) before the index child's birth. In 2009, a woman with longstanding common-variable immunodeficiency was diagnosed with VAPP and died of polio-associated complications. Molecular characterization of the poliovirus isolated suggested that the infection likely occurred approximately 12 years earlier, coinciding with OPV immunization of her child. Circulation of indigenous wild-type poliovirus strains ceased in the United States several decades ago, and the risk of contact with imported wild-type polioviruses has decreased, in parallel with the success of the global eradication program.

Communicability of poliovirus is greatest shortly before and after onset of clinical illness, when the virus is present in the throat and excreted in high concentration in feces. Virus persists in the throat for approximately 2 weeks after onset of illness and is excreted in feces for 3 to 6 weeks. Patients potentially are contagious as long as fecal excretion persists. In recipients of OPV vaccine, virus persists in the throat for 1 to 2 weeks and is excreted in feces for several weeks, although in rare cases, excretion for more than 2 months can occur. Immunocompromised patients with significant B-lymphocyte immune deficiencies have excreted virus for periods of more than 20 years.

Incubation Period

Nonparalytic poliomyelitis, 3 to 6 days;. paralytic poliomyelitis, 7 to 21 days after exposure.

Diagnostic Tests

Poliovirus can be detected in specimens from the pharynx, feces, urine and, rarely, CSE by isolation in cell culture or PCR. Two or more stool and throat swab specimens for enterovirus isolation should be obtained at least 24 hours apart from patients with suspected paralytic poliomyelitis as early in the course of illness as possible, ideally within 14 days of onset of symptoms. Fecal material is most likely to yield virus in cell culture. However, in immunocompromised patients, poliovirus can be excreted intermittently, and a negative test does not rule out infection.

Because OPV vaccine no longer is available in the United States, the chance of exposure to vaccine-type polioviruses has become remote. Therefore, if a poliovirus is isolated in the United States, the isolate should be reported promptly to the state health department and sent to the Centers for Disease Control and Prevention through the state health department for further testing. The diagnostic test of choice for confirming poliovirus disease is viral culture of stool specimens and throat swab specimens obtained as early in the course of illness as possible. Interpretation of acute and convalescent serologic test results can be difficult.

Treatment

Supportive.

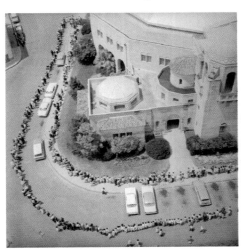

Image 106.1
An aerial view of a crowd surrounding a city auditorium in San Antonio, TX, awaiting polio immunization, 1962. Courtesy of Centers for Disease Control and Prevention/ Mr Stafford Smith.

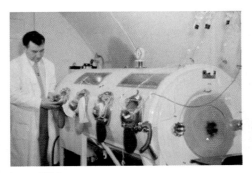

Image 106.2
The physician is shown here examining a tank respirator, also known as an iron lung, during a polio epidemic. The iron lung encased the thoracic cavity externally in an air-tight chamber. The chamber was used to create a negative pressure around the thoracic cavity, thereby causing air to rush into the lungs to equalize intrapulmonary pressure. Courtesy of Centers for Disease Control and Prevention.

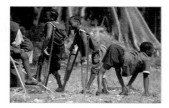

Image 106.3
Cheshire Home for Handicapped Children, Free-town, Sierra Leone. Courtesy of World Health Organization.

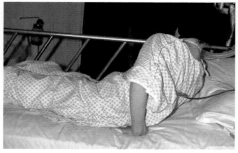

Image 106.5
A young girl with bulbar polio with tripod sign attempts to sit upright. Copyright Martin G. Myers, MD.

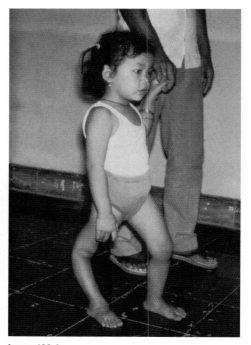

Image 106.4
This child is displaying a deformity of her right lower extremity caused by the poliovirus. Courtesy of Centers for Disease Control and Prevention.

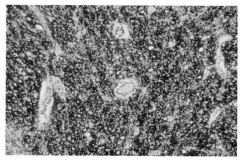

Image 106.6
A photomicrograph of the cervical spinal cord in the region of the anterior horn revealing polio type III degenerative changes. The poliovirus has an affinity for the anterior horn motor neurons of the cervical and lumbar regions of the spinal cord. Death of these cells causes muscle weakness of those muscles once innervated by the now dead neurons. Courtesy of Centers for Disease Control and Prevention/Dr Karp, Emory University.

107

Prion Diseases: Transmissible Spongiform Encephalopathies

Clinical Manifestations

Transmissible spongiform encephalopathies (TSEs or prion diseases) constitute a group of rare, rapidly progressive, universally fatal neurodegenerative diseases of humans and animals that are characterized by neuronal degeneration, spongiform change, gliosis, and accumulation of abnormal misfolded protease-resistant amyloid protein (protease-resistant prion protein, variably called scrapie prion protein or, as suggested by the World Health Organization, TSE-associated PrP [PrP^{TSE}]) that is distributed diffusely throughout the brain and sometimes also in discrete plaques.

Human TSEs include several diseases: Creutzfeldt-Jakob disease (CJD), Gerstmann-Sträussler-Scheinker disease, fatal familial and sporadic insomnia, kuru, and variant CJD (vCJD, caused by the agent of bovine spongiform encephalopathy (BSE), popularly called mad cow disease). Classic CJD can be sporadic (approximately 85% of cases), familial (approximately 15% of cases), or iatrogenic (<1% of cases). Sporadic CJD most commonly is a disease of older adults (median age of death, 68 years in the United States) but also rarely has been described in adolescents older than 13 years and young adults. Iatrogenic CJD has been acquired through intramuscular injection of contaminated cadaveric pituitary hormones (growth hormone and human gonadotropin), dura mater allografts, corneal transplantation, and contaminated instrumentation of the brain at neurosurgery or depth-electrode electro-encephalographic recording. In 1996, an outbreak of vCJD linked to exposure to tissues from BSE-infected cattle was reported in the United Kingdom. Since the end of 2003, 4 presumptive cases of transfusion-transmitted vCJD have been reported: 3 clinical cases as well as 1 probable asymptomatic transfusion-transmitted vCJD infection in which prion protein was detected in spleen and lymph node but not brain. A fifth iatrogenic vCJD infection in the United Kingdom, also preclinical, was attributed to treatment with plasma-derived coagulation factor VIII. The best-known TSEs affecting animals include scrapie of sheep; BSE; and a chronic wasting disease of North American deer, elk, and moose. Except for vCJD, thought to result from infection with the BSE agent, no other human TSE has been attributed convincingly to infection with an agent of animal origin.

CJD manifests as a rapidly progressive, dementia-causing illness with defects in memory, personality, and other higher cortical functions. At presentation, approximately one-third of patients have cerebellar dysfunction, including ataxia and dysarthria. Iatrogenic CJD also may manifest as dementia with cerebellar signs. Myoclonus develops in at least 80% of affected patients at some point in the course of disease. Death usually occurs in weeks to months (median, 4–5 months); approximately 10% to 15% of patients with sporadic CJD survive for more than 1 year.

vCJD is distinguished from classic CJD by younger age of onset, early "psychiatric" manifestations, and other features, such as painful sensory symptoms, delayed onset of overt neurologic signs, absence of diagnostic electroencephalographic changes, and a more prolonged duration of illness. In vCJD, the neuropathologic examination reveals numerous "florid" plaques (surrounded by vacuoles) and exceptionally striking accumulation of PrP^{TSE} in the brain. In addition, PrP^{TSE} often is detectable in lymphoid tissues of patients with vCJD. In vCJD, but not in classic CJD, a high proportion of people exhibit high signal abnormalities on T2-weighted brain magnetic resonance imaging in the pulvinar region of the posterior thalamus (known as the pulvinar sign).

Etiology

The infectious particle or prion responsible for human and animal prion diseases is thought by many authorities to be the abnormal form of normal ubiquitous PrP glycoprotein, without a nucleic acid component. Proponents of the prion hypothesis postulate that sporadic CJD arises from a rare spontaneous structural change of the normal "cellular" protease-sensitive host-encoded glycoprotein (PrP^C or PrP^{sen}) found on the surface of neurons and many other cells in both humans and animals. Conformational changes are postulated to be propagated by a "recruitment" reaction (the nature of which is unknown), in which abnormal PrP^{TSE} serves as a template or lattice for the conversion of neighboring PrP^C molecules.

Epidemiology

Classic CJD is rare, occurring at a rate of approximately 1 case per million people annually. The onset of disease peaks in the 60- through 74-year age group. Familial CJD illnesses, which are associated with a variety of mutations of the PrP-encoding gene (PRNP) on chromosome 20, occur at approximately one-sixth the frequency of sporadic CJD, with onset of disease approximately 10 years earlier than sporadic CJD. Case-control studies of sporadic CJD have not identified any consistent environmental risk factor. No statistically significant increase in cases of sporadic CJD has been observed in people previously treated with blood, blood components, or plasma derivatives. The incidence of sporadic CJD is not increased in patients with several diseases associated with frequent exposure to blood or blood products, specifically hemophilia A and B, thalassemia, and sickle cell disease, suggesting that the risk of transfusion transmission of classic CJD, if any, is very low and appropriately regarded as theoretical. CJD has not been reported in infants born to infected mothers.

As of November 2011, the total number of primary cases of vCJD reported was in 173 patients in the United Kingdom; 25 in France; 5 in Spain; 4 in Ireland; 3 in the United States; 3 in the Netherlands; 2 in Portugal; 2 in Italy; 2 in Canada; and 1 each in Taiwan, Japan, and Saudi Arabia. Two of the 3 patients in the United States, 2 of the 4 in Ireland, and 1 each of the patients in France and Canada are believed to have acquired vCJD during prolonged residence in the United Kingdom. The Centers for Disease Control and Prevention has concluded that the third vCJD patient in the United States probably was infected during his prolonged residence as a child in Saudi Arabia. Authorities suspect that the Japanese patient was infected during a short visit of 24 days to the United Kingdom, 12 years before the onset of vCJD. Most patients with vCJD were younger than 30 years, and several were adolescents. All but 5 of the 174 United Kingdom patients with noniatrogenic vCJD died before 60 years of age, and all but 15 died before 50 (median age at death is 28 years and 87% of cases died before age 40). On the basis of animal inoculation studies, comparative PrP immunoblotting, and epidemiologic investigations, almost all cases of vCJD are believed to have resulted from exposure to tissues from cattle infected with BSE. As noted, 4 patients are believed to have been infected with vCJD through blood transfusion and 1 from injections of human plasma-derived clotting factor.

Incubation Period

Iatrogenic CJD varies by route of exposure and ranges from 1.5 to more than 30 years.

Diagnostic Tests

The diagnosis of human prion diseases can be made with certainty only by neuropathologic examination of affected brain tissue, best obtained at autopsy. In most patients with classic CJD, a characteristic 1 cycle to 2 cycles per second triphasic sharp-wave discharge on electroencephalographic tracing has been described. The likelihood of finding this abnormality is enhanced when serial electroencephalographic recordings are obtained. A protein assay that detects the 14-3-3 protein in cerebrospinal fluid (CSF) has been reported to be reasonably sensitive, although not specific, as a marker for CJD. Measurement of the Tau protein level in addition to the detection of 14-3-3 protein in the CSF has been reported to increase the specificity of CSF testing for CJD. No validated blood test is available. A progressive neurologic syndrome in a person bearing a known pathogenic mutation of the PRNP gene (not a normal polymorphism) is presumed to be prion disease. Because no unique nucleic acid has been detected in the infectious particles of TSEs, genome amplification studies, such as PCR, are not possible. Consideration of brain biopsies for patients with possible CJD should be given when some other potentially treatable disease remains in the differential diagnosis. Complete postmortem examination of the brain is encouraged to confirm the clinical diagnosis and to detect emerging forms of CJD, such as vCJD.

Treatment

No treatment has been shown in humans to slow or stop the progressive neurodegeneration in prion diseases. Experimental treatments are being studied. Supportive therapy is necessary to manage dementia, spasticity, rigidity, and seizures occurring during the course of the illness. Genetic counseling is indicated in familial disease, taking into account that penetrance has been variable in some kindreds in which people with a PRNP mutation survived to an advanced age without neurodegenerative disease.

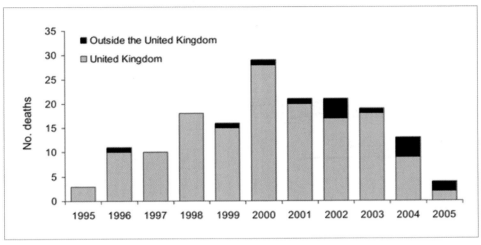

Image 107.1
Number of deceased variant Creutzfeldt-Jakob disease patients worldwide (150 from the United Kingdom and 15 outside the United Kingdom) by year of death, June 2005. Courtesy of Belay ED, Sejvour JJ, Shieh W-J, et al. Variant Creutzfeldt-Jakob disease, death, United States. *Emerg Infect Dis.* 2005;11(9):1351–1354.

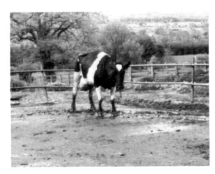

Image 107.2
Cattle such as the one pictured here, which are affected by bovine spongiform encephalopathy (BSE) experience progressive degeneration of the nervous system. Behavioral changes in temperament (eg, nervousness or aggression), abnormal posture, incoordination and difficulty in rising, decreased milk production, and/or loss of weight despite continued appetite are followed by death in cattle affected by BSE. Courtesy of US Department of Agriculture—Animal and Plant Health Inspection Service/Dr Art Davis.

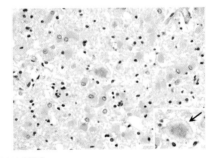

Image 107.3
Histopathologic changes in frontal cerebral cortex of the patient who died of variant Creutzfeldt-Jakob disease in the United States. Marked astroglial reaction is shown, occasionally with relatively large florid plaques surrounded by vacuoles (arrow in inset) (hematoxylin-eosin stain, original magnification x40). Courtesy of Belay ED, Sejvour JJ, Shieh W-J, et al. Variant Creutzfeldt-Jakob disease, death, United States. *Emerg Infect Dis.* 2005;11(9):1351–1354.

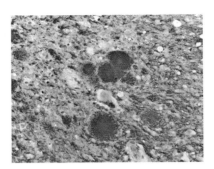

Image 107.4
Immunohistochemical staining of cerebellar tissue of the patient who died of variant Creutzfeldt-Jakob disease in the United States. Stained amyloid plaques are shown with surrounding deposits of abnormal prion protein (immunoalkaline phosphatase stain, naphthol fast red substrate with light hematoxylin counterstain; original magnification x158). Courtesy of Belay ED, Sejvour JJ, Shieh W-J, et al. Variant Creutzfeldt-Jakob disease, death, United States. *Emerg Infect Dis.* 2005;11(9):1351–1354.

108

Q Fever

Clinical Manifestations

Although approximately 50% of infections are asymptomatic, symptomatic Q fever occurs in 2 forms: acute and chronic; each form can present as fever of undetermined origin. Q fever in children typically is characterized by abrupt onset of fever often accompanied by chills, headache, weakness, cough, and other nonspecific systemic symptoms. Illness typically is self-limited, although a relapsing febrile illness lasting for several months has been documented in children. Gastrointestinal tract symptoms, such as diarrhea, vomiting, abdominal pain, and anorexia, are reported in 50% to 80% of children. Rash, although uncommon, can occur in young children. Q fever pneumonia usually manifests as mild cough, respiratory distress, and chest pain. Chest radiographic patterns are variable. More severe manifestations of acute Q fever are rare but include hepatitis, hemolytic uremic syndrome, myocarditis, pericarditis, cerebellitis, encephalitis, meningitis, hemophagocytosis, lymphadenitis, acalculous cholecystitis, and rhabdomyolysis. Chronic Q fever is rare in children but can present as blood culture–negative endocarditis, chronic relapsing or multifocal osteomyelitis, or chronic hepatitis. Children who are immunocompromised or have underlying valvular heart disease may be a higher risk for chronic Q fever.

Etiology

Coxiella burnetii, the cause of Q fever, formerly considered to be a *Rickettsia* organism, is an obligate gram-negative intracellular bacterium that belongs to the order Legionellaceae. The infectious form of *C burnetii* is highly resistant to heat, desiccation, and disinfectant chemicals and can persist for long periods in the environment. *C burnetii* is a potential agent of bioterrorism.

Epidemiology

In 2010 there were 106 reported cases of acute and 25 cases of chronic Q fever in the United States, but this infection is believed to be substantially underreported. Q fever is a zoonotic infection that has been reported worldwide. In animals, *C burnetii* infection usually is asymptomatic. The most common reservoirs for human infection are domestic farm animals (eg, sheep, goats, and cows). Cats, dogs, rodents, marsupials, other mammalian species, and some wild and domestic bird species also may serve as reservoirs. Tick vectors may be important for maintaining animal and bird reservoirs but are not thought to be important in transmission to humans. Humans typically acquire infection by inhalation of *C burnetii* in fine-particle aerosols generated from birthing fluids of infected animals during animal parturition or through inhalation of dust contaminated by these materials. Infection also can occur by exposure to contaminated materials, such as wool, straw, bedding, or laundry. Windborne particles containing infectious organisms can travel a half-mile or more, contributing to sporadic cases for which no apparent animal contact can be demonstrated. Unpasteurized dairy products can contain the organism. Seasonal trends occur in farming areas with predictable frequency, and the disease often coincides with the lambing season in early spring.

Incubation Period

Usually 14 to 22 days, range 9 to 39 days, depending on the inoculum size. Chronic Q fever can develop months or years after initial infection.

Diagnostic Tests

Isolation of *C burnetii* from blood can be performed only in special laboratories because of the potential hazard to laboratory workers. The diagnosis of Q fever is established through serologic testing. Serologic evidence of a fourfold increase in phase II immunoglobulin (Ig) G by indirect immunofluorescent antibody (IFA) assay between paired sera taken 2 to 4 weeks apart establishes the diagnosis of acute infection. A single high serum phase II IgG titer ($\geq$1:128) by IFA may be considered evidence of probable infection. Acute Q fever also is diagnosed by detection of *C burnetii* in infected tissues by using immunohistochemical staining or DNA detection methods. Confirmation of chronic Q fever is based on an increasing phase 1 IgG titer (typically

≥1:800) that often is higher than phase II IgG *and* an identifiable nidus of infection (eg, endocarditis, vascular infection, osteomyelitis, chronic hepatitis).

Treatment

Acute Q fever generally is a self-limited illness, and many patients recover without antimicrobial therapy. Doxycycline is the drug of choice for severe infections in patients of any age, and treatment is recommended for 14 days. Appropriate therapy, if initiated within 3 days of illness onset, can lessen the severity of illness and hasten recovery. Children younger than 8 years with mild illness, pregnant women, and patients allergic to doxycycline can be treated with trimethoprim-sulfamethoxazole. Chronic Q fever is much more difficult to treat, and relapses can occur despite appropriate therapy, necessitating repeated courses of therapy.

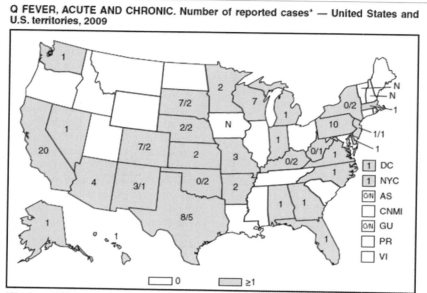

Q FEVER, ACUTE AND CHRONIC. Number of reported cases* — United States and U.S. territories, 2009

* Number of Q fever acute cases/Q fever chronic cases. Numbers displayed with no forward slash are Q fever acute cases.

Q fever, caused by *Coxiella burnetii*, is reported throughout the United States. Human cases occur as a result of human interaction with livestock, especially sheep, goats, and cattle. Although relatively few human cases are reported annually, the disease is believed to be substantially underreported because of its nonspecific presentation and the subsequent failure to suspect infection and request appropriate diagnostic tests.

Image 108.1

Q Fever, acute and chronic. Number of reported cases—United States and US territories, 2009. Courtesy of *Morbidity and Mortality Weekly Report*.

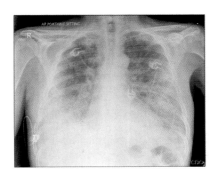

Image 108.2

Chest radiograph of patient at time of admission to hospital, before intubation, demonstrating extensive bilateral airspace disease. Courtesy of Marrie TJ, Campbell N, McNeil SA, Webster D, Hatchette TF. Q fever update, Maritime Canada. *Emerg Infect Dis.* 2008;14(1):67–69.

109

Rabies

Clinical Manifestations

Infection with rabies virus and other lyssaviruses characteristically produces an acute illness with rapidly progressive central nervous system manifestations, including anxiety, radicular pain, dysesthesia or pruritus, hydrophobia, and dysautonomia. Some patients can have paralysis. Illness almost invariably progresses to death. Three unimmunized people have recovered from clinical rabies in the United States. The differential diagnosis of acute encephalitic illnesses of unknown cause with atypical focal neurologic signs or with features of Guillain-Barré syndrome should include rabies.

Etiology

Rabies virus is an RNA virus classified in the Rhabdoviridae family, Lyssavirus genus.

Epidemiology

Understanding the epidemiology of rabies has been aided by viral variant identification using monoclonal antibodies and nucleotide sequencing. In the United States, human cases have decreased steadily since the 1950s, reflecting widespread immunization of dogs and the availability of effective prophylaxis after exposure to a rabid animal. Between 2000 and 2009, 24 of 31 cases of human rabies reported in the United States were acquired indigenously. Among the 24 indigenously acquired cases, 18 were associated with bat rabies virus variants, and 4 had a history of bat exposure and had rabies virus antibodies in serum or cerebrospinal fluid (CSF) samples but had no rabies virus antigens detected. Despite the large focus of rabies in raccoons in the eastern United States, only 1 human death has been attributed to the raccoon rabies virus variant. Historically, 2 cases of human rabies were attributable to probable aerosol exposure in laboratories, and 2 unusual cases have been attributed to possible airborne exposures in caves inhabited by millions of bats, although alternative infection routes cannot be discounted. Transmission also has occurred by transplantation of organs, corneas, and other tissues from patients dying of undiagnosed rabies. Person-to-person transmission by bite has not been documented in the United States, although the virus has been isolated from saliva of infected patients.

Wildlife rabies perpetuates throughout all of the 50 United States except Hawaii, which remains "rabies-free." Wildlife, including bats, raccoons, skunks, foxes, coyotes, and bobcats, are the most important potential sources of infection for humans and domestic animals in the United States. Rabies in small rodents (squirrels, hamsters, guinea pigs, gerbils, chipmunks, rats, and mice) and lagomorphs (rabbits, pikas, and hares) is rare. Rabies can occur in woodchucks or other large rodents in areas where raccoon rabies is common. The virus is present in saliva and is transmitted by bites or, rarely, by contamination of mucosa or skin lesions by saliva or other potentially infectious material (eg, neural tissue). Worldwide, most rabies cases in humans result from dog bites in areas where canine rabies is enzootic. Most rabid dogs, cats, and ferrets may shed virus for a few days before there are obvious signs of illness. No case of human rabies in the United States has been attributed to a dog, cat, or ferret that has remained healthy throughout the standard 10-day period of confinement.

Incubation Period

1 to 3 months; range, days to years.

Diagnostic Tests

Infection in animals can be diagnosed by demonstration of virus-specific fluorescent antigen in brain tissue. Suspected rabid animals should be euthanized in a manner that preserves brain tissue for appropriate laboratory diagnosis. Virus can be isolated in suckling mice or in tissue culture from saliva, brain, and other specimens and can be detected by identification of viral antigens or nucleotides in affected tissues. Diagnosis in suspected human cases can be made postmortem by either immunofluorescent or immunohistochemical examination of brain tissue. Antemortem diagnosis can be made by fluorescent microscopy of skin biopsy specimens from the nape of the neck; by isolation of the virus from saliva; by detection of antibody in serum in unimmunized people or in CSF; and by detection of viral nucleic acid in saliva, skin, or other affected tissues. No single test sufficiently is sensitive. Laboratory personnel should be consulted before submission of specimens to the Centers for Disease Control and Prevention so that appropriate collection and transport of materials can be arranged.

Treatment

Once symptoms have developed, neither rabies vaccine nor rabies immune globulin improves the prognosis. There is no specific treatment. Very few patients with human rabies have survived, even with intensive supportive care. Since 2004, 2 adolescent females and an 8-year-old girl, each of whom had not received rabies postexposure prophylaxis, survived rabies after receipt of a combination of sedation and intensive medical intervention.

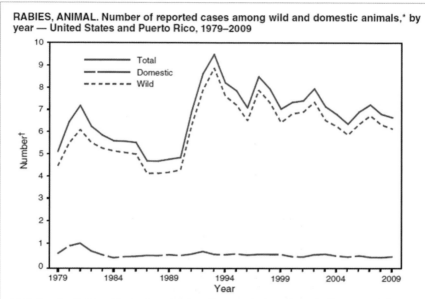

RABIES, ANIMAL. Number of reported cases among wild and domestic animals,* by year — United States and Puerto Rico, 1979–2009

* Data from the Division of Vector-Borne Infectious Diseases, National Center for Emerging and Zoonotic Infectious Diseases (NCZVED).
† In thousands.

The proportion of rabid animals among those tested has demonstrated a downward trend from 6.1% in 2006 to 5.6% in 2009. Despite an overall decrease in the number of rabid animals submitted for testing during 2009, bats remained the second most submitted animals for rabies testing and behind only raccoons in total reported rabid animals. The raccoon rabies virus variant remains responsible for the majority of reported rabid animals, but increases in rabid animals attributable to skunk rabies virus variants were reported during 2009.

Image 109.1

Rabies, animal. Number of reported cases among wild and domestic animals, by year—United States and Puerto Rico 1979–2009. Courtesy of *Morbidity and Mortality Weekly Report.*

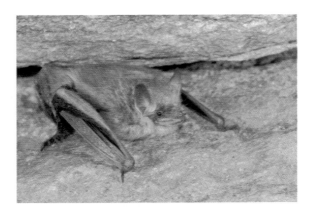

Image 109.2
Bites from wild animals, such as raccoons, bats, and skunks, account for most rabies cases in the United States. Rabies is caused by a virus that invades the central nervous system and disrupts its functioning. The virus is transmitted in the saliva of infected animals. Prompt postexposure treatment is generally effective. Once symptoms appear, the disease is almost always fatal.

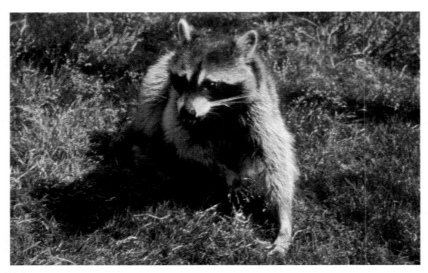

Image 109.3
Raccoons can be vectors of the rabies virus, transmitting the virus to humans and other animals. Rabies virus belongs to the order Mononegavirales. Raccoons continue to be the most frequently reported rabid wildlife species and involved 37.7% of all animal-transmitted cases during 2000. Courtesy of Centers for Disease Control and Prevention.

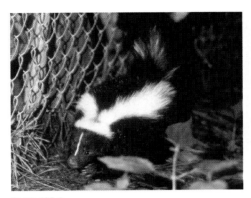

Image 109.4

Approximately a third of reported animal rabies is attributed to the wild skunk population. Wild animals accounted for 93% of reported animal cases of rabies in the year 2000. Skunks were responsible for 30.1% of this number. Courtesy of Centers for Disease Control and Prevention.

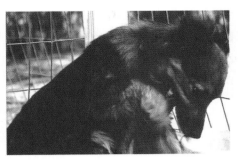

Image 109.5

Here a penned dog is afflicted with "dumb" rabies, manifested as depression, lethargy, and a seemingly overly tame disposition. Domesticated animals afflicted with "dumb" rabies may become increasingly depressed and try to hide in isolated places, while wild animals seem to lose their fear of human beings, often appearing unusually friendly. Courtesy of Centers for Disease Control and Prevention.

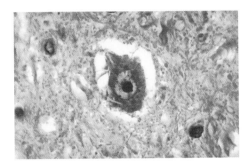

Image 109.6

This micrograph depicts the histopathologic changes associated with rabies encephalitis (hematoxylin-eosin stain). Note the Negri bodies, which are cellular inclusions found most frequently in the pyramidal cells of Ammon's horn, and the Purkinje cells of the cerebellum. They are also found in the cells of the medulla and various other ganglia. Courtesy of Centers for Disease Control and PreventionDr Daniel P. Perl.

110

Rat-Bite Fever

Clinical Manifestations

Rat-bite fever is caused by *Streptobacillus moniliformis* or *Spirillum minus*. *S moniliformis* infection (streptobacillary fever or Haverhill fever) is characterized by fever, rash, and arthritis. There is an abrupt onset of fever, chills, muscle pain, vomiting, headache, and occasionally, lymphadenopathy. A maculopapular or petechial rash develops predominantly on the extremities including the palms and soles, typically within a few days of fever onset. The bite site usually heals promptly and exhibits no or minimal inflammation. Nonsuppurative migratory polyarthritis or arthralgia follows in approximately 50% of patients. Untreated infection usually has a relapsing course for a mean of 3 weeks. Complications include soft tissue and solid-organ abscesses, septic arthritis, pneumonia, endocarditis, myocarditis, and meningitis. The case-fatality rate is 7% to 10% in untreated patients, and fatal cases have been reported in young children. With *S minus* infection ("sodoku"), a period of initial apparent healing at the site of the bite usually is followed by fever and ulceration at the site, regional lymphangitis and lymphadenopathy, and a distinctive rash of red or purple plaques. Arthritis is rare. Infection with *S minus* is rare in the United States.

Etiology

The causes of rat-bite fever are *S moniliformis*, a microaerophilic, gram-negative, pleomorphic bacillus, and *S minus*, a small, gram-negative, spiral organism with bipolar flagellar tufts.

Epidemiology

Rat-bite fever is a zoonotic illness. The natural habitat of *S moniliformis* and *S minus* is the upper respiratory tract of rodents. *S moniliformis* is transmitted by bites or scratches from or exposure to oral secretions of infected rats (eg, kissing the rodent); other rodents (eg, mice, gerbils, squirrels, weasels) and rodent-eating animals, including cats and dogs, also can transmit the infection. Haverhill fever refers to infection after ingestion of unpasteurized milk, water, or food contaminated with *S moniliformis*. *S minus* is transmitted by bites of rats and mice. *S moniliformis* infection accounts for most cases of rat-bite fever in the United States; *S minus* infections occur primarily in Asia.

Incubation Period

For *S moniliformis,* usually 3 to 10 days, but can be as long as 3 weeks; for *S minus,* 7 to 21 days.

Diagnostic Tests

S moniliformis is a fastidious, slow-growing organism isolated from specimens of blood, synovial fluid, aspirates from abscesses, or material from the bite lesion by inoculation into bacteriologic media enriched with blood. Cultures should be held up to 3 weeks if *S moniliformis* is suspected. *S minus* has not been recovered on artificial media but can be visualized by darkfield microscopy in wet mounts of blood, exudate of a lesion, and lymph nodes. Blood specimens also should be viewed with Giemsa or Wright stain. *S minus* can be recovered from blood, lymph nodes, or local lesions by intraperitoneal inoculation of mice or guinea pigs.

Treatment

Penicillin G procaine administered intramuscularly or penicillin G administered intravenously for 7 to 10 days is the drug of choice for treatment for rat-bite fever caused by either agent. Doxycycline, streptomycin or gentamicin can be substituted when a patient has a serious allergy to penicillin. Doxycycline can be given to children older than 8 years if allergic to penicillin. Patients with endocarditis should receive intravenous high-dose penicillin G for at least 4 weeks. The addition of streptomycin or gentamicin for initial therapy may be useful.

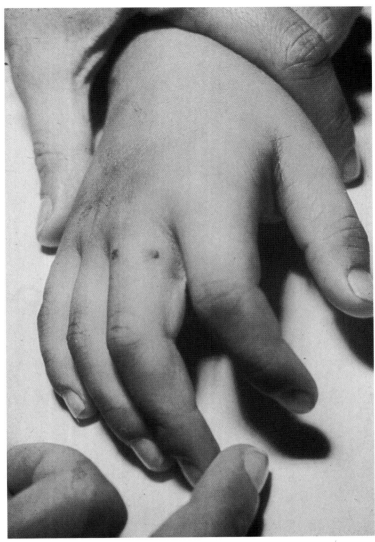

Image 110.1

Rat bite wounds on the finger of a 5-year-old white male 12 hours after the bite appear non-inflammatory. Because of fever, chills, headache, and rash 5 days later, blood cultures were obtained that grew *Streptobacillus moniliformis*. Courtesy of George Nankervis, MD.

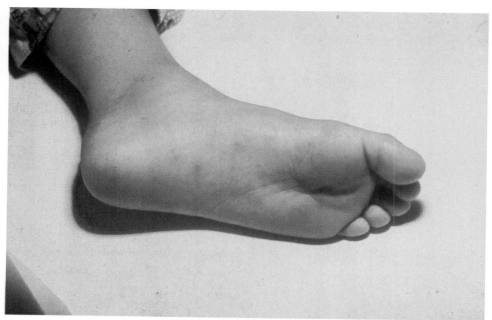

Image 110.2

Five days after being bitten by a rat the child in Image 110.1 developed fever, chills, and headache followed 5 days later by a papulovesicular rash on the hands and feet. *Streptobacillus moniliformis* was isolated from blood cultures and he responded to intravenous penicillin therapy without complication. Courtesy of George Nankervis, MD.

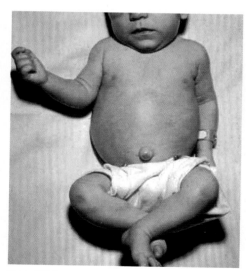

Image 110.3

The rash of rat-bite fever *(Streptobacillus moniliformis)* in an infant bitten by a rat on the right side of the face while sleeping.

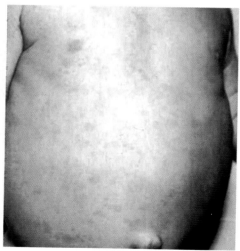

Image 110.4

Close-up view of the rash of an infant who was bitten on the right cheek by a rat. This is the same infant as in Image 110.3. Sodoku, or rat-bite fever caused by *Spirillum minus*, rarely occurs in the United States.

111

Respiratory Syncytial Virus

Clinical Manifestations

Respiratory syncytial virus (RSV) causes acute respiratory tract infections in people of all ages and is one of the most common diseases of early childhood. Most infants are infected during the first year of life, with virtually all having been infected at least once by the second birthday. Most RSV-infected infants experience upper respiratory tract symptoms, and 20% to 30% develop lower respiratory tract disease (eg, bronchiolitis and/or pneumonia) with their first infection. Signs of bronchiolitis may include tachypnea, wheezing, cough, crackles, use of accessory muscles, and nasal flaring. During the first few weeks of life, particularly among preterm infants, infection with RSV can produce minimal respiratory tract signs. Lethargy, irritability, and poor feeding, sometimes accompanied by apneic episodes, may be presenting manifestations in these infants. Most previously healthy infants who develop RSV bronchiolitis do not require hospitalization, and most who are hospitalized improve with supportive care and are discharged in fewer than 5 days. Approximately 1% to 3% of all children in the first 12 months of life will be hospitalized because of RSV lower tract disease. Factors that increase the risk of severe RSV lower respiratory tract illness include preterm birth; cyanotic or complicated congenital heart disease, especially conditions causing pulmonary hypertension; chronic lung disease of prematurity (formerly called bronchopulmonary dysplasia); and immunodeficiency disease or therapy causing immunosuppression at any age. Approximately 400 deaths in young children are attributable to complications of RSV infection annually.

Reinfection with RSV throughout life is common. RSV infection in older children and adults usually manifests as upper respiratory tract illness. More serious disease involving the lower respiratory tract may develop in older children and adults, especially in immunocompromised patients, the elderly, and in people with cardiopulmonary disease.

Etiology

RSV is an enveloped, nonsegmented, negative strand RNA virus of the family Paramyxoviridae. There are 2 major strains (groups A and B) that often circulate concurrently.

Epidemiology

Humans are the only source of infection. Transmission usually is by direct or close contact with contaminated secretions. RSV can persist on environmental surfaces for several hours and for a half-hour or more on hands. Infection among health care personnel and others can occur by hand to eye or hand to nasal epithelium self-inoculation with contaminated secretions. Enforcement of infection-control policies is important to decrease the risk of health care–associated transmission of RSV. Health care–associated spread of RSV to hematopoietic stem cell or solid organ transplant recipients or patients with cardiopulmonary abnormalities or immunocompromised conditions has been associated with severe and fatal disease in children and adults. Children with HIV infection experience extended virus shedding and sometimes prolonged illness but usually do not exhibit greatly enhanced disease.

RSV usually occurs in annual epidemics during winter and early spring in temperate climates. Spread among household and child care contacts, including adults, is common. The period of viral shedding usually is 3 to 8 days, but shedding can last longer, especially in young infants and in immunosuppressed people, in whom shedding may continue for as long as 3 to 4 weeks.

Incubation Period

4 to 6 days, range, 2 to 8 days.

Diagnostic Tests

Rapid diagnostic assays, including immunofluorescent and enzyme immunoassay techniques for detection of viral antigen in nasopharyngeal specimens, are available commercially and generally are reliable in infants and young children. In children, the sensitivity of these assays in comparison with culture varies between 53% and 96%, with most in the 80% to 90% range. The sensitivity may be lower in older children and is quite poor in adults, because adults typically shed low concentrations of RSV. As with all antigen detection assays, the predictive value is high during the peak season, but false-positive test results are more likely to occur when the incidence of disease is low, such as in the summer in temperate areas. Therefore, antigen detection assays should not be the only basis on which the beginning and end of monthly immunoprophylaxis is determined. In most outpatient settings, specific viral testing has little effect on management.

One disadvantage of antigen detection relative to virologic assessment (culture or reverse transcriptase PCR [RT-PCR] assay) is that coinfections may not be detected. Young children with bronchiolitis are often infected with more than one virus. Up to 20% of children with RSV bronchiolitis may be coinfected with another respiratory tract virus, such as human metapneumovirus or rhinovirus. Whether children with bronchiolitis who are coinfected with more than one virus experience more severe disease is not clear.

Viral isolation from nasopharyngeal secretions in cell culture requires 1 to 5 days (shell vial techniques can produce results within 24 to 48 hours), but results and sensitivity vary among laboratories. Experienced viral laboratory personnel should be consulted for optimal methods of collection and transport of specimens, which may include keeping specimens cold and protected from light, rapid specimen processing, and stabilization in virus transport media. Molecular diagnostic tests using RT-PCR assays are commercially available and have increased RSV detection rates substantially over viral isolation or antigen detection. These tests should be interpreted with caution, because they detect viral RNA that may persist in the airway for many weeks after cessation of shedding of detectable infectious virus.

Treatment

Primary treatment is supportive and should include hydration, careful clinical assessment of respiratory status, measurement of oxygen saturation, use of supplemental oxygen as needed, suction of the upper airway and, if necessary, intubation and mechanical ventilation. Continuous measurement of oxygen saturation may detect transient fluctuations in oxygenation; supplemental oxygen is recommended when oxyhemoglobin saturation persistently falls below 90% in a previously healthy infant. Ribavirin has in vitro antiviral activity against RSV, and aerosolized ribavirin therapy has been associated with a small but statistically significant increase in oxygen saturation during the acute infection in several small studies. However, a consistent decrease in need for mechanical ventilation, decrease in length of stay in the pediatric intensive care unit, or reduction in days of hospitalization among ribavirin recipients has not been demonstrated. The aerosol route of administration, concern about potential toxic effects among exposed health care personnel, and conflicting results of efficacy trials have led to infrequent use of this drug. Ribavirin is not recommended for routine use but may be considered for use in selected patients with documented, potentially life-threatening RSV infection.

Beta-adrenergic Agents. Beta-adrenergic agents are not recommended for routine care of first-time wheezing associated with RSV bronchiolitis.

Corticosteroid Therapy. In most randomized clinical trials of hospitalized infants as well as outpatients with RSV bronchiolitis, corticosteroid therapy has not been found to have an effect on disease severity, need for hospitalization among outpatients, or length of hospitalization.

Antimicrobial Therapy. Antimicrobial therapy is not indicated in infants hospitalized with RSV bronchiolitis or pneumonia unless there is evidence of secondary bacterial infection, which is uncommon. Otitis media caused by RSV or bacterial superinfection occurs in infants with RSV bronchiolitis; oral antimicrobial agents can be used if therapy for otitis media is necessary.

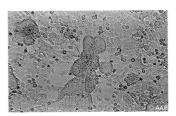

Image 111.1

The characteristic cytopathic effect of respiratory syncytial virus in tissue culture includes the formation of large multinucleated syncytial cells.

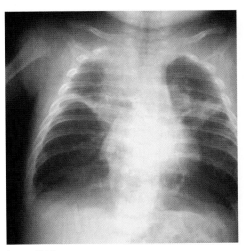

Image 111.2

Respiratory syncytial virus bronchiolitis and pneumonia. Note the bilateral infiltrates and striking hyperaeration. Copyright Martha Lepow.

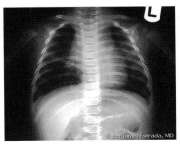

Image 111.3

An anterior-posterior radiograph of a 2-month-old female with respiratory syncytial virus bronchiolitis. Note the wide intercostal spaces, hyperaeration of the lung fields, and flattening of the diaphragm. Copyright Benjamin Estrada, MD.

112

Rickettsial Diseases

Rickettsial diseases comprise infections caused by bacteria of the genera *Rickettsia* (endemic and epidemic typhus and spotted fever group rickettsioses), *Orientia* species (scrub typhus), *Ehrlichia* species (ehrlichiosis), and *Anaplasma* species (anaplasmosis).

Clinical Manifestations

Rickettsial infections have many features in common, including the following:

- Fever, rash (especially in spotted fever and typhus group rickettsiae), headache, myalgia, and respiratory tract symptoms are prominent features.
- Local primary eschars occur with some rickettsial diseases, particularly spotted fever rickettsioses, rickettsialpox, and scrub typhus.
- Systemic capillary and small vessel endothelial damage (ie, vasculitis) with increased microvascular permeability is the primary pathologic feature of spotted fever and typhus group rickettsial infections.
- Rickettsial diseases rapidly can become life-threatening. Risk factors for severe disease include male sex, glucose-6-phosphate dehydrogenase deficiency, and use of sulfonamides.

Immunity against reinfection by the same agent after natural infection usually is of long duration, except in the case of scrub typhus. Among the 4 groups of rickettsial diseases, some cross-immunity usually is conferred by infections within groups but not between groups. Reinfection of humans with *Ehrlichia* species and *Anaplasma* species has not been described.

Etiology

The rickettsiae causing human disease include *Rickettsia* species, *Orientia tsutsugamushi*, *Ehrlichia* species, and *Anaplasma* species. Rickettsiae are small, coccobacillary gram-negative bacteria that are obligate intracellular pathogens and cannot be grown in cell-free media.

Epidemiology

Rickettsial diseases have arthropod vectors including ticks, fleas, mites, and lice. Humans are incidental hosts, except for epidemic (louseborne) typhus, for which humans are the principal reservoir and the human body louse is the vector. Rickettsia life cycles typically involve arthropod and mammalian reservoirs, and transmission occurs as a result of environmental or occupational exposure. Geographic and seasonal occurrence of rickettsial disease is related to arthropod vector life cycles, activity, and distribution.

Diagnostic Tests

Group-specific antibodies are detectable in the serum of many people 7 to 14 days after onset of illness, but slower antibody responses occur commonly in some diseases. Various serologic tests for detecting antirickettsial antibodies are available. The indirect immunofluorescent antibody assay is recommended in most circumstances because of its relative sensitivity and specificity; however, it cannot determine the causative agent to the species level. Treatment early in the course of illness can blunt or delay serologic responses. In laboratories with experienced personnel, immunohistochemical staining and PCR testing of skin biopsy specimens from patients with rash or eschar can help to diagnose rickettsial infections early in the course of disease. The Weil-Felix test is insensitive and nonspecific and is no longer recommended.

Treatment

Prompt and specific therapy is important for optimal outcome. The drug of choice for rickettsioses is doxycycline. Antimicrobial treatment is most effective when children are treated during the first week of illness. If the disease remains untreated during the second week, therapy is less effective in preventing complications. Because confirmatory laboratory tests primarily are retrospective, treatment decisions should be made on the basis of clinical findings and epidemiologic data and should not be delayed until test results are known.

113

Rickettsialpox

Clinical Manifestations

Rickettsialpox is a febrile, eschar-associated illness that is characterized by generalized, relatively sparse, erythematous, papulovesicular eruptions on the trunk, face, and extremities (less often on palms and soles) or mucous membranes of the mouth. The rash develops 1 to 4 days after onset of fever and 3 to 10 days after appearance of an eschar at the site of the bite of a house mouse mite. Regional lymph nodes in the area of the primary eschar typically become enlarged. Without specific antimicrobial therapy, systemic disease lasts approximately 7 to 10 days; manifestations include fever, headache, malaise, and myalgia. Less frequent manifestations include anorexia, vomiting, conjunctivitis, nuchal rigidity, and photophobia. The disease is mild compared with Rocky Mountain spotted fever. No rickettsialpox-associated deaths have been reported, but illness occasionally is severe enough to warrant hospitalization.

Etiology

Rickettsialpox is caused by *Rickettsia akari,* a gram-negative intracellular bacillus, which is classified with the spotted fever group rickettsiae and related antigenically to other members of that group.

Epidemiology

The natural host for *R akari* in the United States is *Mus musculus,* the common house mouse. The disease is transmitted by the house mouse mite, *Liponyssoides sanguineus.* Disease risk is heightened in areas infested with mice and rats. The disease can occur wherever the hosts, pathogens, and humans coexist but most often erupts in large urban settings. In the United States, rickettsialpox has been described predominantly in northeastern metropolitan centers, especially in New York City. It also has been confirmed in many other countries, including Croatia, Ukraine, Turkey, Russia, South Korea, and Mexico. All age groups can be affected. No seasonal pattern of disease occurs. The disease is not communicable but occurs occasionally among families or people cohabiting a house mouse mite–infested dwelling. In Mexico, *R akari* was detected in the brown dog tick, *Rhipicephalus sanguineus.*

Incubation Period

6 to 15 days.

Diagnostic Tests

R akari can be isolated in cell culture from blood and eschar biopsy specimens during the acute stage of disease, but culture is not attempted routinely. Because antibodies to *R akari* have extensive cross-reactivity with antibodies against *Rickettsia rickettsii* (the cause of Rocky Mountain spotted fever), an indirect immunofluorescent antibody assay for *R rickettsii* can demonstrate a fourfold or greater change in antibody titers between acute and convalescent serum specimens taken 4 to 6 weeks apart. Use of *R akari* antigen is recommended for accurate serologic diagnosis. Direct fluorescent antibody or immunohistochemical testing of formalin-fixed, paraffin-embedded eschars or papulovesicle biopsy specimens can detect rickettsiae in the samples and are useful diagnostic techniques.

Treatment

Doxycycline is the drug of choice in all age groups. Doxycycline will shorten the course of illness; symptoms resolve typically within 12 to 48 hours after initiation of therapy. Relapse is rare. Fluoroquinolones and chloramphenicol are alternative drugs.

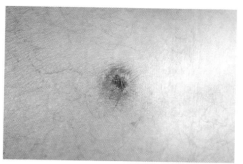

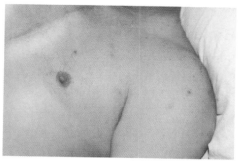

Image 113.1

Eschar on the posterior right calf of a patient with rickettsialpox. This type of lesion is not seen with Rocky Mountain spotted fever. Courtesy of Krusell A, Comer JA, Sexton DJ. Rickettsialpox in North Carolina: a case report. *Emerg Infect Dis.* 2002;8(7):727–728.

Image 113.2

Multiple papulovesicular lesions involving the upper trunk on a patient with rickettsialpox. Courtesy of Krusell A, Comer JA, Sexton DJ. Rickettsialpox in North Carolina: a case report. *Emerg Infect Dis.* 2002;8(7):727–728.

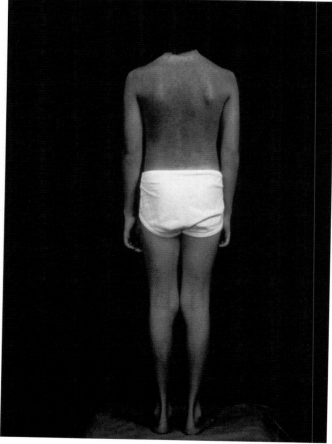

Image 113.3

Rickettsialpox on the trunk and legs. Copyright James Brien, DO.

114

Rocky Mountain Spotted Fever

Clinical Manifestations

Rocky Mountain spotted fever (RMSF) is a systemic, small-vessel vasculitis that often involves a characteristic rash. Fever, myalgia, severe headache, nausea, vomiting, and anorexia are typical presenting symptoms. Abdominal pain and diarrhea often are present and can obscure the diagnosis. The rash usually begins within the first 6 days of symptoms as erythematous macules or maculopapules. Rash usually appears first on the wrists and ankles, often spreading within hours proximally to the trunk and involves the palms and soles. Although early development of a rash is a useful diagnostic sign, rash can be atypical or absent in up to 20% of cases. It can be difficult to visualize in patients with dark skin. A petechial rash typically is a late finding and indicates progression to severe disease. Lack of a typical rash is a risk factor for misdiagnosis and poor outcome. Thrombocytopenia of varying severity and hyponatremia develop in many cases. White blood cell count typically is normal, but leukopenia and anemia can occur. If not treated, illness can last as long as 3 weeks and can be severe, with prominent central nervous system, cardiac, pulmonary, gastrointestinal tract, and renal involvement; disseminated intravascular coagulation; and shock leading to death. RMSF can progress rapidly, even in previously healthy people, and the median time to death is 8 days. Delay in appropriate antimicrobial treatment is associated with severe disease and poor outcomes. Case-fatality rates of untreated RMSF range from 20% to 80%. Significant long-term sequelae are common in patients with severe RMSF, including neurologic (paraparesis; hearing loss; peripheral neuropathy; bladder and bowel incontinence; and cerebellar, vestibular, and motor dysfunction) and non-neurologic (disability from limb or digit amputation). Patients treated early in the course of symptoms may have a mild illness, with fever resolving in the first 48 hours of treatment.

Etiology

Rickettsia rickettsii, an obligate, intracellular, gram-negative bacillus and a member of the spotted fever group of rickettsiae, is the causative agent. The primary targets of infection in mammalian hosts are endothelial cells lining the small blood vessels of all major tissues and organs.

Epidemiology

The pathogen is transmitted to humans by the bite of a tick of the *Ixodes* family (hard ticks). Ticks and their small mammal hosts serve as reservoirs of the pathogen in nature. Other wild animals and dogs have been found with antibodies to *R rickettsii,* but their role as natural reservoirs is not clear. People with occupational or recreational exposure to the tick vector (eg, pet owners, animal handlers, and people who spend more time outdoors) are at increased risk of acquiring the organism. People of all ages can be infected. The period of highest incidence in the United States is from April to September, although RMSF can occur year-round in certain areas with endemic disease. Transmission has occurred on rare occasions by blood transfusion. Mortality is highest in males, people older than 50 years, children aged 5 to 9 years, and people with no recognized tick bite or attachment. In approximately half of pediatric RMSF cases, there is no recall of a recent tick bite. Factors contributing to delayed diagnosis include absence of rash, initial presentation before the fourth day of illness, and onset of illness during months of low incidence.

RMSF is widespread in the United States. Most cases are reported in the south Atlantic and southeastern and south central states, although most states in the contiguous United States record cases each year. The principal recognized vectors of *R rickettsii* are *Dermacentor variabilis* (the American dog tick) in the eastern and central United States and *Dermacentor andersoni* (the Rocky Mountain wood tick) in the western United States. Another common tick throughout the world that feeds on dogs, *Rhipicephalus sanguineus* (the brown dog tick) has been confirmed as a vector of *R rickettsii* in Arizona and Mexico and may play a role in other regions. Transmission parallels the tick season in a given geographic area. RMSF also occurs in Canada, Mexico, Central America, and South America.

Incubation Period

Approximately 1 week; range, 2 to 14 days.

Diagnostic Tests

The gold standard for serologic diagnosis of RMSF is a fourfold or greater change in immunoglobulin (Ig) G-specific antibody titer between acute and convalescent serum specimens determined by indirect immuno-fluorescence antibody assay. The acute sample should be taken early in the course of illness, preferably in the first week of symptoms, and the convalescent sample should be taken 2 to 3 weeks later. Both IgG and IgM antibodies begin to increase around day 7 to 10 after onset of symptoms; therefore, an elevated acute titer can represent past exposure rather than acute infection. A fourfold rise in antibodies is more specific for acute RMSF than a single elevated

titer. IgM antibodies may remain elevated for months and are not highly specific for acute RMSF.

During the first few days of symptoms, *R rickettsii* can be detected by immunohisto-chemical staining or PCR of skin punch biopsy specimens taken from rash sites. Sensitivity of skin biopsy testing decreases greatly after the first 24 hours of appropriate treatment.

Treatment

Doxycycline is the treatment of choice for RMSF in patients of any age. If RMSF is suspected, empirical treatment should be initiated without laboratory confirmation. Chloramphenicol is an alternative treatment, but should be considered only in rare cases, such as severe doxycycline allergies or during pregnancy. Antimicrobial treatment should be continued until the patient has been afebrile for at least 3 days and has demonstrated clinical improvement.

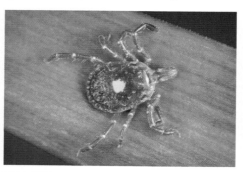

Image 114.1
This is a female Lone Star tick, *Amblyomma americanum,* and is found in the southeastern and midatlantic United States. This tick is a vector of several zoonotic diseases, including human monocytic ehrlichiosis, southern tick-associated rash illness, tularemia, and Rocky Mountain spotted fever. Courtesy of Centers for Disease Control and Prevention/James Gathany.

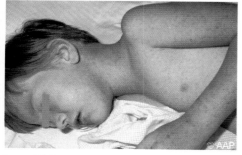

Image 114.2
Rocky Mountain spotted fever in an 8-year-old male. Sixth day of rash without treatment.

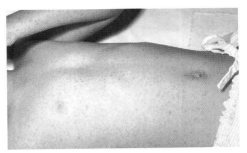

Image 114.3
Rocky Mountain spotted fever. Sixth day of rash without treatment. This is the same patient as in Image 114.2.

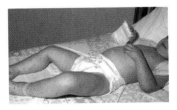

Image 114.5
A 2-year-old boy with obtundation, disorientation, and petechial rash of Rocky Mountain spotted fever, with facial and generalized edema secondary to generalized vasculitis. Rocky Mountain spotted fever is the most severe and frequently reported rickettsial illness in the United States.

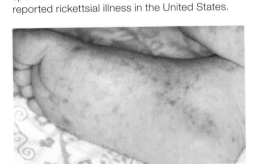

Image 114.7
This is the same patient as in images 114.5 and 114.6 showing petechiae and edema of foot.

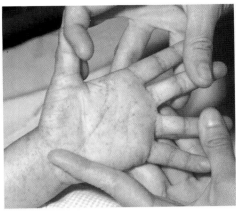

Image 114.4
Rocky Mountain spotted fever. Sixth day of rash without treatment. This is the same patient as in images 114.2 and 114.3.

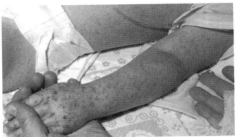

Image 114.6
This is the same patient as in the Image 114.5 showing petechial rash and edema of the upper extremity. The rickettsiae multiply in the endothelial cells of small blood vessels resulting in vasculitis.

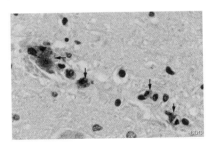

Image 114.8
Immunohistochemical analysis shows the presence of spotted fever group rickettsiae (brown) in vessels of the brain of a patient with fatal Rocky Mountain spotted fever (magnification x400). Courtesy of Hidalgo M, Orejuela L, Fuya P, et al. Rocky Mountain spotted fever, Columbia. *Emerg Infect Dis.* 2007;13(7):1058–1060.

115

Rotavirus Infections

Clinical Manifestations

Infection begins with acute onset of fever and vomiting followed 24 to 48 hours later by watery diarrhea. Symptoms generally persist for 3 to 8 days. In moderate to severe cases, dehydration, electrolyte abnormalities, and acidosis can occur. In certain immunocompromised children, including children with severe congenital immunodeficiencies or children who are hematopoietic stem cell or solid organ transplant recipients, persistent infection and diarrhea can develop.

Etiology

Rotaviruses are segmented, double-stranded RNA viruses belonging to the family Reoviridae, with at least 7 distinct antigenic groups (A through G). Group A viruses are the major causes of rotavirus diarrhea worldwide. Serotyping is based on the 2 surface proteins, VP7 glycoprotein (G) and VP4 protease-cleaved hemagglutinin (P). Prior to introduction of the rotavirus vaccine, G types 1 through 4 and 9 and P types 1A[8] and 1B[4] were most common in the United States.

Epidemiology

Before rotavirus vaccine was introduced in the United States, rotavirus was an important cause of acute gastroenteritis in children attending child care. Rotavirus is present in high titer in stools of infected patients several days before and several days after onset of clinical disease. Transmission is believed to be by the fecal-oral route. Rotavirus can be found on toys and hard surfaces in child care centers, indicating that fomites may serve as a mechanism of transmission. Respiratory transmission likely plays a minor role in disease transmission. Spread within families and child care is common. Rarely, common-source outbreaks from contaminated water or food have been reported.

The epidemiology of rotavirus disease in the United States has changed dramatically since rotavirus vaccines became available in 2006. The rotavirus season now is shorter and relatively delayed, peaking in late spring, and the overall burden of rotavirus disease has declined dramatically. In the first 2 years after the RV5 vaccine became available, emergency department visits and hospitalizations for rotavirus decreased by 85%, such that in the 2008 season, there were an estimated 40,000 to 60,000 fewer gastroenteritis hospitalizations among children younger than 5 years compared with prevaccine seasons. There also were substantial reductions in office visits for gastroenteritis during this period.

Incubation Period

1 to 3 days.

Diagnostic Tests

It is not possible to diagnose rotavirus infection by clinical presentation or nonspecific laboratory tests. Enzyme immunoassays (EIAs), immunochromotography, and latex agglutination assays for group rotavirus antigen detection in stool are available commercially. EIAs are used most widely because of their high sensitivity and specificity. Rotavirus also can be identified in stool by electron microscopy, by electrophoresis and silver staining, and by reverse transcriptase PCR assay for detection of viral genomic RNA.

Treatment

No specific antiviral therapy is available. Oral or parenteral fluids and electrolytes are given to prevent or correct dehydration.

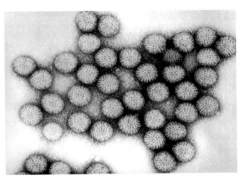

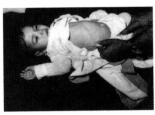

Image 115.2
Doctor examining a child dehydrated from rotavirus infection. In developing countries, rotavirus causes approximately 600,000 deaths each year in children younger than 5 years. Courtesy of World Health Organization.

Image 115.1
Transmission electron micrograph of intact rotavirus particles, double-shelled. Distinctive rim of radiating capsomeres. Courtesy of Centers for Disease Control and Prevention/ Dr Erskine Palmer.

116

Rubella

Clinical Manifestations:

Postnatal Rubella. Many cases of postnatal rubella are subclinical. Clinical disease usually is mild and characterized by a generalized erythematous maculopapular rash, lymphadenopathy, and slight fever. The rash starts on the face, becomes generalized in 24 hours, and lasts a median of 3 days. Lymphadenopathy, which may precede rash, often involves posterior auricular or suboccipital lymph nodes, can be generalized, and lasts between 5 and 8 days. Conjunctivitis and palatal enanthem have been noted. Transient polyarthralgia and polyarthritis rarely occur in children but are common in adolescents and adults, especially females. Encephalitis (1 in 6,000 cases) and thrombocytopenia (1 in 3,000 cases) are complications.

Congenital Rubella Syndrome. Maternal rubella during pregnancy can result in miscarriage, fetal death, or a constellation of congenital anomalies (congenital rubella syndrome [CRS]). The most commonly described anomalies/manifestations associated with CRS are ophthalmologic (cataracts, pigmentary retinopathy, microphthalmos, and congenital glaucoma), cardiac (patent ductus arteriosus, peripheral pulmonary artery stenosis), auditory (sensorineural hearing impairment), or neurologic (behavioral disorders, meningoencephalitis, microcephaly, and mental retardation). Neonatal manifestations of CRS include growth restriction, interstitial pneumonitis, radiolucent bone disease, hepatosplenomegaly, thrombocytopenia, and dermal erythropoiesis (so-called "blueberry muffin" lesions). Congenital defects occur in up to 85% if maternal infection occurs during the first 12 weeks of gestation, 50% during the first 13 to 16 weeks of gestation, and 25% during the end of the second trimester.

Etiology

Rubella virus is an enveloped, positive-stranded RNA virus classified as a *Rubivirus* in the Togaviridae family.

Epidemiology

Humans are the only source of infection. Postnatal rubella is transmitted primarily through direct or droplet contact from nasopharyngeal secretions. The peak incidence of infection is during late winter and early spring. Approximately 25% to 50% of infections are asymptomatic. Immunity from wild-type or vaccine virus usually is prolonged, but reinfection on rare occasions has been demonstrated and rarely has resulted in CRS. Although volunteer studies have demonstrated rubella virus in nasopharyngeal secretions from 7 days before to 14 days after onset of rash, the period of maximal communicability extends from a few days before to 7 days after onset of rash. A small number of infants with congenital rubella continue to shed virus in nasopharyngeal secretions and urine for 1 year or more and can transmit infection to susceptible contacts. Rubella virus has been recovered in high titer from lens aspirates in children with congenital cataracts for several years.

Before widespread use of rubella vaccine, rubella was an epidemic disease, occurring in 6- to 9-year cycles, with most cases occurring in children. In the vaccine era, most cases in the mid-1970s and 1980s occurred in young unimmunized adults in outbreaks on college campuses and in occupational settings. More recent outbreaks have occurred in people born in other countries or underimmunized people. The incidence of rubella in the United States has decreased by more than 99% from the prevaccine era.

The United States was determined no longer to have endemic rubella in 2004. A national serologic survey from 1999–2004 indicated that rubella seroprevalence in the US population remained above the postulated threshold for elimination. Among children and adolescents 6 through 19 years of age, seroprevalence was approximately 95%; however, approximately 10% of adults 20 through 49 years of age lacked antibodies to rubella, although 92% of women were seropositive. In addition, epidemiologic studies of rubella and CRS in the United States have identified that seronegativity is higher among people born outside the

United States or from areas with poor vaccine coverage. The risk of CRS is highest in infants of women born outside the United States, because these women are more likely to be susceptible to rubella.

In 2003, the Pan American Health Organization (PAHO) adopted a resolution calling for elimination of rubella and CRS in the Americas by the year 2010. All countries in the Americas implemented the recommended PAHO strategy by the end of 2008, and the last confirmed endemic rubella case in the Americas was diagnosed in Argentina in February 2009. In September 2010, PAHO announced that the region of the Americas had achieved the rubella and CRS elimination goals on the basis of surveillance data, but documentation of elimination is ongoing.

Incubation Period

16 to 18 days; range, 14 to 21 days.

Diagnostic Tests

Detection of rubella-specific immunoglobulin (Ig) M antibody usually indicates recent postnatal infection or congenital infection in a newborn infant, but both false-negative and false-positive results occur. Most postnatal cases are IgM-positive by 5 days after illness onset, and most congenital cases are IgM-positive at birth until 3 months of age. After this a stable or increasing serum concentration of rubella-specific IgG over several months is diagnostic. Diagnosis of congenital rubella in children older than 1 year is difficult. For diagnosis of postnatally acquired rubella, a fourfold or greater increase in antibody titer or seroconversion between acute and convalescent IgG serum titers also indicates infection. A false-positive IgM test result can be caused by rheumatoid factor, parvovirus IgM, and heterophile antibodies.

Rubella virus can be isolated most consistently from throat or nasal specimens (and less consistently, urine) by inoculation of appropriate cell culture. Detection of rubella virus RNA by reverse transcriptase PCR from a throat/nasal swab or urine sample with subsequent genotyping of strains may be valuable for diagnosis and molecular epidemiology. Most postnatal cases are positive virologically on the day of symptom onset, and most congenital cases are positive virologically at birth. Laboratory personnel should be notified that rubella is suspected, because specialized testing is required to detect the virus. Blood, urine, and cataract specimens also may yield virus, particularly in infants with congenital infection. With the successful elimination of indigenous rubella and CRS in the United States, molecular typing of viral isolates is critical in defining a source in outbreak scenarios and for sporadic cases.

Treatment

Supportive.

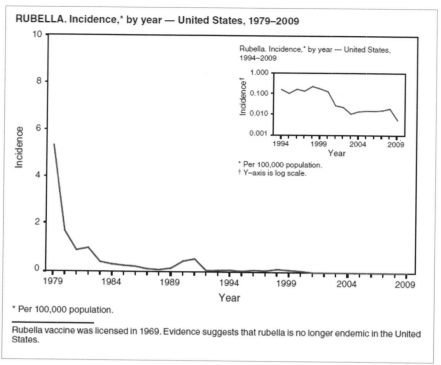

RUBELLA. Incidence,* by year — United States, 1979–2009

Rubella. Incidence,* by year — United States, 1994–2009

† Y-axis is log scale.

* Per 100,000 population.

Rubella vaccine was licensed in 1969. Evidence suggests that rubella is no longer endemic in the United States.

Image 116.1

Rubella. Incidence by year—United States, 1979–2009. Courtesy of *Morbidity and Mortality Weekly Report.*

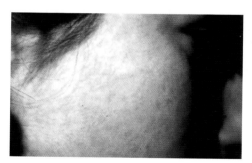

Image 116.2

Rubella rash (face) in a previously unimmunized female. Adenovirus and enterovirus infections can cause exanthema that mimics rubella. Serologic testing is important if the patient is pregnant.

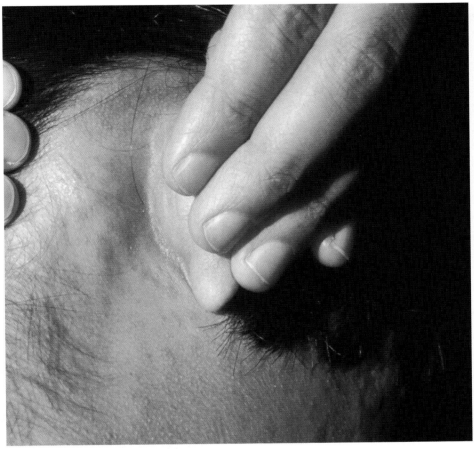

Image 116.3
During a rubella outbreak in Hawaii, this adolescent presented with a 2-day history of fever, malaise, rash, and lymphadenpathy, including these postauricular lymph nodes. Courtesy of Neal Halsey, MD.

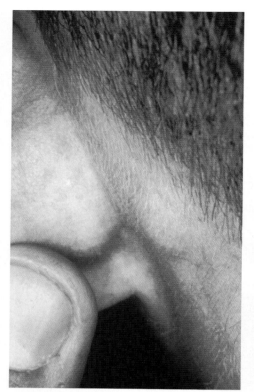

Image 116.4
Postauricular lymphadenopathy in the 17-year-old in Image 116.3 with rubella. Courtesy of George Nankervis, MD.

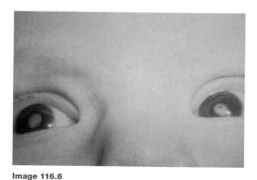

Image 116.6
This photograph shows the cataracts in an infant's eyes due to congenital rubella syndrome. Rubella is a viral disease that can affect susceptible persons of any age. Although generally a mild rash, if contracted in early pregnancy, there can be a high rate of fetal wastage or birth defects, known as congenital rubella syndrome. Courtesy of Centers for Disease Control and Prevention.

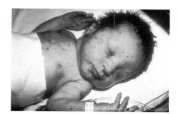

Image 116.5
Newborn with congenital rubella rash. Courtesy Centers for Disease Control and Prevention.

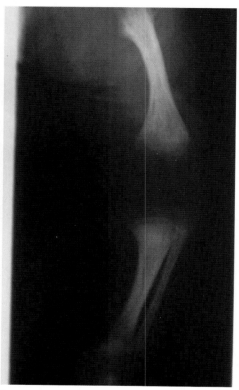

Image 116.7
Radiograph of the lower extremity of the same patient as in Image 116.6 with metaphyseal radiolucent changes, which are found in 10% to 20% of infants with congenital rubella.

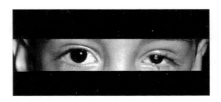

Image 116.8

A 4-year-old boy with congenital rubella syndrome with unilateral microphthalmos and cataract formation in the left eye.

117

Salmonella Infections

Clinical Manifestations

Nontyphoidal *Salmonella* organisms cause a spectrum of illness ranging from asymptomatic gastrointestinal tract carriage to gastroenteritis, bacteremia, and focal infections, including meningitis, brain abscess, and osteomyelitis. The most common illness associated with nontyphoidal *Salmonella* infection is gastroenteritis, in which diarrhea, abdominal cramps, and fever are common manifestations. The site of infection usually is the distal small intestine as well as the colon. Sustained or transient bacteremia can occur, and focal infections are recognized in as many as 10% of patients with nontyphoidal *Salmonella* bacteremia.

Salmonella enterica serotypes Typhi, Paratyphi A, Paratyphi B, and certain other uncommon serotypes can cause a protracted bacteremic illness referred to, respectively, as typhoid and paratyphoid fever and collectively as enteric fevers. The onset of enteric fever typically is gradual, with manifestations such as fever, constitutional symptoms (eg, headache, malaise, anorexia, and lethargy), abdominal pain and tenderness, hepatomegaly, splenomegaly, dactylitis, rose spots typically on the trunk, and change in mental status. In infants and toddlers, invasive infection with enteric fever serotypes can manifest as a mild, nondescript febrile illness accompanied by self-limited bacteremia, or invasive infection can occur in association with more severe clinical symptoms and signs, sustained bacteremia, and meningitis. Constipation can be an early feature.

Etiology

Salmonella organisms are gram-negative bacilli that belong to the family *Enterobacteriaceae.* More than 2,500 *Salmonella* serotypes have been described; most serotypes causing human disease are classified within O serogroups A through E. *Salmonella* serotype Typhi is classified in O serogroup D, along with many other common serotypes including serotype Enteritidis. In 2009, the most commonly reported human isolates in the United States were *Salmonella* serotypes Enteritidis, Typhimurium, Newport, Javiana, and Heidelberg; these 5 serotypes generally account for nearly half of all *Salmonella* infections in the United States (Table 117.1).

Epidemiology

The principal reservoirs for nontyphoidal *Salmonella* organisms include birds, mammals, reptiles, and amphibians. The major food vehicles of transmission to humans include food of animal origin, such as poultry, beef, eggs, and dairy products. Other food vehicles (eg, fruits, vegetables, peanut butter, frozen pot pies, powdered infant formula, cereal, and bakery products) have been implicated in outbreaks, presumably when the food was contaminated by contact with an infected animal product or a human carrier. Other modes of transmission include ingestion of contaminated water and contact with infected reptiles

Table 117.1
Nomenclature for *Salmonella* Organisms

Complete Name[a]	Serotype[b]	Antigenic Formula
S enterica[a] subspecies enterica serotype Typhi	Typhi	9,12,[Vi]:d:-
S enterica subspecies enterica serotype Typhimurium	Typhimurium	[1],4,[5],12:i:1,2
S enterica subspecies enterica serotype Newport	Newport	6,8,[20]:e,h:1,2
S enterica subspecies enterica serotype Paratyphi A	Paratyphi A	[1],2,12:a:[1,5]
S enterica subspecies enterica serotype Enteritidis	Enteritidis	[1],9,12:g,m:-

[a] Species and subspecies are determined by biochemical reactions. Serotype is determined based on antigenic makeup. In the current taxonomy, only 2 species are recognized: *Salmonella enterica* and *Salmonella bongori*. S enterica has 6 subspecies, of which subspecies I (*enterica*) contains the overwhelming majority of all *Salmonella* pathogens that affect humans, other mammals, and birds.
[b] Many *Salmonella* pathogens that previously were considered species (and, therefore, were written italicized with a small case first letter) now are considered serotypes (also called serovars). Serotypes are now written nonitalicized with a capital first letter (eg, Typhi, Typhimurium, Enteritidis). The serotype of *Salmonella* is determined by its O (somatic) and H (flagellar) antigens and whether Vi is expressed.

or amphibians (eg, pet turtles, iguanas, lizards, snakes, frogs, toads, newts, salamanders) and rodents or other mammals.

Unlike nontyphoidal *Salmonella* serotypes, the enteric fever serotypes are restricted to human hosts, in whom they cause clinical and subclinical infections. Chronic human carriers (mostly involving chronic infection of the gall bladder but occasionally involving infection of the urinary tract) constitute the reservoir in areas with endemic infection. Infection with enteric fever serovars implies ingestion of a food or water vehicle contaminated by a chronic carrier or person with acute infection. Although typhoid fever (300–400 cases annually) and paratyphoid fever (~150 cases annually) are uncommon in the United States, these infections are highly endemic in many resource-limited countries, particularly in Asia. Consequently, typhoid fever and paratyphoid fever infections in residents of the United States usually are acquired during international travel.

Age-specific incidences for nontyphoidal *Salmonella* infection are highest in children younger than 4 years. Rates of invasive infections and mortality are higher in infants; elderly people; and people with immunosuppressive conditions, hemoglobinopathies (including sickle cell disease), malignant neoplasms, and HIV infection. Most reported cases are sporadic, but widespread outbreaks, including health care–associated and institutional outbreaks, have been reported. The incidence of nontyphoidal *Salmonella* gastroenteritis has diminished little in recent years, in contrast to other enteric infections of bacterial etiologies.

Every year, nontyphoidal *Salmonella* organisms are one of the most common causes of laboratory-confirmed cases of enteric disease reported by the Foodborne Diseases Active Surveillance Network.

A potential risk of transmission of infection to others persists for as long as the infected person excretes nontyphoidal *Salmonella* organisms. Twelve weeks after infection with the most common nontyphoidal *Salmonella* serotypes, approximately 45% of children younger than 5 years excrete organisms, compared with 5% of older children and adults; antimicrobial therapy can prolong excretion. Approximately 1% of adults continue to excrete *Salmonella* organisms for more than 1 year.

Incubation Period

For nontyphoidal *Salmonella* gastroenteritis, 12 to 36 hours; range, 6 to 72 hours. For enteric fever, 7 to 14 days, range, 3 to 60 days.

Diagnostic Tests

Isolation of *Salmonella* organisms from cultures of stool, blood, urine, bile (including duodenal fluid containing bile), and material from foci of infection is diagnostic. Gastroenteritis is diagnosed by stool culture. Diagnostic tests to detect *Salmonella* antigens by enzyme immunoassay, latex agglutination, and monoclonal antibodies have been developed, as have assays that detect antibodies to antigens of enteric fever serotypes.

If enteric fever is suspected, blood, bone marrow, or bile culture is diagnostic, because organisms often are absent from stool. The sensitivity of blood culture and bone marrow culture in children with enteric fever is approximately 60% and 90%, respectively. The combination of a single blood culture plus culture of bile (collected from a bile-stained duodenal string) is 90% in detecting *Salmonella* serotype Typhi infection in children with clinical enteric fever.

Treatment

Antimicrobial therapy usually is not indicated for patients with either asymptomatic infection or uncomplicated gastroenteritis caused by nontyphoidal *Salmonella* serotypes, because therapy does not shorten the duration of diarrheal disease and can prolong duration of fecal excretion. Although of unproven benefit, antimicrobial therapy is recommended for gastroenteritis caused by nontyphoidal *Salmonella* serotypes in people at increased risk of invasive disease, including infants younger than 3 months and people with chronic gastrointestinal tract disease, malignant neoplasms, hemoglobinopathies, HIV infection, or other immunosuppressive illnesses or therapies.

If antimicrobial therapy is initiated in patients with gastroenteritis, amoxicillin or trimethoprim-sulfamethoxazole is recommended for susceptible strains. Resistance to these antimicrobial agents is becoming more common, especially in resource-limited countries. In areas where ampicillin and trimethoprim-sulfamethoxazole resistance is common, a fluoroquinolone or azithromycin usually is effective.

For patients with localized invasive disease (eg, osteomyelitis, abscess, meningitis) or bacteremia in people infected with HIV, empirical therapy with ceftriaxone is recommended. Once antimicrobial susceptibility test results are available, ampicillin or ceftriaxone for susceptible strains is recommended. For invasive, nonfocal infections, such as bacteremia or septicemia caused by nontyphoidal *Salmonella* or for enteric fever caused by *Salmonella* serotypes Paratyphi A and Paratyphi B, 10 to 14 days of therapy is recommended. Completion of therapy with a fluoroquinolone or azithromycin orally can be considered in patients with uncomplicated infections. Multidrug-resistant isolates of *Salmonella* serotypes Typhi and Paratyphi A and strains with decreased susceptibility to fluoroquinolones are common in Asia and are found increasingly in travelers to areas with endemic infection. Invasive salmonellosis attributable to strains with decreased fluoroquinolone susceptibility is associated with greater risk for treatment failure.

Relapse of nontyphoidal *Salmonella* infection can occur, particularly in immunocompromised patients, who may require longer duration of treatment and re-treatment. Aminoglycosides are not recommended for treatment of invasive *Salmonella* infections. The propensity to become a chronic *Salmonella* serotype Typhi carrier (excretion >1 year) following acute typhoid infection correlates with prevalence of cholelithiasis, increases with age, and is greater in females than males. Chronic carriage in children is uncommon. The chronic carrier state may be eradicated by 4 weeks of oral therapy with ciprofloxacin or norfloxacin, antimicrobial agents that are highly concentrated in bile. High-dose parenteral ampicillin also can be used.

Corticosteroids may be beneficial in patients with severe enteric fever, which is characterized by delirium, obtundation, stupor, coma, or shock. These drugs should be reserved for critically ill patients in whom relief of manifestations of toxemia may be life-saving. The usual regimen is high-dose dexamethasone given intravenously.

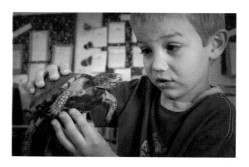

Image 117.1

A young boy holding a box turtle. Turtles carry *Salmonella*. The sale of turtles less than 4 inches in length has been banned in the United States since 1975. The ban by the US Food and Drug Administration has prevented an estimated 100,000 cases of salmonellosis annually in children. Courtesy of Centers for Disease Control and Prevention/James Gathany.

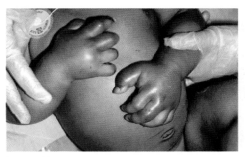

Image 117.2

A young African American child with sickle cell disease and *Salmonella* sepsis with swelling of the hands. Probable diagnosis: acute sickle cell dactylitis with septicemia. Copyright Martin G. Myers, MD.

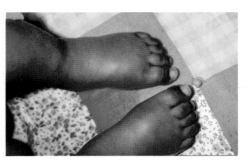

Image 117.3

A young child with sickle cell dactylitis of the foot and *Salmonella* sepsis. This is the same patient as in Image 117.2. Copyright Martin G. Myers, MD.

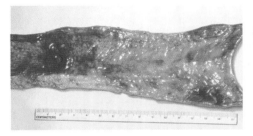

Image 117.4

Typhoid fever cholecystitis with an ulceration and perforation of the gallbladder into the jejunum. *Salmonella* serotype Typhi, the bacterium responsible for causing typhoid fever, has a preference for the gallbladder and, if present, will colonize the surface of gallstones, which is how people become long-term carriers of the disease. Courtesy of Centers for Disease Control and Prevention/Armed Forces Institute—Pathology, Charles N. Farmer.

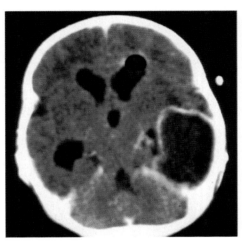

Image 117.5

A computed tomography scan showing a large brain abscess in the posterior parietal region as a complication of *Salmonella* meningitis in a neonate.

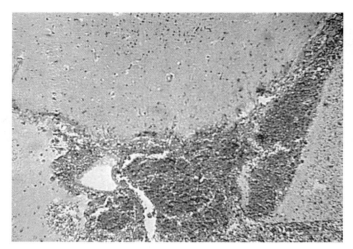

Image 117.6

Histopathologic changes in brain tissue due to *Salmonella typhi* meningitis. *Salmonella* septicemia has been associated with subsequent infection of virtually every organ system, and the nervous system is no exception. Courtesy of Centers for Disease Control and Prevention/Armed Forces Institute—Pathology, Charles N. Farmer.

118

Scabies

Clinical Manifestations

Scabies is characterized by an intensely pruritic, erythematous, papular eruption caused by burrowing of adult female mites in upper layers of the epidermis, creating serpiginous burrows. Itching is most intense at night. In older children and adults, the sites of predilection are interdigital folds, flexor aspects of wrists, extensor surfaces of elbows, anterior axillary folds, waistline, thighs, navel, genitalia, areolae, abdomen, intergluteal cleft, and buttocks. In children younger than 2 years, the eruption generally is vesicular and often occurs in areas usually spared in older children and adults, such as the scalp, face, neck, palms, and soles. The eruption is caused by a hypersensitivity reaction to the proteins of the parasite.

Characteristic scabietic burrows appear as gray or white, tortuous, thread-like lines. Excoriations are common, and most burrows are obliterated by scratching before a patient is seen by a physician. Occasionally, 2- to 5-mm red-brown nodules are present, particularly on covered parts of the body, such as the genitalia, groin, and axilla. These scabies nodules are a granulomatous response to dead mite antigens and feces; the nodules can persist for weeks and even months after effective treatment. Cutaneous secondary bacterial infection can occur.

Crusted (Norwegian) scabies is an uncommon clinical syndrome characterized by a large number of mites and widespread, crusted, hyperkeratotic lesions. Crusted scabies usually occurs in debilitated, developmentally disabled, or immunologically compromised people but has occurred in otherwise healthy children after long-term use of topical corticosteroid therapy.

Etiology

The mite, *Sarcoptes scabiei* subspecies *hominis,* is the cause of scabies. The adult female burrows in the stratum corneum of the skin and lays eggs. *S scabiei* subspecies *canis,* acquired from dogs (with clinical mange), can cause a self-limited and mild infestation usually involving the area in direct contact with the infested animal that will, in humans, resolve without specific treatment.

Epidemiology

Humans are the source of infestation. Transmission usually occurs through prolonged, close, personal contact. Because of the large number of mites in exfoliating scales, even minimal contact with a patient with crusted scabies may result in transmission. Infestation acquired from dogs and other animals is uncommon, and these mites do not replicate in humans. Scabies of human origin can be transmitted as long as the patient remains infested and untreated, including during the interval before symptoms develop. Scabies is endemic in many countries and occurs worldwide in cycles thought to be 15 to 30 years long. Scabies affects people from all socioeconomic levels without regard to age, sex, or standards of personal hygiene. Scabies in adults often is acquired sexually.

Incubation Period

Without previous exposure, 4 to 6 weeks; if previously infested, 2 to 4 days.

Diagnostic Tests

Diagnosis is confirmed by identification of the mite or mite eggs or scybala (feces) from scrapings of papules or intact burrows, preferably from the terminal portion where the mite generally is found. Mineral oil, microscope immersion oil, or water applied to skin facilitates collection of scrapings. A broad-blade scalpel is used to scrape the burrow. Scrapings and oil can be placed on a slide under a glass coverslip and examined microscopically under low power. Adult female mites average 330 to 450 μm in length.

Treatment

Topical permethrin 5% cream or oral ivermectin both are effective agents for treatment of scabies. Most experts recommend starting with topical 5% permethrin cream as the drug of choice, particularly for infants, young children (not approved for children <2 months), and pregnant or nursing women. Permethrin cream should be removed by bathing after 8 to 14 hours. Infested children and adults should apply lotion or cream containing this scabicide over their entire body below the head. Because scabies can affect the face, scalp, and neck in infants and young children, treatment of the entire head, neck, and body in this age group is required. Special attention should be given to trimming fingernails and ensuring application of medication to these areas. A Cochrane review found that ivermectin is effective for treating scabies but less effective than topical permethrin. Because ivermectin is not ovicidal, it is given as 2 doses, 1 week apart. Alternative drugs are precipitated sulfur compounded into petrolatum or 10% crotamiton cream or lotion.

Because scabietic lesions are the result of a hypersensitivity reaction to the mite, itching may not subside for several weeks despite successful treatment. The use of oral antihistamines and topical corticosteroids can help relieve this itching. Topical or systemic antimicrobial therapy is indicated for secondary bacterial infections of the excoriated lesions.

Lindane should not be used for treatment of scabies.

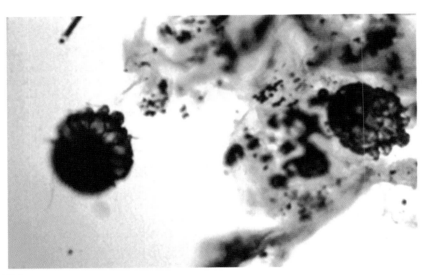

Image 118.1
Linear papulovesicular burrows often contain female scabies mites when examined in mineral oil, which confirms the diagnosis of scabies as shown here. Courtesy of Centers for Disease Control and Prevention.

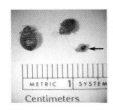

Image 118.2

The 2 most common species of bed bugs implicated in human infestations are *Cimex lectularius* and *Cimex hemipterus,* the former of which is cosmopolitan and the latter being found mostly in the tropics and subtropics. Adults are on average 5 mm long, oval-shaped, and dorso-ventrally flattened. Like other members of the order *Hemiptera,* they possess piercing-sucking mouthparts. Adults are brachypterous; the hindwings are nearly absent and the forewings are reduced to small, leathery pads. Nymphs look like smaller, paler versions of the adults. While *Cimex* spp have been found to be naturally infected with several bloodborne pathogens, they are not effective vectors of disease. The primary medical importance is inflammation associated with their bites. Two adults and one nymph (arrow) of *C lectularius,* collected in a hotel in urban Georgia.

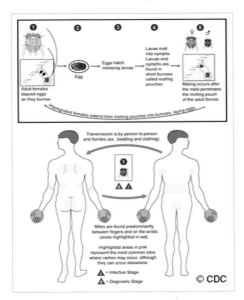

Image 118.3

Life cycle. Female *Sarcoptes scabiei* deposit eggs at 2- to 3-day intervals as they burrow through the skin (1). Eggs are oval and 0.1 to 0.15 mm in length (2), and incubation time is 3 to 8 days. After the eggs hatch, the larvae migrate to the skin surface and burrow into the intact stratum corneum to construct almost invisible, short burrows called molting pouches. The larval stage, which emerges from the eggs, has only 3 pairs of legs (3), and this form lasts 2 to 3 days. After larvae molt, the result-ing nymphs have 4 pairs of legs (4). This form molts into slightly larger nymphs before molting into adults. Larvae and nymphs may often be found in molting pouches or in hair follicles and look similar to adults, only smaller. Adults are round, sac-like eyeless mites. Females are 0.3 to 0.4 mm long and 0.25 to 0.35 mm wide, and males are half that size. Mating occurs after the male penetrates the molt-ing pouch of the adult female (5). Impregnated females create characteristic serpentine burrows, lay-ing eggs in the process, spending the remaining 2 months of their lives in tunnels under the surface of the skin. Males are rarely seen. Transmission occurs by the transfer of ovigerous females during personal contact. Transmission is primarily person-to-person contact, but may also occur via fomites (eg, bedding or clothing). Mites are found predominantly between the fingers and on the wrists. The mites hold onto the skin using suckers attached to the 2 most anterior pairs of legs. Courtesy of Centers for Disease Control and Prevention/Alexander J da Silva, PhD/Melanie Moser.

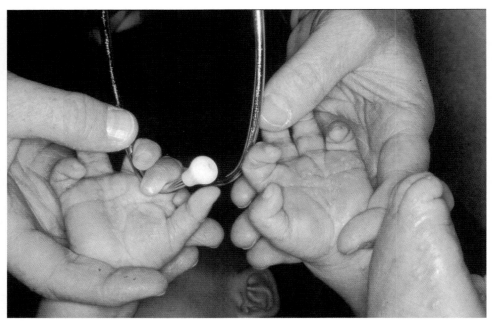

Image 118.4
Scabies. Courtesy of James Brien, DO.

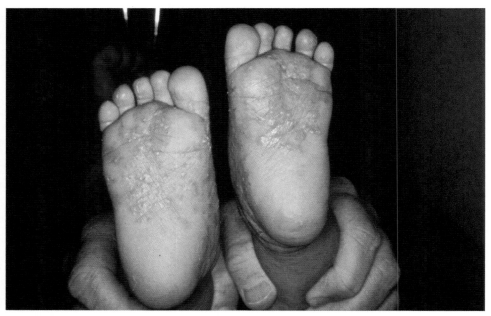

Image 118.5
Scabies. Courtesy of James Brien, DO.

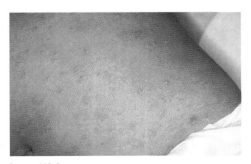

Image 118.6
Scabies rash in an infant. Courtesy of James Brien, DO.

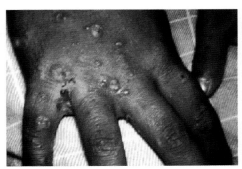

Image 118.7
Older children, adolescents, and adults with scabies exhibit erythematous papules, nodules, or burrows in the interdigital webs, as in this patient.

119

Schistosomiasis

Clinical Manifestations

Infections are established by skin penetration of infecting larvae (cercariae, shed by freshwater snails), which may be accompanied by a transient, pruritic, papular rash (cercarial dermatitis). After penetration, the organism enters the bloodstream, migrates through the lungs, and eventually migrates to the venous plexus that drains the intestines or (in the case of *Schistosoma haematobium*) the bladder, where the adult worms reside. Four to 8 weeks after exposure, an acute illness (Katayama fever) can develop that manifests as fever, malaise, cough, rash, abdominal pain, hepatosplenomegaly, diarrhea, nausea, lymphadenopathy, and eosinophilia. The severity of symptoms associated with chronic disease is related to the worm burden. People with low to moderate worm burdens may never develop overt clinical disease or may develop milder manifestations, such as anemia. Higher worm burdens can have a range of symptoms caused primarily by inflammation and fibrosis triggered by the immune response to eggs produced by adult worms. Severe forms of intestinal schistosomiasis (*Schistosoma mansoni* and *Schistosoma japonicum* infections) can result in hepatosplenomegaly, abdominal pain, bloody diarrhea, portal hypertension, ascites, and esophageal varices and hematemesis. Urinary schistosomiasis (*S haematobium* infections) can result in the bladder becoming inflamed and fibrotic. Symptoms and signs include dysuria, urgency, terminal microscopic and gross hematuria, secondary urinary tract infections, hydronephrosis, and nonspecific pelvic pain. *S haematobium* also is associated with lesions of the lower genital tract (vulva, vagina, and cervix) in women, hematospermia in men, and certain forms of bladder cancer. Other organ systems can be involved—for example, eggs can embolize to the lungs, causing pulmonary hypertension. Less commonly, eggs can localize to the central nervous system, notably the spinal cord in *S mansoni* or *S haematobium* infections and the brain in *S japonicum* infection, causing neurologic complications.

Cercarial dermatitis (swimmer's itch) is caused by larvae of nonhuman schistosome species that penetrate human skin but are unable to complete their life cycle and do not cause systemic disease. Manifestations include pruritus at the penetration site a few hours after water exposure, followed in 5 to 14 days by an intermittent pruritic, sometimes papular, eruption. In previously sensitized people, more intense papular eruptions may occur for 7 to 10 days after exposure.

Etiology

The trematodes (flukes) *S mansoni, S japonicum, Schistosoma mekongi,* and *Schistosoma intercalatum* cause intestinal schistosomiasis, and *S haematobium* causes urinary tract disease. All species have similar life cycles. Swimmer's itch is caused by multiple avian and mammalian species of *Schistosoma.*

Epidemiology

Persistence of schistosomiasis depends on the presence of an appropriate snail as an intermediate host. Eggs excreted in stool (*S mansoni, S japonicum, S mekongi,* and *S intercalatum*) or urine (*S haematobium*) into freshwater hatch into motile miracidia, which infect snails. Children commonly are first infected when they accompany their mothers to lakes, ponds, and other open freshwater sources. School-aged children commonly are the most heavily infected people in the community and are important in maintaining transmission because of behaviors such as uncontrolled defecation and urination and prolonged wading and swimming in infected waters. Communicability lasts as long as infected snails are in the environment or live eggs are excreted in the urine and feces of humans into freshwater sources with appropriate snails. In the case of *S japonicum,* animals play an important zoonotic role (as a source of eggs) in maintaining the life cycle. Infection is not transmissible by person-to-person contact or blood transfusion.

The distribution of schistosomiasis often is local, limited by the presence of appropriate snail vectors, infected human reservoirs, and freshwater sources. *S mansoni* occurs throughout tropical Africa; in parts of several

Caribbean islands; and in areas of Venezuela, Brazil, Suriname, and the Arabian Peninsula. *S japonicum* is found in China, the Philippines, and Indonesia. *S haematobium* occurs in Africa and the Middle East. *S mekongi* is found in Cambodia and Laos. *S intercalatum* is found in West and Central Africa. Adult worms of *S mansoni* can live as long as 30 years in the human host. Thus schistosomiasis can be diagnosed in patients many years after they have left an area with endemic infection. Immunity is incomplete, and reinfection occurs commonly.

Incubation Period

Approximately 4 to 6 weeks for *S japonicum*, 6 to 8 weeks for *S mansoni*, and 10 to 12 weeks for *S haematobium*.

Diagnostic Tests

Eosinophilia is common and may be intense in Katayama syndrome. Infection with *S mansoni* and other species (except *S haematobium*) is determined by microscopic examination of stool specimens to detect characteristic eggs, but results may be negative if performed too early in the course of infection. In light infections, several stool specimens examined by a concentration technique may be needed before eggs are found, or a biopsy of the rectal mucosa

may be necessary. *S haematobium* is diagnosed by examining urine for eggs. Egg excretion in urine often peaks between noon and 3:00 pm. Biopsy of the bladder mucosa may be necessary. Serologic tests are available through the Centers for Disease Control and Prevention and some commercial laboratories. Specific serologic tests may be particularly helpful for detecting light infections. Results of these antibody-based tests remain positive for many years, thus these are not useful in differentiating ongoing from past infection.

Swimmer's itch can be difficult to differentiate from other causes of dermatitis. A skin biopsy may demonstrate larvae, but their absence does not exclude the diagnosis.

Treatment

The drug of choice for schistosomiasis caused by any species is praziquantel; the alternative drug for *S mansoni* is oxamniquine, although this drug is not available in the United States but is used in some areas of Brazil. Praziquantel therapy given within 4 to 8 weeks of exposure should be repeated 1 to 2 months later. Swimmer's itch is a self-limited disease that can require symptomatic treatment of the rash. More intense reactions may require a course of oral corticosteroids.

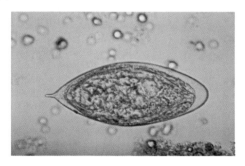

Image 119.1

This micrograph depicts an egg from a *Schistosoma haematobium* trematode parasite (magnification x500). Note the egg's posteriorly protruding terminal spine, unlike the spinal remnant, which protrudes from the lateral wall of the *Schistosoma japonicum* egg. These eggs are eliminated in an infected human's feces or urine, and under optimal conditions in a watery environment, the eggs hatch and release miracidia, which then penetrate a specific snail intermediate host. Once inside the host, the *S haematobium* parasite passes through 2 developmental generations of sporocysts and are released by the snail into its environment as cercariae. Courtesy of Centers for Disease Control and Prevention.

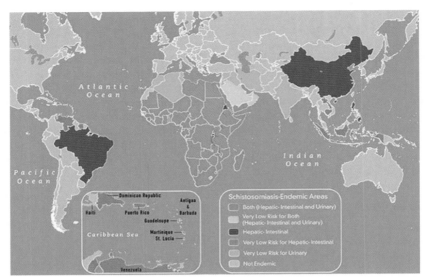

Image 119.2
Geographic distribution of schistosomiasis. Courtesy of Centers for Disease Control and Prevention.

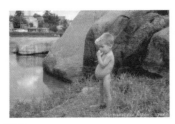

Image 119.3
A boy with swollen abdomen due to schistosomiasis (bilharziasis) with hepatosplenomegaly. Courtesy of Centers for Disease Control and Prevention.

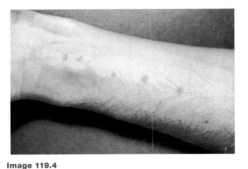

Image 119.4
Schistosome dermatitis, or "swimmers itch," occurs when skin is penetrated by a free-swimming, fork-tailed infective cercaria. On release from the snail host, the infective cercariae swim, penetrate the skin of the human host, and shed their forked tail, becoming schistosomulae. The schistosomulae migrate through several tissues and stages to their residence in the veins. Courtesy of Centers for Disease Control and Prevention.

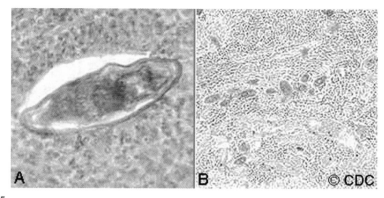

Image 119.5

(A, B) Cross-section of different human tissues showing *Schistosoma* spp eggs. *Schistosoma* spp in liver and bladder, respectively. Courtesy of Centers for Disease Control and Prevention.

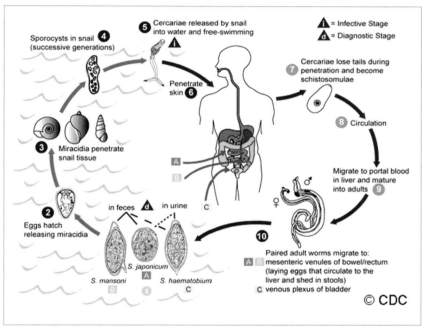

Image 119.6

Life cycle. *Schistosoma haematobium* most often occurs in the venous plexus of the bladder (C), but it can also be found in the rectal venules. The females (size 7–20 mm; males slightly smaller) deposit eggs in the small venules of the portal and perivesical systems. The eggs are moved progressively toward the lumen of the intestine (*Schistosoma mansoni* and *Schistosoma japonicum*) and of the bladder and ureters (*S haematobium*), and are eliminated with feces or urine, respectively (1). Pathology of *S mansoni* and *S japonicum* schistosomiasis includes Katayama fever, presinusoidal egg granulomas, Symmers pipe stem periportal fibrosis, portal hypertension, and occasional embolic egg granulomas in the brain or spinal cord. Pathology of *S haematobium* schistosomiasis includes hematuria, scarring, calcification, squamous cell carcinoma, and occasional embolic egg granulomas in the brain or spinal cord. Human contact with water is thus necessary for infection by schistosomes. Various animals, such as dogs, cats, rodents, pigs, horses, and goats, serve as reservoirs for *S japonicum,* and dogs for *Schistosoma mekongi.* Courtesy of Centers for Disease Control and Prevention/Alexander J. da Silva, PhD/Melanie Moser.

120

Shigella Infections

Clinical Manifestations

Shigella species primarily infect the large intestine, causing clinical manifestations that range from watery or loose stools with minimal or no constitutional symptoms to more severe symptoms, including high fever, abdominal cramps or tenderness, tenesmus, and mucoid stools with or without blood. *Shigella dysenteriae* serotype 1 often causes a more severe illness than other shigellae with a higher risk of complications, including pseudomembranous colitis, toxic megacolon, intestinal perforation, hemolysis, and hemolytic uremic syndrome (HUS). Generalized seizures have been reported among young children with shigellosis; although the pathophysiology and incidence are poorly understood, such seizures usually are self-limited and associated with high fever or electrolyte abnormalities. Septicemia is rare during the course of illness and is caused either by *Shigella* organisms or by other gut flora that gain access to the bloodstream through intestinal mucosa damaged during shigellosis. Septicemia occurs most often in neonates, malnourished children, and people with *S dysenteriae* serotype 1 infection. Reactive arthritis (Reiter syndrome) is a rare complication of *Shigella* infection that can develop weeks or months after shigellosis, especially in patients expressing HLA-B27.

Etiology

Shigella species are facultative aerobic, gram-negative bacilli in the family Enterobacteriaceae. Four species (with >40 serotypes) have been identified. Among *Shigella* isolates reported in industrialized nations including the United States in 2009, approximately 86% were *Shigella sonnei,* 12% were *Shigella flexneri,* 1% were *Shigella boydii,* and less than 1% were *S dysenteriae*. In resource-limited countries, especially in Africa and Asia, *S flexneri* predominates. Shiga toxin is produced by *S dysenteriae* serotype 1, which enhances virulence at the colonic mucosa and can cause small blood vessel and renal damage (HUS).

Epidemiology

Humans are the natural host for *Shigella* organisms, although other primates can be infected. The primary mode of transmission is fecal-oral, although transmission also can occur via contact with a contaminated inanimate object, ingestion of contaminated food or water, or sexual contact. Houseflies also may be vectors through physical transport of infected feces. Ingestion of as few as 10 organisms, depending on the species, is sufficient for infection to occur. Children 5 years of age or younger in child care settings and their caregivers and people living in crowded conditions are at increased risk of infection. Infections attributable to *S flexneri, S boydii,* and *S dysenteriae* are more common in older children and adults than are infections attributable to *S sonnei* in the United States; nonetheless, more than 25% of cases caused by each species are reported among children younger than 5 years. Travel to resource-limited countries with inadequate sanitation can place travelers at risk of infection. Even without antimicrobial therapy, the carrier state usually ceases within 1 to 4 weeks after onset of illness; long-term carriage is uncommon and does not correlate with underlying intestinal dysfunction.

Incubation Period

1 to 3 days; range, 1 to 7 days.

Diagnostic Tests

Isolation of *Shigella* organisms from feces or rectal swab specimens containing feces is diagnostic; sensitivity is improved by testing stool as soon as it is passed. The presence of fecal leukocytes on a methylene-blue stained stool smear is sensitive for the diagnosis of colitis but is not specific for *Shigella* species. Although bacteremia is rare, blood should be cultured in severely ill, immunocompromised, or malnourished children.

Treatment

Although severe dehydration is rare with shigellosis, correction of fluid and electrolyte losses, preferably by oral rehydration solutions, is the mainstay of treatment. Most clinical infections with *S sonnei* are self-limited

(48–72 hours), and mild episodes do not require antimicrobial therapy. Available evidence suggests that antimicrobial therapy is somewhat effective in shortening duration of diarrhea and hastening eradication of organisms from feces. Treatment is recommended for patients with severe disease, dysentery, or underlying immunosuppressive conditions; in these patients, empiric therapy should be given while awaiting culture and susceptibility results. Antimicrobial susceptibility testing of clinical isolates is indicated to guide appropriate therapy. Plasmid-mediated resistance has been identified in all *Shigella* species. In 2009 in the United States, approximately 46% of *Shigella* species were resistant to ampicillin, 40% were resistant to trimethoprim-sulfamethoxazole, and less than 1% were resistant to ciprofloxacin and ceftriaxone. Ciprofloxacin and ceftriaxone resistance is increasing around the world.

For cases in which treatment is required and susceptibility is unknown or an ampicillin- and trimethoprim-sulfamethoxazole–resistant strain is isolated, parenteral azithromycin for 3 days, ceftriaxone for 5 days, or a fluoroquinolone (such as ciprofloxacin) for 3 days should be administered. Oral cephalosporins are not useful for treatment. For susceptible strains, ampicillin or trimethoprim-sulfamethoxazole is effective; amoxicillin is less effective because of its rapid absorption from the gastrointestinal tract. The oral route of therapy is recommended except for seriously ill patients.

Antidiarrheal compounds that inhibit intestinal peristalsis are contraindicated, because they can prolong the clinical and bacteriologic course of disease and increase the rate of complications. Nutritional supplementation, including vitamin A and zinc, can be given to hasten clinical resolution in geographic areas where children are at risk of malnutrition.

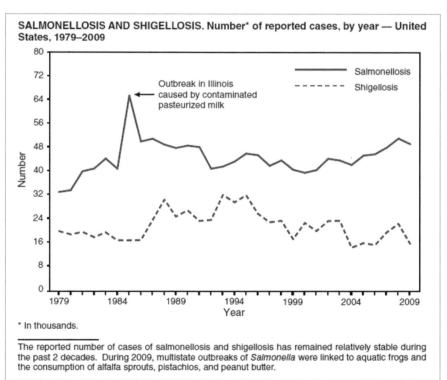

SALMONELLOSIS AND SHIGELLOSIS. Number* of reported cases, by year — United States, 1979–2009

* In thousands.

The reported number of cases of salmonellosis and shigellosis has remained relatively stable during the past 2 decades. During 2009, multistate outbreaks of *Salmonella* were linked to aquatic frogs and the consumption of alfalfa sprouts, pistachios, and peanut butter.

Image 120.1
Salmonellosis and shigellosis, incidence by year in the United States—1976–2006. Courtesy of *Morbidity and Mortality Weekly Report.*

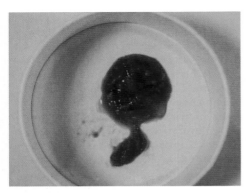

Image 120.2
Characteristic bloody mucoid stool of a child with shigellosis.

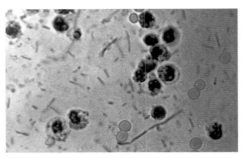

Image 120.3
Fecal leukocytes (shigellosis) (methylene blue stain). The presence of fecal leukocytes suggests a bacterial diarrhea, though not specific for *Shigella* infection. Courtesy of Edgar O. Ledbetter, MD, FAAP.

121

Smallpox (Variola)

The last naturally occurring case of smallpox occurred in Somalia in 1977, followed by 2 cases in 1978 after a photographer was infected during a laboratory exposure and later transmitted smallpox to her mother in the United Kingdom. In 1980, the World Health Assembly declared that smallpox (variola virus) had been eradicated successfully worldwide. The United States discontinued routine childhood immunization against smallpox in 1972. Immunization of US military personnel continued until 1990. As a result of terrorism events on September 11, 2001, and concern that the virus could be used as a weapon of bioterrorism, the smallpox immunization policy was revisited. In 2002, the United States resumed immunization of military personnel deployed to certain areas of the world and initiated a civilian preevent smallpox immunization program in 2003 to facilitate preparedness and response to a smallpox bioterrorism event.

Clinical Manifestations

People infected with variola major strains develop a severe prodromal illness characterized by high fever (102°F–104°F [38.9°C–40.0°C]) and constitutional symptoms, including malaise, severe headache, backache, abdominal pain, and prostration, lasting for 2 to 5 days. Infected children can have vomiting and seizures during this prodromal period. Most patients with smallpox tend to be severely ill and bedridden during the febrile prodrome. The prodrome is followed by development of lesions on mucosa of the mouth or pharynx, which may not be noticed by the patient. This stage occurs less than 24 hours before onset of rash, which usually is the first recognized manifestation of smallpox. With onset of oral lesions, the patient becomes infectious. The rash typically begins on the face and rapidly progresses to involve the forearms, trunk, and legs, with the greatest concentration of lesions on the face and distal extremities. Most patients will have lesions on the palms and soles. With rash onset, fever decreases but does not resolve. Lesions begin as macules that progress to papules, followed by firm vesicles and then deep-seated, hard pustules described

as "pearls of pus." Each stage lasts 1 to 2 days. By day 6 of rash, lesions may begin to umbilicate or become confluent. Lesions increase in size for approximately 8 to 10 days, after which they begin to crust. Once all the crusts have separated, 3 to 4 weeks after rash onset, the patient no longer is infectious. Variola minor strains cause a disease that is indistinguishable clinically from variola major, except that it causes less severe systemic symptoms, more rapid rash, and fewer fatalities.

Variola major in unimmunized people is associated with case-fatality rates of approximately 30% during epidemics of smallpox. The mortality rate is highest in children younger than 1 year and adults older than 30 years. The potential for modern supportive therapy to improve outcome is not known.

In addition to the typical presentation of smallpox (≥90% of cases), there are 2 uncommon forms of variola major: hemorrhagic (characterized either by a hemorrhagic diathesis prior to onset of the typical smallpox rash [early hemorrhagic smallpox] or by hemorrhage into skin lesions and disseminated intravascular coagulation [late hemorrhagic smallpox]) and malignant or flat type (in which the skin lesions do not progress to the pustular stage but remain flat and soft). Each variant occurs in approximately 5% of cases and is associated with a 95% to 100% mortality rate.

Etiology

Variola is a member of the Poxviridae family (genus *Orthopoxvirus*). Other members of this genus that can infect humans include monkeypox virus, cowpox virus, and vaccinia virus.

Epidemiology

Humans are the only natural reservoir for variola virus (smallpox). Smallpox is spread most commonly in droplets from the oropharynx of infected people, although rare transmission from aerosol spread has been reported. Infection from direct contact with lesion material or indirectly via fomites, such as clothing and bedding, also has been reported. Because most patients with smallpox are extremely ill and bedridden, spread generally is limited to household contacts, hospital workers, and other health care professionals.

Incubation Period

7 to 17 days; mean, 12 days.

Diagnostic Tests

Variola virus can be detected in vesicular or pustular fluid by a number of different methods, including electron microscopy, immunohistochemistry, culture, or PCR assay. Only PCR can definitively diagnose infection with variola virus; all other methods simply screen for orthopoxviruses. Diagnostic workup includes exclusion of varicella-zoster virus or other common conditions that cause a vesicular/pustular rash illness.

Treatment

There is no known effective antiviral therapy available to treat smallpox. Infected patients should receive supportive care. Cidofovir has been suggested as having a role in smallpox therapy, but data to support cidofovir use in smallpox are not available.

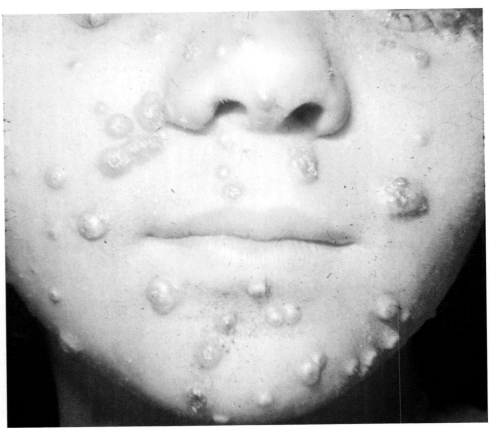

Image 121.1
Variola minor lesions on the face of a 2-year-old Latin American male. Courtesy of Paul Wehrle, MD.

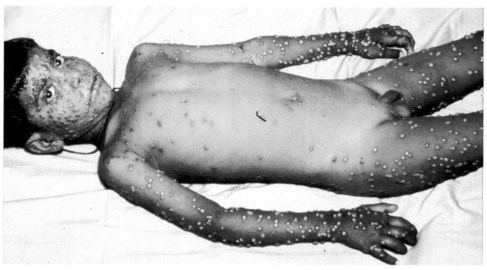

Image 121.2
A 7-year-old male residing in India with smallpox lesions in a typical centripetal distribution. Courtesy of Paul Wehrle, MD.

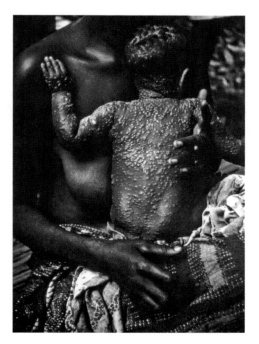

Image 121.3
This photograph reveals the back of a Nigerian child with smallpox. Note the pustules are centripetal in distribution, radiating from their densest area of eruption on the upper back and outward along the extremities. All the skin lesions are at the same stage of development. Courtesy of Centers for Disease Control and Prevention/Dr Lyle Conrad.

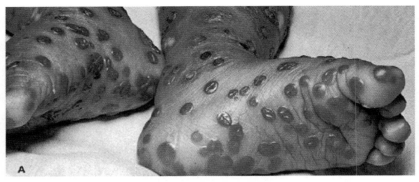

Image 121.4
Numerous healing smallpox lesions on the feet of a young child. Courtesy of Edgar O. Ledbetter, MD, FAAP.

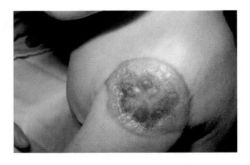

Image 121.5
Due to progressive vaccinia this patient required a graft in order to correct the necrotic vaccination site. What is now referred to as progressive vaccinia, vaccinia gangrenosum is one of the most severe complications of smallpox vaccination, and it is almost always life-threatening. Those who are most susceptible to this condition are the immunosuppressed. Courtesy of Centers for Disease Control and Prevention/Allen W. Mathies, MD.

122

Sporotrichosis

Clinical Manifestations

Sporotrichosis manifests either as cutaneous or extracutaneous disease. The lymphocutaneous manifestation is the most common **cutaneous** form. Inoculation occurs at a site of minor trauma, causing a painless papule that enlarges slowly to become a nodular lesion that can develop a violaceous hue or can ulcerate. Secondary lesions follow the same evolution and develop along the lymphatic distribution proximal to the initial lesion. A localized cutaneous form of sporotrichosis, also called fixed cutaneous form, common in children, presents as a solitary crusted papule or papuloulcerative or nodular lesion in which lymphatic spread is not observed. The extremities and face are the most common sites of infection. A disseminated cutaneous form with multiple lesions is rare, usually occurring in immunocompromised children.

Extracutaneous sporotrichosis is uncommon, with cases occurring primarily in immunocompromised patients. Osteoarticular infection results from hematogenous spread or local inoculation. The most commonly affected joints are the knee, elbow, wrist, and ankle. Pulmonary sporotrichosis clinically resembles tuberculosis and occurs after inhalation or aspiration of aerosolized spores. Disseminated disease generally occurs after hematogenous spread from primary skin or lung infection. Disseminated sporotrichosis can involve multiple foci (eg, eyes, pericardium, genitourinary tract, central nervous system) and occurs predominantly in immunocompromised patients.

Etiology

Sporothrix schenckii is a dimorphic fungus that grows as a mold or mycelial form at room temperature and as a yeast at 37°C (98°F) and in host tissues. *S schenckii* is a complex of at least 6 species. The related species *Sporothrix brasiliensis*, *Sporothrix globosa*, and *Sporothrix mexicana* also cause human infection.

Epidemiology

S schenckii is a ubiquitous organism that has worldwide distribution but is most common in tropical and subtropical regions of Central and South America and parts of North America. The fungus is isolated from soil and plants, including hay, straw, thorny plants (especially roses), sphagnum moss, and decaying vegetation. Cutaneous disease occurs from inoculation of debris containing the organism. People engaging in gardening or farming are at risk of infection. Inhalation of spores can lead to pulmonary disease. Zoonotic spread from infected cats or scratches from digging animals, such as armadillos, has led to cutaneous disease.

Incubation Period

7 to 30 days after cutaneous inoculation.

Diagnostic Tests

Culture of *Sporothrix* species from a tissue, wound drainage, or sputum specimen is diagnostic. Culture of *Sporothrix* species from a blood specimen suggests the disseminated form of infection associated with immunodeficiency. Histopathologic examination of tissue may not be helpful, because the organism seldom is abundant. Special fungal stains to visualize the oval or cigar-shaped organism are required.

Treatment

Sporotrichosis usually does not resolve without treatment. Itraconazole is the drug of choice for children with lymphocutaneous and localized cutaneous disease. Alternative therapies include saturated solution of potassium iodide. Oral fluconazole should only be used if the patient cannot tolerate other agents.

Amphotericin B is recommended as the initial therapy for visceral or disseminated sporotrichosis in children. After clinical response to amphotericin B therapy is documented, itraconazole can be substituted. Serum concentrations of itraconazole should be measured after at least 2 weeks of therapy to ensure adequate drug exposure. Itraconazole can be required for lifelong therapy in children with HIV infection. Surgical débridement or excision may be necessary to resolve cavitary pulmonary disease.

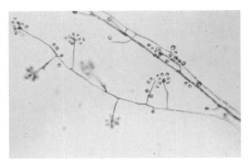

Image 122.1
Sporothrix schenkii, mold phase (48-hour potato dextrose agar, lactophenol cotton blue preparation); small tear-shaped conidia forming rosette-like clusters. Courtesy of Centers for Disease Control and Prevention.

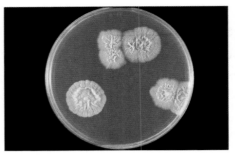

Image 122.2
This is an image of a Sabhi agar plate culture of *Sporothrix schenckii* grown at 20°C. *S schenckii* is the causative agent for the fungal infection sporotrichosis, also known as "rose handler's disease," which affects individuals who handle thorny plants, sphagnum moss, or baled hay. Courtesy of Centers for Disease Control and Prevention/Dr William Kaplan.

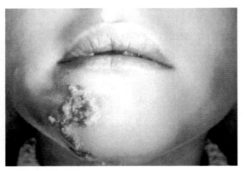

Image 122.3
Cutaneous sporotrichosis of the face in a preschool-aged child. Courtesy of Edgar O. Ledbetter, MD, FAAP.

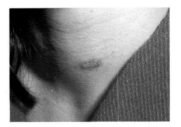

Image 122.4
Anterior cervical sporotrichosis lesions of an adolescent girl.

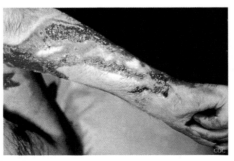

Image 122.5
This patient's arm shows the effects of the fungal disease sporotrichosis, caused by the fungus *Sporothrix schenckii.* Courtesy of Centers for Disease Control and Prevention/Dr Lucille K. Georg.

123

Staphylococcal Infections

Clinical Manifestations

Staphylococcus aureus causes a variety of localized and invasive suppurative infections and 3 toxin-mediated syndromes: toxic shock syndrome, scalded skin syndrome, and food poisoning. Localized infections include hordeola, furuncles, carbuncles, impetigo (bullous and nonbullous), paronychia, mastitis, ecthyma, cellulitis, erythroderma, peritonsillar abscess (Quinsy), retropharyngeal abscess, omphalitis, parotitis, lymphadenitis, and wound infections. *S aureus* also causes infections associated with foreign bodies, including intravascular catheters or grafts, pacemakers, peritoneal catheters, cerebrospinal fluid (CSF) shunts, and prosthetic joints, which can be associated with bacteremia. Bacteremia can be complicated by septicemia; endocarditis; pericarditis; pneumonia; pleural empyema; soft tissue, muscle, or visceral abscesses; arthritis; osteomyelitis; septic thrombophlebitis of small and large vessels; and other foci of infection. Primary *S aureus* pneumonia also can occur after aspiration of organisms from the upper respiratory tract and typically is associated with mechanical ventilation or viral infections in the community (eg, influenza). Meningitis is rare unless accompanied by an intradermal foreign body (eg, ventriculoperitoneal shunt) or a congenital or acquired defect in the dura. *S aureus* infections can be fulminant and commonly are associated with metastatic foci and abscess formation, often requiring prolonged antimicrobial therapy, drainage, and foreign body removal to achieve cure. Risk factors for severe *S aureus* infections include chronic diseases, such as diabetes mellitus and cirrhosis, immunodeficiency, nutritional disorders, surgery, and transplantation.

Staphylococcal toxic shock syndrome (TSS).
TSS is a toxin-mediated disease, usually is caused by strains producing TSS toxin-1 or possibly other related staphylococcal enterotoxins. TSS toxin-1 acts as a superantigen that stimulates production of tumor necrosis factor and other mediators that cause capillary leak, leading to hypotension and multiorgan failure. Staphylococcal TSS is characterized by acute onset of fever, generalized erythroderma, rapid-onset hypotension, and signs of multisystem organ involvement, including profuse watery diarrhea, vomiting, conjunctival injection, and severe myalgia (see Box 123.1). Although approximately 50% of reported cases of staphylococcal TSS occur in menstruating females using tampons, nonmenstrual TSS cases occur after childbirth or abortion, after surgical procedures, and in association with cutaneous lesions. TSS also can occur in males and females without a readily identifiable focus of infection. Prevailing clones (eg, USA300) of community-associated methicillin-resistant *S aureus* (MRSA) rarely produce TSS toxin. People with TSS, especially menses-associated illness, are at risk of a recurrent episode.

Staphylococcal scalded skin syndrome (SSSS).
SSS is a toxin-mediated disease caused by circulation of exfoliative toxins A and B. The manifestations of SSSS are age related and include Ritter disease (generalized exfoliation) in the neonate, a tender scarlatiniform eruption and localized bullous impetigo in older children, or a combination of these with thick white/brown flaky desquamation of the entire skin, especially on the face and neck, in older infants and toddlers. The hallmark of SSSS is the toxin-mediated cleavage of the stratum granulosum layer of the epidermis (ie, Nikolsky sign). Healing occurs without scarring. Bacteremia is rare, but dehydration and superinfection can occur with extensive exfoliation.

Coagulase-Negative Staphylococci. Most coagulase-negative staphylococci (CoNS) isolates from patient specimens represent contamination of culture material. Of the isolates that do not represent contamination, most come from infections that are associated with health care, in patients who have obvious disruptions of host defenses caused by surgery, medical device insertion, immunosuppression, or developmental maturity (eg, very low birth weight infants). CoNS are the most common cause of late-onset bacteremia and septicemia among preterm infants, typically infants weighing less than 1,500 g at birth, and of episodes of health care–associated bacteremia in all age groups. CoNS are responsible for bacteremia in children with intravascular catheters, CSF, peritoneal catheters, vascular grafts or

Box 123.1
Staphylococcus aureus **Toxic Shock Syndrome: Clinical Case Definition**[a]

Clinical Findings
- Fever: temperature ≥38.9°C (102.0°F)
- Rash: diffuse macular erythroderma
- Desquamation: 1–2 wk after onset, particularly on palms, soles, fingers, and toes
- Hypotension: systolic pressure ≤90 mm Hg for adults; lower than fifth percentile for age for children younger than 16 years; orthostatic drop in diastolic pressure of ≥15 mm Hg from lying to sitting; orthostatic syncope or orthostatic dizziness
- Multisystem organ involvement: ≥3 of the following:
  1. Gastrointestinal: vomiting or diarrhea at onset of illness
  2. Muscular: severe myalgia or creatinine phosphokinase concentration greater than twice the upper limit of normal
  3. Mucous membrane: vaginal, oropharyngeal, or conjunctival hyperemia
  4. Renal: serum urea nitrogen or serum creatinine concentration greater than twice the upper limit of normal or urinary sediment with 5 white blood cells/high-power field or greater in the absence of urinary tract infection
  5. Hepatic: total bilirubin, aspartate transaminase, or alanine transaminase concentration greater than twice the upper limit of normal
  6. Hematologic: platelet count ≤100,000/mm^3
  7. Central nervous system: disorientation or alterations in consciousness without focal neurologic signs when fever and hypotension are absent

Laboratory Criteria
- *Negative* results on the following tests, if obtained:
  — Blood, throat, or cerebrospinal fluid cultures; blood culture may be positive for *S aureus*
  — Serologic tests for Rocky Mountain spotted fever, leptospirosis, or measles

Case Classification
- ***Probable:*** a case that meets the laboratory criteria and in which 4 of 5 clinical findings are present
- ***Confirmed:*** a case that meets laboratory criteria and all 5 of the clinical findings, including desquamation, unless the patient dies before desquamation occurs

[a] Adapted from Wharton M, Chorba TL, Vogt RL, Morse DL, Buehler JW. Case definitions for public health surveillance. *MMWR Recomm Rep.* 1990;39(RR-13):1–43.

intracardiac patches, prosthetic cardiac valves, pacemaker wires, or prosthetic joints. Mediastinitis after open-heart surgery, endophthalmitis after intraocular trauma, and omphalitis and scalp abscesses in preterm neonates have been described. CoNS also can enter the bloodstream from the respiratory tract of mechanically ventilated preterm infants or from the gastrointestinal tract of infants with necrotizing enterocolitis. Some species of CoNS are associated with urinary tract infection, including *Staphylococcus saprophyticus* in adolescent females and young adult women, often after sexual intercourse, and *Staphylococcus epidermidis* and *Staphylococcus haemolyticus* in hospitalized patients with urinary tract catheters. In general, CoNS infections have an indolent clinical course in children with intact immune function and even in children who are immunocompromised.

Etiology

Staphylococci are catalase-positive, gram-positive cocci that appear microscopically as grape-like clusters. There are 32 species that are related closely on the basis of DNA base composition, but only 17 species are indigenous to humans. *S aureus* is the only species that produces coagulase. Of the 16 CoNS species, *S epidermidis, S haemolyticus, S saprophyticus, Staphylococcus schleiferi,* and *Staphylococcus lugdunensis* most often are associated with human infections. Staphylococci are ubiquitous and can survive extreme conditions of drying, heat, and low-oxygen and high-salt environments. *S aureus* has many surface proteins, including the microbial surface components recognizing adhesive matrix molecule receptors, which allow the organism to bind to tissues and foreign bodies coated with fibronectin, fibrinogen, and collagen. This permits a low inoculum of organisms to adhere to sutures, catheters, prosthetic valves, and other devices. Many CoNS produce an exopolysaccharide slime biofilm that makes these organisms, as they bind to medical devices (eg, catheters), relatively inaccessible to host defenses and antimicrobial agents.

Epidemiology

Staphylococcus aureus. *S aureus,* which is second only to CoNS as a cause of health care–associated bacteremia, is equal to *Pseudomonas aeruginosa* as the most common cause of health care–associated pneumonia in adults and is responsible for most health care–associated surgical site infections. *S aureus* colonizes the skin and mucous membranes of 30% to 50% of healthy adults and children. The anterior nares, throat, axilla, perineum, vagina, or rectum are usual sites of colonization. Rates of carriage of more than 50% occur in children with desquamating skin disorders or burns and in people with frequent needle use (eg, diabetes mellitus, hemodialysis, illicit drug use, allergy shots).

S aureus–mediated TSS was recognized in 1978, and many early cases were associated with tampon use. Although changes in tampon composition and use have resulted in a decreased proportion of cases associated with menses, menstrual and nonmenstrual cases of TSS continue to occur and are reported with similar frequency. Risk factors for TSS include absence of antibody to TSS toxin-1 and focal *S aureus* infection with a TSS toxin-1–producing strain. TSS toxin-1 producing strains can be part of normal flora of the anterior nares or vagina, and colonization at these sites is believed to result in protective antibody in more than 90% of adults. Health care–associated TSS can occur and most often follows surgical procedures. In postoperative cases, the organism generally originates from the patient's own flora.

***Transmission of* S aureus.** *S aureus* is transmitted most often by direct contact in community settings and indirectly from patient to patient via transiently colonized hands of health care professionals in health care settings. Health care professionals and family members who are colonized with *S aureus* in the nares or on skin also can serve as a reservoir for transmission. Contaminated environmental surfaces and objects also can play a role in transmission of *S aureus,* although their contribution to spread probably is minor. Although not transmitted by the droplet route routinely, *S aureus* can be dispersed into the air over short distances. Dissemination of *S aureus* from people, including infants, with nasal carriage is related to density of colonization, and increased dissemination occurs during viral upper respiratory tract infections. Additional risk factors for health care–associated acquisition of *S aureus* include illness requiring care in neonatal or pediatric intensive care or burn units, surgical procedures, prolonged hospitalization, local epidemic of *S aureus* infection, and the presence of indwelling catheters or prosthetic devices.

Staphylococcus aureus *Colonization and Disease.* Nasal, skin, vaginal, and rectal carriage are the primary reservoirs for *S aureus.* Although domestic animals can be colonized, data suggest that colonization is acquired from humans. Adults who carry MRSA in the nose preoperatively are more likely to develop surgical site infections after general, cardiac, orthopedic, or solid organ transplant surgery than are patients who are not carriers. Heavy cutaneous colonization at an insertion site is the single most important predictor of intravenous catheter-related infections for short-term percutaneously inserted catheters. For hemodialysis patients with *S aureus* skin colonization, the incidence of central line–associated bloodstream infection is sixfold higher than for patients without skin colonization. After head trauma, adults who are nasal carriers of *S aureus* are more likely to develop *S aureus* pneumonia than are noncolonized patients.

Health Care–Associated MRSA. MRSA has been endemic in most US hospitals since the 1980s, recently accounting for more than 60%

of health care–associated *S aureus* infections in intensive care units reported to the Centers for Disease Control and Prevention (CDC). Health care–associated MRSA strains are resistant to all beta-lactamase–resistant (BLR) beta-lactam antimicrobial agents and cephalosporins as well as to antimicrobial agents of several other classes (multidrug resistance). Methicillin-susceptible *S aureus* (MSSA) strains can be heterogeneous for methicillin resistance.

Risk factors for nasal carriage of health care–associated MRSA include hospitalization within the previous year, recent (within the previous 60 days) antimicrobial use, prolonged hospital stay, frequent contact with a health care environment, presence of an intravascular or peritoneal catheter or tracheal tube, increased number of surgical procedures, or frequent contact with a person with one or more of the preceding risk factors. A discharged patient known to have had colonization with MRSA should be assumed to have continued colonization when rehospitalized, because carriage can persist for years.

MRSA, both health care– and community-associated strains, and methicillin-resistant CoNS are responsible for a large portion of infections acquired in health care settings. A review of 25 pediatric hospitals demonstrated a 10-fold increase in MRSA infections since 1999 without change in the frequency of MSSA infections. Health care–associated MRSA strains are difficult to treat, because they usually are multidrug resistant and predictably susceptible only to vancomycin, linezolid, and agents not approved by the US Food and Drug Administration for use in children.

Community-Associated MRSA. Unique clones of MRSA are responsible for community-associated infections in healthy children and adults without typical risk factors for health care–associated MRSA infections. The most frequent manifestation of community-associated (CA) MRSA infections is skin and soft tissue infection, but invasive disease also occurs. Antimicrobial susceptibility patterns of these strains differ from those of health care–associated MRSA strains. Although CA MRSA are resistant to all beta-lactam antimicrobial agents, they typically are susceptible

to multiple other antimicrobial agents, including trimethoprim-sulfamethoxazole, gentamicin, and doxycycline; clindamycin susceptibility is variable. A review of prescribing patterns among 25 pediatric hospitals has demonstrated clindamycin to be the most commonly prescribed antimicrobial agent for non–life-threatening MRSA infections. However, attention to local resistance rates of *S aureus* to clindamycin is imperative, because CA MRSA and MSSA with intrinsic resistance to clindamycin exceeding 20% have been reported by some institutions. CA MRSA infections have occurred in settings where there is crowding; frequent skin-to-skin contact; body piercing; sharing of personal items, such as towels and clothing; and poor personal hygiene, such as occurs among athletic teams, in correctional facilities, and in military training facilities. However, most CA MRSA infections occur in people without direct links to those settings. Transmission of CA MRSA from an infected classmate or team member has been described in child care centers and among sports teams. Although CA MRSA arose from the community, in many health care settings, these clones are overtaking health care–associated MRSA strains as a cause of health care–associated MRSA infections, making the terms "health care–associated" and "community-associated" less useful.

Vancomycin–Intermediately Susceptible S aureus. Strains of MRSA with intermediate susceptibility to vancomycin (minimum inhibitory concentration [MIC], 4–8 μg/mL) have been isolated from people (historically, dialysis patients) who had received multiple courses of vancomycin for a MRSA infection. Strains of MRSA can be heterogeneous for vancomycin resistance. Extensive vancomycin use allows vancomycin–intermediately susceptible *S aureus* (VISA) strains to grow. These strains can emerge during therapy. Recommended control measures from the CDC have included using proper methods to detect VISA, using appropriate infection-control measures, and adopting measures to ensure appropriate vancomycin use. Although rare, outbreaks of VISA and heteroresistant VISA have been reported in France, Spain, and Japan.

Vancomycin-Resistant S aureus. In 2002, 2 isolates of vancomycin-resistant *S aureus* (VRSA [MIC, ≥16 µg/mL]) were identified in adults from 2 different states. As of November 2011, VRSA had been isolated from 12 adults from 4 states. Each of these adults with VRSA infections had underlying medical conditions, a history of MRSA infections, and prolonged exposure to vancomycin. No spread of VRSA beyond case patients has been documented. A concern is that most automated antimicrobial susceptibility testing methods commonly used in the United States were unable to detect vancomycin resistance in these isolates.

Coagulase-Negative Staphylococci. CoNS are common inhabitants of the skin and mucous membranes. Virtually all infants have colonization at multiple sites by 2 to 4 days of age. The most frequently isolated CoNS organism is *S epidermidis*. Different species colonize specific areas of the body. *S haemolyticus* is found on areas of skin with numerous apocrine glands. The frequency of health care–associated CoNS infections increased steadily until 2000, when these infections seem to have plateaued. Infants and children in intensive care units, including neonatal intensive care units, have the highest incidence of CoNS bloodstream infections. CoNS can be introduced at the time of medical device placement, through mucous membrane or skin breaks, through loss of bowel wall integrity (eg, necrotizing enterocolitis in very low birth weight neonates), or during catheter manipulation. Less often, health care professionals with environmental CoNS colonization on hands transmit the organism.

Methicillin-resistant CoNS. Methicillin-resistant CoNS account for most health care–associated CoNS infections. Methicillin-resistant strains are resistant to all beta-lactam drugs, including cephalosporins, and usually several other drug classes.

Incubation Period

Variable. For toxin-mediated SSSS, 1 to 10 days; postoperative SSSS, as short as 12 hours.

Diagnostic Tests

Gram-stained smears of material from skin lesions or pyogenic foci showing gram-positive cocci in pairs and clusters can provide presumptive evidence of infection. Isolation of organisms from culture of otherwise sterile body fluid is the method for definitive diagnosis. *S aureus* almost never is a contaminant when isolated from a blood culture. CoNS isolated from a single blood culture commonly are dismissed as "contaminants." In very preterm neonates, immunocompromised persons, or patients with an indwelling catheter or prosthetic device, repeated isolation of the same strain of CoNS (by antimicrobial susceptibility results or molecular techniques) from blood cultures or another normally sterile body fluid suggests true infection, but genotyping more strongly supports the diagnosis. For central line–association bloodstream infection, quantitative blood cultures from the catheter will have 5 to 10 times more organisms than cultures from a peripheral blood vessel. Criteria that suggest CoNS as pathogens rather than contaminants include the following:

- Two or more positive blood cultures from different collection sites
- A single positive culture from blood and another sterile site (eg, CSF, joint) with identical antimicrobial susceptibility patterns for each isolate
- Growth in a continuously monitored blood culture system within 15 hours of incubation
- Clinical findings of infection
- An intravascular catheter that has been in place for 3 days or more
- Similar or identical genotypes among all isolates

S aureus-mediated TSS is a clinical diagnosis. *S aureus* grows in culture of blood specimens from fewer than 5% of patients. Specimens for culture should be obtained from an identified site of infection, because these sites usually will yield the organism. Because approximately one-third of isolates of *S aureus* from nonmenstrual cases produce toxins other than TSS toxin-1, and TSS toxin-1-producing organisms can be present as normal flora, TSS-1 production by an isolate is not useful diagnostically.

Quantitative antimicrobial susceptibility testing should be performed for all staphylococci, including CoNS, isolated from normally sterile sites. Health care–associated MRSA heterogeneous or heterotypic strains appear susceptible by disk testing. However, when a parent strain is cultured on methicillin-containing media, resistant subpopulations are apparent.

A large proportion of CA *S aureus* strains are methicillin resistant, and more than 90% of health care–associated *S aureus* as well as CoNS strains are methicillin and multidrug resistant. Because of the high rates of CA MRSA infections in the United States, clindamycin has become an often-used drug for treatment of non–life-threatening presumed *S aureus* infections. Routine antimicrobial susceptibility testing of *S aureus* strains historically did not include a method to detect strains susceptible to clindamycin that rapidly become clindamycin resistant when exposed to this agent. This clindamycin-inducible resistance can be detected by the D zone test. When a MRSA isolate is determined to be erythromycin resistant and clindamycin susceptible by routine methods, the D zone test is performed. Patients with MRSA isolates that demonstrate clindamycin-inducible resistance should not receive clindamycin routinely. All *S aureus* strains with an MIC to vancomycin

of 4 μg/mL or greater should be confirmed and further characterized. Early detection of VISA is critical to trigger aggressive infection-control measures.

S aureus and CoNS strain genotyping has become a necessary adjunct for determining whether several isolates from one patient or from different patients are the same. Typing, in conjunction with epidemiologic information, can facilitate identification of the source, extent, and mechanism of transmission in an outbreak. Antimicrobial susceptibility testing is the most readily available method for typing by a phenotypic characteristic. A number of molecular typing methods are available for *S aureus* (Box 123.2).

Treatment

The most frequent manifestation of CA MRSA infection is skin and soft tissue infection. The figure shows the initial management of skin and soft tissue infections suspected to be caused by CA MRSA. Serious MSSA infections require intravenous therapy with a BLR beta-lactam antimicrobial agent, such as nafcillin or oxacillin, because most *S aureus* strains produce beta-lactamase enzymes and are resistant to penicillin and ampicillin (see Table 123.1). First- or second-generation cephalosporins (eg, cefazolin or cefuroxime)

Box 123.2
Recommendations for Detecting *Staphylococcus aureus* With Decreased Susceptibility to Vancomycin[a]

Definitions
- **Vancomycin-susceptible *S aureus***
  MIC ≤2 μg/mL
- **Vancomycin-intermediately susceptible *S aureus* (VISA)**
  MIC 4–8 μg/mL
  Not transferable to susceptible strains
- **Vancomycin-resistant *S aureus* (VRSA)**
  MIC ≥16 μg/mL
  Potentially transferable to susceptible strains
- **Confirmation of VISA and VRSA**
  Possible VISA and VRSA isolates should be retested using vancomycin screen plates or a validated MIC method.
  VISA and VRSA isolates should be reported to the local health department or CDC.

Abbreviations: CDC, Centers for Disease Control and Prevention; MIC, minimum inhibitory concentration.
[a] Hageman JC, Patel JB, Carey RC, Tenover FC, McDonald LC. *Investigation and Control of Vancomycin-Intermediate and –Resistant Staphylococcus aureus (VISA/VRSA): A Guide for Health Departments and Infection Control Personnel*. Atlanta, GA: Centers for Disease Control and Prevention; 2006.

Table 123.1

Parenteral Antimicrobial Agent(s) for Treatment of Bacteremia and Other Serious *Staphylococcus aureus* Infections

Susceptibility	Antimicrobial Agents	Comments
I. Initial empirical therapy (organism of unknown susceptibility)		
Drugs of choice	Vancomycin (15 mg/kg q6h)+ nafcillin or oxacillin	For life-threatening infections (ie, septicemia, endocarditis, CNS infection); linezolid could be substituted for vancomycin if the patient has received several recent courses of vancomycin
	Vancomycin (15 mg/kg q8h)	For non–life-threatening infection without signs of sepsis (eg, skin infection, cellulitis, osteomyelitis, pyarthrosis) when rates of MRSA colonization and infection in the community are substantial
	Clindamycin	For non–life-threatening infection without signs of sepsis when rates of MRSA colonization and infection in the community are substantial and prevalence of clindamycin resistance is low
II. Methicillin-susceptible, penicillin-resistant S aureus (MSSA)		
Drugs of choice	Nafcillin or oxacillin[a]	
Alternatives	Cefazolin	
	Clindamycin	Only for patients with a serious penicillin allergy and clindamycin-susceptible strain
	Vancomycin	Only for patients with a serious penicillin and cephalosporin allergy
	Ampicillin + sulbactam	
III. MRSA (oxacillin MIC, ≥4 µg/mL)		
A. Health care–associated (multidrug resistant)		
Drugs of choice	Vancomycin + gentamicin[a]	
Alternatives: susceptibility testing results available before alternative drugs are used	Trimethoprim-sulfamethoxazole	
	Linezolid[b]	
	Quinupristin-dalfopristin[b]	
	Fluoroquinolones	Not recommended for people <18 years or as monotherapy

Table 123.1
Parenteral Antimicrobial Agent(s) for Treatment of Bacteremia and Other Serious *Staphylococcus aureus* Infections, continued

Susceptibility	Antimicrobial Agents	Comments
III. MRSA (oxacillin MIC, ≥4 μg/mL), continued		
B. Community-associated (not multidrug resistant)		
Drugs of choice	Vancomycin + gentamicin	For life-threatening infections
	Clindamycin (if strain susceptible)	For pneumonia, septic arthritis, osteomyelitis, skin or soft tissue infections
	Trimethoprim-sulfamethoxazole	For skin or soft tissue infections
Alternative	Vancomycin	
IV. Vancomycin-intermediately susceptible S aureus (MIC, 4–16 μg/mL)b		
Drugs of choice	Optimal therapy is not known	Dependent on in vitro susceptibility test results
	Linezolid[b]	
	Daptomycin[c]	
	Quinupristin-dalfopristin[b]	
	Tigecycline[b]	
Alternatives	Vancomycin + linezolid ± gentamicin	
	Vancomycin + trimethoprim-sulfa-methoxazole[a]	

Abbreviations: CNS, central nervous system; MIC, minimum inhibitory concentration; MRSA, methicillin-resistant *S aureus*.

[a] One of the adjunctive agents, gentamicin or rifampin, should be added to the therapeutic regimen for life-threatening infections such as endocarditis or CNS infection or infections with a vancomycin-intermediate *S aureus* strain. Consultation with an infectious diseases specialist should be considered to determine which agent to use and duration of use.

[b] Linezolid, quinupristin-dalfopristin, and tigecycline are agents with activity in vitro and efficacy in adults with multidrug-resistant, gram-positive organisms, including *S aureus*. Because experience with these agents in children is limited, consultation with an infectious diseases specialist should be considered before use.

[c] Daptomycin is active in vitro against multidrug-resistant, gram-positive organisms, including *S aureus*, but has not been evaluated in children. Daptomycin is approved by the US Food and Drug Administration only for treatment of complicated skin and skin structure infections and for *S aureus* bloodstream infections. Daptomycin is ineffective for treatment of pneumonia and is not indicated in patients 18 years of age and older.

or vancomycin are effective but less so than nafcillin or oxacillin, especially for some sites of infection (eg, endocarditis, meningitis). Furthermore, nafcillin or oxacillin, rather than vancomycin (or clindamycin if the S aureus strain is susceptible to this agent), is recommended for treatment of serious MSSA infections to minimize emergence of vancomycin- or clindamycin-resistant strains. Treatment of serious MRSA infections in adults does not support addition of gentamicin or rifampin to vancomycin because of an increase in adverse effects and lack of greater efficacy of the combination versus monotherapy. A patient who has a nonserious allergy to penicillin can be treated with a first- or second-generation cephalosporin, and if the patient is not also allergic to cephalosporins, with vancomycin or with clindamycin, if endocarditis or central nervous system infection is not a consideration and the S aureus strain is susceptible.

Intravenous vancomycin is recommended for treatment of serious infections caused by staphylococcal strains resistant to BLR beta-lactam antimicrobial agents (eg, MRSA and all CoNS). For empirical therapy of life-threatening S aureus infections, initial therapy should include vancomycin and a BLR beta-lactam antimicrobial agent (eg, nafcillin, oxacillin) if the isolate is MSSA. For hospital-acquired CoNS infections, vancomycin is the drug of choice. Subsequent therapy should be determined by antimicrobial susceptibility results.

Duration of therapy for serious MSSA or MRSA infections depends on the site and severity of infection but usually is 4 weeks or more for endocarditis, osteomyelitis, necrotizing pneumonia, or disseminated infection. After initial parenteral therapy and documented clinical improvement, completion of the course with an oral drug can be considered in older children if adherence can be ensured and endocarditis or central nervous system (CNS) infection is not a consideration. For endocarditis and CNS infection, parenteral therapy is recommended for the entire treatment. Drainage of abscesses and removal of foreign bodies is desirable and almost always is required for medical treatment to be effective.

As summarized in Box 123.3, the first priority in management of S aureus TSS is aggressive fluid management as well as management of respiratory or cardiac failure, if present. Initial antimicrobial therapy should include a parenterally administered beta-lactam antistaphylococcal antimicrobial agent and a protein synthesis-inhibiting drug, such as clindamycin, at maximum dosages. Vancomycin should be substituted for BLR penicillins or cephalosporins in regions where CA MRSA infections are common. Once the organism is identified and susceptibility is known, therapy for S aureus should be modified, but an active antimicrobial agent should be continued for 10 to 14 days. Administration of antimicrobial agents can be changed to the oral route once the patient is tolerating oral alimentation. The total duration of therapy is based on the usual duration of established foci of infection (eg, pneumonia, osteomyelitis). Aggressive drainage and irrigation of accessible sites of purulent infection should be per-

Box 123.3
Management of Staphylococcal Toxic Shock Syndrome

- Fluid management to maintain adequate venous return and cardiac filling pressures to prevent end-organ damage
- Anticipatory management of multisystem organ failure
- Parenteral antimicrobial therapy at maximum doses
    - Kill organism with bactericidal cell wall inhibitor (eg, beta-lactamase–resistant antistaphylococcal antimicrobial agent)
    - Reduce enzyme or toxin production with protein synthesis inhibitor (eg, clindamycin)
- Immune Globulin Intravenous may be considered for infection refractory to several hours of aggressive therapy or in the presence of an undrainable focus or persistent oliguria with pulmonary edema

formed as soon as possible. All foreign bodies, including those recently inserted during surgery, should be removed if possible. Immune globulin intravenous (IGIV) can be considered in patients with severe staphylococcal TSS unresponsive to all other therapeutic measures, because IGIV may neutralize circulating toxin. The optimal IGIV regimen is unknown. SSSS in infants should be treated with a parenteral BLR beta-lactam antimicrobial agent or, if MRSA is a consideration, vancomycin. In older children, depending on severity, oral agents can be considered. Skin and soft tissue infections, such as impetigo or cellulitis attributable to S aureus, can be treated with oral penicillinase-resistant beta-lactam drugs, such as cloxacillin, dicloxacillin, or a first- or second-generation cephalosporin. However, the continued increase in prevalence of CA MRSA throughout the United States may limit the utility of these agents. In this situation, or for the penicillin-allergic patient, trimethoprim-sulfamethoxazole, doxycycline in children 8 years of age and older, or clindamycin can be used if the isolate is susceptible. Trimethoprim-sulfamethoxazole should not be used as a single agent in the initial treatment of cellulitis, because it is not active against group A streptococci.

Duration of therapy for central line–associated bloodstream infections is controversial and depends on consideration of a number of factors, including the organism (S aureus vs CoNS), the type and location of the catheter, the site of infection (exit site vs tunnel vs line), the feasibility of using an alternative vessel at a later date, and the presence or absence of a catheter-related thrombus. Infections are more difficult to treat when associated with a thrombus, thrombophlebitis, or intra-atrial thrombus. If a central line can be removed, there is no demonstrable thrombus, and bacteremia resolves promptly, a short course of therapy seems appropriate for CoNS infections in the immunocompetent host. A longer course is suggested if the patient is immunocompromised or the organism is S aureus; experts differ on recommended duration. If the patient needs a new central line, waiting 48 to 72 hours after bacteremia apparently has resolved before insertion is optimal. If a tunneled catheter is needed for ongoing care, in situ treatment of the infection can be attempted. If the patient responds to antimicrobial therapy with immediate resolution of the S aureus bacteremia, treatment should be continued for 10 to 14 days parenterally. Antimicrobial lock therapy of tunneled central lines may result in a higher rate of catheter salvage in adults with CoNS infections, but experience with this approach is limited in children. If blood cultures remain positive for staphylococci for more than 3 to 5 days or if the clinical illness fails to improve, the central line should be removed, parenteral therapy should be continued, and the patient should be evaluated for metastatic foci of infection. Vegetations or a thrombus in the heart or great vessels always should be considered when a central line becomes infected. Transesophageal echocardiography, if feasible, is the most sensitive technique for identifying vegetations.

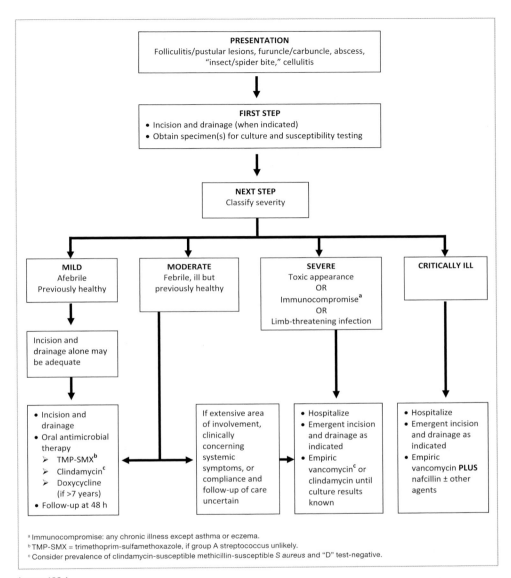

PRESENTATION
Folliculitis/pustular lesions, furuncle/carbuncle, abscess, "insect/spider bite," cellulitis

FIRST STEP
- Incision and drainage (when indicated)
- Obtain specimen(s) for culture and susceptibility testing

NEXT STEP
Classify severity

MILD
Afebrile
Previously healthy

MODERATE
Febrile, ill but previously healthy

SEVERE
Toxic appearance
OR
Immunocompromise[a]
OR
Limb-threatening infection

CRITICALLY ILL

Incision and drainage alone may be adequate

- Incision and drainage
- Oral antimicrobial therapy
  - TMP-SMX[b]
  - Clindamycin[c]
  - Doxycycline (if >7 years)
- Follow-up at 48 h

If extensive area of involvement, clinically concerning systemic symptoms, or compliance and follow-up of care uncertain

- Hospitalize
- Emergent incision and drainage as indicated
- Empiric vancomycin[c] or clindamycin until culture results known

- Hospitalize
- Emergent incision and drainage as indicated
- Empiric vancomycin **PLUS** nafcillin ± other agents

[a] Immunocompromise: any chronic illness except asthma or eczema.
[b] TMP-SMX = trimethoprim-sulfamethoxazole, if group A streptococcus unlikely.
[c] Consider prevalence of clindamycin-susceptible methicillin-susceptible S aureus and "D" test-negative.

Image 123.1
Algorithm for initial management of skin and soft tissue infections caused by community-associated *Staphylococcus aureus*.

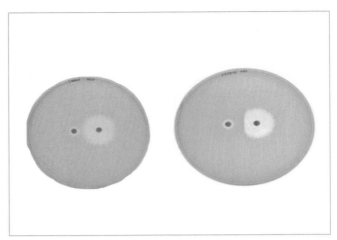

Image 123.2
D zone test for clindamycin-induced resistance by *Staphylococcus aureus*. The left shows a negative result and the right shows a positive one. Courtesy of Sarah Long, MD, FAAP.

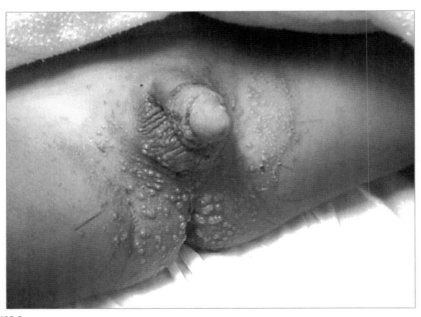

Image 123.3
Infant with pustulosis of the perineum and genitalia due to *Staphylococcus aureus*. Copyright Michael Rajnik, MD, FAAP.

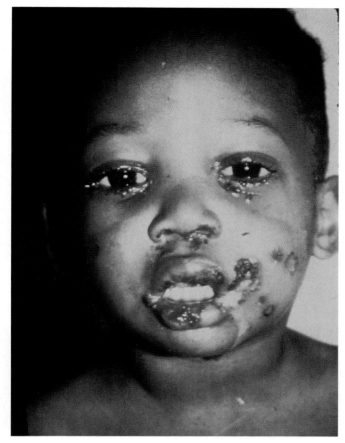

Image 123.4
Staphylococcal bullous impetigo lesions about the eyes, nose, and mouth in a 6-year-old black male. Also note the secondary anterior cervical lymphadenopathy. Courtesy of George Nankervis, MD.

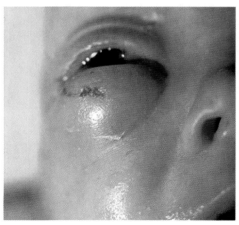

Image 123.5
An infant with orbital cellulitis and ethmoid sinusitis due to *Staphylococcus aureus*. Copyright Martin G. Myers, MD.

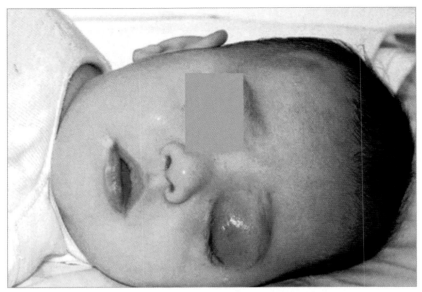

Image 123.6
Periorbital cellulitis due to *Staphylococcus aureus*.

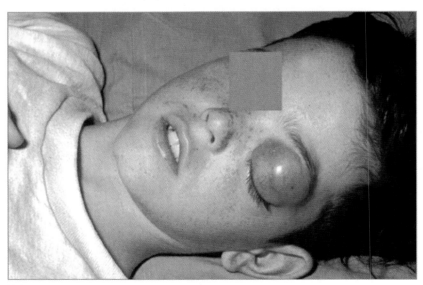

Image 123.7
Orbital abscess with proptosis of the globe due to *Staphylococcus aureus* in a 12-year-old boy. Delayed surgical drainage contributed to permanent visual impairment due to central retinal vascular involvement. The patient also had left ethmoid and maxillary sinusitis.

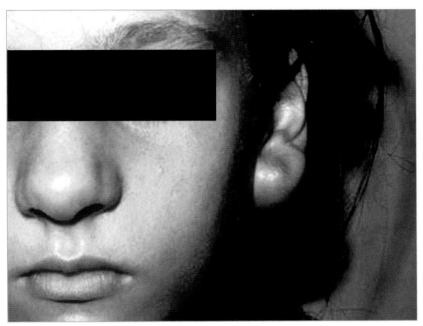

Image 123.8
Staphylococcus aureus abscess of left earlobe secondary to ear piercing. Courtesy of Edgar O. Ledbetter, MD, FAAP.

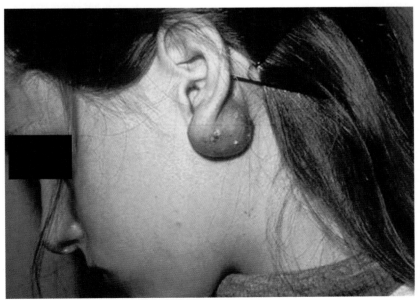

Image 123.9
Staphylococcus aureus abscess of the lobe of the left ear secondary to ear piercing in an adolescent girl. This is the same patient as in Image 123.8. Courtesy of Edgar O. Ledbetter, MD, FAAP.

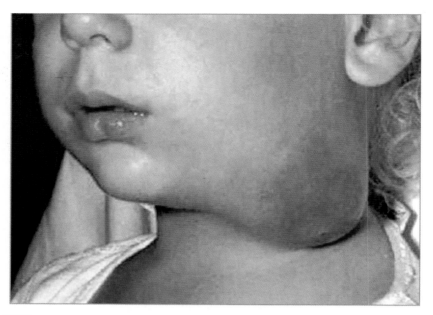

Image 123.10
Cervical adenitis with abscess formation due to *Staphylococcus aureus.* Delay in seeking medical care resulted in spontaneous drainage of the abscess.

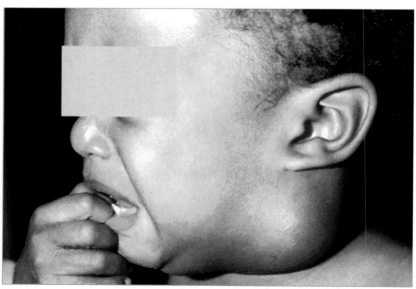

Image 123.11
Subauricular cervical adenitis *Staphylococcus aureus* in a 2-year-old boy. Copyright Neal Halsey, MD.

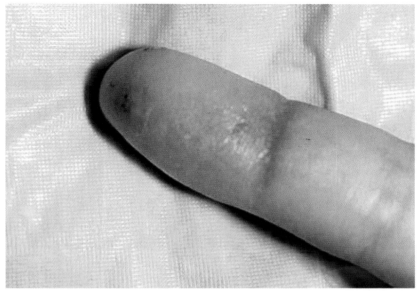

Image 123.12
A 15-year-old with Fanconi anemia with *Staphylococcus aureus* infection at the finger-stick site. Copyright Martin G. Myers, MD.

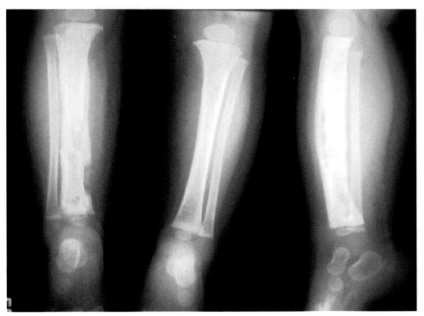

Image 123.13
Chronic osteomyelitis of the right tibia due to *Staphylococcus aureus*.

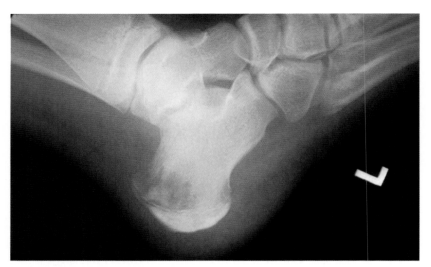

Image 123.14
Osteomyelitis of the calcaneus due to *Staphylococcus aureus* with no history of injury.

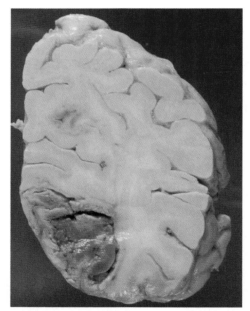

Image 123.15
Cerebral infarct in a patient with bacterial endocarditis.
Courtesy of Dimitris P. Agamanolis, MD.

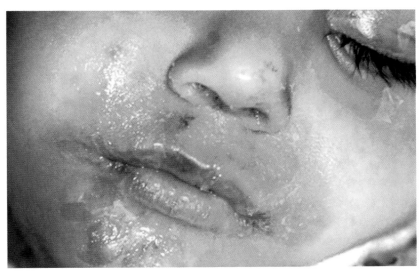

Image 123.16
Staphylococcal scalded skin syndrome. Epidermolytic toxins A and B are the components of *Staphylococcus aureus* thought to cause this syndrome.

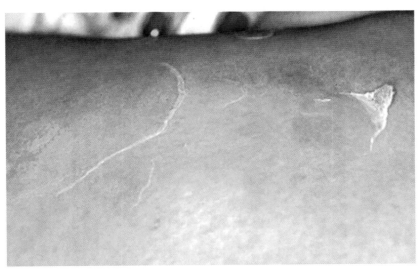

Image 123.17
Staphylococcal scalded skin syndrome with a positive Nikolsky sign.

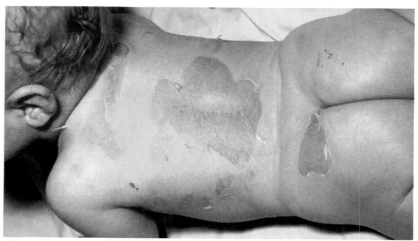

Image 123.18
Infant with staphylococcal scalded skin syndrome with sheets of skin desquamation.

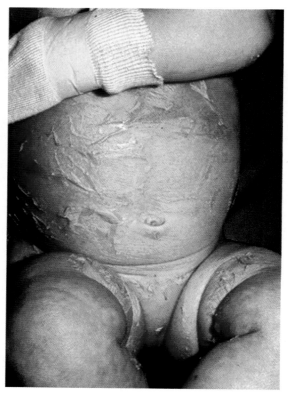

Image 123.19
Staphylococcal scalded skin syndrome. Epidermolytic exotoxin results in superficial, generalized desquamation. Courtesy of Edgar O. Ledbetter, MD, FAAP.

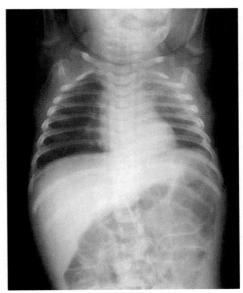

Image 123.20
Staphylococcal pneumonia, primary, with rapid progression and with empyema. The infant had only mild respiratory distress and paralytic ileus without fever when first examined.

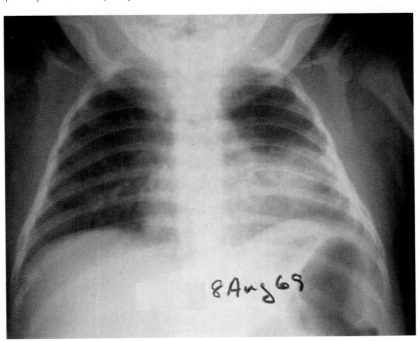

Image 123.21
Pneumonia (primary) with pneumatoceles due to *Staphylococcus aureus* in a 3-week-old infant.

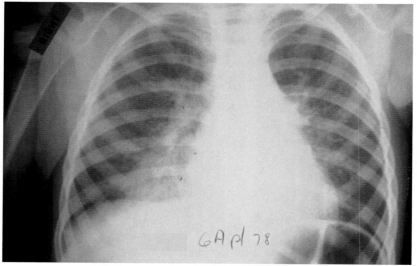

Image 123.22
Pneumonia due to *Staphylococcus aureus* with right lower lobe infiltrate in a preschool-aged child (Day 1). Courtesy of Edgar O. Ledbetter, MD, FAAP.

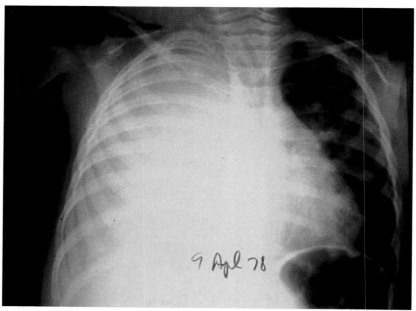

Image 123.23
Staphylococcal pneumonia with massive empyema demonstrating the rather rapid progression typical of staphylococcal infection. This is the same patient as in Image 123.22 (Day 4). Courtesy of Edgar O. Ledbetter, MD, FAAP.

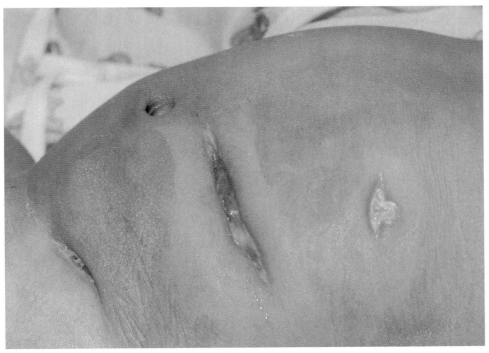

Image 123.24
Staphylococcus aureus necrotizing fasciitis in an 8-month-old female. Copyright Benjamin Estrada, MD.

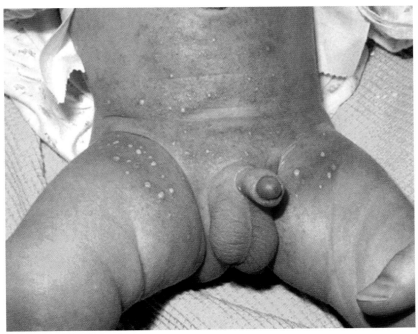

Image 123.25
Pyoderma due to *Staphylococcus aureus* in a young infant.

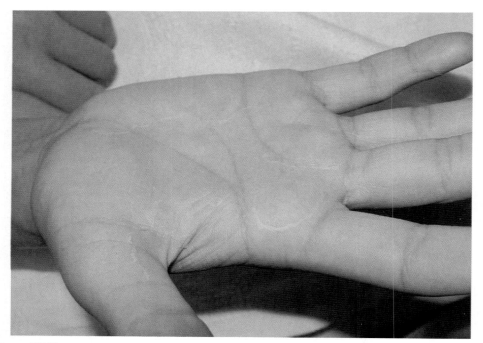

Image 123.26
Digit and palm desquamation in a 15-year-old male during staphylococcal toxic shock syndrome convalescence. Copyright Benjamin Estrada, MD.

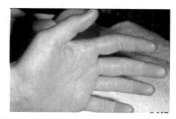

Image 123.27
Characteristic erythroderma of the hand of the patient in Image 123.26 with staphylococcal toxic shock syndrome.

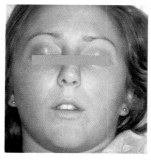

Image 123.28
Facial erythroderma secondary to *Staphylococcus aureus* toxic shock syndrome in a woman who was obtunded and hypotensive on admission.

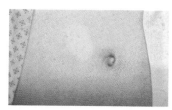

Image 123.29
Erythroderma that blanches on pressure in a patient with toxic shock syndrome. The mortality rate for staphylococcal toxic shock syndrome is lower than that of streptococcal toxic shock syndrome.

124

Group A Streptococcal Infections

Clinical Manifestations

The most common group A streptococcal (GAS) infection is acute pharyngotonsillitis. Purulent complications of pharyngotonsillitis, including otitis media, sinusitis, peritonsillar and retropharyngeal abscesses, and suppurative cervical adenitis, develop in some patients, usually those who are untreated. Nonsuppurative sequelae include acute rheumatic fever (ARF) and acute glomerulonephritis. The goals of antimicrobial therapy for GAS upper respiratory tract disease are to reduce acute morbidity, nonsuppurative sequelae (acute rheumatic fever and acute glomerulonephritis), and transmission to close contacts.

Scarlet fever occurs most often in association with pharyngitis and, rarely, with pyoderma or an infected wound. Scarlet fever has a characteristic confluent erythematous sandpaper-like rash that is caused by one or more of several erythrogenic exotoxins produced by group A streptococci. Severe scarlet fever occurs rarely. Other than occurrence of rash, the epidemiologic features, symptoms, signs, sequelae, and treatment of scarlet fever are the same as those of streptococcal pharyngitis. Toddlers (1–3 years of age) with GAS respiratory tract infection initially can have serous rhinitis and then develop a protracted illness with moderate fever, irritability, and anorexia (streptococcal fever or streptococcosis). Acute pharyngotonsillitis is uncommon in children younger than 3 years.

The second most common site of GAS infection is the skin. Streptococcal skin infections (ie, pyoderma or impetigo) can result in acute glomerulonephritis, which occasionally occurs in epidemics. ARF is not a sequela of GAS skin infection.

Other manifestations of GAS infections include erysipelas, perianal cellulitis, vaginitis, bacteremia, pneumonia, endocarditis, pericarditis, septic arthritis, cellulitis, necrotizing fasciitis, purpura fulminans, osteomyelitis, myositis, puerperal sepsis, surgical wound infection, acute otitis media, sinusitis, retropharyngeal abscess, peritonsillar abscess, mastoiditis, and neonatal omphalitis. Invasive GAS infections can be severe, may or may not be associated with an identified focus of local infection, and can be associated with streptococcal toxic shock syndrome (STSS) or necrotizing fasciitis. Severe infection can follow minor or unrecognized trauma. An association between GAS infection and sudden onset of obsessive-compulsive or tic disorders—pediatric autoimmune neuropsychiatric disorders associated with streptococcal infections—has been proposed but is unproven.

STSS is caused by toxin-producing GAS strains and typically manifests as an acute illness characterized by fever, generalized erythroderma, rapid-onset hypotension, and signs of multiorgan involvement, including rapidly progressive renal failure (see Box 124.1). Evidence of local soft tissue infection (eg, cellulitis, myositis, or necrotizing fasciitis) associated with severe, rapidly increasing pain is common, but STSS can occur without an identifiable focus of infection. STSS also can be associated with invasive infections, such as bacteremia, pneumonia, pleural empyema, osteomyelitis, pyarthrosis, or endocarditis.

Etiology

More than 120 distinct serotypes or genotypes of group A beta-hemolytic streptococci (*Streptococcus pyogenes*) have been identified based on M-protein serotype or M-protein gene sequence (*emm* types). Most cases of STSS are caused by strains producing at least 1 of several different pyrogenic exotoxins, most commonly streptococcal pyrogenic exotoxin A. These toxins act as superantigens that stimulate production of tumor necrosis factor and other inflammatory mediators that cause capillary leak and other physiologic changes, leading to hypotension and organ damage.

Epidemiology

Pharyngitis usually results from contact with a person who has GAS pharyngitis. Fomites and household pets, such as dogs, are not vectors of GAS infection. Transmission of GAS infection, including in school outbreaks of pharyngitis, almost always follows contact with respiratory

Box 124.1
Streptococcal Toxic Shock Syndrome: Clinical Case Definition[a,b]

I. Isolation of group A streptococcus *(Streptococcus pyogenes)*
   A. From a normally sterile site (eg, blood, cerebrospinal fluid, peritoneal fluid, or tissue biopsy specimen)
   B. From a nonsterile site (eg, throat, sputum, vagina, open surgical wound, or superficial skin lesion)
II. Clinical signs of severity
   A. Hypotension: systolic pressure ≤90 mm Hg in adults or lower than the fifth percentile for age in children

AND

   B. ≥2 of the following signs:
   - Renal impairment: creatinine concentration ≥177 μmol/L (2 mg/dL) for adults or at least 2 times the upper limit of normal for age
   - Coagulopathy: platelet count ≤100,000/mm³ or disseminated intravascular coagulation
   - Hepatic involvement: elevated alanine transaminase, aspartate transaminase, or total bilirubin concentrations at least 2 times the upper limit of normal for age
   - Adult respiratory distress syndrome
   - A generalized erythematous macular rash that may desquamate
   - Soft tissue necrosis, including necrotizing fasciitis or myositis, or gangrene

[a] Adapted from The Working Group on Severe Streptococcal Infections. Defining the group A streptococcal toxic shock syndrome: rationale and consensus definition. *JAMA.* 1993;269(3):390–39.

[b] An illness fulfilling criteria IA and IIA and IIB can be defined as a definite case. An illness fulfilling criteria IB and IIA and IIB can be defined as a *probable* case if no other cause for the illness is identified.

tract secretions. Pharyngitis and impetigo (and their nonsuppurative complications) can be associated with crowding, which often is present in socioeconomically disadvantaged populations. The close contact that occurs in schools, child care centers, contact sports (eg, wrestling), boarding schools, and military installations facilitates transmission. Foodborne outbreaks of pharyngitis occur rarely and are a consequence of human contamination of food in conjunction with improper food preparation or improper refrigeration procedures. Streptococcal pharyngitis occurs at all ages but is most common among school-aged children and adolescents. GAS pharyngitis and pyoderma are less common in adults than in children.

Geographically, GAS pharyngitis and pyoderma are ubiquitous. Pyoderma is more common in tropical climates and warm seasons, presumably because of antecedent insect bites and other minor skin trauma. Streptococcal pharyngitis is more common during late autumn, winter, and spring in temperate climates, presumably because of close person-to-person contact in schools. Communicability of patients with streptococcal pharyngitis is highest during acute infection and untreated gradually diminishes over a period of weeks. Patients are not considered to be contagious beginning 24 hours after initiation of appropriate antimicrobial therapy.

Throat culture surveys of healthy asymptomatic children during school outbreaks of pharyngitis have yielded GAS prevalence rates as high as 20%. These surveys identified children who were pharyngeal carriers. Carriage of GAS can persist for months, but risk of transmission to others is low.

The incidence of acute rheumatic fever in the United States decreased sharply during the 20th century. Rates of this nonsuppurative sequela likely still are low, although the true incidence in the United States is unknown, because ARF no longer is a nationally reportable condition. Focal outbreaks of ARF in school-aged children occurred in several areas throughout the 1990s, and small clusters continue to be reported periodically. Although reasons for these focal outbreaks are not completely clear, they most likely relate to increased circulation of rheumatogenic strains, and their occurrence reemphasizes the importance of diagnosing GAS pharyngitis and treating with a recommended antimicrobial regimen.

In streptococcal impetigo, the organism usually is acquired by direct contact from another person with impetigo. GAS colonization of healthy skin usually precedes development of impetigo, but group A streptococci do not penetrate intact skin. Impetiginous lesions occur at the site of breaks in skin (eg, insect bites, burns, traumatic wounds, varicella). After development of impetiginous lesions, the upper respiratory tract often becomes colonized with GAS. Infection of surgical wounds and postpartum (puerperal) sepsis usually result from contact transmission. Anal or vaginal carriers and people with skin infection can transmit GAS to surgical and obstetrical patients, resulting in health care–associated outbreaks. Infections in neonates result from intrapartum or contact transmission; in the latter situation, infection can begin as omphalitis, cellulitis, or necrotizing fasciitis.

The incidence of invasive GAS infections is highest in infants and the elderly. Before use of varicella vaccine, varicella was the most commonly identified predisposing factor in children with GAS infection. Other factors increasing risk for invasive GAS disease among children include exposure to other children and household crowding. The portal of entry is unknown in most invasive GAS infections; and the entry site is presumed to be skin or mucous membranes. Such infections rarely follow symptomatic GAS pharyngitis.

The incidence of GAS-mediated TSS is highest among young children, although STSS can occur at any age. Of all cases of invasive streptococcal infections in children, fewer than 5% are associated with documented STSS. Among children, STSS has been reported with focal lesions (eg, varicella, cellulitis, trauma, osteomyelitis), pneumonia, and bacteremia without a defined focus. Mortality rates are substantially lower for children than for adults with GAS-mediated STSS.

Incubation Period

Pharyngitis, 2 to 5 days; impetigo, 7 to 10 days; STSS, unknown.

Diagnostic Tests

Laboratory confirmation of GAS pharyngitis is recommended for children, because accurate clinical differentiation of viral and GAS pharyngitis is difficult, except in children with obvious viral symptoms (eg, rhinorrhea, cough, hoarseness). A specimen should be obtained by vigorous swabbing of both tonsils and the posterior pharynx for culture and/or rapid antigen testing. Culture on sheep blood agar can confirm GAS infection, with latex agglutination differentiating group A streptococci from other beta-hemolytic streptococci. False-negative culture results occur in fewer than 10% of symptomatic patients when an adequate throat swab specimen is obtained and cultured by trained personnel. Recovery of group A streptococci from the pharynx does not distinguish patients with true streptococcal infection (defined by a serologic response to extracellular antigens [eg, streptolysin O]) from streptococcal carriers who have an intercurrent viral pharyngitis. The number of colonies of group A streptococci on an agar culture plate also does not differentiate true infection from carriage. Cultures that are negative for group A streptococci after 18 to 24 hours should be incubated for a second day to optimize recovery of group A streptococci.

Several rapid diagnostic tests for GAS pharyngitis are available. Most are based on nitrous acid extraction of group A carbohydrate antigen from organisms obtained by throat swab. Specificities of these tests generally are high, but the reported sensitivities vary considerably (ie, false-negative results occur). As with throat swab cultures, sensitivity of these tests is highly dependent on the quality of the throat swab specimen, the experience of the person performing the test, and the rigor of the culture method used for comparison. Rapid tests for use in home settings are available, but their use should be discouraged. Because of high specificity of rapid tests, a positive test result does not require throat culture confirmation. Rapid diagnostic tests using techniques such as optical immunoassay and chemiluminescent DNA probes have been developed. These tests may be as sensitive as standard throat cultures on sheep blood agar. The diagnosis of ARF is based on the Jones criteria (Box 124.2).

Indications for GAS Testing. Factors to be considered in the decision to obtain a throat swab specimen for testing children with pharyngitis are the patient's age; signs and symptoms; season; and family and community epidemiology, including contact with a case of GAS infection or presence in the family of a person with a history of ARF or with poststreptococcal glomerulonephritis. GAS pharyngitis is uncommon in children younger than 3 years, but outbreaks of GAS pharyngitis have been reported in young children in child care settings. The risk of ARF is so remote in young children in industrialized countries that diagnostic studies for GAS pharyngitis often are not indicated for children younger than 3 years. Children with manifestations highly suggestive of viral infection, such as coryza, conjunctivitis, hoarseness, cough, anterior stomatitis, discrete ulcerative lesions, or diarrhea, are unlikely to have GAS pharyngitis and generally should not be tested. In contrast, children with acute onset of sore throat and clinical signs and symptoms such as pharyngeal exudate, pain on swallowing, fever, and enlarged tender anterior cervical lymph nodes or exposure to a person with GAS pharyngitis are more likely to have GAS infection and should have a rapid antigen test and/or throat culture performed.

Testing Contacts for GAS Infection. Indications for testing contacts for GAS infection vary according to circumstances. Testing asymptomatic household contacts for GAS is not recommended except when contacts are at increased risk of developing sequelae of GAS infection, ARF, or acute glomerulonephritis; if test results are positive, contacts should be treated.

Follow-up Throat Cultures. Post-treatment throat swab cultures are indicated only for patients who are at particularly high risk of ARF or have active symptoms compatible with GAS pharyngitis. Repeated courses of antimicrobial therapy are not indicated for asymptomatic patients with GAS-positive cultures; the exceptions are people who have had or whose family members have had ARF or other uncommon epidemiologic circumstances, such as outbreaks of rheumatic fever or acute poststreptococcal glomerulonephritis.

Patients who have repeated episodes of pharyngitis at short intervals and in whom GAS infection is documented by culture or antigen detection test present a special problem. Most often, these people are chronic GAS carriers who are experiencing frequent viral illnesses and for whom repeated testing and use of antimicrobial agents are unnecessary. In assessing such patients, inadequate adherence to oral treatment also should be considered. Although relatively uncommon, macrolide and azalide resistance among GAS strains occurs, resulting in erythromycin, clarithromycin, or azithromycin treatment failures. Testing asymptomatic household contacts usually is not helpful. However, if multiple household members have pharyngitis or other GAS infections, simulta-

Box 124.2

Jones Criteria for Diagnosis of Acute Rheumatic Fever[a]

Major Criteria	Minor Criteria	Supporting Evidence
Carditis Polyarthritis Chorea Erythema marginatum Subcutaneous nodules	Clinical findings: Fever, arthralgia[b] Laboratory findings: Elevated acute phase reactants; prolonged PR interval	Positive throat culture or rapid test for GAS antigen OR Elevated or rising streptococcal antibody test

[a] Diagnosis requires 2 major criteria or 1 major and 2 minor criteria with supporting evidence of antecedent group A streptococcal infection.
[b] Arthralgia is not a minor criterion in a patient with arthritis as a major criterion.

neous cultures of all household members and treatment of all people with positive cultures or rapid antigen test results may be of value.

Testing for GAS in Nonpharyngitis Infections. Cultures of impetiginous lesions often yield both streptococci and staphylococci, and determination of the primary pathogen is not possible. In suspected invasive GAS infections, cultures of blood and focal sites of possible infection are indicated. In necrotizing fasciitis, imaging studies often delay, rather than facilitate, the diagnosis. Clinical suspicion of necrotizing fasciitis should prompt surgical evaluation with intervention, including debridement of deep tissues with Gram stain and culture of surgical specimens.

STSS is diagnosed on the basis of clinical findings and isolation of group A streptococci (Box 124.3). Blood culture results are positive for *S pyogenes* in approximately 50% of patients with STSS. Culture results from a focal site of infections also usually are positive and can remain so for several days after appropriate antimicrobial agents have been initiated. *S pyogenes* uniformly is susceptible to beta-lactam antimicrobial agents, and susceptibility testing is needed only for non–beta-lactam agents, such as erythromycin or clindamycin, to which *S pyogenes* can be resistant. A significant increase in antibody titers to streptolysin O, deoxyribonuclease B, or other streptococcal extracellular enzymes 4 to 6 weeks after infection can help to confirm the diagnosis if culture results are negative.

Treatment

Although penicillin V is the drug of choice for treatment of GAS pharyngitis, amoxicillin equally is effective. A clinical GAS isolate resistant to penicillin or cephalosporin never has been documented. Prompt administration of penicillin therapy shortens the clinical course, decreases risk of suppurative sequelae and transmission, and prevents acute rheumatic fever, even when given up to 9 days after illness onset. For all patients with ARF, a complete course of penicillin or another appropriate antimicrobial agent for GAS pharyngitis should be given to eradicate GAS organisms from the throat, even if GAS organisms are not recovered in the initial throat culture.

Intramuscular penicillin G benzathine is appropriate therapy. It ensures adequate blood concentrations and avoids the problem of adherence, but administration is painful. Discomfort is less if the preparation of penicillin G benzathine is brought to room temperature before intramuscular injection. Mixtures containing shorter-acting penicillins (eg, penicillin G procaine) in addition to penicillin G benzathine have not been demonstrated to be more effective than penicillin G benzathine alone but are less painful when administered.

For some patients who are allergic to penicillin, a narrow-spectrum (first-generation) oral cephalosporin is indicated. However, as many as 5% to 10% of penicillin-allergic people also are allergic to cephalosporins. Patients with immediate or type I hypersensitivity to peni-

---

Box 124.3
Management of Streptococcal Toxic Shock Syndrome Without Necrotizing Fasciitis

- Fluid management to maintain adequate venous return and cardiac filling pressures to prevent end-organ damage
- Anticipatory management of multisystem organ failure
- Parenteral antimicrobial therapy at maximum doses with the capacity to
  - Kill organism with bactericidal cell wall inhibitor (eg, beta-lactamase–resistant antimicrobial agent)
  - Decrease enzyme, toxin, or cytokine production with protein synthesis inhibitor (eg, clindamycin)
- Immune globulin intravenous may be considered for infection refractory to several hours of aggressive therapy or in the presence of an undrainable focus or persistent oliguria with pulmonary edema

Box 124.4
Management of Streptococcal Toxic Shock Syndrome With Necrotizing Fasciitis

- Principles outlined in Box 124.3
- Immediate surgical evaluation
  - Exploration or incisional biopsy for diagnosis and culture
  - Resection of all necrotic tissue
- Repeated resection of tissue may be needed if infection persists or progresses

cillin should not be treated with a cephalosporin. Oral clindamycin is an acceptable alternative to penicillin in people with intermediate or type I hypersensitivity to penicillin. An oral macrolide or azalide (eg, erythromycin, clarithromycin, or azithromycin) is acceptable for patients allergic to penicillins. In recent years, macrolide resistance rates in most areas of the United States have been 5% to 8%, but resistance rates need continued monitoring. Tetracyclines, sulfonamides (including trimethoprim-sulfamethoxazole), and fluoroquinolones should not be used for treating GAS pharyngitis.

Children who have a recurrence of GAS pharyngitis shortly after completing a full course of a recommended oral antimicrobial agent can be re-treated with the same antimicrobial agent, an alternative oral drug, or an intramuscular dose of penicillin G benzathine, especially if inadequate adherence to oral therapy is likely. Alternative drugs include a narrow-spectrum cephalosporin (ie, cephalexin), amoxicillin-clavulanate, clindamycin, a macrolide, or azalide. Expert opinions differ about the most appropriate therapy in this circumstance.

Management of a patient who has repeated and frequent episodes of acute pharyngitis associated with positive laboratory tests for group A streptococci is problematic. To determine whether the patient is a long-term streptococcal pharyngeal carrier who is experiencing repeated episodes of intercurrent viral pharyngitis (which is the situation in most cases), the following should be determined: (1) whether the clinical findings are more suggestive of a GAS or a viral cause, (2) whether epidemiologic factors in the community support a GAS or a viral cause, (3) the nature of the clinical response to the antimicrobial therapy (in true GAS pharyngitis, response to therapy usually is ≤24 hours), (4) whether laboratory test results are positive for GAS infection between episodes of acute pharyngitis, and (5) whether a serologic response to GAS extracellular antigens (eg, antistreptolysin O) has occurred. Serotyping of GAS isolates generally is available only in research laboratories, but if performed, repeated isolation of the same serotype suggests carriage, and isolation of differing serotypes indicates repeated infections.

Pharyngeal Carriers. Antimicrobial therapy is not indicated for most GAS pharyngeal carriers. The few specific situations in which eradication of carriage may be indicated include the following: (1) a local outbreak of ARF or poststreptococcal glomerulonephritis, (2) an outbreak of GAS pharyngitis in a closed or semiclosed community, (3) a family history of ARF, or (4) multiple ("ping-pong") episodes of documented symptomatic GAS pharyngitis occurring within a family for many weeks despite appropriate therapy.

Streptococcal carriage can be difficult to eradicate with conventional antimicrobial therapy. A number of antimicrobial agents, including clindamycin, cephalosporins, amoxicillin-clavulanate, azithromycin, and a combination of rifampin for the last 4 days of treatment with either penicillin V or penicillin G benzathine have been demonstrated to be more effective than penicillin in eliminating chronic streptococcal carriage. Of these drugs, oral clindamycin has been reported to be most effective. Documented eradication of the carrier state is helpful in the evaluation of subsequent episodes of acute pharyngitis; however, carriage can recur after reacquisition of GAS infection, as some individuals appear to be "carrier prone."

Nonbullous Impetigo. Local mupirocin or retapamulin ointment may be useful for limiting person-to-person spread of nonbullous impetigo and for eradicating localized disease. With multiple lesions or with nonbullous impetigo in multiple family members, child care groups, or athletic teams, impetigo should be treated with antimicrobial regimens administered systemically. Because episodes of nonbullous impetigo may be caused by *Staphylococcus aureus* or *S pyogenes,* children with nonbullous impetigo usually should be treated with an antimicrobial agent active against both GAS and *S aureus* infections.

Toxic Shock Syndrome. As outlined in boxes 124.3 and 124.4), most aspects of management are the same for toxic shock syndrome caused by group A streptococci or by *S aureus.* Paramount are immediate aggressive fluid replacement and management of respiratory and cardiac failure, if present, and aggressive surgical debridement of any deep-seated GAS infection. Because *S pyogenes* and *S aureus* toxic shock syndrome are difficult to distinguish clinically, initial antimicrobial therapy should include an antistaphylococcal agent and a protein synthesis–inhibiting antimicrobial agent, such as clindamycin. The addition of clindamycin is more effective than penicillin alone for treating well-established GAS infections, because the antimicrobial activity of clindamycin is not affected by inoculum size, has a long postantimicrobial effect, and acts on bacteria by inhibiting protein synthesis. Inhibition of protein synthesis results in suppression of synthesis of the *S pyogenes* antiphagocytic M-protein and bacterial toxins. Clindamycin should not be used alone as initial antimicrobial therapy in life-threatening situations, because in the United States, 1% to 2% of GAS strains are resistant to clindamycin.

Once GAS infection has been identified, antimicrobial therapy can be changed to penicillin and clindamycin. Intravenous therapy should be continued until the patient is afebrile and stable hemodynamically and blood culture results are negative. The total duration of therapy is based on duration established for the primary site of infection.

Aggressive drainage and irrigation of accessible sites of infection should be performed as soon as possible. If necrotizing fasciitis is suspected, immediate surgical exploration or biopsy is crucial to identify deep soft tissue infection that should be debrided immediately.

The use of immune globulin intravenous can be considered as adjunctive therapy of STSS or necrotizing fasciitis if the patient is severely ill, although randomized trials to assess efficacy have not been performed.

Other Infections. Parenteral antimicrobial therapy is required for severe infections, such as endocarditis, pneumonia, septicemia, meningitis, arthritis, osteomyelitis, erysipelas, necrotizing fasciitis, neonatal omphalitis, and STSS. Treatment often is prolonged.

Prevention of Sequelae. ARF and acute glomerulonephritis are serious nonsuppurative sequelae of GAS infections. During epidemics of GAS infections on military bases in the 1950s, rheumatic fever developed in 3% of untreated patients with acute GAS pharyngitis. The current incidence after endemic infections is not known but is believed to be substantially less than 1%. The risk of ARF virtually can be eliminated by adequate treatment of the antecedent GAS infection; however, rare cases have occurred even after apparently appropriate therapy. The effectiveness of antimicrobial therapy for preventing acute poststreptococcal glomerulonephritis after pyoderma or pharyngitis has not been established. Suppurative sequelae, such as peritonsillar abscesses and cervical adenitis, usually are prevented by treatment of the primary infection.

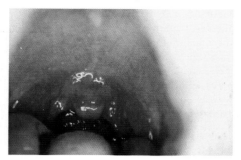

Image 124.1
Group A streptococcal pharyngitis with inflammation of the tonsils and uvula. Courtesy of Centers for Disease Control and Prevention.

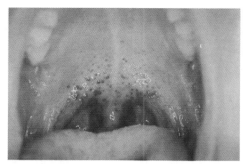

Image 124.2
Note inflammation of the oropharynx with petechiae on the soft palate, small red spots caused by group A streptococcal pharyngitis. Courtesy of Centers for Disease Control and Prevention/ Dr Heinz F. Eichenwald.

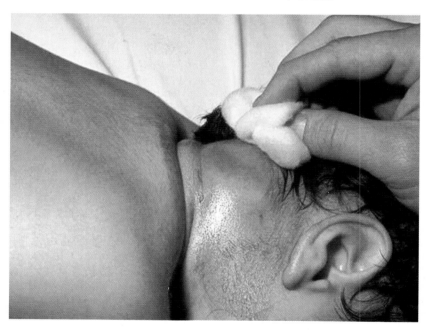

Image 124.3
Fluctuant, abscessed posterior cervical lymph node in a 4-year-old boy with impetigo of the scalp, prepped with povidone-iodine for needle aspiration for drainage and culture. Aspirate culture was positive for group A streptococci. Courtesy of Edgar O. Ledbetter, MD, FAAP.

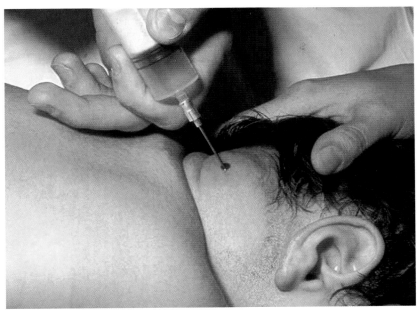

Image 124.4
Posterior cervical lymph node aspiration in the same patient as in Image 124.3. Culture was positive for group A streptococci. Courtesy of Edgar O. Ledbetter, MD, FAAP.

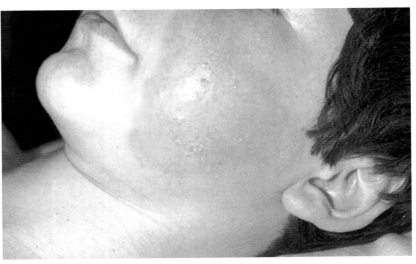

Image 124.5
A 13-year-old white male with group A streptococcal erysipelas of the left cheek. Copyright Martin G. Myers, MD.

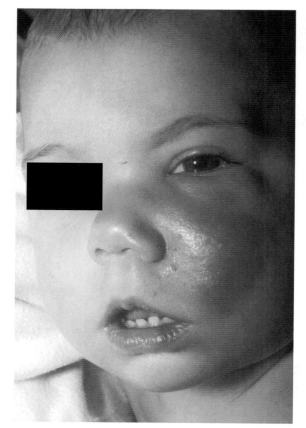

Image 124.6
Facial erysipelas in a 1-year-old white male. Courtesy of George Nankervis, MD.

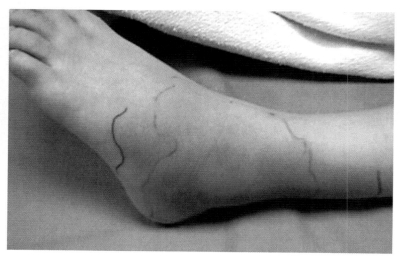

Image 124.7
Group A streptococcal cellulitis and arthritis of the left ankle in a 4-year-old white female. Copyright Michael Rajnik, MD, FAAP.

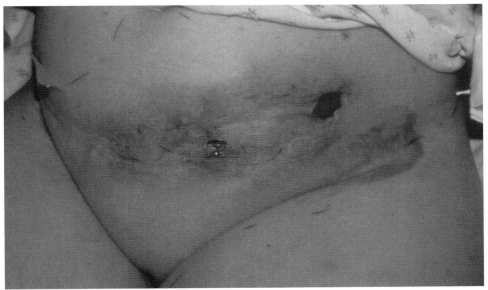

Image 124.8
Group A streptococcal necrotizing fasciitis complicating varicella in a 3-year-old white female.
Courtesy of George Nankervis, MD.

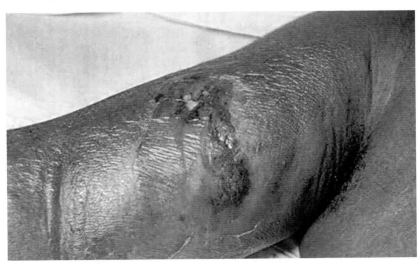

Image 124.9
Necrotizing fasciitis of the left upper arm and shoulder secondary to group A streptococcus. Copyright
Charles Prober, MD.

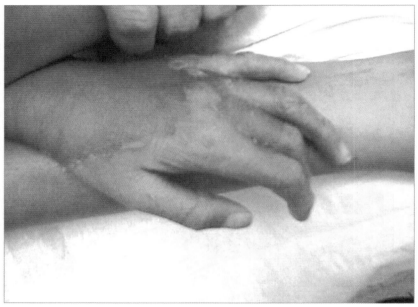

Image 124.10
Desquamation of the skin of the hand following a group A streptococcal infection (pharyngitis) in a 13-year-old black female. Copyright Michael Rajnik, MD, FAAP.

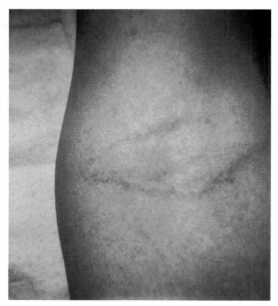

Image 124.11
Pastia lines in the antecubital space of a 12-year-old white male with scarlet fever. Courtesy of George Nankervis, MD.

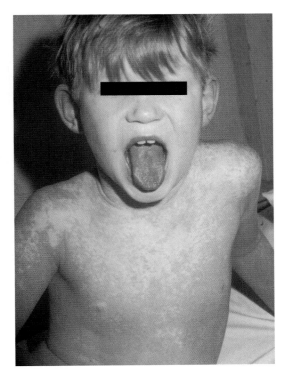

Image 124.12
A 4½-year-old white male with the rash and strawberry tongue of scarlet fever. Courtesy of George Nankervis, MD.

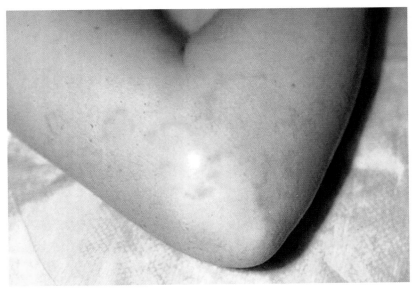

Image 124.13
Erythema marginatum in a 12-year-old white female. Although a characteristic rash of rheumatic fever, it is noted in fewer than 3% of cases. Its serpiginous border and evanescent nature serve to distinguish it from erythema migrans lesions of Lyme disease. Copyright Martin G. Myers, MD.

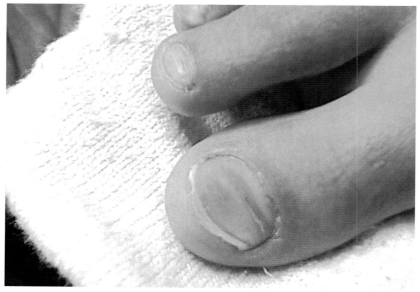

Image 124.14
Beau lines in the toenails of a child following a severe, protracted group A streptococcal illness.
Copyright Michael Rajnik, MD, FAAP.

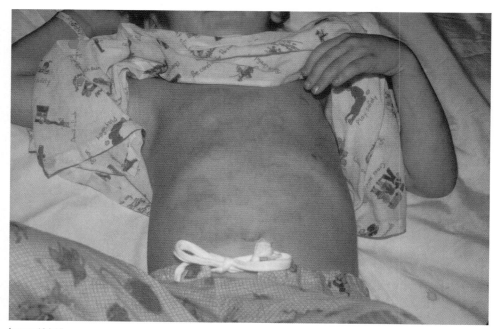

Image 124.15
Erythema marginatum lesions on the anterior trunk of a 5-year-old white male with acute post-streptococcal rheumatic fever. Courtesy of George Nankervis, MD.

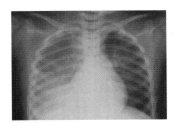

Image 124.16
Streptococcus pyogenes pneumonia in a 3-year-old female. Copyright Benjamin Estrada, MD.

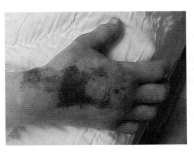

Image 124.17
Purpura fulminans in a 6-year-old female with *Streptococcus pyogenes* septicemia. Copyright Benjamin Estrada, MD.

125

Group B Streptococcal Infections

Clinical Manifestations

Group B streptococci are a major cause of perinatal infections, including bacteremia, endometritis, and chorioamnionitis, urinary tract infections in pregnant women; and systemic and focal infections in young infants. Invasive disease in infants is categorized on the basis of chronologic age at onset. Early-onset disease usually occurs within the first 24 hours of life (range, 0–6 days) and is characterized by signs of systemic infection, respiratory distress, apnea, shock, pneumonia and, less often, meningitis (5%–10% of cases). Late-onset disease, which typically occurs at 3 to 4 weeks of age (range, 7–89 days), commonly manifests as occult bacteremia or meningitis; other focal infections, such as osteomyelitis, septic arthritis, necrotizing fasciitis, pneumonia, adenitis, and cellulitis, occur less commonly. Late late-onset disease occurs beyond 89 days of age, usually in very preterm infants requiring prolonged hospitalization. Group B streptococci also cause systemic infections in nonpregnant adults with underlying medical conditions, such as diabetes mellitus, chronic liver or renal disease, malignancy, or other immunocompromising conditions and in adults 65 years of age and older.

Etiology

Group B streptococci (Streptococcus agalactiae) are gram-positive, aerobic diplococci that typically produce a narrow zone of beta hemolysis on 5% sheep blood agar. These organisms are divided into 10 types on the basis of capsular polysaccharides (Ia, Ib, II, and III–IX). Types Ia, Ib, II, III, and V account for approximately 95% of cases in infants in the United States. Type III is the predominant cause of early-onset meningitis and most late-onset infections in infants. Pilus-like structures are important virulence factors and potential vaccine candidates.

Epidemiology

Group B streptococci are common inhabitants of the human gastrointestinal and genitourinary tracts. Less commonly, they colonize the pharynx. The colonization rate in pregnant women ranges from 15% to 35%. Colonization during pregnancy can be constant or intermittent. Before recommendations for prevention of early-onset group B streptococcal (GBS) disease through maternal intrapartum antimicrobial prophylaxis were made, the incidence was 1 to 4 cases per 1,000 live births; early-onset disease accounted for approximately 75% of cases in infants and occurred in approximately 1 to 2 infants per 100 colonized women. Associated with implementation of widespread maternal intrapartum antimicrobial prophylaxis, the incidence of early-onset disease has decreased by approximately 80% to an estimated 0.28 cases per 1,000 live births in 2008. The use of intrapartum chemoprophylaxis has had no measurable impact on late-onset GBS disease, which nearly equals that of early-onset disease (an estimated 0.25 cases per 1,000 live births in 2010). The case-fatality ratio in term infants ranges from 1% to 3% but is higher in preterm neonates (20% for early-onset disease and 5% for late-onset disease). Approximately 50% of early-onset cases still afflict term neonates.

Transmission from mother to infant occurs shortly before or during delivery. After delivery, person-to-person transmission can occur. Although uncommon, GBS infection can be acquired in the nursery from health care professionals (probably via breaks in hand hygiene) or visitors and more commonly in the community (colonized family members or caregivers). The risk of early-onset disease is increased in preterm infants (<37 weeks' gestation), infants born after the amniotic membranes have been ruptured 18 hours or more, and infants born to women with high genital GBS inoculum, intrapartum fever (temperature ≥38°C [100.4°F]), chorioamnionitis, GBS bacteriuria during the current pregnancy, or a previous infant with invasive GBS disease. A low or undectable maternal concentration of type-specific serum antibody to capsular polysaccharide of the infecting strain also is a predisposing factor. Other risk factors are intrauterine fetal monitoring and maternal age younger than 20 years. Black race is an independent risk factor for both early-onset and late-onset disease. Although the incidence of early-onset disease has declined in all racial groups since the 1900s, rates consistently have been higher among black infants (0.52–0.83 cases per 1,000 live births from 2002–2007) compared with white infants (0.24–0.33 cases per 1,000 live births from 2002–2007), with the highest incidence observed among preterm black infants. The reason for this racial/ethnic disparity is not known. The period of communicability is unknown but can extend throughout the duration of colonization or disease. Infants can remain colonized for several months after birth and after treatment for systemic infection. Recurrent GBS disease affects an estimated 1% to 3% of appropriately treated infants.

Incubation Period

Early-onset disease, fewer than 7 days. Late-onset and late late-onset disease, unknown.

Diagnostic Tests

Gram-positive cocci in pairs or short chains by Gram stain of body fluids that typically are sterile (eg, cerebrospinal [CSF], pleural, or joint fluid) provide presumptive evidence of infection. Cultures of blood, CSF and, if present, a suppurative focus are necessary to establish the diagnosis. Rapid tests that identify group B streptococcal antigen in body fluids other than CSF are not recommended for diagnosis because of poor specificity.

Treatment

- Ampicillin plus an aminoglycoside is the initial treatment of choice for a newborn infant with presumptive invasive GBS infection.
- Penicillin G alone can be given when group B streptococcus has been identified as the cause of the infection and when clinical and microbiologic responses have been documented.

- For infants with meningitis attributable to group B streptococcus, the recommended dosage of penicillin G for infants 7 days of age or younger is 250,000 to 450,000 U/kg per day, intravenously, in 3 divided doses; for infants older than 7 days, 450,000 to 500,000 U/kg per day, intravenously, in 4 divided doses is recommended. For ampicillin, the recommended dosage for infants with meningitis 7 days of age or younger is 200 to 300 mg/kg per day, intravenously, in 3 divided doses; the recommended dosage for infants older than 7 days is 300 mg/kg per day, intravenously, in 4 divided doses.
- For meningitis, some experts believe that a second lumbar puncture approximately 24 to 48 hours after initiation of therapy assists in management and prognosis. If CSF sterility is not achieved, a complicated course (eg, cerebral infarcts) can be expected; also, an increasing protein concentration suggests an intracranial complication (eg, infarction, ventricular obstruction). Additional lumbar punctures and diagnostic imaging studies are indicated if response to therapy is in doubt, neurologic abnormalities persist, or focal neurologic deficits occur. Consultation with a specialist in pediatric infectious diseases often is useful.
- For infants with bacteremia without a defined focus, treatment should be continued for 10 days. For infants with uncomplicated meningitis, 14 days of treatment is satisfactory, but longer periods of treatment may be necessary for infants with prolonged or complicated courses. Septic arthritis or osteomyelitis requires treatment for 3 to 4 weeks; endocarditis or ventriculitis requires treatment for at least 4 weeks.
- Because of the reported increased risk of infection, the sibling of a multiple birth index case with early- or late-onset disease should be observed carefully and evaluated and treated empirically for suspected systemic infection if signs of illness occur.

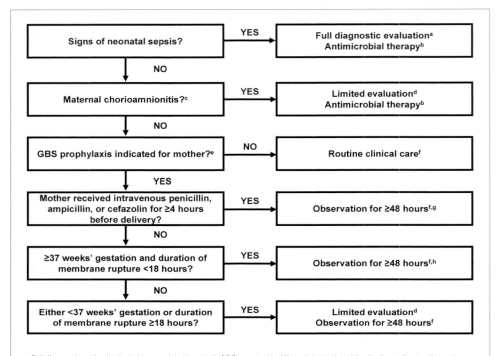

^a Full diagnostic evaluation includes complete blood cell (CBC) count with differential, platelets, blood culture, chest radiograph (if respiratory abnormalities are present), and lumbar puncture (if patient stable enough to tolerate procedure and sepsis is suspected).

^b Antimicrobial therapy should be directed toward the most common causes of neonatal sepsis, including GBS and other organisms (including gram-negative pathogens), and should take into account local antimicrobial resistance patterns.

^c Consultation with obstetric providers is important to determine the level of clinical suspicion for chorioamnionitis. Chorioamnionitis is diagnosed clinically, and some of the signs are nonspecific.

^d Limited evaluation includes blood culture (at birth) and CBC count with differential and platelets (at birth and/or at 6–12 hours of life).

^e GBS prophylaxis indicated if one or more of the following: (1) mother GBS positive at 35 to 37 weeks' gestation; (2) GBS status unknown with one or more intrapartum risk factors, including <37 weeks' gestation, rupture of membranes ≥18 hours or temperature ≥100.4°F (38.0°C), or intrapartum nucleic acid amplification test results positive for GBS; (3) GBS bacteriuria during current pregnancy; (4) history of a previous infant with GBS disease.

^f If signs of sepsis develop, a full diagnostic evaluation should be performed and antimicrobial therapy should be initiated.

^g If ≥37 weeks' gestation, observation may occur at home after 24 hours if other discharge criteria have been met, if there is a knowledgeable observer and ready access to medical care.

^h Some experts recommend a CBC with differential and platelets at 6 to 12 hours of age.

Image 125.1

Management of neonates for prevention of early-onset group B streptococcal (GBS) disease.

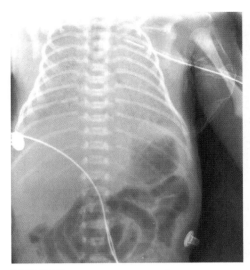

Image 125.2
Bilateral, severe group B streptococcal pneumonia in a neonate. Copyright David Clark, MD.

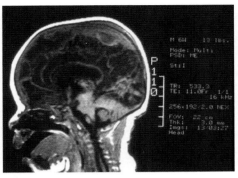

Image 125.3
Magnetic resonance imaging after group B streptococcal meningitis revealing extensive encephalomalacia.

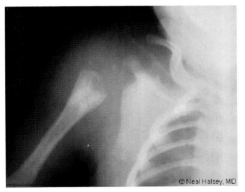

Image 125.4
Neonatal group B streptococcal septic arthritis of the right shoulder joint and osteomyelitis of the right proximal humerus. Copyright Neal Halsey, MD.

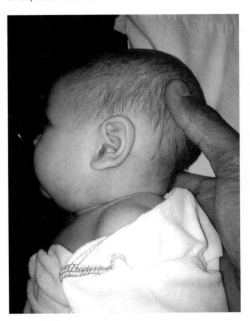

Image 125.5
A 3-week-old term neonate who had poor feeding and irritability followed 2 hours later by fever to 100.6°F (38.1°C). On admission to the hospital 3 hours later, he required fluid resuscitation and intravenous antibiotic therapy. His spinal fluid was within normal limits, but the blood culture grew group B streptococcus (GBS). At admission the physical examination revealed the classic facial and submandibular erythema, tenderness, and swelling characteristic of GBS cellulitis. Courtesy of Nate Serazin, MD, and C. Mary Healy, MD.

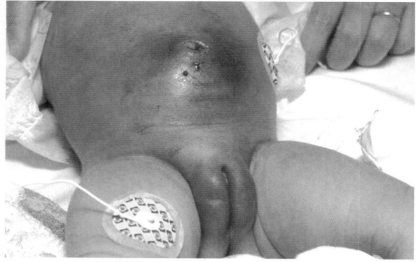

Image 125.6
Necrotizing fasciitis of the periumbilical area. Group B streptococcus, *Staphylococcus aureus,* and anaerobic streptococci were isolated at the time of surgical debridement. Courtesy of Edgar O. Ledbetter, MD, FAAP.

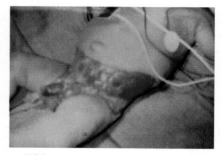

Image 125.7
Streptococcus agalactiae necrotizing fasciitis in a 3-month-old infant. Copyright Benjamin Estrada, MD.

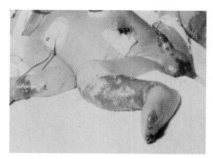

Image 125.8
A 3-day-old term neonate with fatal group B streptococcus sepsis and peripheral gangrene. Courtesy of Carol J. Baker, MD.

126

Non–Group A or B Streptococcal and Enterococcal Infections

Clinical Manifestations

Streptococci other than Lancefield groups A or B can be associated with invasive disease in infants, children, adolescents, and adults. The principal clinical syndromes of groups C and G streptococci are septicemia, upper and lower respiratory tract infections, skin and soft tissue infections, septic arthritis, meningitis with a parameningeal focus, brain abscess, and endocarditis with various clinical manifestations. Group F is an infrequent cause of invasive infection. Viridans streptococci are the most common cause of bacterial endocarditis in children, especially children with congenital or valvular heart disease, and these organisms have become a common cause of bacteremia in neutropenic patients with cancer. Among the viridans streptococci, organisms from the *Streptococcus anginosus* group often cause localized infections, such as brain or dental abscess or abscesses in other sites, including lymph nodes, liver, and lung. Enterococci are associated with bacteremia in neonates and bacteremia, device-associated infections, intra-abdominal abscesses, and urinary tract infections in older children and adults.

Etiology

Changes in taxonomy and nomenclature of the *Streptococcus* genus have evolved with advances in molecular technology. Among gram-positive organisms that are catalase negative and display chains by Gram stain, the genera associated most often with human disease, are *Streptococcus* and *Enterococcus*. Members of the *Streptococcus* genus that are beta-hemolytic on blood agar plates include *Streptococcus pyogenes, S agalactiae,* and groups C and G streptococci. *S agalactiae* subspecies *equisimilis* is the group C species most often associated with human infections. Streptococci that are non–beta-hemolytic (alpha-hemolytic or nonhemolytic) on blood agar plates include (1) *Streptococcus pneumoniae,* a member of the *mitis* group; (2) the

bovis group; and (3) species of viridans streptococci commonly isolated from humans, which can be divided into 4 groups by use of 16S rRNA gene sequencing (the *anginosus* group, the *mitis* group, the *salivarius* group, and the *mutans* group). Nutritionally variant streptococci, once thought to be viridans streptococci, now are classified in the genera *Abiotrophia* and *Granulicatella*.

The genus *Enterococcus* (previously included with Lancefield group D streptococci) contains at least 18 species, with *Enterococcus faecalis* and *Enterococcus faecium* accounting for most human enterococcal infections. Outbreaks and nosocomial spread in association with *Enterococcus gallinarum* also have occurred occasionally. Nonenterococcal group D streptococci include *Streptococcus bovis* and *Streptococcus equinus,* both members of the *bovis* group.

Epidemiology

The habitats that nongroup A and B streptococci and enterococci occupy in humans include skin (groups C and G), oropharynx (groups C and G and the *mutans* group), gastrointestinal tract (groups C and G, the *bovis* group, and *Enterococcus* species), and vagina (groups C, D, and G and *Enterococcus* species). Typical human habitats of different species of viridans streptococci are the oropharynx, epithelial surfaces of the oral cavity, teeth, skin, and gastrointestinal and genitourinary tracts. Intrapartum transmission is responsible for most cases of early-onset neonatal infection caused by non–group A and B streptococci and enterococci. Groups C and G streptococci have been known to cause foodborne outbreaks of pharyngitis.

Incubation Period

Unknown.

Diagnostic Tests

Diagnosis is established by culture of usually sterile body fluids with appropriate biochemical testing and serologic analysis for definitive identification. Antimicrobial susceptibility testing of isolates from usually sterile sites should be performed to guide treatment of infections caused by viridans streptococci or enterococci. The proportion of vancomycin-resistant enterococci among hospitalized patients can be as high as 30%.

Treatment

Penicillin G is the drug of choice for groups C and G streptococci. Other agents with good activity include ampicillin, cefotaxime, vancomycin, and linezolid. The combination of gentamicin with a beta-lactam antimicrobial agent (eg, penicillin or ampicillin) or vancomycin may enhance bactericidal activity needed for treatment of life-threatening infections (eg, endocarditis or meningitis).

Many viridans streptococci remain fully susceptible to penicillin (minimal inhibitory concentration [MIC], ≤0.1 µg/mL). Strains with an MIC greater than 0.1 µg/mL and less than 0.5 µg/mL are considered relatively resistant by criteria in the American Heart Association guidelines for determining treatment of streptococcal endocarditis. Strains with a penicillin MIC 0.5 µg/mL or greater are considered resistant. The Clinical Laboratory Standards Institute defines susceptible viridans streptococci as having an MIC of 0.12 µg/mLor less, intermediate isolates as having an MIC of 0.25 µg/mL to 2 µg/mL, and those exhibiting resistance as having an MIC of 4 µg/mL or greater. Nonpenicillin antimicrobial agents with good activity against viridans streptococci include cephalosporins (especially ceftriaxone), vancomycin, and linezolid. *Abiotrophia* and *Granulicatella* organisms can exhibit relative or high-level resistance to penicillin. The combination of high-dose penicillin or vancomycin and an aminoglycoside can enhance bactericidal activity.

Enterococci exhibit uniform resistance to cephalosporins and isolates resistant to vancomycin, especially *E faecium*, are increasing in prevalence. In general, children with a central line–associated bloodstream infection caused by enterococci should have the device removed promptly.

Invasive enterococcal infections, such as endocarditis or meningitis, should be treated with ampicillin (if the isolate is susceptible) or vancomycin in combination with an aminoglycoside. Gentamicin is the aminoglycoside recommended for achieving synergy. Gentamicin should be discontinued if in vitro susceptibility testing demonstrates high-level resistance, in which case synergy cannot be achieved. The role of combination therapy for treating central line–associated bloodstream infections is uncertain. Linezolid is approved for use in children, including neonates, only for treatment of infections caused by vancomycin-resistant *E faecium*. Isolates of vancomycin-resistant enterococci (VRE) that also are resistant to linezolid have been described. Resistance to linezolid among VRE isolates also can develop during prolonged treatment. Although most vancomycin-resistant isolates of *E faecalis* and *E faecium* are daptomycin susceptible, daptomycin is approved for use only in adults for treatment of infections attributable to vancomycin-resistant *E faecalis*.

Endocarditis. Guidelines for antimicrobial therapy in adults have been formulated by the American Heart Association and should be consulted for regimens that are appropriate for children and adolescents.

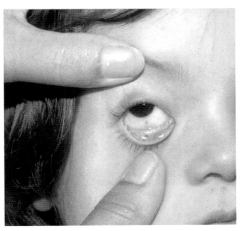

Image 126.1
Conjunctival (palpebral) petechiae in an adolescent girl with *Streptococcus viridans* subacute bacterial endocarditis.

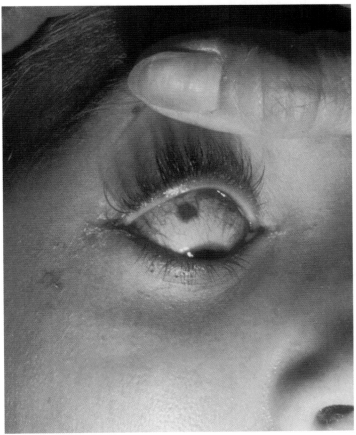

Image 126.2
A conjunctival hemorrhage in an adolescent female with enterococcal endocarditis. Courtesy of George Nankervis, MD.

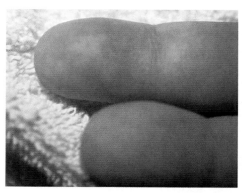

Image 126.3
A patient with Osler nodes from *Streptococcus viridans* bacterial endocarditis. Copyright Martin G. Myers, MD.

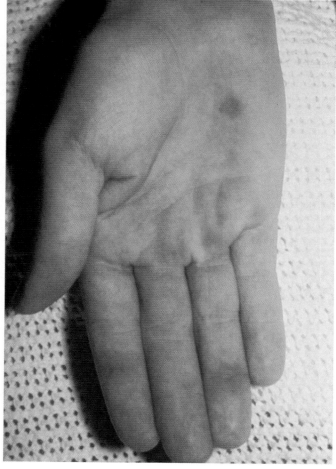

Image 126.4
Osler nodes on the fingers and a Janeway lesion in the palm of the previous patient with enterococcal endocarditis. Courtesy of George Nankervis, MD.

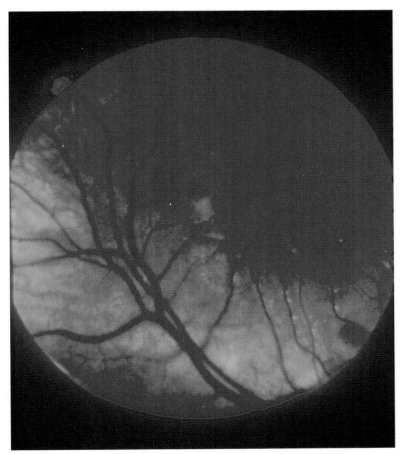

Image 126.5
Hemorrhagic retinitis with Roth spots in the previous adolescent female with enterococcal endocarditis. Courtesy of George Nankervis, MD.

127

Strongyloidiasis
(Strongyloides stercoralis)

Clinical Manifestations

Most infections with *Strongyloides stercoralis* are asymptomatic. When symptoms occur, they are most often related to larval skin invasion, tissue migration, or the presence of adult worms in the intestine. Infective (filariform) larvae are acquired from skin contact with contaminated soil, producing transient pruritic papules at the site of penetration. Larvae migrate to the lungs and can cause a transient pneumonitis or Löffler-like syndrome. After ascending the tracheobronchial tree, larvae are swallowed and mature into adults within the gastrointestinal tract. Symptoms of intestinal infection include nonspecific abdominal pain, malabsorption, vomiting, and diarrhea. Larval migration from defecated stool can result in migratory pruritic skin lesions in the perianal area, buttocks, and upper thighs, which is called "larva currens." Immunocompromised people, most often those receiving glucocorticoids for underlying malignancy or autoimmune disease, people receiving biologic response modifiers, and people infected with human T-lymphotropic virus 1 are at risk of *Strongyloides* hyperinfection syndrome and disseminated disease with involvement of brain, liver, heart, and skin. This condition, which frequently is fatal, is characterized by fever, abdominal pain, diffuse pulmonary infiltrates, and septicemia or meningitis caused by enteric gram-negative bacilli.

Etiology

S stercoralis is a nematode (roundworm).

Epidemiology

Strongyloidiasis is endemic in the tropics and subtropics, including the southeastern United States, wherever suitable moist soil and improper disposal of human waste coexist. Humans are the principal hosts, but dogs, cats, and other animals can serve as reservoirs. Transmission involves penetration of skin by infective (filariform) larvae. Infections rarely can be acquired from intimate skin contact or

from inadvertent coprophagy, such as from ingestion of contaminated food. Adult females release eggs in the small intestine, where they hatch as first-stage (rhabditiform) larvae that are excreted in feces. A small percentage of larvae molt to the infective (filariform) stage during intestinal transit, at which point they can penetrate the bowel mucosa or perianal skin, thus maintaining the life cycle within a single person. Because of this capacity for autoinfection, people can remain infected for decades.

Incubation Period

Unknown.

Diagnostic Tests

Strongyloidiasis can be difficult to diagnose in immunocompetent people, because excretion of larvae in feces is often of low intensity. At least 3 consecutive stool specimens should be examined microscopically for characteristic larvae, but stool concentration techniques may be required to establish the diagnosis. The use of agar plate culture methods may have greater sensitivity than fecal microscopy, and examination of duodenal contents obtained using the string test (Enterotest), or a direct aspirate through a flexible endoscope also may demonstrate larvae. Eosinophilia (blood eosinophil count >500/μL) is common in chronic infection. Serodiagnosis is sensitive and should be considered in all people with unexplained eosinophilia.

In disseminated strongyloidiasis, filariform larvae can be isolated from sputum or bronchoalveolar lavage fluid as well as cerebrospinal fluid. Gram-negative bacillary meningitis is a common associated finding in disseminated disease.

Treatment

Ivermectin is the treatment of choice for both chronic strongyloidiasis and hyperinfection with disseminated disease. Alternative agents include thiabendazole and albendazole, although both drugs are associated with lower cure rates. Prolonged or repeated treatment may be necessary in people with hyperinfection and disseminated strongyloidiasis, and relapse can occur.

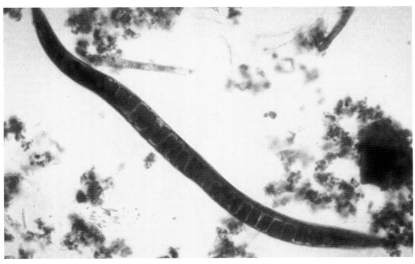

Image 127.1
Strongyloides stercoralis larvae (oil-immersion magnification). Copyright James Brien, DO.

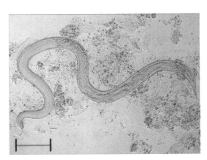

Image 127.2
Adult female of *Strongyloides stercoralis* collected in bronchial fluid of a patient with disseminated disease (scale bar = 400 μm). Courtesy of Abrescia FF, FAlda A, Caramaschi G, et al. Reemergence of strongyloidiasis, Northern Italy [letter]. *Emerg Infect Dis.* 2009;15(9):1531–1533.

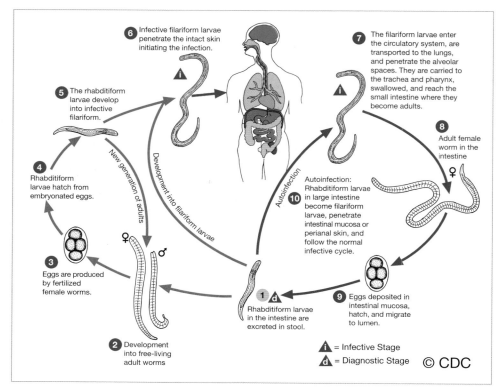

Image 127.3

The *Strongyloides* life cycle is complex among helminths with its alternation between free-living and parasitic cycles, and its potential for autoinfection and multiplication within the host.

In the case of *Strongyloides,* autoinfection may explain the possibility of persistent infections for many years in persons who have not been in an endemic area and of hyperinfections in immunodepressed individuals. Courtesy of Centers for Disease Control and Prevention/Alexander J. da Silva, PhD/Melanie Moser.

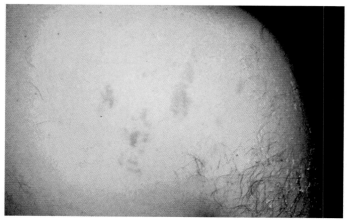

Image 127.4

Cutaneous migration sites of *Strongyloides stercoralis* over the left shoulder area. Copyright Neal Halsey, MD.

128

Syphilis

Clinical Manifestations

Congenital Syphilis. Intrauterine infection with *Treponema pallidum* can result in stillbirth, hydrops fetalis, or preterm birth or can be asymptomatic at birth. Infected infants can have hepatosplenomegaly, snuffles (copious nasal secretions), lymphadenopathy, mucocutaneous lesions, pneumonia, osteochondritis and pseudoparalysis, edema, rash, hemolytic anemia, or thrombocytopenia at birth or within the first 4 to 8 weeks of age. Skin lesions or moist nasal secretions of congenital syphilis are highly infectious. However, organisms rarely are found in lesions more than 24 hours after treatment has begun. Untreated infants, regardless of whether they have manifestations in early infancy, can develop late manifestations, which usually appear after 2 years of age and involve the central nervous system (CNS), bones and joints, teeth, eyes, and skin. Some consequences of intrauterine infection may not become apparent until many years after birth, such as interstitial keratitis (5–20 years of age), eighth cranial nerve deafness (10–40 years of age), Hutchinson teeth (peg-shaped, notched central incisors), anterior bowing of the shins, frontal bossing, mulberry molars, saddle nose, rhagades (perioral fissures), and Clutton joints (symmetric, painless swelling of the knees). The first 3 manifestations are referred to as the Hutchinson triad. Late manifestations can be prevented by treatment of early infection.

Acquired Syphilis. Infection with *T pallidum* in childhood or adulthood can be divided into 3 stages. The **primary stage** appears as one or more painless indurated ulcers (chancres) of the skin or mucous membranes at the site of inoculation. Lesions most commonly appear on the genitalia but can appear elsewhere, depending on the sexual contact responsible for transmission. These lesions appear, on average, 3 weeks after exposure (10–90 days) and heal spontaneously in a few weeks. Chancres sometimes are not recognized clinically. The **secondary stage,** beginning 1 to 2 months later, is characterized by rash, mucocutaneous lesions, and lymphadenopathy. The polymorphic maculopapular rash is generalized and

typically includes the palms and soles. In moist areas around the vulva or anus, hypertrophic papular lesions (condylomata lata) can occur and can be confused with condyloma acuminata secondary to human papillomavirus (HPV) infection. Generalized lymphadenopathy, fever, malaise, splenomegaly, sore throat, headache, and arthralgia can be present. This stage also resolves spontaneously without treatment in approximately 3 to 12 weeks, leaving the infected person completely asymptomatic. A variable latent period follows but sometimes is interrupted during the first few years by recurrences of symptoms of secondary syphilis. **Latent syphilis** is defined as the period after infection when patients are seroreactive but demonstrate no clinical manifestations of disease. Latent syphilis acquired within the preceding year is referred to as **early latent syphilis**; all other cases of latent syphilis are **late latent syphilis** (>1 year's duration) or **syphilis of unknown duration.** The **tertiary stage** of infection occurs 15 to 30 years after the initial infection and can include gumma formation, cardiovascular involvement, or neurosyphilis. Neurosyphilis is defined as infection of the CNS with *T pallidum.* Manifestations of neurosyphilis can occur at any stage of infection, especially in people infected with HIV and neonates with congenital syphilis.

Etiology

T pallidum is a thin, motile spirochete that is extremely fastidious, surviving only briefly outside the host. The organism has not been cultivated successfully on artificial media.

Epidemiology

Syphilis, which is rare in much of the industrialized world, persists in the United States and in resource-limited countries. The incidence of acquired and congenital syphilis increased dramatically in the United States during the late 1980s and early 1990s but decreased subsequently, and in 2000, the incidence was the lowest since reporting began in 1941. Since 2001, however, the rate of primary and secondary syphilis has increased, primarily among men who have sex with men. Among women, the rate of primary and secondary syphilis has increased since 2005, with a concomitant increase in cases of congenital syphilis. Rates of infection remain disproportionately high in large urban areas and in the southern United States. In adults, syphilis is more common among people with HIV infection. Primary and secondary rates of syphilis are highest in black, non-Hispanic people and in males compared with females.

Congenital syphilis is contracted from an infected mother via transplacental transmission of T pallidum at any time during pregnancy or possibly at birth from contact with maternal lesions. Among women with untreated early syphilis, as many as 40% of pregnancies result in spontaneous abortion, stillbirth, or perinatal death. Infection can be transmitted to the fetus at any stage of maternal disease. The rate of transmission is 60% to 100% during primary and secondary syphilis and slowly decreases with later stages of maternal infection (approximately 40% with early latent infection and 8% with late latent infection).

Acquired syphilis almost always is contracted through direct sexual contact with ulcerative lesions of the skin or mucous membranes of infected people. Open, moist lesions of the primary or secondary stages are highly infectious. Relapses of secondary syphilis with infectious mucocutaneous lesions can occur up to 4 years after primary infection. Sexual abuse must be suspected in any young child with acquired syphilis. In most cases, identification of acquired syphilis in children must be reported to state child protective services agencies. Physical examination for signs of sexual abuse and forensic interviews may be conducted under the auspices of a pediatrician with expertise in child abuse or at a local child advocacy center.

Incubation Period

Primary syphilis, 3 weeks; range, 10 to 90 days.

Diagnostic Tests

Definitive diagnosis is made when spirochetes are identified by microscopic darkfield examination or direct fluorescent antibody (DFA) tests of lesion exudate, nasal discharge, or tissue, such as placenta, umbilical cord, or autopsy specimens. Specimens should be scraped from moist mucocutaneous lesions or aspirated from a regional lymph node. Specimens from mouth lesions are best examined by DFA techniques to distinguish T pallidum from nonpathogenic treponemes that may be seen on darkfield microscopy. Although such testing can provide definitive diagnosis, in most instances, serologic testing is necessary. PCR tests and immunoglobulin (Ig) M immunoblotting have been developed but are not yet available commercially.

Presumptive diagnosis is possible using nontreponemal and treponemal serologic tests. Use of only 1 type of test is insufficient for diagnosis, because false-positive nontreponemal test results occur with various medical conditions, and treponemal test results remain positive long after syphilis has been treated adequately and can be falsely positive with other spirochetal diseases.

Standard nontreponemal tests for syphilis include the Venereal Disease Research Laboratory (VDRL) slide test and the rapid plasma reagin (RPR) test. These tests measure antibody directed against lipoidal antigen from T pallidum, antibody interaction with host tissues, or both. These tests are inexpensive and performed rapidly and provide semiquantitative results. Quantitative results help define disease activity and monitor response to therapy. Nontreponemal test results (eg, VDRL or RPR) may be falsely negative (ie, nonreactive) with early primary syphilis, latent acquired syphilis of long duration, and late congenital syphilis. Occasionally, a nontreponemal test performed on serum samples containing high concentrations of antibody against T pallidum will be weakly reactive or falsely negative, a reaction termed the *prozone* phenomenon. Diluting serum results in a positive test. When nontreponemal tests are used to monitor treatment response, the same specific test (eg, VDRL or RPR) must be used throughout the follow-up period, preferably performed by the same laboratory, to ensure comparability of results.

A reactive nontreponemal test result from a patient with typical lesions indicates a presumptive diagnosis of syphilis and the need for treatment. However, any reactive nontreponemal test result must be confirmed by one of the specific treponemal tests to exclude a false-positive test result. False-positive results can be caused by certain viral infections (eg, Epstein-Barr virus infection, hepatitis, varicella, and measles), lymphoma, tuberculosis, malaria, endocarditis, connective tissue disease, pregnancy, abuse of injection drugs, laboratory or technical error, or Wharton jelly contamination when umbilical cord blood specimens are used. Treatment should not be delayed while awaiting the results of the treponemal test results if the patient is symptomatic or at high risk of infection. A sustained fourfold decrease in titer, equivalent to a change of 2 dilutions (eg, from 1:32 to 1:8), of the nontreponemal test result after treatment usually demonstrates adequate therapy, whereas a sustained fourfold increase in titer (eg, from 1:8 to 1:32) after treatment suggests reinfection or relapse. The nontreponemal test titer usually decreases fourfold within 6 to 12 months after therapy for primary or secondary syphilis and usually becomes nonreactive within 1 year after successful therapy if the infection (primary or secondary syphilis) was treated early. The patient usually becomes seronegative within 2 years even if the initial titer was high or the infection was congenital. Some people will continue to have low stable nontreponemal antibody titers despite effective therapy. This serofast state is more common in patients treated for latent or tertiary syphilis.

Treponemal tests in use include fluorescent treponemal antibody absorption (FTA-ABS), microhemagglutination test for antibodies to *T pallidum* (MHA-TP), *T pallidum* enzyme immunoassay (TP-EIA), and *T pallidum* particle agglutination (TP-PA). People who have reactive treponemal test results usually remain reactive for life, even after successful therapy. However, 15% to 25% of patients treated during the primary stage revert to being serologically nonreactive after 2 to 3 years. Treponemal test antibody titers correlate poorly with disease activity and should not be used to assess response to therapy.

Treponemal tests also are not 100% specific for syphilis; positive reactions occur variably in patients with other spirochetal diseases, such as yaws, pinta, leptospirosis, rat-bite fever,

relapsing fever, and Lyme disease. Nontreponemal tests can be used to differentiate Lyme disease from syphilis, because the VDRL test is nonreactive in Lyme disease.

The Centers for Disease Control and Prevention (CDC) recommends syphilis serologic screening with a nontreponemal test, such as the RPR or VDRL test, to identify people with possible untreated infection; this screening is followed by confirmation using one of several treponemal tests. Some clinical laboratories and blood banks have begun to screen samples using treponemal enzyme immunoassay (EIA) tests, rather than beginning with a nontreponemal test; the reasons for this change in sequence of the screening relates to cost and manpower issues. However, this "reverse sequence screening" approach is associated with high rates of false-positive results, and in 2011, the CDC reaffirmed its longstanding recommendation that nontreponemal tests be used to screen for syphilis and that treponemal testing be used to confirm syphilis as the cause of nontreponemal reactivity. The traditional algorithm performs well in identifying people with active infection who require further evaluation and treatment while minimizing false-positive results in low prevalence populations.

Cerebrospinal Fluid Tests. For evaluation of possible neurosyphilis, the VDRL test should be performed on cerebrospinal fluid (CSF). The CSF VDRL is highly specific but is insensitive. In addition, evaluation of CSF protein and white blood cell count is used to assess the likelihood of CNS involvement. The CSF leukocyte count usually is elevated in neurosyphilis (>5 white blood cells [WBCs]/mm^3). Although the FTA-ABS test of CSF is less specific than the VDRL test, some experts recommend using the FTA-ABS test, believing it to be more sensitive than the VDRL test. Results from the VDRL test should be interpreted cautiously, because a negative result on a VDRL test of CSF does not exclude a diagnosis of neurosyphilis. Alternatively, a reactive VDRL test in the CSF of neonates can be the result of nontreponemal IgG antibodies that cross the blood-brain barrier. Fewer data exist for the TP-PA test for CSF, and none exist for the RPR test; these tests should not be used for CSF evaluation.

Testing During Pregnancy. All women should be screened serologically for syphilis early in pregnancy with a nontreponemal test (eg, RPR or VDRL) and preferably again at delivery. In areas of high prevalence of syphilis and in patients considered at high risk of syphilis, a nontreponemal serum test at the beginning of the third trimester (28 weeks of gestation) and at delivery is indicated. For women treated during pregnancy, follow-up serologic testing is necessary to assess the efficacy of therapy. Low-titer false-positive nontreponemal antibody test results occasionally occur in pregnancy. The result of a positive nontreponemal antibody test should be confirmed with a treponemal antibody test (eg, FTA-ABS, MHA-TP, TP-EIA, or TP-PA). When a pregnant woman has a reactive nontreponemal test result and a persistently negative treponemal test result, a false-positive test result is confirmed. As noted previously, some laboratories are screening pregnant women using an EIA treponemal test, but this reverse sequence screening approach is not recommended. Pregnant women with reactive treponemal EIA screening tests should have confirmatory testing with a nontreponemal test; subsequent evaluation and possible treatment of the infant should follow the infant's RPR or VDRL result, as outlined in Image 128.1. Any woman who delivers a stillborn infant after 20 weeks' gestation should be tested for syphilis.

Evaluation of Infants for Congenital Infection During the First Month of Age. No newborn infant should be discharged from the hospital without determination of the mother's serologic status for syphilis at least once during pregnancy and also at delivery in communities and populations in which the risk of congenital syphilis is high. Testing of umbilical cord blood or an infant serum sample is inadequate for screening, because these can be nonreactive if the mother's serologic test result is of low titer or if she was infected late in pregnancy. All infants born to seropositive mothers require a careful examination and a nontreponemal syphilis test. The test performed on the infant should be the same as that performed on the mother to enable comparison of titer results. A negative maternal RPR or VDRL test result at delivery does not rule out the

possibility of the infant having congenital syphilis, although such a situation is rare. The diagnostic and therapeutic approach to infants being evaluated for congenital syphilis is summarized in Image 128.1 and depends on (1) identification of maternal syphilis; (2) adequacy of maternal therapy; (3) maternal response to therapy; (4) comparison of maternal and infant serologic titers; and (5) evaluation of results of the infant's nontreponemal serologic test, physical examination, ophthalmologic examination, long-bone and chest radiography, and laboratory tests (liver function tests; complete blood cell [CBC] and platelet counts; and CSF cell count, protein, and quantitative VDRL). Infants born to mothers who are coinfected with syphilis and HIV do not require different evaluation, therapy, or follow-up for syphilis than is recommended for all infants.

Evaluation and Treatment of Older Infants and Children. Children who are identified as having reactive serologic tests for syphilis after the neonatal period (ie, ≥1 month of age) should have maternal serologic test results and records reviewed to assess whether they have congenital or acquired syphilis. The recommended evaluation includes (1) CSF analysis for VDRL testing, cell count, and protein concentration; (2) CBC, differential, and platelet counts; and (3) other tests as indicated clinically (eg, long-bone or chest radiography, liver function tests, abdominal ultrasonography, ophthalmologic examination, auditory brain stem response testing, and neuroimaging studies).

Cerebrospinal Fluid Testing. Guidance for examination of CSF in the evaluation for possible congenital syphilis is provided under Evaluation of Newborn Infants for Congenital Infection During the First Month of Age. CSF test results obtained during the neonatal period can be difficult to interpret; normal values differ by gestational age and are higher in preterm infants. Values as high as 18 WBCs/mm^3 and/or protein up to 130 mg/dL might occur among normal term neonates; some specialists, however, recommend that lower values (ie, 5 WBCs/mm^3 and protein of 40 mg/dL) be considered the upper limits of normal when assessing a term infant for congenital syphilis. Other causes of elevated values should be considered when an infant is being evaluated for congenital syphilis.

CSF should be examined in all patients with neurologic or ophthalmic signs or symptoms, evidence of active tertiary syphilis (eg, aortitis and gumma), treatment failure, or HIV infection with late latent syphilis or syphilis of unknown duration. Abnormalities in CSF in patients with neurosyphilis include increased protein concentration, increased WBC count, and/or a reactive VDRL test result. Some experts also recommend performing the FTA-ABS test on CSF, believing it to be more sensitive but less specific than VDRL testing of CSF for neurosyphilis.

Treatment

Parenteral penicillin G remains the drug of choice for treatment of syphilis at any stage. Recommendations for penicillin G use and duration of therapy vary, depending on the stage of disease and clinical manifestations. Parenteral penicillin G is the only documented effective therapy for patients who have neurosyphilis, congenital syphilis, or syphilis during pregnancy and is recommended for HIV-infected patients. Such patients always should be treated with penicillin, even if desensitization for penicillin allergy is necessary.

Congenital Syphilis: Infants in the First Month of Age. The diagnostic and therapeutic approach to neonates delivered to mothers with syphilis is outlined in Image 128.1. Management decisions are based on the 3 possible maternal situations: (1) maternal treatment before pregnancy, (2) adequate maternal treatment and response during pregnancy, or (3) inadequate maternal treatment or inadequate maternal response to treatment (or reinfection) during pregnancy.

For proven or probable congenital syphilis (based on the neonate's physical examination and radiographic and laboratory testing), the preferred treatment is aqueous crystalline penicillin G, administered intravenously. Alternatively, procaine penicillin G intramuscularly can be administered; no treatment failures have occurred with this formulation despite its low CSF concentrations. When the

neonate is at risk of congenital syphilis because of inadequate maternal treatment or response to treatment (or reinfection) during pregnancy but the neonate's physical examination, radiographic imaging, and laboratory analyses are normal (including infant RPR/VDRL either the same as or less than fourfold the maternal RPR/VDRL), some experts would treat with a single dose of penicillin G benzathine intramuscularly, but most still would prefer 10 days of treatment. If more than 1 day of therapy is missed, the entire course should be restarted. Use of agents other than penicillin requires close serologic follow-up to assess adequacy of therapy.

Infants who have a normal physical examination and a serum quantitative nontreponemal serologic titer either the same as or less than fourfold (eg, 1:4 is fourfold lower than 1:16) the maternal titer are at minimal risk of syphilis if (1) they are born to mothers who completed appropriate penicillin treatment for syphilis during pregnancy and more than 4 weeks before delivery and (2) the mother had no evidence of reinfection or relapse. Although a full evaluation may be unnecessary, these infants should be treated with a single intramuscular injection of penicillin G benzathine, because fetal treatment failure can occur despite adequate maternal treatment during pregnancy. Alternatively, these infants may be examined carefully, preferably monthly, until their nontreponemal serologic test results are negative.

Infants who have a normal physical examination and a serum quantitative nontreponemal serologic titer either the same as or less than fourfold the maternal titer and (1) whose mother's treatment was adequate before pregnancy and (2) whose mother's nontreponemal serologic titer remained low and stable before and during pregnancy and at delivery (VDRL <1:2; RPR <1:4) require no evaluation. Some experts, however, would treat with penicillin G benzathine as a single intramuscular injection if follow-up is uncertain.

Congenital Syphilis: Older Infants and Children. Because establishing the diagnosis of neurosyphilis is difficult, infants older than 1 month who possibly have congenital syphilis or who have neurologic involvement should be treated with intravenous aqueous crystalline penicillin for 10 days (Table 128.1). This regimen also should be used to treat children older than 2 years who have late and previously untreated congenital syphilis. If the patient has no clinical manifestations of disease, the CSF examination is normal, and the result of the VDRL test of CSF is negative, some experts would treat with 3 weekly doses of penicillin G benzathine intramuscularly.

Syphilis in Pregnancy. Regardless of stage of pregnancy, women should be treated with penicillin according to the dosage schedules appropriate for the stage of syphilis as recommended for nonpregnant patients (see Table 128.1). For penicillin-allergic patients, no proven alternative therapy has been established. A pregnant woman with a history of penicillin allergy should be treated with penicillin after desensitization. Desensitization should be performed in consultation with a specialist and only in facilities in which emergency assistance is available.

Erythromycin, azithromycin, or any other nonpenicillin treatment of syphilis during pregnancy cannot be considered reliable to cure infection in the fetus. Tetracycline is not recommended for pregnant women because of potential adverse effects on the fetus.

Early Acquired Syphilis (Primary, Secondary, Early Latent Syphilis). A single intramuscular dose of penicillin G benzathine is the preferred treatment for children and adults (see Table 128.1). All children should have a CSF examination before treatment to exclude a diagnosis of neurosyphilis. Evaluation of CSF in adolescents and adults is necessary only if clinical signs or symptoms of neurologic or ophthalmic involvement are present. Neurosyphilis should be considered in the differential diagnosis of neurologic disease in HIV-infected people.

For nonpregnant patients who are allergic to penicillin, doxycycline or tetracycline should be given. Clinical studies, along with biologic and pharmacologic considerations, suggest ceftriaxone should be effective for early-acquired syphilis. Because efficacy of ceftriaxone is not well documented, close follow-up is essential. Single-dose therapy with ceftriaxone is not effective. Preliminary data suggest that azithromycin might be effective as a single oral dose. However, several cases of azithromycin treatment failures have been reported, and resistance to azithromycin has been documented in several geographic areas. When follow-up cannot be ensured, especially for children younger than 8 years, consideration must be given to hospitalization and desensitization followed by administration of penicillin G.

Syphilis of More Than 1 Year's Duration (Late Latent Syphilis, Except Neurosyphilis) or of Unknown Duration. Penicillin G benzathine should be given intramuscularly weekly for 3 successive weeks (see Table 128.1). In patients who are allergic to penicillin, doxycycline or tetracycline for 4 weeks should be given only with close serologic and clinical follow-up. Limited clinical studies suggest that ceftriaxone might be effective, but the optimal dose and duration have not been defined. Patients who have syphilis and who demonstrate any of the following criteria should have a prompt CSF examination:

1. Neurologic or ophthalmic signs or symptoms
2. Evidence of active tertiary syphilis (eg, aortitis, gumma, iritis, uveitis)
3. Treatment failure
4. HIV infection with late latent syphilis or syphilis of unknown duration

If dictated by circumstances and patient or parent preferences, a CSF examination may be performed for patients who do not meet these criteria. Some experts recommend performing a CSF examination on all patients who have latent syphilis and a nontreponemal serologic test result of 1:32 or greater or if the patient is HIV infected and has a serum CD4+ T-lymphocyte count 350 or less. The risk of asymptomatic neurosyphilis in these circumstances is increased approximately threefold. If a CSF examination is performed and the results indicate abnormalities consistent with neurosyphilis, the patient should be treated for neurosyphilis (see Neurosyphilis below).

Neurosyphilis. The recommended regimen for adults is aqueous crystalline penicillin G, intravenously (see Table 128.1). If adherence to

Table 128.1
Recommended Treatment for Syphilis in People Older Than 1 Month

Status	Children	Adults
Congenital syphilis	Aqueous crystalline penicillin G, 200,000–300,000 U/kg/day, IV, administered as 50,000 U/kg, every 4–6 h for 10 days[a]	
Primary, secondary, and early latent syphilis[b]	Penicillin G benzathine,[c] 50,000 U/kg, IM, up to the adult dose of 2.4 million U in a single dose	Penicillin G benzathine, 2.4 million U, IM, in a single dose **OR** *If allergic to penicillin and not pregnant,* doxycycline, 100 mg, orally, twice a day for 14 days **OR** Tetracycline, 500 mg, orally, 4 times/day for 14 days
Late latent syphilis[d] or latent syphilis of unknown duration	Penicillin G benzathine, 50,000 U/kg, IM, up to the adult dose of 2.4 million U, administered as 3 single doses at 1-wk intervals (total 150,000 U/kg, up to the adult dose of 7.2 million U)	Penicillin G benzathine, 7.2 million U total, administered as 3 doses of 2.4 million U, IM, each at 1-wk intervals **OR** *If allergic to penicillin and not pregnant,* doxycycline, 100 mg, orally, twice a day for 4 wk **OR** Tetracycline, 500 mg, orally, 4 times/day for 4 wk
Tertiary	…	Penicillin G benzathine 7.2 million U total, administered as 3 doses of 2.4 million U, IM, at 1-wk intervals *If allergic to penicillin and not pregnant, same as for late latent syphilis*
Neurosyphilis[e]	Aqueous crystalline penicillin G, 200,000–300,000 U/kg/day, IV, every 4–6 h for 10–14 days, in doses not to exceed the adult dose	Aqueous crystalline penicillin G, 18–24 million U per day, administered as 3–4 million U, IV, every 4 h for 10–14 days[f] **OR** Penicillin G procaine,[c] 2.4 million U, IM, once daily **PLUS** probenecid, 500 mg, orally, 4 times/day, both for 10–14 days[f]

Abbreviations: IM, intramuscularly; IV, intravenously.

[a] If the patient has no clinical manifestations of disease, the cerebrospinal fluid (CSF) examination is normal, and the CSF Venereal Disease Research Laboratory test result is negative, some experts would treat with up to 3 weekly doses of penicillin G benzathine, 50,000 U/kg, IM. Some experts also suggest giving these patients a single dose of penicillin G benzathine, 50,000 U/kg, IM, after the 10-day course of intravenous aqueous penicillin.

[b] Early latent syphilis is defined as being acquired within the preceding year.

[c] Penicillin G benzathine and penicillin G procaine are approved for intramuscular administration only.

[d] Late latent syphilis is defined as syphilis beyond 1 year's duration.

[e] Patients who are allergic to penicillin should be desensitized.

therapy can be ensured, patients may be treated with an alternative regimen of daily intramuscular penicillin G procaine plus oral probenecid. For children, intravenous aqueous crystalline penicillin G for 10 to 14 days is recommended. If the patient has a history of allergy to penicillin, consideration should be given to desensitization, and the patient should be managed in consultation with an allergy specialist.

Other Considerations. Mothers of infants with congenital syphilis should be tested for other sexually transmitted infections (STIs), including *Neisseria gonorrhoeae, Chlamydia trachomatis,* HIV, and hepatitis B infections. If injection drug use is suspected, the mother also may be at risk of hepatitis C virus infection. All recent sexual contacts of people with acquired syphilis should be evaluated for other STIs as well as syphilis. Partners who were exposed within 90 days preceding the diagnosis of primary, secondary, or early latent syphilis in the index patient should be treated presumptively for syphilis, even if they are seronegative. All patients with syphilis should be tested for other STIs, including HIV, and hepatitis B infection. Patients who have primary syphilis should be retested for HIV after 3 months if the first HIV test result is negative. For HIV-infected patients with syphilis, careful follow-up is essential. Patients infected with HIV who have early syphilis may be at increased risk of neurologic complications and higher rates of treatment failure with currently recommended regimens. Children with acquired primary, secondary, or latent syphilis should be evaluated for possible sexual assault or abuse.

Follow-up and Management.

Congenital syphilis. All infants who have reactive serologic tests for syphilis or were born to mothers who were seroreactive at delivery should receive careful follow-up evaluations during regularly scheduled well-child care visits at 2, 4, 6, and 12 months of age. Serologic nontreponemal tests should be performed every 2 to 3 months until the nontreponemal test becomes nonreactive or the titer has decreased at least fourfold (ie, 1:16 to 1:4). Nontreponemal antibody titers should decrease by 3 months of age and should be nonreactive by 6 months of age if the infant was infected and adequately treated or was not infected and initially seropositive because of transplacentally acquired maternal antibody. The serologic response after therapy may be slower for infants treated after the neonatal period. Patients with increasing titers or with persistent stable titers 6 to 12 months after initial treatment should be reevaluated, including a CSF examination, and treated with a 10-day course of parenteral penicillin G, even if they were treated previously.

Treponemal tests should not be used to evaluate treatment response, because results for an infected child can remain positive despite effective therapy. Passively transferred maternal treponemal antibodies can persist in an infant until 15 months of age. A reactive treponemal test after 18 months of age is diagnostic of congenital syphilis. If the nontreponemal test is nonreactive at this time, no further evaluation or treatment is necessary. If the nontreponemal test is reactive at 18 months of age, the infant should be evaluated (or reevaluated) fully and treated for congenital syphilis.

Treated infants with congenital neurosyphilis and initially positive results of VDRL tests of CSF or abnormal CSF cell counts and/or protein concentrations should undergo repeated clinical evaluation and CSF examination at 6-month intervals until their CSF examination is normal. A reactive result of VDRL testing of CSF at the 6-month interval is an indication for re-treatment. Abnormal CSF indices that cannot be attributed to another ongoing illness also require retreatment. Neuroimaging studies, such as magnetic resonance imaging, should be considered in these children.

Acquired syphilis. Treated pregnant women with syphilis should have quantitative nontreponemal serologic tests repeated at 28 to 32 weeks of gestation, at delivery, and according to recommendations for the stage of disease. Serologic titers may be repeated monthly in women at high risk of reinfection or in geographic areas where the prevalence of syphilis is high. The clinical and antibody response should be appropriate for stage of disease. Most women will deliver before their serologic response to treatment can be assessed definitively. Therapy should be judged inadequate if the maternal antibody titer has not decreased fourfold by delivery. Inadequate maternal treatment is likely if clinical signs of infection are present at delivery or if maternal antibody titer is fourfold higher than the pretreatment titer. Fetal treatment is considered inadequate if delivery occurs within 28 days of maternal therapy.

Indications for Retreatment.

Primary/secondary syphilis: If clinical signs or symptoms persist or recur or if a fourfold increase in titer of a nontreponemal test occurs, evaluate CSF and HIV status and repeat therapy. If the nontreponemal titer fails to decrease fourfold within 6 months after therapy, evaluate for HIV; repeat therapy unless follow-up for continued clinical and serologic assessment can be ensured. Some experts recommend CSF evaluation.

Latent syphilis: In the following situations, CSF examination should be performed and retreatment should be provided: Re-treatment should be provided if titers increase at least fourfold (ie, 1:4 to 1:16), an initially high titer (>1:32) fails to decrease at least fourfold (ie, 1:32 to 1:8) within 12 to 24 months, or signs or symptoms attributable to syphilis develop.

In all these instances, re-treatment, when indicated, should be performed with 3 weekly injections of penicillin G benzathine intramuscularly unless CSF examination indicates that neurosyphilis is present, at which time treatment for neurosyphilis should be initiated. Re-treated patients should be treated with the schedules recommended for patients with syphilis for more than 1 year. In general, only 1 re-treatment course is indicated. The possibility of reinfection or concurrent HIV infection always should be considered when re-treating patients with early syphilis, and repeat HIV testing should be performed in such cases.

Patients with neurosyphilis must have periodic serologic testing, clinical evaluation at 6-month intervals, and repeat CSF examinations. If the CSF cell count has not decreased after 6 months or CSF is not entirely normal after 2 years, re-treatment should be considered. CSF abnormalities may persist for extended periods in HIV-infected people with neurosyphilis. Close follow-up is warranted.

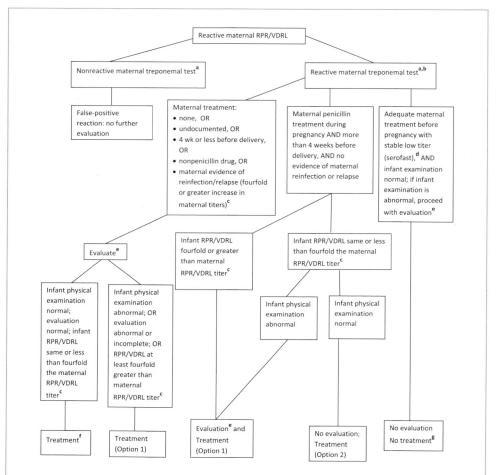

Abbreviations: FTA-ABS, fluorescent treponemal antibody absorption; MHA-TP, Microhemagglutination test for antibodies to *T pallidum*; RPR, rapid plasma reagin; TP-EIA, T pallidum enzyme immunoassay; TP-PA, *Treponema pallidum* particle agglutination; VDRL, Venereal Disease Research Laboratory.

[a] TP-PA, FTA-ABS, TP-EIA, or MHA-TP.

[b] Test for HIV antibody. Infants of HIV-infected mothers do not require different evaluation or treatment.

[c] A fourfold change in titer is the same as a change of 2 dilutions. For example, a titer of 1:64 is fourfold greater than a titer of 1:16, and a titer of 1:4 is fourfold lower than a titer of 1:16.

[d] Women who maintain a VDRL titer ≤1:2 or an RPR ≤1:4 beyond 1 year after successful treatment are considered serofast.

[e] Complete blood cell and platelet count; cerebrospinal fluid (CSF) examination for cell count, protein, and quantitative VDRL; other tests as clinically indicated (eg, chest radiographs, long-bone radiographs, eye examination, liver function tests, neuroimaging, and auditory brainstem response).

[f] Treatment (Option 1 or Option 2, below), with many experts recommending Treatment Option 1. If a single dose of benzathine penicillin G is used, then the infant must be fully evaluated, full evaluation must be normal, and follow-up must be certain. If any part of the infant's evaluation is abnormal or not performed, or if the CSF analysis is rendered uninterpretable, then a 10-day course of penicillin is required.

[g] Some experts would consider a single intramuscular injection of benzathine penicillin (Treatment Option 2), particularly if follow-up is not certain.

Treatment Options

(1) Aqueous penicillin G, 50,000 U/kg, intravenously, every 12 hours (≤1 week of age) or every 8 hours (>1 week); or procaine penicillin G, 50,000 U/kg, intramuscularly, as a single daily dose for 10 days. If ≥24 hours of therapy are missed, the entire course must be restarted.

(2) Benzathine penicillin G, 50,000 U/kg, intramuscularly, single dose.

Image 128.1

Algorithm for evaluation and treatment of infants born to mothers with reactive serologic tests for syphilis.

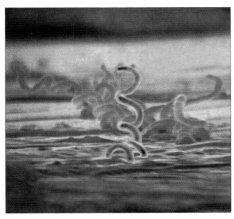

Image 128.2
This electron micrograph shows *Treponema pallidum* on cultures of cotton-tail rabbit epithelium cells (Sf1Ep). Courtesy of Centers for Disease Control and Prevention.

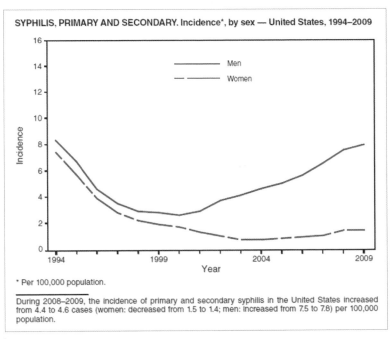

Image 128.3
Syphilis, primary and secondary. Incidence by sex—United States, 1994–2009. Courtesy of *Morbidity and Mortality Weekly Report.*

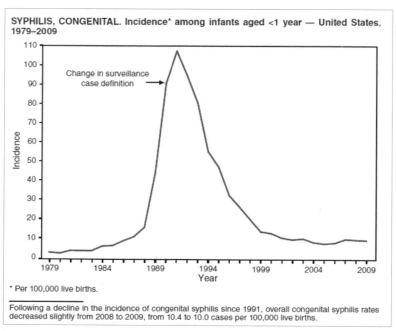

SYPHILIS, CONGENITAL. Incidence* among infants aged <1 year — United States, 1979–2009

* Per 100,000 live births.

Following a decline in the incidence of congenital syphilis since 1991, overall congenital syphilis rates decreased slightly from 2008 to 2009, from 10.4 to 10.0 cases per 100,000 live births.

Image 128.4

Syphilis, congenital. Incidence among infants <1 year—United States. 1979–2009. Courtesy of *Morbidity and Mortality Weekly Report.*

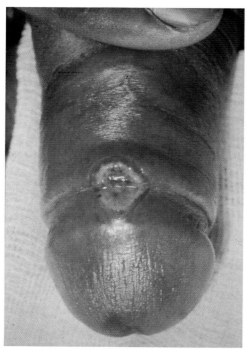

Image 128.5

Syphilis chancre. Copyright James Brien, DO.

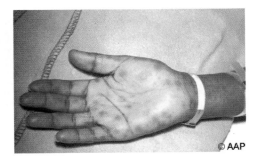

Image 128.6
A 16-year-old girl with rash of secondary syphilis noticed at 3 months' gestation of her pregnancy. The signs and symptoms of secondary syphilis generally occur 6 to 8 weeks after the primary infection when primary lesions have usually healed.

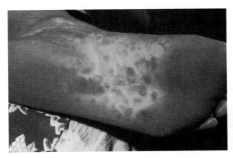

Image 128.7
This patient presented with a papular rash on the sole of the foot due to secondary syphilis. The second stage of syphilis starts when one or more areas of the skin break into a rash that appears as rough red or reddish brown spots both on the palms of hands and on the bottoms of feet. Even without treatment, the rash clears up spontaneously. Courtesy of Centers for Disease Control and Prevention/Susan Lindsley.

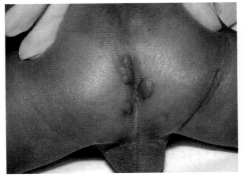

Image 128.8
Cutaneous syphilis in a 6-month-old infant. Copyright Neal Halsey, MD.

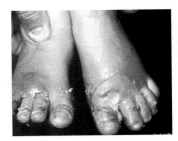

Image 128.10
Newborn with congenital syphilis with cutaneous ulceration (luetic gumma). These lesions are highly infectious.

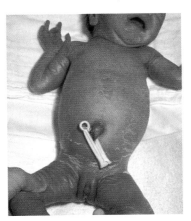

Image 128.9
A newborn with congenital syphilis. Note the marked generalized desquamation.

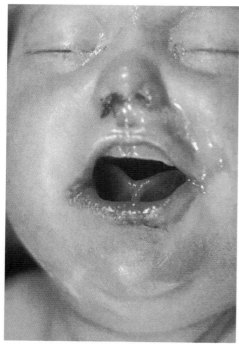

Image 128.11
The face of a newborn infant displaying pathologic morphology indicative of congenital syphilis
with striking mucous membrane involvement.
Courtesy of Centers for Disease Control
and Prevention/Dr Norman Cole.

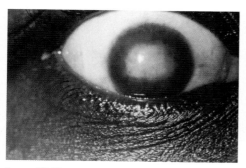

Image 128.15
This photograph depicts the presence of a diffuse stromal haze in the cornea of a female
patient, known as interstitial keratitis (IK), which
was due to her late-staged congenital syphilitic
condition. IK, which is an inflammation of the
cornea's connective tissue elements, and usually
affects both eyes, can occur as a complication
brought on by congenital or acquired syphilis.
IK usually occurs in children older than 2 years.
Courtesy of Centers for Disease Control
and Prevention/Susan Lindsley.

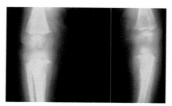

Image 128.12
Congenital syphilis with proximal tibial metaphys-
itis (Wimberger sign).

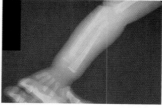

Image 128.13
Congenital syphilis with metaphyseal destruction
of distal humerus, radius, and ulna.

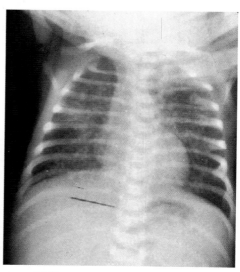

Image 128.14
Congenital syphilis with pneumonia alba. The
infant survived with penicillin treatment.

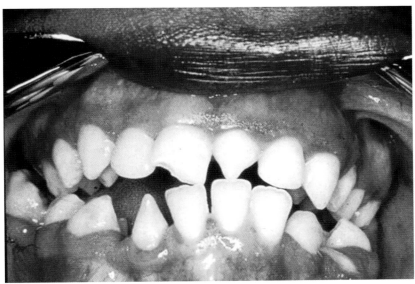

Image 128.16
Hutchinson teeth, a late manifestation of congenital syphilis. Changes occur in secondary dentition. The central incisors are smaller than normal and have sloping sides. Courtesy of Edgar O. Ledbetter, MD, FAAP.

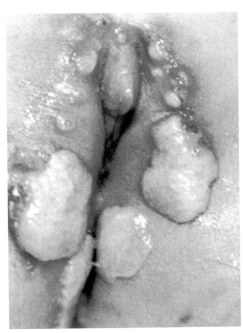

Image 128.17
Condyloma latum in a 7-year-old girl who has been sexually abused. These moist lesions are whitish gray caused by *Treponema pallidum,* and are highly contagious.

129

Tapeworm Diseases

(Taeniasis and Cysticercosis)

Clinical Manifestations

Taeniasis. Infection often is asymptomatic; however, mild gastrointestinal tract symptoms, such as nausea, diarrhea, and pain, can occur. Tapeworm segments can be seen migrating from the anus or in feces.

Cysticercosis. Manifestations depend on the location and number of pork tapeworm larval cysts (cysticerci) and the host response. Cysticerci may be found anywhere in the body. The most common and serious manifestations are caused by cysticerci in the central nervous system. Larval cysts of *Taenia solium* in the brain (neurocysticercosis) can cause seizures, behavioral disturbances, obstructive hydrocephalus, and other neurologic signs and symptoms. In some countries, including parts of the southwest United States, neurocysticercosis is a leading cause of epilepsy. The host reaction to degenerating cysticerci can produce signs and symptoms of meningitis. Cysts in the spinal column can cause gait disturbance, pain, or transverse myelitis. Subcutaneous cysticerci produce palpable nodules, and ocular involvement can cause visual impairment.

Etiology

Taeniasis is caused by intestinal infection by the adult tapeworm, *Taenia saginata* (beef tapeworm) or *T solium* (pork tapeworm). *Taenia asiatica* causes taeniasis in Asia. Human cysticercosis is caused only by the larvae of *T solium* (*Cysticercus cellulosae*).

Epidemiology

These tapeworm diseases have worldwide distribution. Prevalence is high in areas with poor sanitation and human fecal contamination in areas where cattle graze or swine are fed. Most cases of *T solium* infection in the United States are imported from Latin America or Asia. High rates of *T saginata* infection occur in Mexico, parts of South America, East Africa, and central Europe. *T asiatica* is common in China, Taiwan, and Southeast Asia. Taeniasis is acquired by eating undercooked beef *(T saginata)* or pork *(T solium)*. *T asiatica* is acquired by eating viscera of infected pigs that contain encysted larvae. Infection often is asymptomatic.

Cysticercosis in humans is acquired by ingesting eggs of the pork tapeworm *(T solium)*, through fecal-oral contact with a person harboring the adult tapeworm, or by autoinfection. Eggs are found only in human feces because humans are the obligate definitive host. Eggs liberate oncospheres in the intestine that migrate through the blood and lymphatics to tissues throughout the body, including the central nervous system; the oncospheres develop into cysticerci. Although most cases of cysticercosis in the United States have been imported, cysticercosis can be acquired in the United States from tapeworm carriers who emigrated from an area with endemic infection and still have *T solium* intestinal stage infection.

Incubation Period

Taeniasis (the time from ingestion of the larvae until segments are passed in the feces), 2 to 3 months; cysticercosis, several years.

Diagnosis

Diagnosis of taeniasis (adult tapeworm infection) is based on demonstration of the proglottids in feces or the perianal region. However, these techniques are insensitive. Species identification of the parasite is based on the different structures of gravid proglottids and scolex. Diagnosis of neurocysticercosis is made primarily on the basis of computed tomography (CT) scanning or magnetic resonance imaging (MRI) of the brain or spinal cord. Antibody assays that detect specific antibody to larval *T solium* in serum and cerebrospinal fluid (CSF) are the confirmatory tests of choice. In the United States, antibody tests are available through the Centers for Disease Control and Prevention and several commercial laboratories. In general, antibody tests are more sensitive with serum specimens than with CSF specimens. Serum antibody assay results often are negative in children with solitary parenchymal lesions but usually are positive in patients with multiple lesions.

Treatment

Taeniasis. Praziquantel is highly effective for eradicating infection with the adult tapeworm, and niclosamide is an alternative but is not available in the United States.

Cysticercosis. Neurocysticercosis treatment should be individualized on the basis of the number and viability of cysticerci as assessed by neuroimaging studies (MRI or CT scan) and where they are located. For patients with only a single nonviable cyst (eg, only calcifications on CT scan), management generally is aimed at symptoms and should include anticonvulsants for patients with seizures and insertion of shunts for patients with hydrocephalus. Two antiparasitic drugs—albendazole and praziquantel—are available. Although both drugs are cysticercidal and hasten radiologic resolution of cysts, most symptoms result from the host inflammatory response and may be exacerbated by treatment. Most experts recommend therapy with albendazole or praziquantel for patients with nonenhancing or multiple cysticerci. Albendazole is preferred over praziquantel, because it has fewer drug-drug interactions with anticonvulsants. Coadministration of corticosteroids for the first 2 to 3 days of therapy may decrease adverse effects if more extensive viable central nervous system cysticerci are suspected. Arachnoiditis, vasculitis, or diffuse cerebral edema (cysticercal encephalitis) is treated with corticosteroid therapy until cerebral edema is controlled and albendazole or praziquantel therapy is completed.

Seizures can recur for months or years. Anticonvulsant therapy is recommended until there is neuroradiologic evidence of resolution and seizures have not occurred for 1 to 2 years. Calcification of cysts may require prolonged or indefinite use of anticonvulsants. Intraventricular cysts and hydrocephalus usually require surgical therapy. Intraventricular cysticerci often can be removed by endoscopic surgery, which is the treatment of choice. If cysticerci cannot be removed easily, hydrocephalus should be corrected with placement of intraventricular shunts. Ocular cysticercosis is treated by surgical excision of the cysticerci. Ocular and spinal cysticerci generally are not treated with anthelmintic drugs, which can exacerbate inflammation. An ophthalmic examination should be performed before treatment to rule out intraocular cysticerci.

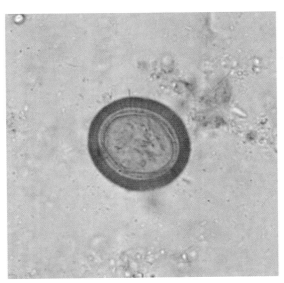

Image 129.1

The eggs of *Taenia solium* and *Taenia saginata* are indistinguishable from each other, as well as from other members of the Taeniidae family. The eggs measure 30 to 35 μm in diameter and are radially striated. The internal oncosphere contains 6 refractile hooks. *Taenia* spp eggs in unstained wet mounts. Courtesy of Centers for Disease Control and Prevention/Dr Mae Melvin.

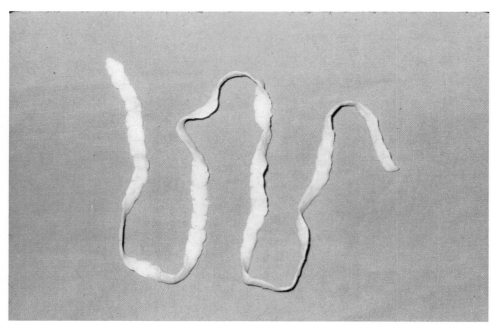

Image 129.2
Taenia saginata. Courtesy of Gary Overturf, MD.

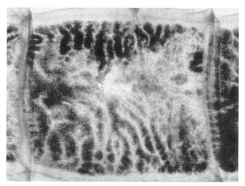

Image 129.3
Taenia solium. Gravid proglottid. Copyright
James Brien, DO.

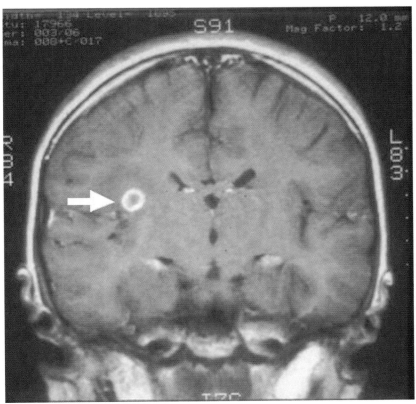

Image 129.4
A young male with a seizure. Magnetic resonance imaging of the brain revealed a ring-like lesion characteristic of neurocysticercosis. Copyright Barbara Ann Jantausch, MD, FAAP.

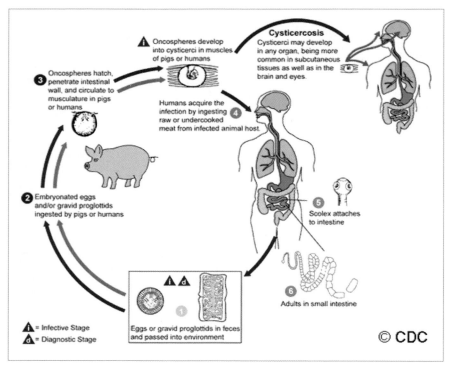

Image 129.5

Cysticercosis is an infection of both humans and pigs with the larval stages of the parasitic cestode, *Taenia solium*. This infection is caused by ingestion of eggs shed in the feces of a human tapeworm carrier (1). Pigs and humans become infected by ingesting eggs or gravid proglottids (2). Humans are infected either by ingestion of food contaminated with feces or by autoinfection. In the latter case, a human infected with adult *T solium* can ingest eggs produced by that tapeworm either through fecal contamination or, possibly, from proglottids carried into the stomach by reverse peristalsis. Once eggs are ingested, oncospheres hatch in the intestine (3), invade the intestinal wall, and migrate to striated muscles, as well as the brain, liver, and other tissues, where they develop into cysticerci. In humans, cysts can cause serious sequelae if they localize in the brain, resulting in neurocysticercosis. The parasite life cycle is completed, resulting in human tapeworm infection when humans ingest undercooked pork containing cysticerci (4). Cysts evaginate and attach to the small intestine by their scolex (5). Adult tapeworms develop (up to 2–7 m in length and produce <1,000 proglottids, each with approximately 50,000 eggs) and reside in the small intestine for years (6). Courtesy of Centers for Disease Control and Prevention/Alexander J. da Silva, PhD/Melanie Moser.

130

Other Tapeworm Infections
(Including Hydatid Disease)

Most infections are asymptomatic, but nausea, abdominal pain, and diarrhea have been observed in people who are heavily infected.

Etiologies, Diagnosis, and Treatment

Hymenolepis nana. This tapeworm, also called dwarf tapeworm because it is the smallest of the adult human tapeworms, can complete its entire cycle within humans. New infection may be acquired by ingestion of eggs passed in feces of infected people or of infected arthropods (fleas). More problematic is autoinfection, which tends to perpetuate infection in the host, because eggs can hatch within the intestine and reinitiate the cycle, leading to development of new worms and a large worm burden. Diagnosis is made by recognition of the characteristic eggs passed in stool. Praziquantel is the treatment of choice, with nitazoxanide as an alternative drug. If infection persists after treatment, re-treatment with praziquantel is indicated.

Dipylidium caninum. This tapeworm is the most common and widespread adult tapeworm of dogs and cats. *D caninum* infects children when they inadvertently swallow a dog or cat flea, which serves as the intermediate host. Diagnosis is made by finding the characteristic eggs or motile proglottids in stool. Proglottids resemble rice kernels. Therapy with praziquantel is effective. Niclosamide is an alternative therapeutic option.

Diphyllobothrium latum *(and related species).* The *D latum* tapeworm, also called fish tapeworm, has fish as one of its intermediate hosts. Consumption of infected, raw freshwater fish (including salmon) leads to infection. Three to 5 weeks are needed for the adult tapeworm to mature and begin to lay eggs. The worm sometimes causes mechanical obstruction of the bowel or diarrhea, abdominal pain or, rarely, megaloblastic anemia secondary to vitamin B_{12} deficiency. Diagnosis is made by recognition of the characteristic pro-

glottids or eggs passed in stool. Therapy with praziquantel is effective; niclosamide is an alternative.

Echinococcus granulosus *and* Echinococcus multilocularis. The larval forms of these tapeworms are the causes of hydatid disease. The distribution of *E granulosus* is related to sheep or cattle herding. Areas of high prevalence include parts of Central and South America, East Africa, Eastern Europe, the Middle East, the Mediterranean region, China, and Central Asia. The parasite also is endemic in Australia and New Zealand. In the United States, small foci of endemic transmission have been reported in Arizona, California, New Mexico, and Utah, and a strain adapted to wolves, moose, and caribou occurs in Alaska and Canada. Dogs, coyotes, wolves, dingoes, and jackals can become infected by swallowing protoscolices of the parasite within hydatid cysts in the organs of sheep or other intermediate hosts. Dogs pass embryonated eggs in their stools, and sheep become infected by swallowing the eggs. If humans swallow *Echinococcus* eggs, they can become inadvertent intermediate hosts, and cysts can develop in various organs, such as the liver, lungs, kidney, and spleen. These cysts usually grow slowly and eventually can contain several liters of fluid. If a cyst ruptures, anaphylaxis and multiple secondary cysts from seeding of protoscolices can result. Clinical diagnosis often is difficult. A history of contact with dogs in an area with endemic infection is helpful. Cystic lesions can be demonstrated by radiography, ultrasonography, or computed tomography of various organs. Serologic tests, available at the Centers for Disease Control and Prevention, are helpful, but false-negative results occur. In uncomplicated cases, treatment of choice is **p**uncture **a**spiration, **i**njection of protoscolicidal agents, and **r**easpiration (PAIR). Contraindications to PAIR include communication of the cyst with the biliary tract (eg, bile staining after initial aspiration), superficial cysts, and heavily septated cysts. Surgical therapy is indicated for complicated cases and requires meticulous care to prevent spillage, including preparations such as soaking of surgical drapes in hypertonic saline. In general, the cyst should be removed intact, because leakage of contents is associated with a higher rate of complications. Patients are at risk of anaphylactic reactions to cyst contents. Treatment with albendazole generally should be initiated days to weeks before surgery or PAIR and continued for several weeks to months afterward.

E multilocularis, a species for which the life cycle involves foxes, dogs, and rodents, causes the alveolar form of hydatid disease, which is characterized by invasive growth of the larvae in the liver with occasional metastatic spread. The alveolar form of hydatid disease is limited to the northern hemisphere and usually is diagnosed in people 50 years of age or older. The preferred treatment is surgical removal of the entire larval mass. In nonresectable cases, continuous treatment with albendazole has been associated with clinical improvement.

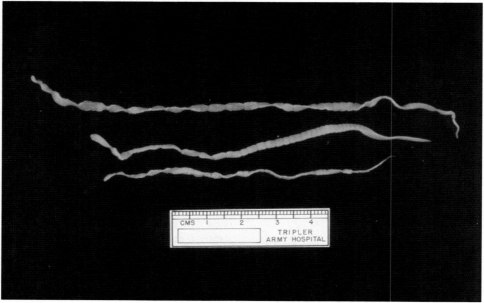

Image 130.1
Dipylidium caninum. Dog tapeworm. Copyright James Brien, DO.

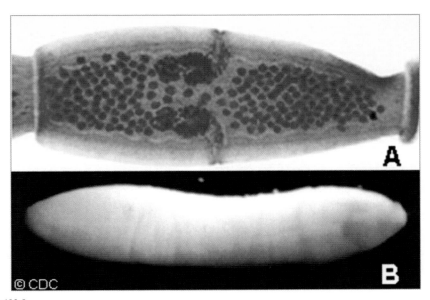

Image 130.2
Proglottids of *Dipylidium caninum*. Such proglottids (average mature size 12 mm x 3 mm) have 2 genital pores, one in the middle of each lateral margin. Proglottids may be passed singly or in chains, and occasionally may be seen dangling from the anus. They are pumpkin seed–shaped when passed and often resemble rice grains when dried. Courtesy of Centers for Disease Control and Prevention.

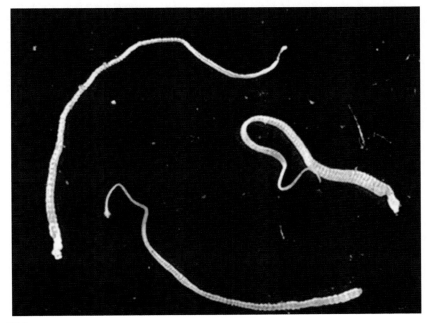

Image 130.3
Three adult *Hymenolepis nana* tapeworms. Each tapeworm (length, 15–40 mm) has a small, rounded scolex at the anterior end, and proglottids can be distinguished at the posterior, wider end. Courtesy of Centers for Disease Control and Prevention.

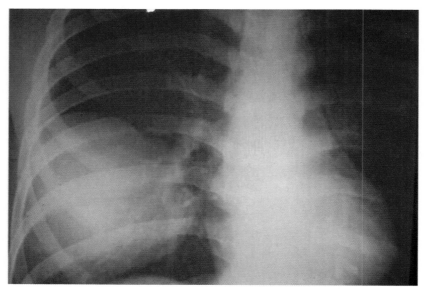

Image 130.4
Fluid-filled echinococcus cyst in the lungs of an adolescent male. Courtesy of Edgar O. Ledbetter, MD, FAAP.

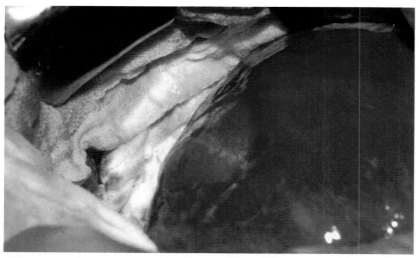

Image 130.5
Echinococcus abscess of liver in an adult, the most common site of abscess formation.

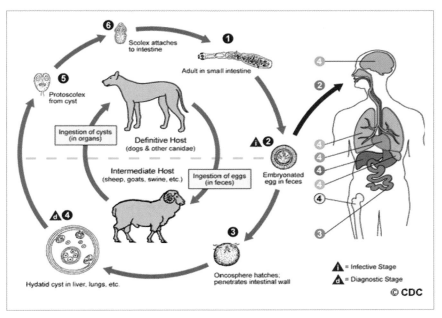

Image 130.6

The adult *Echinococcus granulosus* (3–6 mm long) (1) resides in the small bowel of the definitive hosts (dogs or other canids). Gravid proglottids release eggs (2) that are passed in the feces. After ingestion by a suitable intermediate host (under natural conditions: sheep, goat, swine, cattle, horses, camel), the egg hatches in the small bowel and releases an oncosphere (3) that penetrates the intestinal wall and migrates through the circulatory system into various organs, especially the liver and lungs. In these organs, the oncosphere develops into a cyst (4) that enlarges gradually, producing protoscolices and daughter cysts that fill the cyst interior. The definitive host becomes infected by ingesting the cyst-containing organs of the infected intermediate host. After ingestion, the protoscolices (1) evaginate, attach to the intestinal mucosa (6), and develop into adult stages (1) in 32 to 80 days

The same life cycle occurs with *Echinococcus multilocularis* (1.2–3.7 mm), with the following differences: the definitive hosts are foxes, and to a lesser extent dogs, cats, coyotes, and wolves; the intermediate host are small rodents; and larval growth (in the liver) remains indefinitely in the proliferative stage, resulting in invasion of the surrounding tissues. With *Echinococcus vogelii* (up to 5.6 mm long), the definitive hosts are bush dogs and dogs; the intermediate hosts are rodents; and the larval stage (in the liver, lungs, and other organs) develops both externally and internally, resulting in multiple vesicles. *Echinococcus oligarthrus* (up to 2.9 mm long) has a life cycle that involves wild felids as definitive hosts and rodents as intermediate hosts. Humans become infected by ingesting eggs (2), with resulting release of oncospheres (3) in the intestine and the development of cysts (4) in various organs. Courtesy of Centers for Disease Control and Prevention.

131

Tetanus
(Lockjaw)

Clinical Manifestations

Tetanus can manifest in 1 of 4 clinical forms: generalized, local, neonatal, and cephalic. **Generalized tetanus (lockjaw)** is a neurologic disease manifesting as trismus and severe muscular spasms, including risus sardonicus. Onset is gradual, occurring over 1 to 7 days, and symptoms progress to severe generalized muscle spasms, which often are aggravated by any external stimulus. Severe spasms persist for 1 week or more and subside over several weeks in people who recover. **Local tetanus** manifests as local muscle spasms in areas contiguous to a wound. Localized tetanus most often progresses to generalized tetanus. **Neonatal tetanus** is a form of generalized tetanus occurring in newborn infants lacking protective passive immunity because their mothers are not immune. **Cephalic tetanus** is a dysfunction of cranial nerves associated with infected wounds on the head and neck. Cephalic tetanus can precede generalized tetanus.

Etiology

Clostridium tetani is a spore-forming, obligate anaerobic, gram-positive bacillus. This organism is a wound contaminant that causes neither tissue destruction nor an inflammatory response. The vegetative form of *C tetani* produces a potent plasmid-encoded exotoxin (tetanospasmin), which binds to gangliosides at the myoneural junction of skeletal muscle and on neuronal membranes in the spinal cord, blocking inhibitory impulses to motor neurons.

Epidemiology

Tetanus occurs worldwide and is more common in warmer climates and during warmer months, in part because of higher frequency of contaminated wounds associated with those locations and seasons. The organism, a normal inhabitant of soil and animal and human intestines, is ubiquitous in the environment, especially where contamination by excreta is common. Organisms multiply in wounds, recognized or unrecognized, and elaborate toxins in the presence of anaerobic conditions. Contaminated wounds, especially wounds with devitalized tissue and deep-puncture trauma, are at greatest risk. Neonatal tetanus is common in many developing countries where pregnant women are not immunized appropriately against tetanus and nonsterile umbilical cord care practices are followed. Widespread active immunization against tetanus has modified the epidemiology of disease in the United States, where 40 or fewer cases have been reported annually since 1999. Tetanus is not transmissible from person to person.

Incubation Period

Approximately 8 days (range, 3–21 days); neonatal tetanus, mean 7 days (range, 4–14 days after birth).

Diagnostic Tests

The diagnosis of tetanus is made clinically by excluding other causes of tetanic spasms, such as hypocalcemic tetany, phenothiazine reaction, strychnine poisoning, and conversion disorder. A protective serum antitoxin concentration should not be used to exclude the diagnosis of tetanus.

Treatment

Human tetanus immune globulin (TIG), given in a single dose, is recommended for treatment; however, the optimal therapeutic dose has not been established. Infiltration of part of the dose locally around the wound is recommended, although the efficacy of this approach has not been proven. In countries where TIG is not available, equine tetanus antitoxin may be available. This product no longer is available in the United States. Equine antitoxin is administered after appropriate testing for sensitivity and desensitization. All wounds should be cleaned and debrided properly, especially if extensive necrosis is present. In neonatal tetanus, wide excision of the umbilical stump is not indicated. Supportive care and pharmacotherapy to control tetanic spasms are of major importance. Oral (or intravenous) metronidazole is effective in decreasing the number of vegetative forms of *C tetani* and is the antimicrobial agent of choice. Parenteral penicillin is an alternative treatment.

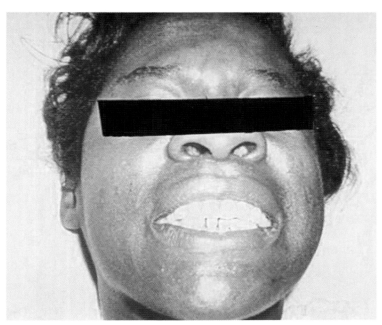

Image 131.1
Trismus in an adult with tetanus. Copyright Charles Prober, MD.

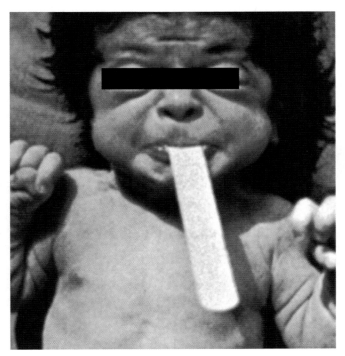

Image 131.2
Severe muscular spasms with trismus in an infant who acquired neonatal tetanus from contamination of the umbilical stump.

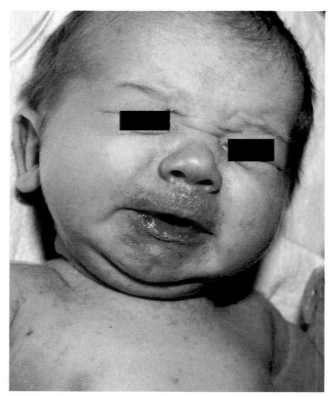

Image 131.3
The face of an infant with neonatal tetanus with risus sardonicus. Copyright Martin G. Myers, MD.

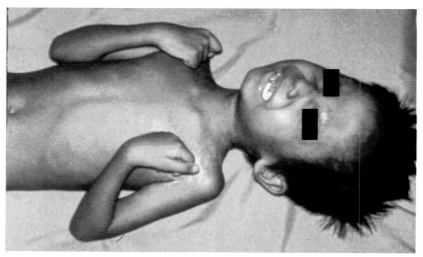

Image 131.4
A preschool-aged boy with tetanus with severe muscle contractions, generalized, caused by tetano-spasmin action in the central nervous system. Courtesy of Centers for Disease Control and Prevention.

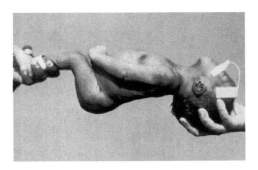

Image 131.5

This neonate is displaying a bodily rigidity produced by *Clostridium tetani* exotoxin. Neonatal tetanus may occur in infants born without protective passive immunity when the mother is not immune. It usually occurs through infection of the unhealed umbilical stump, particularly when the stump is cut with an unsterile instrument. Courtesy of Centers for Disease Control and Prevention.

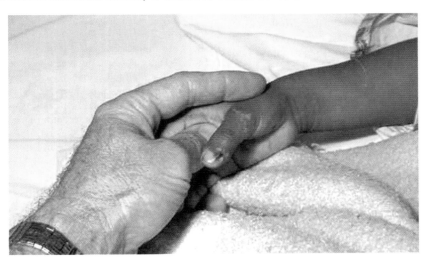

Image 131.6

A preschool-aged boy with localized tetanus secondary to the parent attempting to drain an impetigo lesion with a mesquite thorn contaminated with tetanus spores. Courtesy of Edgar O. Ledbetter, MD, FAAP.

132

Tinea Capitis
(Ringworm of the Scalp)

Clinical Manifestations

Fungal infection of the scalp may manifest as one of the following distinct clinical syndromes: **patchy areas** of dandruff-like scaling, with subtle or extensive hair loss, which may be confused with dandruff, seborrheic dermatitis, or atopic dermatitis; head/neck lymphadenopathy; **discrete areas** of hair loss studded by stubs of broken hairs, which is referred to as *black-dot ringworm*; **numerous discrete pustules** or excoriations with little hair loss or scaling or **kerion,** a boggy inflammatory mass surrounded by follicular pustules, which is a hypersensitivity reaction to the fungal infection; and a **pruritic, fine, papulovesicular eruption** (dermatophytid or id reaction) involving the trunk, extremities, and/or face caused by a hypersensitivity response to the infecting fungus. Kerion can be accompanied by fever and local lymphadenopathy and commonly is misdiagnosed as impetigo, cellulitis, or an abscess of the scalp.

Tinea capitis may be confused with many other diseases, including seborrheic dermatitis, atopic dermatitis, psoriasis, alopecia areata, trichotillomania, folliculitis, impetigo, head lice, and lupus erythematosus.

Etiology

Trichophyton tonsurans is the cause of tinea capitis in more than 90% of cases in North and Central America. *Microsporum canis, Microsporum audouinii, Trichophyton violaceum,* and *Trichophyton mentagrophytes* are less common.

Epidemiology

Infection of the scalp with *T tonsurans* is thought to result primarily from person-to-person transmission. The organism remains viable on combs, hairbrushes, and other fomites for long periods, and the role of fomites in transmission is a concern but has not been defined. *T tonsurans* often is cultured from the scalp of family members or asymptomatic children in close contact with an index case. Asymptomatic carriers are thought to have a significant role as reservoirs for infection and reinfection within families, schools, and communities. Tinea capitis attributable to *T tonsurans* occurs most commonly in children between 3 and 9 years of age and appears to be more common in black children. Cases in young infants have been documented.

M canis infection results primarily from animal-to-human transmission, although person-to-person transmission can occur. Infection often is the result of contact with household cats or dogs.

Incubation Period

Unknown; thought to be 1 to 3 weeks.

Diagnostic Tests

Potassium hydroxide wet mount and cultures confirms the diagnosis before treatment. Wood light examination is helpful if the pathogen is *Microsporum* species. Hairs and scale obtained by gentle scraping of a moistened area of the scalp with a blunt scalpel, toothbrush, brush, tweezers, or a moistened cotton swab are used for potassium hydroxide wet mount examination and culture. In cases of *T tonsurans* infection, microscopic examination of a potassium hydroxide wet mount preparation will disclose numerous arthroconidia within the hair shaft. In *Microsporum* infection, spores surround the hair shaft. Use of dermatophyte test medium also is a reliable, simple, and inexpensive method of diagnosing tinea capitis. Skin scrapings, brushings, or hairs from lesions are inoculated directly onto culture medium and incubated at room temperature.

Examination of hair of patients with *Microsporum* infection under Wood light results in brilliant green fluorescence. However, because *T tonsurans* does not fluoresce under Wood light, this diagnostic test is not helpful for most patients with tinea capitis.

Treatment

Because topical antifungal medications are not effective for treatment of tinea capitis, systemic antifungal therapy is required. Microsize griseofulvin or ultramicrosize griseofulvin is administered orally once daily. Optimally, griseofulvin is given after a meal containing fat (eg, peanut butter or ice cream). Treatment typically is necessary for 4 to 6 weeks and should be continued for 2 weeks beyond clinical resolution. Prolonged therapy (beyond 8 weeks) may be associated with a greater risk of hepatotoxicity. A 6-week course of terbinafine in the form of oral granules has been shown to be as effective as a 6-week course of griseofulvin for treatment of tinea capitis. Baseline serum transaminase (alanine transaminase and aspartate transaminase) testing is advised. In addition, off-label treatment with oral itraconazole or fluconazole may be effective for tinea capitis. *Microsporum* infections are more likely to respond to griseofulvin, and *Trichophyton* infections are more likely to respond to terbinafine. Selenium sulfide shampoo, either 1% or 2.5%, used twice a week, decreases fungal shedding and may help curb spread of infection.

Kerion can be treated with griseofulvin; terbinafine may be used if a *Trichophyton* species is the pathogen. Corticosteroid therapy consisting of prednisone or prednisolone administered occasionally is needed for optimal therapeutic response. Treatment with a corticosteroid should be continued for approximately 2 weeks, with tapering doses toward the end of therapy. Antibacterial agents generally are not needed, except if there is suspected secondary infection. Surgery is not indicated.

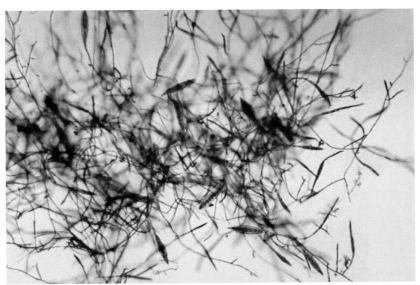

Image 132.1

Microsporum audouinii. Microsporum canis, a zoophilic dermatophyte often found in cats and dogs, is a common cause of tinea corporis and tinea capitis in humans. Other dermatophytes are included in the genera *Epidermophyton* and *Trichophyton.* Courtesy of Centers for Disease Control and Prevention/Dr Leanor Haley.

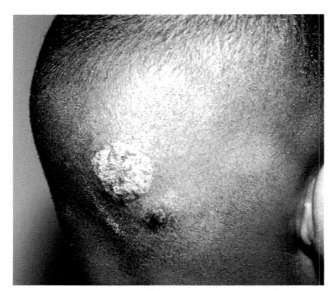

Image 132.2
A 3-year-old male with a Tinea capitis lesion on the occiput for 1 month. The mother had been applying a topical antifungal agent but the lesion became progressively larger. The patient was treated successfully with griseofulvin. Copyright Larry I. Corman.

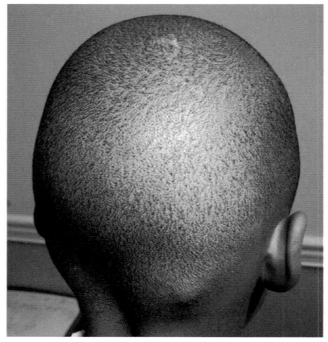

Image 132.3
An 8-year-old boy with a bald spot, hair loss, and enlarging posterior cervical lymph node for 2 weeks. The node was described as tender, not fluctuant, and without erythema of the overlying scalp. The area of hair loss was boggy and fluctuant. The patient responded well to treatment with griseofulvin. Copyright Stan Block, MD, FAAP.

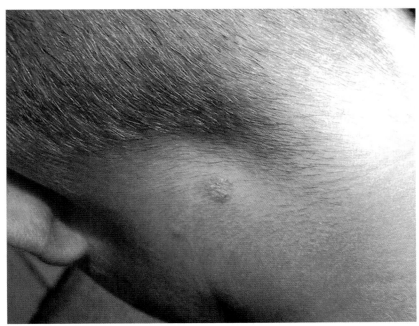

Image 132.4
Tinea capitis in the hairline of an 8-year-old boy. Copyright Stan Block, MD, FAAP.

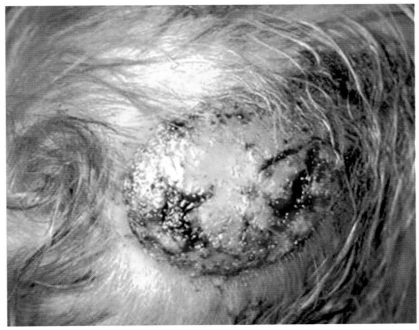

Image 132.5
A 2½-year-old boy with a kerion secondary to chronic, progressive tinea capitis. Copyright Martin G. Myers, MD.

133

Tinea Corporis
(Ringworm of the Body)

Clinical Manifestations

Superficial tinea infections of the nonhairy (glabrous) skin termed tinea corporis involve the face, trunk, or limbs. The lesion often is ring-shaped or circular (hence, the term "ringworm," slightly erythematous, and well demarcated with a scaly, vesicular, or pustular border. Small confluent plaques or papules as well as multiple lesions can occur, particularly in wrestlers (tinea gladiatorum). Lesions can be mistaken for psoriasis, pityriasis rosea, or atopic, seborrheic, or contact dermatitis. A frequent source of confusion is an alteration in the appearance of lesions as a result of application of a topical corticosteroid preparation, termed tinea incognito. Such patients also can develop Majocchi granuloma, a follicular fungal infection associated with a granulomatous dermal reaction. In patients with diminished T-lymphocyte function (eg, HIV infection), skin lesions may appear as grouped papules or pustules unaccompanied by scaling or erythema.

A pruritic, fine, papulovesicular eruption (dermatophytic or id reaction) involving the trunk, hands, or face, caused by a hypersensitivity response to infecting fungus, can accompany skin lesions. Tinea corporis can occur in association with tinea capitis, and examination of the scalp should be performed, particularly in affected wrestlers and people who have lesions on the neck and face.

Etiology

The causes of disease are fungi of the genus *Trichophyton,* especially *Trichophyton tonsurans, Trichophyton rubrum,* and *Trichophyton mentagrophytes*; the genus *Microsporum,* especially *Microsporum canis*; and *Epidermophyton floccosum. Microsporum gypseum* also occasionally can cause infection.

Epidemiology

These causative fungi occur worldwide and are transmissible by direct contact with infected humans, animals, soil, or fomites. Fungi in lesions are communicable.

Incubation Period

1 to 3 weeks but can be shorter.

Diagnostic Tests

Fungi responsible for tinea corporis can be detected by microscopic examination of a potassium hydroxide wet mount of skin scrapings. Use of dermatophyte test medium also is a reliable, simple, and inexpensive method of diagnosis. Histopathologic diagnosis using periodic acid-Schiff staining and PCR diagnostic tools are available but are expensive and generally unnecessary.

Treatment

Topical application of a miconazole, clotrimazole, terbinafine (≥12 years of age), tolnaftate, naftifine, or ciclopirox (≥10 years of age) preparation twice a day or of a ketoconazole, econazole, oxiconazole, butenafine (≥12 years of age), or sulconazole preparation once a day is recommended. If significant clinical improvement is not seen after 4 to 6 weeks of treatment, an alternate diagnosis should be considered. Topical preparations of antifungal medication mixed with high-potency corticosteroids should not be used. If lesions are extensive or unresponsive to topical therapy, griseofulvin is administered orally for 4 weeks. Oral itraconazole, fluconazole, and terbinafine are alternative effective options for more severe cases.

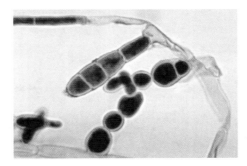

Image 133.1
This photomicrograph reveals a number of macroconidia of the dermatophytic fungus *Epidermophyton floccosum. E floccosum* is known to be a cause of dermatophytosis leading to tinea corporis (ringworm), tinea cruris (jock itch), tinea pedis (athlete's foot), and onychomycosis or tinea unguium, a fungal infection of the nail bed. Courtesy of Centers for Disease Control and Prevention/Dr Libero Ajello.

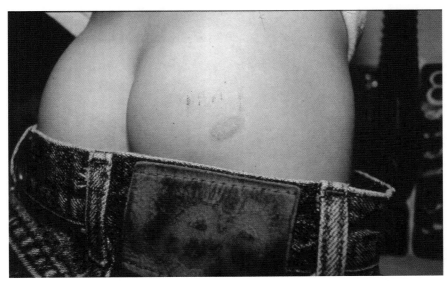

Image 133.2
Ringworm. Copyright James Brien, DO.

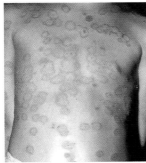

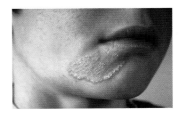

Image 133.4
Tinea corporis of the face. These annular erythematous lesions have a scaly center. Copyright Charles Prober, MD.

Image 133.3
Generalized tinea corporis in a 5-year-old female.

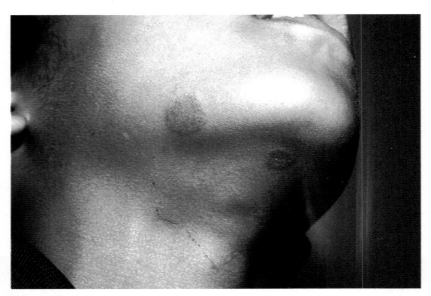

Image 133.5
Tinea corporis of the chin on a 6-year-old girl with enlarging lesions. The patient was successfully treated with clotrimazole. Copyright Larry I. Corman.

134

Tinea Cruris
(Jock Itch)

Clinical Manifestations

Tinea cruris is a common superficial fungal disorder of the groin and upper thighs. The eruption usually is bilaterally symmetric and sharply marginated, often with polycyclic borders. Involved skin is erythematous and scaly and varies from red to brown; occasionally, the eruption is accompanied by central clearing and a vesiculopapular border. In chronic infections, the margin may be subtle, and lichenification may be present. Tinea cruris skin lesions may be extremely pruritic. These lesions should be differentiated from candidiasis, intertrigo, seborrheic dermatitis, psoriasis, atopic dermatitis, irritant or allergic contact dermatitis (generally caused by therapeutic agents applied to the area), and erythrasma. The latter is a superficial bacterial infection of the skin caused by *Corynebacterium minutissimum*.

Etiology

The fungi *Epidermophyton floccosum, Trichophyton rubrum,* and *Trichophyton mentagrophytes* are the most common causes. *Trichophyton tonsurans* also has been identified.

Epidemiology

Tinea cruris occurs predominantly in adolescent and adult males, mainly via indirect contact from desquamated epithelium or hair. Moisture, close-fitting garments, friction, and obesity are predisposing factors. Direct or indirect person-to-person transmission can occur. This infection commonly occurs in association with tinea pedis, and all infected patients should be evaluated for this possibility.

Incubation Period

Approximately 1 to 3 weeks.

Diagnostic Tests

Fungi responsible for tinea cruris may be detected by microscopic examination of a potassium hydroxide wet mount of scales. Use of dermatophyte test medium also is a reliable, simple, and inexpensive method of diagnosing tinea cruris. Skin scrapings from lesions are inoculated directly onto culture medium and incubated at room temperature. A characteristic coral-red fluorescence under Wood light can identify the presence of erythrasma (an eruption of reddish brown patches attributable to the presence of *C minutissimum*) and, thus, exclude tinea cruris.

Treatment

Twice-daily topical application of a clotrimazole, miconazole, terbinafine (≥12 years of age), tolnaftate, or ciclopirox (≥10 years of age) preparation rubbed or sprayed onto the affected areas and surrounding skin is effective. Once-daily therapy with topical econazole, ketoconazole, naftifine, oxiconazole, butenafine (≥12 years of age), or sulconazole preparation also is effective. Tinea pedis, if present, should be treated concurrently.

Topical preparations of antifungal medication mixed with high-potency corticosteroids should be avoided because of the potential for prolonged infections and local and systemic adverse corticosteroid-induced events. Loose-fitting, washed cotton underclothes to decrease chafing as well as the use of an absorbent powder can be helpful adjuvants to therapy. Griseofulvin, given orally for 2 to 6 weeks, may be effective in unresponsive cases. Because many conditions mimic tinea cruris, a differential diagnosis should be considered if primary treatments fail.

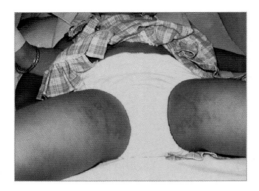

Image 134.1
Symmetric, confluent, annular, scaly red, and hyperpigmented plaques. This 10-year-old girl developed a chronic itchy eruption on the groin that spread to the anterior thighs. A potassium hydroxide preparation showed hyphae, and she was treated successfully with topical antifungal cream.

135

Tinea Pedis and Tinea Unguium
(Athlete's Foot, Ringworm of the Feet)

Clinical Manifestations

Tinea pedis manifests as a fine scaly or vesiculopustular eruption that commonly is pruritic. Lesions can involve all areas of the foot but usually are patchy in distribution, with a predisposition to fissures and scaling between toes, particularly in the third and fourth interdigital spaces or distributed around the sides of the feet. Toenails can be infected and can be dystrophic (tinea unguium). Tinea pedis must be differentiated from dyshidrotic eczema, atopic dermatitis, contact dermatitis, juvenile plantar dermatosis, palmoplantar keratoderma, and erythrasma (an eruption of reddish brown patches caused by *Corynebacterium minutissimum*). Tinea pedis commonly occurs in association with tinea cruris and onychomycosis (tinea unguium), a nail infection by any fungus. Dermatophyte infections commonly affect otherwise healthy people, but immunocompromised people have increased susceptibility.

Tinea pedis and many other fungal infections can be accompanied by a hypersensitivity reaction to the fungi (the dermatophytid or id reaction), with resulting papular or papulovesicular eruptions on the palms and the sides of fingers and, occasionally, by an erythematous vesicular eruption on the extremities and trunk.

Etiology

The fungi *Trichophyton rubrum, Trichophyton mentagrophytes,* and *Epidermophyton floccosum* are the most common causes of tinea pedis.

Epidemiology

Tinea pedis is a common infection worldwide in adolescents and adults but is less common in young children. Fungi are acquired by contact with skin scales containing fungi or with fungi in damp areas, such as swimming pools, locker rooms, and showers. Tinea pedis can spread throughout the household among family members and is communicable for as long as infection is present.

Incubation Period

Unknown.

Diagnostic Tests

Tinea pedis usually is diagnosed by clinical manifestations and may be confirmed by microscopic examination of a potassium hydroxide wet mount of the cutaneous scrapings. Use of dermatophyte test medium is a reliable, simple, and inexpensive method of diagnosis in complicated or unresponsive cases but must be interpreted by an experienced observer. Skin scrapings are inoculated directly onto the culture medium and incubated at room temperature. Infection of the nail can be verified by direct microscopic examination with potassium hydroxide, fungal culture of desquamated subungual material, or fungal stain of a nail clipping fixed in formalin.

Treatment

Topical application of terbinafine, twice daily; ciclopirox; or an azole agent (clotrimazole, miconazole, econazole, oxiconazole, sertaconazole, ketoconazole), once or twice daily, usually is adequate for milder cases. Acute vesicular lesions may be treated with intermittent use of open wet compresses (eg, with Burrow solution, 1:80). Dermatophyte infections in other locations, if present, should be treated concurrently.

Tinea pedis that is severe, chronic, or refractory to topical treatment can be treated with oral therapy. Oral itraconazole or terbinafine is the most effective, with griseofulvin next and fluconazole least effective. Hypersensitivity response reactions are treated by wet compresses, topical corticosteroids, occasionally systemic corticosteroids, and eradication of the primary source of infection.

Recurrence is prevented by proper foot hygiene, which includes keeping the feet dry and cool, gentle cleaning, drying between the toes, use of absorbent antifungal foot powder, frequent airing of affected areas, and avoidance of occlusive footwear and nylon socks or other fabrics that interfere with dissipation of moisture.

In people with onychomycosis (tinea unguium), topical therapy should be used only when the infection is confined to the distal ends of the nail. Studies in adults have demonstrated the best cure rates after therapy with oral itraconazole or terbinafine; however, safety and effectiveness in children has not been established. Recurrences are common. Removal of the nail plate followed by use of oral therapy during the period of regrowth can help to affect a cure in resistant cases.

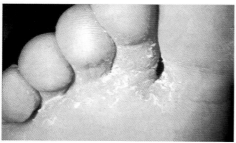

Image 135.1
Tinea pedis.

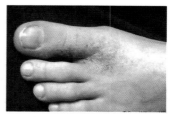

Image 135.2
Tinea pedis and tinea unguium. Copyright Gary Williams, MD.

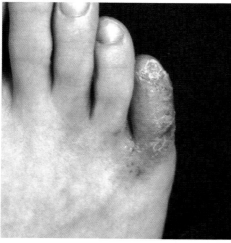

Image 135.3
Tinea pedis and tinea unguium infection. This is the same patient as in Image 135.2. Copyright Gary Williams, MD.

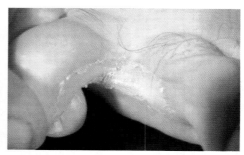

Image 135.4
This patient presented with ringworm or tinea pedis of the toes, which is also known as athlete's foot. Tinea pedis is a fungal infection of the feet, principally involving the toe webs and soles. Athlete's foot can be caused by the fungi *Epidermophyton floccosum* or by numerous members of the *Trichophyton* genus. Courtesy of Centers for Disease Control and Prevention/Dr Lucille K. Georg.

136

Toxocariasis

(Visceral Larva Migrans, Ocular Larva Migrans)

Clinical Manifestations

The severity of symptoms depends on the number of larvae ingested and the degree of allergic response. Most people who are infected lightly are asymptomatic. Toxocariasis can manifest only as wheezing or eosinophilia. Characteristic manifestations of visceral toxocariasis include fever, leukocytosis, eosinophilia, hypergammaglobulinemia, and hepatomegaly. Other manifestations may include malaise, anemia, cough and, in rare instances, pneumonia, myocarditis, and encephalitis. When ocular invasion (resulting in endophthalmitis or retinal granulomas) occurs, other evidence of infection usually is lacking, suggesting that visceral and ocular manifestations are distinct syndromes. Atypical manifestations include hemorrhagic rash and seizures.

Etiology

Toxocariasis is caused by *Toxocara* species, which are common roundworms of dogs and cats (especially puppies or kittens), specifically *Toxocara canis* and *Toxocara cati*. In the United States, most cases are caused by *T canis*. Other nematodes of animals also can cause this syndrome, although rarely.

Epidemiology

On the basis of a nationally representative survey, 14% of the US population has serologic evidence of *Toxocara* infection, and infection is concentrated among the poor. Visceral toxocariasis typically occurs in children 2 to 7 years of age often with a history of pica but can occur in older children and adults. Ocular larva migrans usually occurs in older children and adolescents. Humans are infected by ingestion of soil containing infective eggs of the parasite. Eggs may be found wherever dogs and cats defecate, often in sandboxes and playgrounds. Direct contact with dogs is of secondary importance, because eggs are not infective immediately when shed in the feces. Infection risk is highest in hot, humid regions where eggs persist in soil.

Incubation Period

Unknown.

Diagnostic Tests

Hypereosinophilia and hypergammaglobulinemia associated with increased titers of isohemagglutinin to the A and B blood group antigens are presumptive evidence of infection. Microscopic identification of larvae in a liver biopsy specimen is diagnostic, but this finding is rare and a negative biopsy does not exclude the diagnosis. An enzyme immunoassay for *Toxocara* antibodies in serum, available at the Centers for Disease Control and Prevention and some commercial laboratories, can provide confirmatory evidence of toxocariasis but does not distinguish between past and current, active infection. This assay is specific and sensitive for diagnosis of visceral larva migrans but is less sensitive for diagnosis of ocular larva migrans.

Treatment

Albendazole is the drug of choice for treatment of toxocariasis. In severe cases with myocarditis or involvement of the central nervous system, corticosteroid therapy is indicated. Correcting the underlying causes of pica helps prevent reinfection.

Antiparasitic treatment of ocular larva migrans may not be effective. Inflammation may be decreased by topical or systemic corticosteroids, and secondary damage decreased with surgery.

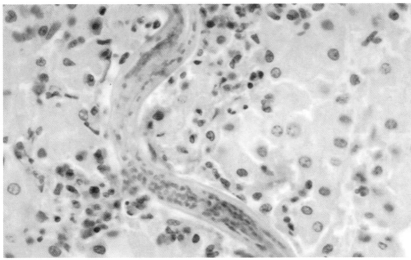

Image 136.1
Toxocariasis (visceral larva migrans) with *Toxocara canis* larvae on liver biopsy.

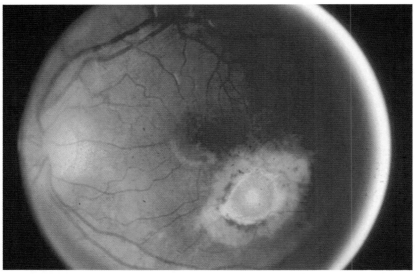

Image 136.2
Toxocara canis. Fundus damage from larval invasion. Courtesy of Hugh Moffet, MD.

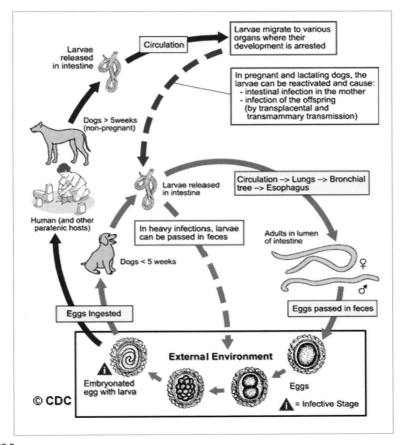

Image 136.3

Toxocara canis accomplishes its life cycle in dogs, with humans acquiring the infection as accidental hosts. Following ingestion by dogs, the infective eggs yield larvae that penetrate the gut wall and migrate into various tissues, where they encyst if the dog is older than 5 weeks. In younger dogs, the larvae migrate through the lungs, bronchial tree, and esophagus; adult worms develop and oviposit in the small intestine. In the older dogs, the encysted stages are reactivated during pregnancy and infect by the transplacental and transmammary routes of the puppies, in whose small intestine adult worms become established. Thus infective eggs are excreted by lactating adult female dogs and puppies. Humans are paratenic hosts who become infected by ingesting infective eggs in contaminated soil. After ingestion, the eggs yield larvae that penetrate the intestinal wall and are carried by the circulation to a wide variety of tissues (liver, heart, lungs, brain, muscle, eyes).

While the larvae do not undergo any further development in these sites, they can cause severe local reactions that are the basis of toxocariasis. Courtesy of Centers for Disease Control and Prevention/ Alexander J. da Silva, PhD/Melanie Moser.

137

Toxoplasma gondii Infections
(Toxoplasmosis)

Clinical Manifestations

Infants with congenital infection are asymptomatic at birth in 70% to 90% of cases, although visual or hearing impairment, learning disabilities, or mental retardation will become apparent in a large proportion of children several months to years later. Signs of congenital toxoplasmosis at birth can include a maculopapular rash, generalized lymphadenopathy, hepatosplenomegaly, jaundice, pneumonitis, diarrhea, hypothermia, petechiae, and thrombocytopenia. As a consequence of intrauterine infection, meningoencephalitis, cerebrospinal fluid (CSF) abnormalities, hydrocephalus, microcephaly, chorioretinitis, seizures, and deafness can develop. Some severely affected fetuses/infants die in utero or within a few days of birth. Cerebral calcifications can be demonstrated by ultrasonography or computed tomography (CT) of the head. CT is the radiologic technique of choice because it is the most sensitive for calcifications and can reveal brain abnormalities when ultrasonographic studies are normal. The classical triad of cerebral calcifications, chorioretinitis, and hydrocephalus is rare but it is highly suggestive of congenital toxoplasmosis, and it is seen primarily in babies whose mothers were not treated for toxoplasmosis during gestation.

Toxoplasma gondii infection acquired after birth can be asymptomatic, except in immunocompromised people. When symptoms develop, they are nonspecific and include malaise, fever, headache, sore throat, arthralgia, and myalgia. Lymphadenopathy, frequently cervical, is the most common sign. Occasionally, patients may have a mononucleosis-like illness associated with a macular rash and hepatosplenomegaly. The clinical course usually is benign and self-limited. Myocarditis, myositis, hepatitis, pericarditis, pneumonia, and skin lesions are rare complications in the United States and Europe. However, these manifestations and more aggressive disease, including brain abscesses, life-threatening syndromes, and death, have been observed in immunocompetent people infected in certain tropical countries in South America, such as French Guiana, Brazil, and Colombia.

Isolated ocular toxoplasmosis commonly results from reactivation of congenital infection but also occurs in people with acquired infection. In Brazil and Canada, up to 17% of patients diagnosed with postnatally acquired toxoplasmosis have been found to have toxoplasmic chorioretinitis. Characteristic retinal lesions (chorioretinitis) develop in up to 85% of young adults after untreated congenital infection. Acute ocular involvement manifests as blurred vision, eye pain, decreased visual acuity, floaters, scotoma, photophobia, or epiphora. The most common late finding is chorioretinitis, which can result in unilateral vision loss. Ocular disease can become reactivated years after the initial infection in healthy and immunocompromised people.

In chronically infected immunodeficient patients, including people with HIV infection, reactivation of *T gondii* can result in life-threatening encephalitis, pneumonitis, fever of unknown origin, or disseminated toxoplasmosis. In patients with AIDS, toxoplasmic encephalitis (TE) is the most common syndrome and typically presents with acute to subacute neurologic or psychiatric symptoms and multiple ring-enhancing brain lesions. In these patients, a clear improvement in their symptoms and signs within 7 to 10 days of beginning empirical antitoxoplasma drugs is considered diagnostic of TE. However, immunocompromised patients without AIDS (eg, transplant or cancer patients, patients taking immunosuppressive drugs) who are chronically infected with *T gondii* and who present with multiple ring-enhancing brain lesions, the differential diagnosis should be widened to other pathogens, such as molds and *Nocardia*. TE also can present as single brain lesion by magnetic resonance imaging (MRI) or as a diffuse and rapidly progressive process in the setting of apparently negative brain MRI studies. MRI is superior to CT for the diagnosis of toxoplasmic encephalitis.

Seropositive hematopoietic stem cell and solid organ transplant patients are at risk of their latent *T gondii* infection being reactivated. In these patients, toxoplasmosis can manifest as pneumonia, unexplained fever, myocarditis, hepatosplenomegaly, lymphadenopathy, or skin lesions in addition to brain abscesses and diffuse encephalitis. *T gondii*–seropositive solid organ donors (D+) can transmit the parasite via the allograft to seronegative recipients (R-). Thirty percent of D+/R- heart transplant recipients develop toxoplasmosis in the absence of anti–*T gondii* prophylaxis.

Etiology

T gondii is a protozoan and obligate intracellular parasite. *T gondii* exists in nature in 3 primary clonal lineages (types I, II, and III) and several infectious forms (tachyzoite, tissue cysts containing bradyzoites, and oocysts containing sporozoites. The tachyzoite and the host immune response are responsible for symptoms observed during the acute infection in humans or during the reactivation of a latent infection in immunocompromised patients. The tissue cyst is responsible for latent infection and usually is present in skeletal muscle, cardiac tissue, brain, and eyes of humans and other vertebrate animals. It is the tissue cyst form that is transmitted through undercooked or raw meat. The oocyst is present in the small intestine of cats and other members of the feline family; it is responsible for transmission through soil, water, or food contaminated with infected cat feces.

Epidemiology

T gondii is worldwide in distribution and infects most species of warm-blooded animals. The seroprevalence of *T gondii* infection (a reflection of the chronic infection and measured by the presence of *T gondii*–specific immunoglobulin [Ig] antibodies) varies by geographic locale and the socioeconomic strata of the population. The age-adjusted seroprevalence of the parasite in the United States has been estimated at 11%. Members of the feline family are definitive hosts. Cats generally acquire the infection by feeding on infected animals (eg, mice), uncooked household meats, or water or food contaminated with their own oocysts. The parasite replicates sexually in the

feline small intestine. Cats may begin to excrete millions of oocysts in their stools 3 to 30 days after primary infection and may shed oocysts for 7 to 14 days. After excretion, oocysts require a maturation phase (sporulation) of 24 to 48 hours in temperate climates before they are infective by the oral route. Sporulated oocysts survive for long periods under most ordinary environmental conditions and can survive in moist soil, for example, for months and even years. Intermediate hosts (including sheep, pigs, and cattle) can have tissue cysts in the brain, myocardium, skeletal muscle, and other organs. These cysts remain viable for the lifetime of the host. Humans usually become infected by consumption of raw or undercooked meat that contains cysts or by accidental ingestion of sporulated oocysts from soil or in contaminated food or water. A recent epidemiologic study revealed the following risk factors associated with acute infection in the United States: eating raw ground beef; eating rare lamb; eating locally produced cured, dried, or smoked meat; working with meat; drinking unpasteurized goat milk; and having 3 or more kittens. In this study, eating raw oysters, clams, or mussels also was identified as novel risk factor. Untreated water also was found to have a trend toward increased risk for acute infection in the United States. Although the risk factors for acute infection have been reported in studies from Europe, South America, and the United States, up to 50% of acutely infected people do not have identifiable risk factors or symptoms. Thus *T gondii* infection and toxoplasmosis may occur even in patients without a suggestive epidemiologic history or illness. Only appropriate laboratory testing can establish or rule out the diagnosis of *T gondii* infection or toxoplasmosis.

Transmission of *T gondii* has been documented to result from solid organ (eg, heart, kidney, liver) or hematopoietic stem cell transplantation from a seropositive donor with latent infection to a seronegative recipient. Rarely, infection has occurred as a result of a laboratory accident or from blood or blood product transfusion. In most cases, congenital transmission occurs as a result of primary maternal infection during gestation. Rarely, in utero infection may occur as a result of reactivated parasitemia during pregnancy in chronically infected immunocompromised women. There is no evidence of any other type of human-to-human transmission. The incidence of congenital toxoplasmosis in the United States has been estimated to be 1 in 1,000 to 1 in 10,000 live births.

Incubation Period

Approximately 7 days; range, 4 to 21 days.

Diagnostic Tests

Serologic tests are the primary means of diagnosing primary and latent infection. PCR assays of body fluids and staining of a biopsy specimen with *T gondii*–specific immunoperoxidase are valuable for confirming the diagnosis of toxoplasmosis. Laboratories with special expertise in *Toxoplasma* serologic assays and their interpretation, such as the Palo Alto Medical Foundation Toxoplasma Serology Laboratory (PAMF-TSL, **www.pamf. org/serology**), are useful to clinicians and nonreference laboratories.

IgG G-specific antibodies achieve a peak concentration 1 to 2 months after infection and remain positive lifelong. To determine the approximate time of infection in IgG-positive adults, specific IgM antibody determinations should be performed. The lack of *T gondii*–specific IgM antibodies in a person with low titers of IgG antibodies (eg, a Dye test at PAMF-TSL ≤512) indicates infection of at least 6 months' duration. The presence of *T gondii*–specific IgM antibodies can indicate recent infection, can be detected in chronically infected people, or can result from a false-positive reaction. Sera with positive *T gondii*–specific IgM test results may be sent to PAMF-TSL for confirmatory testing and to establish whether the patient has an acute or a chronic infection. Enzyme immunoassays (EIAs) are the most sensitive tests for IgM, and indirect fluorescent antibody tests are the least sensitive tests for detecting IgM. IgM-specific antibodies can be detected 2 weeks after infection (IgG-specific antibodies usually are negative during this period), achieve peak

concentrations in 1 month, decrease thereafter, and usually become undetectable within 6 to 9 months. However, in some people, a positive IgM test result may persist for years and without an apparent clinical significance. In adults, a positive IgM test should be followed by confirmatory testing at a laboratory with special expertise in *Toxoplasma* serology when determining the timing of infection is important clinically (eg, in a pregnant woman).

Laboratory tests that have been found to be helpful in determining timing of infection include an IgG avidity test, the AC/HS or differential agglutination test, and IgA- and IgE-specific antibody tests. The presence of high-avidity IgG antibodies indicates that infection occurred at least 12 to 16 weeks prior. However, the presence of low-avidity antibodies is not a reliable indication of recent infection, and treatment may affect the maturation of IgG avidity and prolong the presence of low-avidity antibodies. A nonacute pattern in the AC/HS test usually is indicative of an infection that was acquired at least 12 months before serum was obtained. Tests to detect IgA and IgE antibodies, which decrease to undetectable concentrations sooner than IgM antibodies do, are useful for diagnosis of congenital infections and infections in pregnant women, for whom more precise information about the duration of infection is needed. *T gondii*–specific IgA and IgE antibody tests are available in *Toxoplasma* reference laboratories but generally not in other laboratories. Diagnosis of *Toxoplasma* infection during pregnancy should be made on the basis of results of serologic assays performed in a reference laboratory.

PCR and *T gondii*–specific immunoperoxidase staining can be attempted in virtually any body fluid or tissue, depending on the clinical scenario. A positive test result for presence of *T gondii* DNA in any body fluid is diagnostic of toxoplasmosis. Essentially any tissue can be stained with *T gondii*–specific immunoperoxidase; the presence of extracellular antigens and a surrounding inflammatory response are diagnostic of toxoplasmosis.

Special Situations.

Prenatal. A definitive diagnosis of congenital toxoplasmosis can be made prenatally by detecting parasite DNA by PCR in amniotic fluid. Serial fetal ultrasonographic examinations can be performed in cases of suspected congenital infection to detect any increase in size of the lateral ventricles of the central nervous system or other signs of fetal infection, such as brain, hepatic, or splenic calcifications.

Postnatal. Infants who are born to women suspected of having or who have been diagnosed with primary *T gondii* infection during gestation should be assessed for congenital toxoplasmosis. Women infected shortly before conception (eg, within 3 months of conception) also may be at risk. In addition, infants born to immunocompromised women (HIV-infected or otherwise) with serologic evidence of past infection with *T gondii* should be evaluated for the possibility of congenital toxoplasmosis.

If an infant's *Toxoplasma* infection status is unclear at the time of delivery, *Toxoplasma*-specific laboratory tests for IgG, IgM (by the immunosorbent agglutination assay [ISAGA] method), and IgA in newborn serum samples should be performed at a laboratory with special expertise in *Toxoplasma* serologic assays. Detection of *Toxoplasma*-specific IgA antibodies is more sensitive than IgM detection in congenitally infected infants. A maternal serum sample also should be tested for IgG, IgM, and AC/HS. Peripheral blood white blood cells, CSF, urine, and amniotic fluid specimens should be assayed for *T gondii* by PCR assay in a reference laboratory. Evaluation of the infant should include ophthalmologic, auditory, and neurologic examinations; lumbar puncture; and CT of the head. An attempt may be made to isolate *T gondii* by mouse inoculation from placenta, umbilical cord, CSF, urine, or blood specimens.

Congenital infection is confirmed serologically by persistently positive IgG titers beyond the first 12 months of life. Before 12 months of age, a persistently positive or increasing IgG antibody concentration in the infant compared with the mother and/or a positive *Toxoplasma*-specific IgM or IgA assay in the infant indicate congenital infection. Although placental leak occasionally can lead to false-positive IgM or IgA reactions in the newborn infant, repeat testing after approximately 10 days of life can help confirm the diagnosis, because the half-life of these Igs is short and the titers in an infant who is not infected should decrease rapidly. The sensitivity of *T gondii*–specific IgM by an ISAGA is 87% in newborn infants born to mothers not treated during gestation; sensitivity for IgA antibodies is 77%; and when both are taken into consideration, the sensitivity increases to 93%. The indirect fluorescent assay or EIA for IgM should not be relied on to diagnose congenital infection. In an uninfected infant, a continuous decrease in IgG titer without detection of IgM or IgA antibodies will occur. Transplacentally transmitted IgG antibody usually will become undetectable by 6 to 12 months of age.

Immunocompromised patients. Immunocompromised patients (eg, patients with AIDS, solid organ transplant recipients, patients with cancer, or people taking immunosuppressive drugs) who are infected latently with *T gondii* have variable titers of IgG antibody to *T gondii* but rarely have IgM antibody. Immunocompromised patients should be tested for *T gondii*–specific IgG before commencing immunosuppressive therapy or as soon as their status of immunosuppression is diagnosed to determine whether they are chronically infected with *T gondii* and at risk of reactivation of latent infection. Active disease in immunosuppressed patients may or may not result in seroconversion and a fourfold increase in IgG antibody titers; consequently, serologic diagnosis in these patients often is difficult. Previously seropositive patients may have changes in their IgG titers in any direction (increase, decrease, or no change) without any clinical relevance. In these patients, PCR testing, histologic examination, and attempts to isolate the parasite become the laboratory methods of choice to diagnose toxoplasmosis.

In HIV-infected patients who are seropositive for *T gondii* IgG, reactivation of their latent infection usually is manifested by TE. TE can be diagnosed presumptively on the basis of characteristic clinical and radiographic findings. MRI usually reveals the presence of multiple brain-occupying and ring-enhancing lesions. If there is no clinical response within 10 days to an empirical trial of anti–*T gondii* therapy, demonstration of *T gondii* organisms, antigen, or DNA in specimens such as blood, CSF, or bronchoalveolar fluid may be necessary to confirm the diagnosis. TE also can present as diffuse encephalitis without space-occupying lesions on brain MRI. Prompt recognition of this syndrome and confirmation of the diagnosis by PCR testing in CSF is crucial, because these patients usually exhibit a rapidly progressive and fatal clinical course.

Diagnosis of TE in immunocompromised patients other than HIV-infected people requires confirmation by brain biopsy or PCR testing of CSF. In this group of patients, other organisms, such as invasive mold infections and *Nocardia,* should be considered before beginning an empiric trial of anti–*T gondii* therapy.

Infants born to women who are infected simultaneously with HIV and *T gondii* should be evaluated for congenital toxoplasmosis because of an increased likelihood of maternal reactivation and congenital transmission in this setting. Expert advice is available at the PAMF-TSL and National Collaborative Chicago-Based Congenital Toxoplasmosis Study (**www.uchospitals. edu/specialties/infectious-diseases/ toxoplasmosis**).

Ocular toxoplasmosis. Toxoplasmic chorioretinitis usually is diagnosed on the basis of characteristic retinal lesions in conjunction with serum *T gondii*–specific IgG. Confirmatory testing for IgM may yield positive results in situations in which eye lesions are the result of a concomitant acute *T gondii* infection rather than reactivation of a chronic infection. Patients who have atypical retinal lesions or who fail to respond to anti–*T gondii* therapy should undergo examination of vitreous fluid or aqueous humor by PCR, and immune load (Goldmann-Witmer coefficient) should be considered.

Treatment

Most cases of acquired infection in an immunocompetent host do not require specific antimicrobial therapy unless infection occurs during pregnancy or symptoms are severe or persistent. When indicated (eg, chorioretinitis or significant organ damage), the combination of pyrimethamine and sulfadiazine, with supplemental leucovorin (folinic acid) to minimize pyrimethamine-associated hematologic toxicity, is the regimen most widely accepted for children and adults with acute symptomatic disease. Trimethoprim-sulfamethoxazole, also available in the intravenous form, has been reported to be equivalent to pyrimethamine/sulfadiazine in the treatment of patients with toxoplasmic chorioretinitis. In addition, pyrimethamine can be used in combination with clindamycin, atovaquone, or azithromycin if the patient does not tolerate sulfonamide compounds. Corticosteroids appear to be useful in management of ocular complications, central nervous system disease (CSF protein >1,000 mg/dL), and focal lesions with substantial mass effects in certain patients.

HIV-infected adolescents and children 6 years of age or older who have completed initial therapy (at least 6 weeks and clinical response) for toxoplasmic encephalitis should receive suppressive therapy to prevent recurrence until their CD4+ T-lymphocyte count recovers above 200 cells/μL and their HIV viral load is nondetectable for at least 6 months. HIV-infected children 1 through 5 years of age also should receive suppressive therapy after completion of initial therapy; discontinuation may be considered after they have been on stable antiretroviral therapy for longer than 6 months, are asymptomatic, and have demonstrated an increase in CD4+ T-lymphocyte percentage above 15% for more than 3 consecutive months. Prophylaxis should be reinstituted whenever these parameters are not met. Regimens for primary treatment also are effective for suppressive therapy.

For symptomatic and asymptomatic congenital infections, pyrimethamine combined with sulfadiazine (supplemented with folinic acid) is recommended as initial therapy. Duration of therapy is prolonged and often is 1 year. However, the optimal dosage and duration are not established definitively and should be determined in consultation with an infectious diseases specialist. For children who have mild congenital toxoplasmosis, some experts alternate pyrimethamine/sulfadiazine/folinic acid monthly with spiramycin during months 7 through 12 of treatment. Children with moderate or severe congenital toxoplasmosis should receive pyrimethamine/sulfadiazine for the full 12 months.

Treatment of primary *T gondii* infection in pregnant women, including women with HIV infection, is recommended. Appropriate specialists should be consulted for manage-

ment. Spiramycin treatment of primary infection during gestation is used in an attempt to decrease transmission of *T gondii* from the mother to the fetus. Spiramycin treatment in pregnant women may reduce congenital transmission but does not treat the fetus if in utero infection has already occurred. Maternal therapy can decrease the severity of sequelae in the fetus once congenital toxoplasmosis has occurred. Spiramycin is available only as an investigational drug in the United States. If fetal infection is confirmed at or after 18 weeks of gestation or if the mother acquires infection during the third trimester, consideration should be given to starting therapy with pyrimethamine and sulfadiazine.

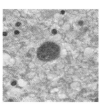

Image 137.1
Toxoplasma gondii cyst in brain tissue stained with hematoxylin and eosin. Cysts of *Toxoplasma gondii* usually range in size from 5 to 50 μm in diameter. Cysts are usually spherical in the brain but more elongated in cardiac and skeletal muscles. They may be found in various sites throughout the body of the host, but are most common in the brain and skeletal and cardiac muscles. Courtesy of Centers for Disease Control and Prevention/Dr Edwin P. Ewing, Jr.

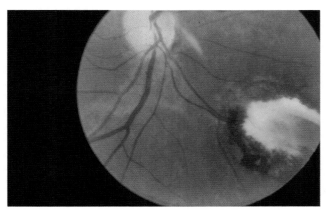

Image 137.2
A neonate with congenital toxoplasmosis with choreoretinitis. Courtesy of Larry Frenkel, MD.

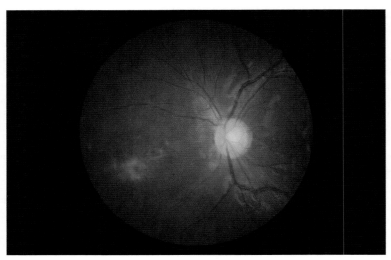

Image 137.3

A 12-year-old male with chorioretinal scar with surrounding retinitis in the left eye nasal to the disk measuring a one-quarter disk diameter adjacent to the scar with mild overlying mild vitritis. No lesions in the macula. Findings typical of toxoplasmosis. Courtesy of Vicki Chen, MD.

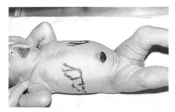

Image 137.4

Infant girl with congenital toxoplasmosis with hepatosplenomegaly. Courtesy of Edgar O. Ledbetter, MD, FAAP.

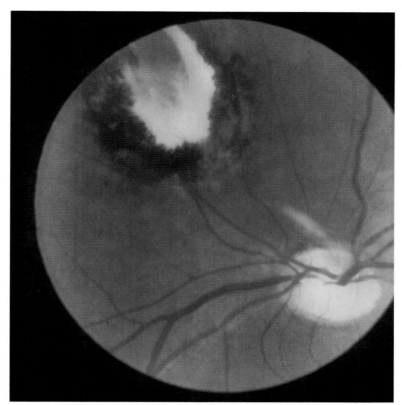

Image 137.5
Peripheral chorioretinitis in an infant with congenital toxoplasmosis. Courtesy of George Nankervis, MD.

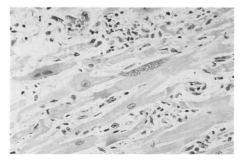

Image 137.6
Histopathology of toxoplasmosis of the heart in fatal AIDS. Within a myocyte is a pseudocyst containing numerous tachyzoites of *Toxoplasma gondii*. Several myocardial contraction bands and scattered inflammatory cells are visible. Courtesy of Centers for Disease Control and Prevention.

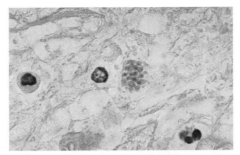

Image 137.7
Histopathology of toxoplasmosis of the brain in fatal AIDS. Pseudocyst contains numerous tachyzoites of *Toxoplasma gondii.* Courtesy of Centers for Disease Control and Prevention/Dr Edwin P. Ewing, Jr.

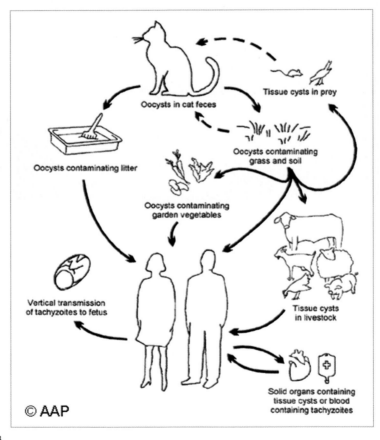

Image 137.8
Pathways for infection with *Toxoplasma gondii.* The only source for the production of *T gondii* oocysts is the feline intestinal tract. Humans usually acquire the disease by direct ingestion of oocysts from contaminated sources (eg, soil, cat litter, garden vegetables) or the ingestion of tissue cysts present in undercooked tissues from infected animals. Fetal infection occurs most commonly following acute maternal infection in pregnancy, but it also can occur following reactivation of latent infection in immunocompromised women. Pathways leading to human disease, solid arrow; pathways leading to feline infection, dashed arrow.

138

Trichinellosis
(Trichinella spiralis)

Clinical Manifestations

The clinical spectrum of infection ranges from inapparent to fulminant and fatal illness, but most infections are asymptomatic. The severity of disease is proportional to the infective dose. During the first week after ingesting infected meat, a person may experience abdominal discomfort, nausea, vomiting, and/or diarrhea as excysted larvae invade the intestine. Two to 8 weeks later, as progeny larvae migrate into tissues, fever (54%), myalgia (70%), periorbital edema (25%), urticarial rash, and conjunctival and subungual hemorrhages can develop. In severe infections, myocarditis, neurologic involvement, and pneumonitis can follow in 1 or 2 months. Larvae may remain viable in tissues for years; calcification of some larvae in skeletal muscle usually occurs within 6 to 24 months.

Etiology

Infection is caused by nematodes (roundworms) of the genus *Trichinella*. At least 5 species capable of infecting only warm-blooded animals have been identified. Worldwide, *Trichinella spiralis* is the most common cause of human infection.

Epidemiology

Infection is enzootic worldwide in carnivores and omnivores, especially scavengers. Infection occurs as a result of ingestion of raw or insufficiently cooked meat containing encysted larvae of *Trichinella* species. Commercial and home-raised pork remains a source of human infections, but meats other than pork, such as venison, horse meat, and particularly meats from wild carnivorous or omnivorous game (bear, boar, seal, and walrus) now are common sources of infection. The disease is not transmitted from person to person.

Incubation Period

Usually less than 1 month.

Diagnostic Tests

Eosinophilia approaching 70%, in conjunction with compatible symptoms and dietary history, suggests the diagnosis. Increases in concentrations of muscle enzymes, such as creatinine phosphokinase and lactic dehydrogenase, occur. Identification of larvae in suspect meat can be the most rapid source of diagnostic information. Encapsulated larvae in a skeletal muscle biopsy specimen (particularly deltoid and gastrocnemius) can be visualized microscopically beginning 2 weeks after infection by examining hematoxylin-eosin stained slides or sediment from digested muscle tissue. Serologic tests are available through commercial and state laboratories and the Centers for Disease Control and Prevention. Serum antibody titers rarely become positive before the second week of illness. Testing paired acute and convalescent serum specimens is diagnostic.

Treatment

Albendazole and mebendazole have comparable efficacy for treatment of trichinellosis. However, albendazole and mebendazole are less effective for *Trichinella* larvae already in the muscles. Coadministration of corticosteroids with mebendazole or albendazole often is recommended when systemic symptoms are severe. Corticosteroids can be lifesaving when the central nervous system or heart is involved.

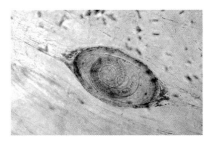

Image 138.1
Trichinella larvae in a sample of infected meat (light microscopy, x100). Courtesy of Marva E, Markovics A, Gdalevich M, Asor N, Sadik C, Leventhal A. Trichinellosis outbreak [letter]. *Emerg Infect Dis.* 2005;11(12):1979–1981.

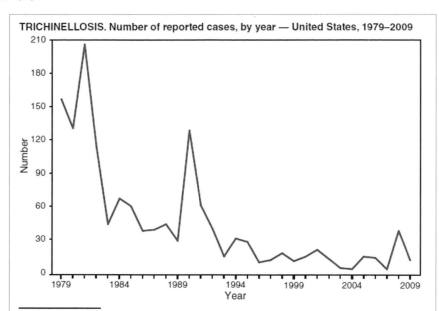

TRICHINELLOSIS. Number of reported cases, by year — United States, 1979–2009

Five of the cases reported in 2009 were associated with a shared meal containing raw bear meat. The outbreak occurred among persons of the same ethnic background as the raw bear meat-associated outbreak in 2008 that sickened approximately 30 persons. This highlights the continued need for public health prevention messages aimed at consumers of wild game meat, particularly bear, and for prevention messages targeted to cultural groups whose food choices might put them at a higher risk for *Trichinella* infection.

Image 138.2
Trichinellosis. Number of reported cases, by year—United States, 1979–2009. Courtesy of *Morbidity and Mortality Weekly Report.*

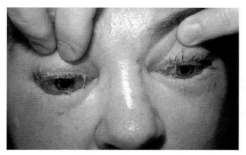

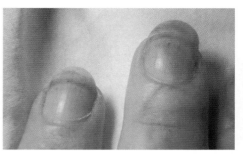

Image 138.3
This patient with trichinosis had periorbital swelling, muscle pain, diarrhea, and 28% eosinophils. Courtesy of Centers for Disease Control and Prevention/Dr Thomas F. Sellers, Emory University.

Image 138.4
Here the parasitic disease trichinosis is manifested by splinter hemorrhages under the fingernails. Trichinosis, or trichinellosis, is caused by eating raw or undercooked pork infected with the larvae of a species of worm called *Trichinella*. Initial symptoms include nausea, diarrhea, vomiting, fatigue, fever, and abdominal discomfort. Courtesy of Centers for Disease Control and Prevention/Dr Thomas F. Sellers, Emory University.

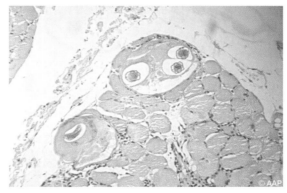

Image 138.5
Trichinella spiralis organisms on cross-section of muscle biopsy of the patient in images 138.3 and 138.4. Courtesy of Edgar O. Ledbetter, MD, FAAP.

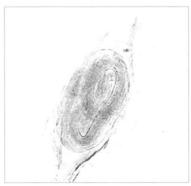

Image 138.6
Larvae of *Trichinella spiralis* in skeletal muscle biopsy.

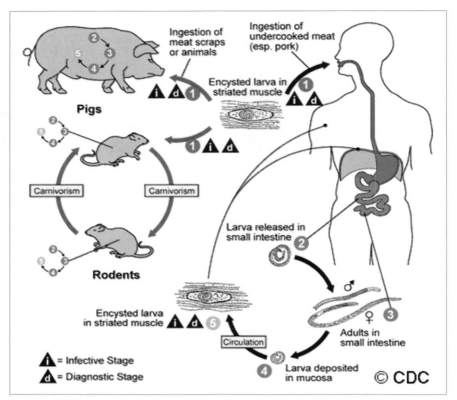

Image 138.7

Life cycle. Trichinosis is acquired by ingesting meat containing cysts (encysted larvae) (1) of *Trichinella*. After exposure to gastric acid and pepsin, the larvae are released (2) from the cysts and invade the small bowel mucosa, where they develop into adult worms (3) (females, 2.2 mm in length; males, 1.2 mm in length; life span in the small bowel, 4 weeks). After 1 week, the females release larvae (4) that migrate to the striated muscles where they encyst (5). *Pseudospiralis,* however, does not encyst. Encystment is completed in 4 to 5 weeks and the encysted larvae may remain viable for several years. Ingestion of the encysted larvae perpetuates the cycle. Rats and rodents are primarily responsible for maintaining the endemicity of this infection. Carnivorous/omnivorous animals, such as pigs or bears, feed on infected rodents or meat from other animals. Different animal hosts are implicated in the life cycle of the different species of *Trichinella.* Humans are accidentally infected when eating improperly processed meat of these carnivorous animals (or eating food contaminated with such meat). Courtesy of Centers for Disease Control and Prevention.

139

Trichomonas vaginalis Infections
(Trichomoniasis)

Clinical Manifestations

Trichomonas vaginalis infection is asymptomatic in up to 90% of infected men and 85% of infected women. Clinical manifestations in symptomatic pubertal or postpubertal female patients consist of a diffuse vaginal discharge, odor, and vulvovaginal pruritus and irritation. Dysuria and, less often, lower abdominal pain can occur. Vaginal discharge usually is yellow-green in color and can have a disagreeable odor. The vulva and vaginal mucosa can be erythematous and even edematous. The cervix can appear inflamed and sometimes is covered with numerous punctate cervical hemorrhages and swollen papillae, referred to as strawberry cervix. Clinical manifestations in symptomatic men include urethritis and, more rarely, epididymitis or prostatitis. Reinfection is common, and resistance to treatment is rare but possible. *T vaginalis* infection can increase both the acquisition and transmission of HIV.

Etiology

T vaginalis is a flagellated protozoan that is the size of a leukocyte. It requires adherence to host cells for survival.

Epidemiology

T vaginalis infection is the most common "curable" sexually transmitted infection (STI) in the United States and globally and commonly coexists with other conditions, particularly with *Neisseria gonorrhoeae* and *Chlamydia trachomatis* infections and bacterial vaginosis. The presence of *T vaginalis* in a child or preadolescent should raise suspicion of sexual abuse. *T vaginalis* acquired during birth by female newborn infants can cause vaginal discharge during the first weeks of life but usually resolves as maternal hormones are metabolized.

Incubation Period

Averages 1 week; range, 5 to 28 days.

Diagnostic Tests

Diagnosis in a symptomatic female usually is established by careful and immediate examination of a wet-mount preparation of vaginal discharge. The jerky motility of the protozoan and the movement of the flagella are distinctive. Microscopy has 60% to 70% sensitivity for diagnosis of *T vaginalis* in vaginal secretions of a symptomatic female. The presence of symptoms and the identification of the organism are related directly to the number of organisms. Culture of the organism is the most sensitive and specific method of diagnosis in females but demonstrates low sensitivity in males. Two point-of-care tests are available when no microscope is available: an immunochromatographic capillary flow dipstick and a nucleic acid probe test. These tests are reported to be more sensitive (79%–83% when compared with culture) than microscopy, but because of specificity of 97% to 99%, these tests may result in more false-positive results in populations with a low prevalence of disease (ie, adolescents). They have not been approved for use in men.

Treatment

Treatment of adults with metronidazole, in a single dose, results in cure rates of approximately 90% to 95%. Treatment with tinidazole appears to be similar or even superior to metronidazole. Topical vaginal preparations should not be used, because they do not achieve therapeutic concentrations in the urethra or perivaginal glands. Sexual partners should be treated concurrently, even if asymptomatic, because reinfection is a major factor in treatment failures. If treatment failure occurs with metronidazole and reinfection is excluded, either metronidazole for 7 days or tinidazole, in a single dose, can be used. In the event of continued treatment failure, consultation with an expert in STIs is advised.

People infected with *T vaginalis* should be evaluated for other STIs, including syphilis, gonorrhea, chlamydia, and HIV infection. For newborn infants, infection with *T vaginalis* acquired maternally is self-limited, and treatment generally is not recommended.

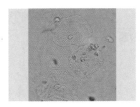

Image 139.1

An asymptomatic vaginal discharge in a premenarcheal girl who has other signs of the effects of estrogen most likely is due to physiologic leukorrhea. The discharge is caused by the desquamation of vaginal epithelial cells in response to the effect of estrogen on the vaginal mucosa. Prior to puberty, the vaginal mucosa is atrophic, the pH of vaginal secretions is 6.5 to 7.5, and the bacterial flora are mixed. Following the onset of puberty, *Lactobacillus* becomes the predominant organism in the vagina. These gram-positive bacilli metabolize sloughed epithelial cells, producing lactic acid and decreasing the pH of the vagina to less than 4.5. Courtesy of H. Cody Meissner, MD, FAAP.

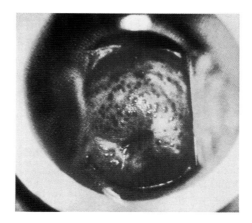

Image 139.2

This patient presented with a strawberry cervix due to a *Trichomonas vaginalis* infection, or trichomoniasis. The term strawberry cervix is used to describe the appearance of the cervix due to the presence of *T vaginalis* protozoa. The cervical mucosa reveals punctate hemorrhages along with accompanying vesicles or papules. Courtesy of Centers for Disease Control and Prevention.

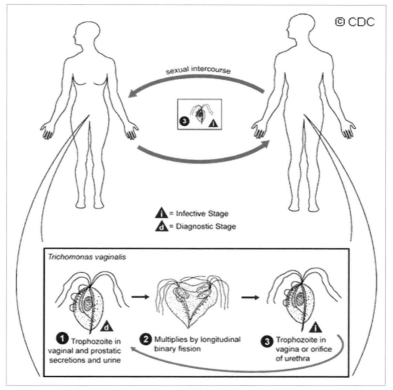

Image 139.3

Trichomonas vaginalis resides in the female lower genital tract and the male urethra and prostate (1), where it replicates by binary fission (2). The parasite does not appear to have a cyst form and does not survive well in the external environment. *T vaginalis* is transmitted among humans, its only known host, primarily by sexual intercourse (3). Courtesy of Centers for Disease Control and Prevention/Alexander J. da Silva, PhD/Melanie Moser.

140

Trichuriasis

(Whipworm Infection)

Clinical Manifestations

Disease is proportional to the intensity of the infection. Most infected children are asymptomatic. Children with heavy infestations can develop *Trichuris trichiura* colitis that mimics inflammatory bowel disease and leads to anemia, physical growth restriction, and clubbing. *T trichiura* dysentery syndrome is more intense and consists of abdominal pain, tenesmus, and bloody diarrhea with mucus; it can be associated with rectal prolapse.

Etiology

T trichiura, the human whipworm, is the causative agent. Adult worms are 30 to 50 mm long with a large, thread-like anterior end that is embedded in the mucosa of the large intestine.

Epidemiology

The parasite is the second most common soil-transmitted helminth in the world and is more common in the tropics and in areas of poor sanitation. It is coendemic with ascaris and hookworm species. Humans are the natural reservoir. In the United States, trichuriasis no longer is a public health problem, although migrants from tropical areas may be infected. Eggs require a minimum of 10 days of incubation in the soil before they are infectious. The disease is not transmissible from person to person.

Incubation Period

Approximately 12 weeks.

Diagnostic Tests

Eggs may be found on direct examination of stool or, preferably, by using concentration techniques.

Treatment

Mebendazole, albendazole, or ivermectin provides moderate rates of cure, with mebendazole being the treatment of choice. In mass treatment efforts involving entire communities, a single dose of either mebendazole or albendazole will reduce worm burdens.

141

African Trypanosomiasis
(African Sleeping Sickness)

Clinical Manifestations

The disease appears in 2 stages: the first is the hemolymphatic stage, and the second is the meningoencephalitis stage, which is characterized by invasion of the central nervous system. The rapidity and severity of clinical manifestations vary with the infecting subspecies. With *Trypanosoma brucei gambiense* (West African) infection, a cutaneous nodule or chancre may appear at the site of parasite inoculation within a few days of a bite by an infected tsetse fly. Systemic illness is chronic, occurring months to years later, and is characterized by intermittent fever, posterior cervical lymphadenopathy (Winterbottom sign), and multiple nonspecific complaints, including malaise, weight loss, arthralgia, rash, pruritus, and edema. If the central nervous system (CNS) is involved, chronic meningoencephalitis with behavioral changes, cachexia, headache, hallucinations, delusions, and somnolence can occur. In contrast, *Trypanosoma brucei rhodesiense* (East African) infection is an acute, generalized illness that develops days to weeks after parasite inoculation, with manifestations including high fever, thrombocytopenia, hepatitis, cutaneous chancre, anemia, myocarditis and, rarely, laboratory evidence of disseminated intravascular coagulopathy. Clinical meningoencephalitis can develop as early as 3 weeks after onset of the untreated systemic illness. Both forms of African trypanosomiasis have high fatality rates; without treatment, infected patients usually die within weeks to months after clinical onset of disease caused by *T brucei rhodesiense* and within a few years from disease caused by *T brucei gambiense.*

Etiology

Human African trypanosomiasis (sleeping sickness) is caused by the protozoan parasite *Trypanosoma brucei.* The west and central African (Gambian) form is caused by *T brucei gambiense.* The east and southern African (Rhodesian) form is caused by *T brucei rhodesiense.* Both are extracellular protozoan hemoflagellates that live in blood and tissue of the human host.

Epidemiology

Approximately 10,000 human cases are reported annually worldwide, although only a few cases, which are acquired in Africa, are reported every year in the United States. Transmission is confined to an area in Africa between the latitudes of 15 degrees north and 20 degrees south, corresponding precisely with the distribution of the tsetse fly vector (*Glossina* species). In East Africa, wild animals, such as antelope, bush buck, and hartebeest, constitute the major reservoirs for sporadic infections with *T brucei rhodesiense,* although cattle serve as reservoir hosts in local outbreaks. Domestic pigs and dogs have been found as incidental reservoirs of *T brucei gambiense;* however, humans are the only important reservoir in West and Central Africa.

Incubation Period

T brucei rhodesiense infection, 3 to 21 days; *T brucei gambiense* infection, 5 to 14 days.

Diagnostic Tests

Diagnosis is made by identification of trypomastigotes in specimens of blood, cerebrospinal fluid (CSF), or fluid aspirated from a chancre or lymph node or by inoculation of susceptible laboratory animals (mice) with heparinized blood. Examination of CSF is critical to management and should be performed using the double-centrifugation technique. Concentration and Giemsa staining of the buffy coat layer of peripheral blood also can be helpful and is easier for *T brucei rhodesiense,* because the density of organisms in blood circulating is higher than for *T brucei gambiense. T brucei gambiense* is more likely to be found in lymph node aspirates. Although an increased concentration of immunoglobulin M in serum or CSF is considered characteristic of African trypanosomiasis, polyclonal hyperglobulinemia is common. There is no serologic screening test for *T brucei rhodesiense.*

Treatment

When no evidence of CNS involvement is present (including absence of trypanosomes and CSF pleocytosis), the drug of choice for the acute hemolymphatic stage of infection is pentamidine for *T brucei gambiense* infection and suramin for *T brucei rhodesiense* infection.

For treatment of infection with CNS involvement, the drug of choice is eflornithine for *T brucei gambiense* infection and melarsoprol for *T brucei rhodesiense* infection. Suramin, eflornithine, and melarsoprol can be obtained from the Centers for Disease Control and Prevention Drug Service.

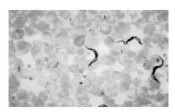

Image 141.1
Trypanosoma gambiense in blood smear (Giemsa stain).

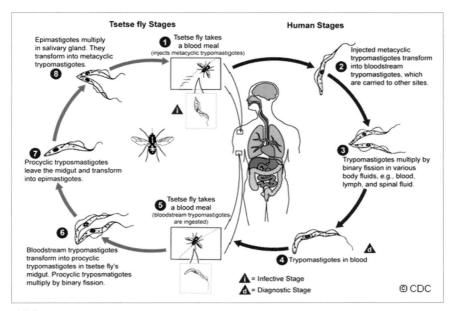

Image 141.2

Life cycle. During a blood meal on the mammalian host, an infected tsetse fly (genus *Glossina*) injects metacyclic trypomastigotes into skin tissue. The parasites enter the lymphatic system and pass into the bloodstream (1). Inside the host, they transform into bloodstream trypomastigotes (2), are carried to other sites throughout the body, reach other body fluids (eg, lymph, spinal fluid), and continue the replication by binary fission (3). The entire life cycle of African trypanosomes is represented by extra-cellular stages. The tsetse fly becomes infected with bloodstream trypomastigotes when taking a blood meal on an infected mammalian host (4, 5). In the fly's midgut, the parasites transform into procyclic trypomastigotes, multiply by binary fission (6), leave the midgut, and transform into epi-mastigotes (7). The epimastigotes reach the fly's salivary glands and continue multiplication by binary fission (8). The cycle in the fly takes approximately 3 weeks. Humans are the main reservoir for *Trypanosoma brucei gambiense,* but this species can also be found in animals. Wild game animals are the main reservoir of *T brucei rhodesiense.* Courtesy of Centers for Disease Control and Prevention/Alexander J. da Silva, PhD/Melanie Moser.

142

American Trypanosomiasis
(Chagas Disease)

Clinical Manifestations

The acute phase of *Trypanosoma cruzi* infection lasts 2 to 3 months, followed by the chronic phase, which in the absence of successful antiparasitic treatment, lasts lifelong. The acute phase commonly is asymptomatic or characterized by mild, nonspecific symptoms. Young children are more likely to exhibit symptoms than are adults. In some patients, a red, indurated nodule known as a *chagoma* develops at the site of the original inoculation, usually on the face or arms. Unilateral edema of the eyelids, known as the Romaña sign, may occur if the portal of entry was the conjunctiva; it is not always present. The edematous skin may be violaceous and associated with conjunctivitis and enlargement of the ipsilateral preauricular lymph node. Fever, malaise, generalized lymphadenopathy, and hepatosplenomegaly may develop. In rare instances, acute myocarditis and/or meningoencephalitis can occur. The symptoms of acute Chagas disease resolve without treatment within 3 months, and patients pass into the chronic phase of the infection. Most people with chronic *T cruzi* infection have no signs or symptoms and are said to have the indeterminate form. In 20% to 30% of cases, serious progressive sequelae affecting the heart and/or gastrointestinal tract develop years to decades after the initial infection (sometimes called determinate forms of chronic *T cruzi* infection). Chagas cardiomyopathy is characterized by conduction system abnormalities, especially right bundle branch block, and ventricular arrhythmias and can progress to dilated cardiomyopathy and congestive heart failure. Patients with Chagas cardiomyopathy can die suddenly from ventricular arrhythmias, complete heart block, or emboli phenomena; death also may occur from intractable congestive heart failure. Congenital Chagas disease may be characterized by low birth weight, hepatosplenomegaly, myocarditis, or meningoencephalitis with seizures and tremors, but most infants with congenital *T cruzi* infection have no signs or symptoms of disease. Reactivation of chronic *T cruzi* infection can occur in immunocompromised people, including people infected with HIV and those who are immunosuppressed after transplantation.

Etiology

T cruzi, a protozoan hemoflagellate, is the cause.

Epidemiology

Parasites are transmitted in feces of infected triatomine insects (sometimes called "kissing bugs"; local Spanish names include *vinchuca, chinche picuda*). The bugs defecate during or after taking blood. The bitten person is inoculated through inadvertently rubbing the insect feces containing the parasite into the site of the bite or mucous membranes of the eye or the mouth. The parasite also can be transmitted congenitally, during solid organ transplantation, through blood transfusion, and by ingestion of food or drink contaminated by the vector's excreta. Vectorborne transmission of the disease is limited to the Western hemisphere, predominantly Mexico and Central and South America. The southern United States has established enzootic cycles of *T cruzi* involving several triatomine vector species and mammalian hosts, such as raccoons, opossums, rodents, and domestic dogs. Nevertheless, most *T cruzi*–infected individuals in the United States are immigrants from areas of Latin America with endemic infection.

Several transfusion- and transplantation-associated cases have been documented in the United States. The disease is an important cause of morbidity and death in Latin America, where an estimated 8 to 10 million people are infected, of whom 30% to 40% either have or will develop cardiomyopathy.

Incubation Period

Acute phase, 1 to 2 weeks or longer; chronic manifestations, years to decades.

Diagnostic Tests

During the acute phase of disease, the parasite is demonstrable in blood specimens by Giemsa staining after a concentration technique or in direct wet-mount or buffy coat preparations.

Molecular techniques and hemoculture in special media (available at the Centers for Disease Control and Prevention) also have high sensitivity in the acute phase. The chronic phase of *T cruzi* infection is characterized by low-level parasitemia; the sensitivity of culture and PCR generally is less than 50%. Diagnosis in the chronic phase relies on serologic tests to demonstrate immunoglobulin (Ig) G antibodies against *T cruzi*. Serologic tests to detect anti–*T cruzi* IgG antibodies include indirect immunofluorescent and enzyme immunosorbent assays. Samples should be tested in 2 assays based on different formats before diagnostic decisions are made. Two blood donor screening assays (Ortho *T cruzi* test system and the Abbott Prism Chagas assay) are available for blood donor screening. Confirmation of positive serologic test by radioimmune precipitation assay (Chagas RIPA) or an in vitro enzyme strip assay (Abbott ESA Chagas [*T cruzi* {*E coli* recombinant} antigen]) is recommended.

The diagnosis of congenital Chagas disease can be made during the first 3 months of life by identification of motile trypomastigotes by direct microscopy of fresh anticoagulated blood specimens. PCR assay has higher sensitivity than microscopy. All infants born to seropositive mothers should be screened using conventional serologic testing after 9 months of age, when IgG measurements reflect infant response.

Treatment

Antitrypanosomal treatment is recommended for all cases of acute and congenital Chagas disease, reactivated infection, and chronic *T cruzi*–infection in children younger than 18 years. Treatment of chronic *T cruzi* infection in adults without advanced cardiomyopathy also generally is recommended. The only drugs with proven efficacy are benznidazole and nifurtimox.

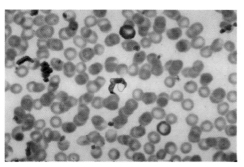

Image 142.1

This is a photomicrograph of *Trypanosoma cruzi* in a blood smear using Giemsa staining technique. This protozoan parasite, *T cruzi,* is the causative agent for Chagas disease, also known as American trypanosomiasis. It is estimated that 16 to 18 million people are infected with Chagas disease, and of those infected, 50,000 will die each year. Courtesy of Centers for Disease Control and Prevention/Dr Mae Melvin.

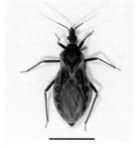

Image 142.2

Adult female kissing bug of the species *Triatoma rubida,* the most abundant triatomine species in southern Arizona (scale bar = 1 cm). Chagas disease is endemic throughout Mexico and Central and South America, with 7.7 million persons infected, 108.6 million persons considered at risk, 33.3 million symptomatic cases, an annual incidence of 42,500 cases (through vectorial transmission), and 21,000 deaths every year. This disease is caused by the protozoan parasite *Trypanosoma cruzi,* which is transmitted to humans by bloodsucking insects of the family Reduviidae (Triatominae). Although mainly a vector-borne disease, Chagas disease also can be acquired by humans through blood transfusions and organ transplantation, congenitally (from a pregnant woman to her baby), and through oral contamination (eg, foodborne). Courtesy of *Emerging Infectious Diseases*/C. Hedgcock.

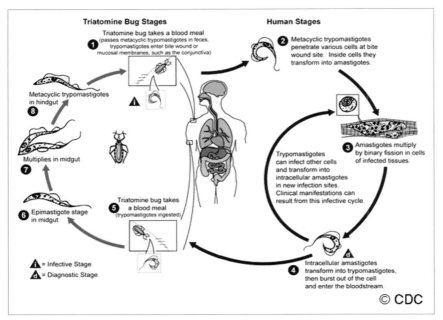

Image 142.3

Life cycle. An infected triatomine insect vector (or "kissing bug") takes a blood meal and releases try-pomastigotes in its feces near the site of the bite wound. Trypomastigotes enter the host through the wound or through intact mucosal membranes, such as the conjunctiva (1). Common triatomine vector species for trypanosomiasis belong to the genera *Triatoma, Rhodinius,* and *Panstrongylus.* Inside the host, the trypomastigotes invade cells, where they differentiate into intracellular amastigotes (2). The amastigotes multiply by binary fission (3), differentiate into trypomastigotes, and then are released into the circulation as bloodstream trypomastigotes (4). Trypomastigotes infect cells from a variety of tis-sues and transform into intracellular amastigotes in new infection sites. Clinical manifestations can result from this infective cycle. The bloodstream trypomastigotes do not replicate (different from the African trypanosomes). Replication resumes only when the parasites enter human or animal blood that contains circulating parasites (5). The ingested trypomastigotes transform into epimastigotes in the vector's midgut (6). The parasites multiply and differentiate in the midgut (7) and differentiate into infec-tive metacyclic trypomastigotes in the hindgut (8). *Trypanosoma cruzi* can also be transmitted through blood transfusions, organ transplantation, transplacentally, and in laboratory accidents. Courtesy of Centers for Disease Control and Prevention/Alexander J. da Silva, PhD/Melanie Moser.

143

Tuberculosis

Clinical Manifestations

Tuberculosis disease is caused by infection with organisms of the *Mycobacterium tuberculosis* complex, which includes *M tuberculosis, Mycobacterium bovis,* and *Mycobacterium africanum. M africanum* is rare in the United States, and clinical laboratories do not distinguish it routinely. *M bovis* can be distinguished routinely from *M tuberculosis,* and although the spectrum of illness that is caused by *M bovis* is similar to that of *M tuberculosis,* the epidemiology, treatment, and prevention are distinct. Most infections caused by *M tuberculosis* complex in children and adolescents are asymptomatic. When tuberculosis disease does occur, clinical manifestations most often appear 1 to 6 months after infection and include fever, weight loss, or poor weight gain and possibly growth delay, cough, night sweats, and chills. Chest radiographic findings after infection range from normal to diverse abnormalities, such as lymphadenopathy of the hilar, subcarinal, paratracheal, or mediastinal nodes; atelectasis or infiltrate of a segment or lobe; pleural effusion; cavitary lesions; or miliary disease. Extrapulmonary manifestations include meningitis and granulomatous inflammation of the lymph nodes, bones, joints, skin, and middle ear and mastoid. Gastrointestinal tuberculosis can mimic inflammatory bowel disease. Renal tuberculosis and progression to disease from latent tuberculosis infection (adult-type pulmonary tuberculosis) are unusual in younger children but can occur in adolescents. In addition, chronic abdominal pain with intermittent partial intestinal obstruction can be present in disease caused by *M bovis.* Clinical findings in patients with drug-resistant tuberculosis disease are indistinguishable from manifestations in patients with drug-susceptible disease.

Etiology

The agent is *M tuberculosis* complex, a group of closely related acid-fast bacilli (AFB): *M tuberculosis, M bovis,* and *M africanum.*

Definitions:

- **Positive tuberculin skin test (TST).**
  A positive TST result (Box 143.1) indicates possible infection with *M tuberculosis* complex. Tuberculin reactivity appears 2 to 10 weeks after initial infection; the median interval is 3 to 4 weeks (see Diagnostic Tests on page 570).
- **Positive interferon-gamma release assay (IGRA).** A positive IGRA result indicates possible infection with *M tuberculosis* complex.
- **Exposed person** refers to a person who has had recent contact with another person with suspected or confirmed contagious pulmonary tuberculosis disease and who has a negative TST or IGRA result, normal physical examination findings, and chest radiographic findings that are not compatible with tuberculosis. Some exposed people become infected (and subsequently develop a positive TST or IGRA result); others do not become infected after exposure; the 2 groups cannot be distinguished initially.
- **Source case** is defined as the person who has transmitted infection with *M tuberculosis* complex to another person who subsequently has either latent tuberculosis infection (LTBI) or tuberculosis disease.
- **LTBI** is defined as *M tuberculosis* complex infection in a person who has a positive TST or IGRA result, no physical findings of disease, and chest radiograph findings that are normal or reveal evidence of healed infection (eg, calcification in the lung, hilar lymph nodes, or both).
- **Tuberculosis disease** is defined as disease in a person with infection in whom symptoms, signs, or radiographic manifestations caused by *M tuberculosis* complex are apparent; disease may be pulmonary, extrapulmonary, or both. Infectious tuberculosis refers to tuberculosis disease of the lungs or larynx in a person who has the potential to transmit the infection to other people.
- **Directly observed therapy (DOT)** is defined as an intervention by which medication is administered directly to the patient by a health care professional or trained third party (not a relative or friend) who observes and documents that the patient ingests each dose of medication.

Box 143.1
Definitions of Positive Tuberculin Skin Test (TST) Results in Infants, Children, and Adolescents[a]

Induration ≥5 mm

Children in close contact with known or suspected contagious people with tuberculosis disease

Children suspected to have tuberculosis disease
- Findings on chest radiograph consistent with active or previous tuberculosis disease
- Clinical evidence of tuberculosis disease[b]

Children receiving immunosuppressive therapy[c] or with immunosuppressive conditions, including HIV infection

Induration ≥10 mm

Children at increased risk of disseminated tuberculosis disease
- Children <4 years
- Children with other medical conditions, including Hodgkin disease, lymphoma, diabetes mellitus, chronic renal failure, or malnutrition (see Box 143.2)

Children with likelihood of increased exposure to tuberculosis disease
- Children born in high-prevalence regions of the world
- Children who travel to high-prevalence regions of the world
- Children frequently exposed to adults who are HIV infected, homeless, users of illicit drugs, residents of nursing homes, incarcerated or institutionalized persons

Induration ≥15 mm

Children ≥4 years without any risk factors

[a] These definitions apply regardless of previous bacille Calmette-Guérin (BCG) immunization (see also Interpretation of TST Results in Previous Recipients of BCG Vaccine, p 572); erythema alone at TST site does not indicate a positive test result. Tests should be read at 48 to 72 hours after placement.
[b] Evidence by physical examination or laboratory assessment that would include tuberculosis in the working differential diagnosis (eg, meningitis).
[c] Including immunosuppressive doses of corticosteroids or tumor necrosis factor-alpha antagonists.

- **Multiply drug-resistant (MDR) tuberculosis** is defined as tuberculosis infection or disease caused by a strain of *M tuberculosis* complex that is resistant to at least isoniazid and rifampin, the 2 first-line drugs with greatest efficacy.
- **Extensively drug-resistant (XDR) tuberculosis** is a subset of MDR tuberculosis. It is defined as infection or disease caused by a strain of *M tuberculosis* complex that is resistant to isoniazid and rifampin, at least 1 fluoroquinolone, and at least 1 of the following parenteral drugs: amikacin, kanamycin, or capreomycin.
- **Bacille Calmette-Guérin (BCG)** is an attenuated live vaccine strain of *M bovis*. BCG vaccine rarely is administered to children in the United States but is one of the most widely used vaccines in the world.

An isolate of BCG can be distinguished from wild-type *M bovis* only in a reference laboratory.

Epidemiology

Case rates of tuberculosis for all ages are higher in urban, low-income areas and in nonwhite racial and ethnic groups; 80% of reported cases in the United States occur in Hispanic and nonwhite people. In recent years, foreign-born children have accounted for more than one-quarter of newly diagnosed cases in children age 14 years or younger. Specific groups with greater LTBI and disease rates include immigrants, international adoptees, and refugees from or travelers to high-prevalence regions (eg, Asia, Africa, Latin America, and countries of the former Soviet Union); homeless people; and residents of correctional facilities.

Box 143.2
Tuberculin Skin Test (TST) Recommendations for Infants, Children, and Adolescents[a]

Children for whom immediate TST or IGRA is indicated[b]
- Contacts of people with confirmed or suspected contagious tuberculosis (contact investigation)
- Children with radiographic or clinical findings suggesting tuberculosis disease
- Children emigrating from countries with endemic infection (eg, Asia, Middle East, Africa, Latin America, countries of the former Soviet Union), including international adoptees
- Children with travel histories to countries with endemic infection and substantial contact with indigenous people from such countries[c]

Children who should have annual TST or IGRA
- Children infected with HIV infection (TST only)

Children at increased risk of progression of LTBI to tuberculosis disease: Children with other medical conditions, including diabetes mellitus, chronic renal failure, malnutrition, congenital or acquired immunodeficiencies, and children receiving tumor necrosis factor (TNF) antagonists deserve special consideration. Without recent exposure, these people are not at increased risk of acquiring tuberculosis infection. Underlying immune deficiencies associated with these conditions theoretically would enhance the possibility for progression to severe disease. Initial histories of potential exposure to tuberculosis should be included for all of these patients. If these histories or local epidemiologic factors suggest a possibility of exposure, immediate and periodic TST or IGRA should be considered. **An initial TST or IGRA should be performed before initiation of immunosuppressive therapy, including prolonged steroid administration, use of TNF-alpha antagonists, or other immunosuppressive therapy in any child requiring these treatments.**

Abbreviations: HIV, human immunodeficiency virus; IGRA, interferon-gamma release assay; LTBI, latent tuberculosis infection.
[a] Bacille Calmette-Guérin immunization is not a contraindication to a TST.
[b] Beginning as early as 3 months of age.
[c] If the child is well and has no history of exposure, the TST or IGRA should be delayed for up to 10 weeks after return.

Infants and postpubertal adolescents are at increased risk of progression of LTBI to tuberculosis disease. Other predictive factors for development of disease include recent infection (within the past 2 years); immunodeficiency, especially from HIV infection; use of immunosuppressive drugs, such as prolonged or high-dose corticosteroid therapy or chemotherapy; intravenous drug use; and certain diseases or medical conditions, including Hodgkin disease, lymphoma, diabetes mellitus, chronic renal failure, and malnutrition. There have been reports of tuberculosis disease in adolescents and adults being treated for arthritis, inflammatory bowel disease, and other conditions with tumor necrosis factor-alpha (TNF-alpha) antagonists, such as infliximab and etanercept. Before use of TNF-alpha antagonists, patients should be screened for risk factors for *M tuberculosis* complex infec-

tion and have a TST or IGRA performed before the initiation of systemic steroids, antimetabolite agents, or these monoclonal antibodies.

A diagnosis of LTBI or tuberculosis disease in a young child is a public health sentinel event usually representing recent transmission. Transmission of *M tuberculosis* complex is airborne, with inhalation of droplet nuclei usually produced by an adult or adolescent with contagious pulmonary or laryngeal tuberculosis disease. *M bovis* is transmitted most often by unpasteurized dairy products, but airborne transmission can occur. The duration of contagiousness of an adult receiving effective treatment depends on drug susceptibilities of the organism, the number of organisms in sputum, and frequency of cough. Although contagiousness usually lasts only a few days to weeks after initiation of effective drug therapy, it can last longer, especially when the adult patient has cavitary disease, does not adhere to medical therapy, or is infected with a drug-resistant strain. If the sputum smear is negative for AFB organisms on 3 separate specimens at least 8 hours apart and the patient has improved clinically with resolution of cough, the treated person can be considered at low risk of disease transmission. Children younger than age 10 years with pulmonary tuberculosis rarely are contagious, because their pulmonary lesions are small (paucibacillary disease), cough is nonproductive, and few or no bacilli are expelled. Unusual cases of adult-form pulmonary disease in young children and cases of congenital tuberculosis can be highly contagious.

Incubation Period

LTBI, 2 to 10 weeks after exposure; tuberculosis disease, highest risk is 6 to 24 months after infection, but can be years.

Diagnostic Tests

Laboratory isolation of *M tuberculosis* complex by culture from specimens of gastric aspirates, sputum, bronchial washings, pleural fluid, cerebrospinal fluid (CSF), urine, or other body fluids or a tissue biopsy specimen establishes the diagnosis. Children older than 5 years and adolescents frequently can produce sputum spontaneously or by induction with aerosolized hypertonic saline. Studies have demonstrated successful collections of induced sputum from infants with pulmonary tuberculosis, but this requires special expertise. The best specimen for diagnosis of pulmonary tuberculosis in any child or adolescent in whom the cough is absent or nonproductive and sputum cannot be induced is an early morning gastric aspirate. Gastric aspirate specimens should be obtained with a nasogastric tube on awakening the child and before ambulation or feeding. Aspirates collected on 3 separate days should be submitted for testing. Results of AFB smears of gastric aspirates usually are negative, and false-positive smear results caused by the presence of nontuberculous mycobacteria can occur. Gastric aspirates have the highest culture yield in young children on the first day of collection. Fluorescent staining methods for gastric aspirate smears are more sensitive than AFB smears and, if available, are preferred. The overall diagnostic yield of gastric aspirates is less than 50%. Histologic examination for and demonstration of AFB and granulomas in biopsy specimens from lymph node, pleura, mesentery, liver, bone marrow, or other tissues can be useful, but *M tuberculosis* complex organisms cannot be distinguished reliably from other mycobacteria in stained specimens. Regardless of results of the AFB smears, each specimen should be cultured.

Because *M tuberculosis* complex organisms are slow growing, detection of these organisms may take as long as 10 weeks using solid media; use of liquid media allows detection within 1 to 6 weeks and usually within 3 weeks. Even with optimal culture techniques, *M tuberculosis* complex organisms are isolated from fewer than 50% of children and 75% of infants with pulmonary tuberculosis diagnosed by other clinical criteria. Species identification of isolates from culture can be more rapid if a DNA probe or high-pressure liquid chromatography is used. The differentiation between *M tuberculosis* and *M bovis* usually is based on pyrazinamide resistance, which is characteristic of almost all *M bovis* isolates.

One nucleic acid amplification test (NAAT) for rapid diagnosis is approved by the US Food and Drug Administration (FDA) for acid-fast stain positive respiratory tract specimens only, and another NAAT is approved for any respiratory tract specimens. These NAATs have decreased sensitivity for gastric aspirate, CSF, and tissue specimens, with false-negative and false-positive results reported. Further research is needed before NAATs can be recommended for the diagnosis of extrapulmonary tuberculosis or pulmonary tuberculosis in children who cannot produce sputum.

Identification of the culture-positive source case supports the child's presumptive diagnosis and provides the likely drug susceptibility of the child's organism. Culture material should be collected from children with evidence of tuberculosis disease, especially when (1) an isolate from a source case is not available, (2) the presumed source case has drug-resistant tuberculosis, (3) the child is immunocompromised (eg, HIV infection), or (4) the child has extrapulmonary disease. Drug resistance cannot be confirmed without a bacterial isolate.

Testing for M tuberculosis *Infection.* The TST is the most common method for diagnosing LTBI in asymptomatic people. The Mantoux method consists of 5 tuberculin units of purified protein derivative (0.1 mL) injected intradermally using a 27-gauge needle and a 1.0-mL syringe into the volar aspect of the forearm. Creation of a palpable induration 6 to 10 mm in diameter is crucial to accurate testing. Multiple puncture tests are not recommended, because they lack adequate sensitivity and specificity.

A TST should be performed in children who are at increased risk of infection with *M tuberculosis* (Box 143.2). Routine TST performance, including programs based at schools, child care centers, and camps that include populations at low risk, is discouraged, because it results in either a low yield of positive results or a large proportion of false-positive results, leading to an inefficient use of health care resources. Simple questionnaires can identify children with risk factors for LTBI who then should have a TST performed (Box 143.3). Risk assessment for tuberculosis should be performed at first contact with a child and every 6 months thereafter for the first year of life (eg, 2 weeks and 6 and 12 months of age). If, at any time, tuberculosis disease is suspected, a TST should be performed, although a negative result should be considered as especially unreliable in infants younger than 3 months. After 1 year of age, risk assessment for tuberculosis should be performed annually, if possible.

Recommendations for use of the TST are independent of those for immunization. Tuberculin testing at any age is not required before administration of live-virus vaccines. Measles vaccine temporarily can suppress tuberculin reactivity for at least 4 to 6 weeks. A TST can be applied at the same visit during which these vaccines are administered. The effect of live-virus varicella, yellow fever, and live-attenuated influenza vaccines on TST reactivity and IGRA results is not known. In the absence of data, the same TST spacing recommendation should be applied to these vaccines as described for measles-mumps-rubella vaccine. There is no evidence that inactivated vaccines, polysaccharide vaccines, or recombinant or subunit vaccines or toxoids interfere with immune response to TST.

Administration of TSTs and interpretation of results should be performed by experienced health care professionals who have been trained in the proper methods, because administration and interpretation by unskilled people and family members are unreliable. The recommended time for assessing the TST result is 48 to 72 hours after administration. However, induration that develops at the site of administration more than 72 hours later should be measured, and some experts advise that this should be considered the result. The diameter of induration in millimeters is measured transversely to the long axis of the forearm. Positive TST results, as defined in Box 143.1 can persist for several weeks.

A negative TST result does not exclude LTBI or tuberculosis disease. Approximately 10% to 40% of immunocompetent children with culture-documented tuberculosis disease do not react initially to a TST. Host factors, such as young age, poor nutrition, immunosuppression, other viral infections (especially measles, varicella, and influenza), recent tuberculosis infection, and disseminated tuberculosis disease can decrease TST reactivity. Many children and adults coinfected with HIV and *M tuberculosis* complex do not react to a TST. Control skin tests to assess cutaneous anergy are not recommended routinely.

Interpretation of TST Results (see Box 143.1). Classification of TST results is based on epidemiologic and clinical factors. The size of induration (millimeter) for a positive result varies with the person's risk of LTBI and progression to tuberculosis disease.

Interpretation is aided by knowledge of the child's risk factors for LTBI and tuberculosis disease and is summarized in Box 143.1. Current guidelines from the Centers for Disease Control and Prevention (CDC), American Thoracic Society, and American Academy of Pediatrics accept 15 mm or greater of induration as a positive TST result for any person who has not received BCG vaccine. Prompt clinical and radiographic evaluation of all children and adolescents with a positive TST reaction is recommended.

Interpretation of TST Results in Previous Recipients of BCG Vaccine. Generally, interpretation of TST results in BCG recipients who are known contacts of a person with tuberculosis disease or at high risk for tuberculosis disease is the same as for people who have not received BCG vaccine. After BCG immunization, distinguishing between a positive TST result caused by pathogenic *M tuberculosis* complex infection and that caused by BCG is difficult. Reactivity of the TST after receipt of BCG vaccine does not occur in some patients. The size of the TST reaction (ie, millimeters of induration) attributable to BCG immunization depends on many factors, including age at BCG immunization, quality and strain of BCG vaccine used, number of doses of BCG vaccine received, nutritional and immunologic status of the vaccine recipient, frequency of TST administration, and time lapse between immunization and TST. Because IGRAs do not cross-react with BGC, an IGRA is the preferred test by many experts for the diagnosis of LTBI in a BCG-immunized child older than 4 years.

Tuberculosis disease should be suspected strongly in any symptomatic person regardless of a TST or IGRA result and history of BCG immunization. When evaluating an asymptomatic child who has a positive TST result and who possibly received BCG vaccine, certain factors, such as documented receipt of multiple BCG immunizations (as evidenced by BCG scars), decrease the likelihood that the positive TST result is attributable to LTBI. Evidence that increases the probability that a positive TST result is attributable to LTBI includes known contact with a person with contagious tuberculosis, a family history of tuberculosis disease, a long interval (>5 years) since neonatal BCG immunization, and a TST reaction 15 mm or greater.

Prompt clinical and radiographic evaluation of all children with a positive TST reaction is recommended. Chest radiographic findings of a granuloma, calcification, or adenopathy can be caused by infection with *M tuberculosis* complex but not by BCG immunization. BCG can cause suppurative lymphadenitis in the regional lymph node drainage of the infectious site of a healthy child and can cause disseminated disease in children with some forms of immunodeficiency.

Recommendations for TST Use. The most reliable strategies for preventing LTBI and tuberculosis disease in children are based on thorough and expedient contact investigations rather than nonselective skin testing of large populations. Contact investigations are public health interventions that should be coordinated through the local public health department. Specific recommendations for TST use are given in Box 143.2. All children need routine health care evaluations that include an assessment of their risk of exposure to tuberculosis. Only children deemed to have increased risk of contact with people with contagious tuberculosis or children with suspected tuberculosis disease should be considered for a TST. Household investigation is indicated whenever a TST result of a household member converts from negative to positive (indicating recent infection).

Box 143.3
Validated Questions for Determining Risk of LTBI in Children in the United States

- Has a family member or contact had tuberculosis disease?
- Has a family member had a positive tuberculin skin test result?
- Was your child born in a high-risk country (countries other than the United States, Canada, Australia, New Zealand, or Western and North European countries)?
- Has your child traveled (had contact with resident populations) to a high-risk country for more than 1 week?

Abbreviation: LTBI, latent tuberculosis infection.

Immunologic-Based Testing. QuantiFERON-TB Gold, T-SPOT.TB, and Gold In-Tube are IGRAs and are the preferred tests in asymptomatic children older than 4 years who have been immunized against BCG. These FDA-approved tests measure ex vivo interferon-gamma production from T-lymphocytes in response to stimulation with antigens that are fairly specific to *M tuberculosis* complex. As with TSTs, IGRAs cannot distinguish between latent infection and disease, and a negative result from these tests cannot exclude the possibility of tuberculosis disease in a patient with findings that raise suspicion for these conditions. The sensitivity of these blood IGRA tests is similar to that of TSTs for detecting infection in adults and children who have untreated culture-confirmed tuberculosis. The specificity of IGRAs is higher than that for TSTs, because the antigens used are not found in BCG or most pathogenic nontuberculous mycobacteria (eg, are not found in *M avium* complex but are found in *Mycobacterium kansasii*, *Mycobacterium szulgai*, and *Mycobacterium marinum*). IGRAs are recommended by the CDC, and some experts prefer IGRAs for use in adults in all circumstances in which a TST would have been used. The published experience testing children with IGRAs is less extensive than for adults, but a number of studies have demonstrated that IGRAs perform well in children 5 years of age and older. Some children who received BCG vaccine can have a false-positive TST result, and LTBI is overestimated by use of the TST in these circumstances. The negative predictive value of IGRAs is not clear, but in general, if the IGRA result is negative and the TST result is positive in an asymptomatic child, the diagnosis of LTBI is unlikely.

At this time, neither an IGRA nor the TST can be considered a gold standard for diagnosis of LTBI. Current recommendations for use of IGRAs in children are in Box 143.4.

- Children with a positive result from an IGRA should be considered infected with *M tuberculosis* complex. A negative IGRA result cannot be interpreted universally as absence of infection.
- Indeterminate IGRA results do not exclude tuberculosis infection and may necessitate repeat testing and should not be used to make clinical decisions.

Serologic tests for tuberculosis disease are not recommended; although they are used in some Asian and African countries, they have

---

Box 143.4
Recommendations for Use of the Tuberculin Skin Test (TST) and an Interferon-Gamma Release Assay (IGRA) in Children

TST preferred, IGRA acceptable
- Children <5 years[a]

IGRA preferred, TST acceptable
- Children >5 years who have received BCG vaccine
- Children >5 years who are unlikely to return for TST reading

TST and IGRA should be considered when
- The initial and repeat IGRA are indeterminate
- The initial test (TST or IGRA) is *negative* and
  - Clinical suspicion for tuberculosis disease is moderate to high[b]
  - Risk of progression and poor outcome is high[b]
- The initial TST is *positive* and
  - ≥5 years and history of BCG vaccination
  - Additional evidence needed to increase compliance
  - Nontuberculous mycobacterial disease is suspected

[a] Positive result of either test is considered significant in these groups.
[b] IGRAs should not be used in children <2 years unless tuberculosis disease is suspected. In children 2–4 years of age, there are limited data about the usefulness of IGRAs in determining tuberculosis infection, but IGRA testing can be performed if tuberculosis disease is suspected.

unsatisfactory sensitivity and specificity, and none of them have been approved for use in the United States.

HIV Infection. Children with HIV infection are considered at high risk of tuberculosis, and an annual TST beginning at 3 through 12 months of age is recommended or, if older, when HIV infection is diagnosed. Children who have tuberculosis disease should be tested for HIV infection.

Treatment (Table 143.1)

Specific Drugs. Antituberculosis drugs kill *M tuberculosis* complex organisms or inhibit multiplication of the organism, thereby arresting progression of LTBI and preventing most complications of early tuberculosis disease. Chemotherapy does not cause rapid disappearance of already caseous or granulomatous lesions (eg, mediastinal lymphadenitis). Dosage recommendations and the more commonly reported adverse reactions of major antituberculosis drugs are summarized in tables 143.1 and 143.2. For treatment of tuberculosis disease, these drugs always must be used in recommended combination given as single doses to minimize emergence of drug-resistant strains. Use of nonstandard regimens for any reason (eg, drug allergy or drug resistance) should be undertaken only in consultation with an expert in treating tuberculosis.

Isoniazid is bactericidal, rapidly absorbed, and well tolerated and penetrates into body fluids, including CSF. Isoniazid is metabolized in the liver and excreted primarily through the kidneys. Hepatotoxic effects are rare in children but can be life-threatening. In children and adolescents given recommended doses, peripheral neuritis or seizures caused by inhibition of pyridoxine metabolism are rare, and most do not need pyridoxine supplements. Pyridoxine supplementation is recommended for exclusively breastfed infants and for children and adolescents on meat- and milk-deficient diets; children with nutritional deficiencies, including all symptomatic HIV-infected children; and pregnant adolescents and women. For infants and young children, isoniazid tablets can be pulverized or made into a suspension by a pharmacy.

Rifampin is a bactericidal agent in the rifamycin class of drugs that is absorbed rapidly and penetrates into body fluids, including CSF. Other drugs in this class approved for treating tuberculosis are rifabutin and rifapentine. Rifampin is metabolized by the liver and can alter the pharmacokinetics and serum concentrations of many other drugs. Rare adverse effects include hepatotoxicity, influenza-like symptoms, and pruritus. Rifampin is excreted in bile and urine and can cause orange urine, sweat, and tears and discoloration of soft contact lenses. Rifampin can make oral contraceptives ineffective, so other birth control methods should be adopted when rifampin is administered to sexually active female adolescents and adults. For infants and young children, the contents of the capsules can be suspended in wild cherry–flavored syrup or sprinkled on semisoft foods (eg, pudding). *M tuberculosis* complex isolates that are resistant to rifampin are uncommon in the United States. Rifabutin is a suitable alternative to rifampin in children with HIV infection receiving antiretroviral therapy that proscribes the use of rifampin; however, experience in children is limited. Major toxicities of rifabutin include leukopenia, gastrointestinal tract upset, polyarthralgia, rash, increased transaminase concentrations, and skin and secretion discoloration (pseudojaundice). Anterior uveitis has been reported among children receiving rifabutin as prophylaxis or as part of a combination regimen for treatment, usually when administered at high doses. Rifabutin also increases hepatic metabolism of many drugs but is a less potent inducer of cytochrome P450 enzymes than rifampin and has fewer problematic drug interactions than rifampin. However, adjustments in doses of rifabutin and coadministered antiretroviral drugs may be necessary for certain combinations. Rifapentine is a long-acting rifamycin that permits weekly dosing in selected adults and adolescents, but its evaluation in younger pediatric patients has been limited.

Pyrazinamide attains therapeutic CSF concentrations, is detectable in macrophages, is administered orally, and is metabolized by the liver. Administration of pyrazinamide for the first 2 months with isoniazid and rifampin

Table 143.1

Recommended Treatment Regimens for Drug-Susceptible Tuberculosis in Infants, Children, and Adolescents

Infection or Disease Category	Regimen	Remarks
Latent tuberculosis infection (positive TST or IGRA result, no disease)		
• Isoniazid susceptible	9 mo of isoniazid, once a day	If daily therapy is not possible, DOT twice a week can be used for 9 mo.
• Isoniazid resistant	6 mo of rifampin, once a day	If daily therapy is not possible, DOT twice a week can be used for 6 mo.
• Isoniazid-rifampin resistant[a]	Consult a tuberculosis specialist	
Pulmonary and extrapulmonary (except meningitis)	2 mo of isoniazid, rifampin, pyrazinamide, and ethambutol daily or twice weekly, followed by 4 mo of isoniazid and rifampin[b] by DOT[c] for drug-susceptible *Mycobacterium tuberculosis*	If possible drug resistance is a concern (see text), some experts recommend a 3-drug initial regimen (isoniazid, rifampin, and pyrazinamide) if the risk of drug resistance is low. DOT is highly desirable.
	9–12 mo of isoniazid and rifampin for drug-susceptible *Mycobacterium bovis*	If hilar adenopathy only, a 6-mo course of isoniazid and rifampin is sufficient. Drugs can be given 2 or 3 times/wk under DOT in the initial phase if nonadherence is likely.
Meningitis	2 mo of isoniazid, rifampin, pyrazinamide, and an aminoglycoside or ethambutol or ethionamide, once a day, followed by 7–10 mo of isoniazid and rifampin, once a day or twice a week (9–12 mo total) for drug-susceptible *M tuberculosis*	For patients who may have acquired tuberculosis in geographic areas where resistance to streptomycin is common, kanamycin, amikacin, or capreomycin can be used instead of streptomycin.
	At least 12 mo of therapy without pyrazinamide for drug-susceptible *M bovis*	

Abbreviations: DOT, directly observed therapy; IGRA, interferon-gamma release assay; TST, tuberculin skin test.

[a] Duration of therapy is longer for HIV-infected people, and additional drugs may be indicated (see Tuberculosis Disease and HIV Infection, p 582).

[b] Medications should be administered daily for the first 2 weeks to 2 months of treatment and then can be administered 2 to 3 times per week by DOT.

[c] If initial chest radiograph shows cavitary lesions and sputum after 2 months of therapy remains positive, duration of therapy is extended to 9 months.

Table 143.2

Commonly Used Drugs for Treatment of Tuberculosis in Infants, Children, and Adolescents

Drugs	Dosage Forms	Daily Dosage, mg/kg	Twice a Week Dosage, mg/kg per Dose	Maximum Dose	Adverse Reactions
Ethambutol	Tablets 100 mg 400 mg	20	50	2.5 g	Optic neuritis (usually reversible), decreased red-green color discrimination, gastrointestinal tract disturbances, hypersensitivity
Isoniazid[a]	Scored tablets 100 mg	10–15[b]	20–30	Daily, 300 mg	Mild hepatic enzyme elevation, hepatitis,[b] peripheral neuritis, hypersensitivity
	300 mg			Twice a week, 900 mg	
	Syrup 10 mg/mL				Diarrhea and gastric irritation caused by vehicle in the syrup
Pyrazinamide[a]	Scored tablets 500 mg	30–40	50	2 g	Hepatotoxic effects, hyperuricemia, arthralgia, gastrointestinal tract upset
Rifampin[a]	Capsules 150 mg 300 mg Syrup-formulated capsules	10–20	10–20	600 mg	Orange discoloration of secretions or urine, staining of contact lenses, vomiting, hepatitis, influenza-like reaction, thrombocytopenia, pruritus; oral contraceptives may be ineffective

[a]Rifamate is a capsule containing 150 mg of isoniazid and 300 mg of rifampin. Two capsules provide the usual adult (>50 kg) daily doses of each drug. Rifater, in the United States, is a capsule containing 50 mg of isoniazid, 120 mg of rifampin, and 300 mg of pyrazinamide. Isoniazid and rifampin also are available for parenteral administration.
[b]When isoniazid in a dosage exceeding 10 mg/kg/day is used in combination with rifampin, the incidence of hepatotoxic effects may be increased.

allows for 6-month regimens in immunocompetent patients with drug-susceptible tuberculosis. Almost all isolates of *M bovis* are resistant to pyrazinamide, precluding 6-month therapy for this pathogen. In daily doses of 40 mg/kg per day or less, pyrazinamide seldom has hepatotoxic effects and is well tolerated by children. Some adolescents and many adults develop arthralgia and hyperuricemia because of inhibition of uric acid excretion. Pyrazinamide must be used with caution in people with underlying liver disease; when administered with rifampin, pyrazinamide is associated with somewhat higher rates of hepatotoxicity.

Ethambutol is well absorbed after oral administration, diffuses well into tissues, and is excreted in urine. However, concentrations in CSF are low. At 20 mg/kg per day, ethambutol is bacteriostatic, and its primary therapeutic role is to prevent emergence of drug resistance. Ethambutol can cause reversible or irreversible optic neuritis, but reports in children with normal renal function are rare. Children who are receiving ethambutol should be monitored monthly for visual acuity and red-green color discrimination if they are old enough to cooperate. Use of ethambutol in young children whose visual acuity cannot be monitored requires consideration of risks and benefits, but should be used routinely to treat tuberculosis disease in infants and children unless otherwise contraindicated.

Streptomycin is regarded as a "second-line" drug and is available only on a limited basis. It is administered intramuscularly. When streptomycin is not available, kanamycin, amikacin, or capreomycin are alternatives that can be prescribed by intravenous administration for the initial 4 to 8 weeks of therapy. Patients who receive any of these drugs should be monitored for otic, vestibular, and renal toxicity.

The less commonly used (eg, "second-line") antituberculosis drugs, their doses, and adverse effects are listed in Table 143.3. These drugs have limited usefulness because of decreased effectiveness and greater toxicity and should be used only in consultation with a specialist familiar with childhood tuberculosis. Ethionamide is an orally administered antituberculosis drug that is well tolerated by children,

achieves therapeutic CSF concentrations, and may be useful for treatment of people with meningitis or drug-resistant tuberculosis. Fluoroquinolones have antituberculosis activity and can be used in special circumstances, including drug-resistant organisms but are not FDA approved for this indication. Because some fluoroquinolones are approved by the FDA for use only in people 18 years of age and older, their use in younger patients necessitates careful assessment of the potential risks and benefits (Table 143.2).

Occasionally, a patient cannot tolerate oral medications. Isoniazid, rifampin, streptomycin and related drugs, and fluoroquinolones can be administered parenterally.

Isoniazid Therapy for LTBI. Isoniazid given to adults who have LTBI (ie, no clinical or radiographic abnormalities suggesting tuberculosis disease) provides substantial protection (54%–88%) against development of tuberculosis disease for at least 20 years. Among children, efficacy approaches 100% with adherence to therapy. All infants, children, and adolescents who have a positive TST or IGRA result but no evidence of tuberculosis disease and who never have received antituberculosis therapy should be considered for isoniazid unless resistance to isoniazid is suspected (ie, known exposure to a person with isoniazid-resistant tuberculosis) or a specific contraindication exists. Isoniazid, in this circumstance, is therapeutic and prevents development of disease. A physical examination and chest radiograph should be performed at the time isoniazid therapy is initiated to exclude tuberculosis disease; if the radiograph is normal, the child remains asymptomatic, and treatment is completed, radiography need not be repeated.

Duration of Isoniazid Therapy for LTBI. For infants, children, and adolescents, including those with HIV infection or other immunocompromising conditions, the recommended duration of isoniazid therapy is 9 months. Isoniazid is given daily in a single dose. Physicians who treat LTBI should educate patients and their families about the adverse effects of isoniazid, provide written information about adverse drug effects, and prescribe it in monthly allocations, with clinic visits sched-

Table 143.3
Less Commonly Used Drugs for Treatment of Drug-Resistant Tuberculosis in Infants, Children, and Adolescents[a]

Drugs	Dosage, Forms	Daily Dosage	Maximum Dose	Adverse Reactions
Amikacin[b]	Vials, 500 mg and 1 g	15–30 mg/kg (intravenous or intramuscular administration)	1 g	Auditory and vestibular toxic effects, nephrotoxic effects
Capreomycin[b]	Vials, 1 g	15–30 mg/kg (intramuscular administration)	1 g	Auditory and vestibular toxicity and nephrotoxic effects
Cycloserine	Capsules, 250 mg	10–20 mg/kg, given in 2 divided doses	1 g	Psychosis, personality changes, seizures, rash
Ethionamide	Tablets, 250 mg	15–20 mg/kg, given in 2–3 divided doses	1 g	Gastrointestinal tract disturbances, hepatotoxic effects, hypersensitivity reactions, hypothyroid
Kanamycin	Vials 75 mg/2 mL 500 mg/2 mL 1 g/3 mL	15–30 mg/kg (intramuscular or intravenous administration)	1 g	Auditory and vestibular toxic effects, nephrotoxic effects
Levofloxacin[c]	Tablets 250 mg 500 mg 750 mg Vials 25 mg/mL	Adults: 750–1,000 mg (once daily) Children: not routinely recommended	1 g	Theoretical effect on growing cartilage, gastrointestinal tract disturbances, rash, headache, restlessness, confusion
Ofloxacin	Tablets 200 mg 300 mg 400 mg Vials 20 mg/mL 40 mg/mL	Adults and adolescents: 800 mg Children: 15–20 mg/kg daily	800 mg	Arthropathy, arthritis

Table 143.3

Less Commonly Used Drugs for Treatment of Drug-Resistant Tuberculosis in Infants, Children, and Adolescents[a], continued

Drugs	Dosage, Forms	Daily Dosage	Maximum Dose	Adverse Reactions
Moxifloxacin	Tablets 400 mg Intravenous solution 400 mg/ 250 mL in 0.8% saline	Adults and adolescents: 400 mg Children: 7.5–10 mg/kg daily	400 mg	Arthropathy, arthritis
Para-aminosalicylic acid	Packets, 3 g	200–300 mg/kg (2–4 times a day)	10 g	Gastrointestinal tract disturbances, hypersensitivity, hepatotoxic effects
Streptomycin[b]	Vials 1 g 4 g	20–40 mg/kg (intramuscular administration)	1 g	Auditory and vestibular toxic effects, nephrotoxic effects, rash

[a]These drugs should be used in consultation with a specialist in tuberculosis.

[b]Dose adjustment in renal insufficiency.

[c]Levofloxacin is not approved for use in children younger than 18 years; its use in younger children necessitates assessment of the potential risks and benefits.

uled for periodic face-to-face monitoring. Successful completion of therapy is based on total number of doses taken. When adherence with daily therapy with isoniazid cannot be ensured, twice-a-week DOT can be considered. The twice-weekly regimen should not be prescribed unless each dose is documented by DOT. Routine determination of serum transaminase values during the 9 months of therapy for LTBI is not indicated. If therapy is completed successfully, there is no need to perform additional tests or chest radiographs unless a new exposure to tuberculosis is documented or the child develops a clinical illness consistent with tuberculosis.

Isoniazid-Rifapentine Therapy for LTBI. In 2011, on the basis of a large clinical trial, the CDC recommended a 12-week, once-weekly dose of isoniazid and rifapentine, **given under DOT by a health department,** as an alternative regimen for treating LTBI in people 12 years and age or older. This regimen was shown to be at least as effective as 9 months of isoniazid given by self-supervision. Although children between 2 and 12 years of age were enrolled in the trial, data for safety, tolerability, and efficacy of this regimen in this group currently are not available, and the regimen is not recommended for children younger than 12 years.

Therapy for Contacts of Patients With Isoniazid-Resistant M tuberculosis. The incidence of isoniazid resistance among M tuberculosis complex isolates from US patients is approximately 9%. Risk factors for drug resistance are listed in Box 143.5. However, most experts recommend that isoniazid be used to treat LTBI in children unless the child has had contact with a person known to have isoniazid-resistant tuberculosis. If the source case is found to have isoniazid-resistant, rifampin-susceptible organisms, isoniazid should be discontinued and rifampin should be given for a total course of 6 months. Optimal therapy for children with LTBI caused by organisms with resistance to isoniazid and rifampin (ie, MDR) is not known. In these circumstances, multidrug regimens have been used. Drugs to consider include pyrazinamide, a fluoroquinolone, and ethambutol, depending on susceptibility of the isolate. Consultation with a tuberculosis specialist is indicated.

Treatment of Tuberculosis Disease. The goal of treatment is to achieve killing of replicating organisms in the tuberculous lesion in the shortest possible time. Achievement of this goal minimizes the possibility of development of resistant organisms. The major problem limiting successful treatment is poor adherence to prescribed treatment regimens. The use of DOT decreases the rates of relapse, treatment failures, and drug resistance; therefore, DOT is recommended strongly for treatment of all children and adolescents with tuberculosis disease in the United States.

For tuberculosis disease, a 6-month, 4-drug regimen consisting of isoniazid, rifampin, pyrazinamide, and ethambutol for the first 2 months and isoniazid and rifampin for the remaining 4 months is recommended for treatment of pulmonary disease, pulmonary disease with hilar adenopathy, and hilar adenopathy disease in infants, children, and adolescents when an MDR case is not suspected as the source of infection or when drug susceptibility results are available. Some experts would administer 3 drugs (isoniazid, rifampin, and pyrazinamide) as the initial regimen if a source case has been identified with known pansusceptible M tuberculosis, if the presumed source case has no risk factors for drug-resistant M tuberculosis, or if the source case is unknown but the child resides in an area with low rates of isoniazid resistance. If the chest radiograph shows one or more cavitary lesions and sputum culture remains positive after 2 months of therapy, the duration of therapy should be extended to 9 months. For children with hilar adenopathy in whom drug resistance is not a consideration, a 6-month regimen of only isoniazid and rifampin is considered adequate by some experts.

In the 6-month regimen with 4-drug therapy, isoniazid, rifampin, pyrazinamide, and ethambutol are given once a day for at least the first 2 weeks by daily (at least 5 days per week) DOT. An alternative to daily dosing between 2 weeks and 2 months of treatment is to give these drugs twice or 3 times a week by DOT. After the initial 2-month period, a DOT regimen of isoniazid and rifampin given 2 or 3 times a week is acceptable (see Table 143.1 for doses). Several alternative regimens with differing

Box 143.5
People at Increased Risk of Drug-Resistant Tuberculosis Infection or Disease

- People with a history of treatment for tuberculosis disease (or whose source case for the contact received such treatment)
- Contacts of a patient with drug-resistant contagious tuberculosis disease
- People from countries with high prevalence of drug-resistant tuberculosis
- Infected people whose source case has positive smears for acid-fast bacilli or cultures after 2 months of appropriate antituberculosis therapy and patients who do not respond to a standard treatment regimen
- Residence in geographic area with a high percentage of drug-resistant isolates

durations of daily therapy and total therapy have been used successfully in adults and children. These alternative regimens should be prescribed and managed by a specialist in tuberculosis.

When **drug resistance** is possible (Box 143.5), initial therapy should be adjusted by adding at least 2 drugs to match the presumed drug susceptibility pattern until drug susceptibility results are available. If an isolate from the pediatric case under treatment is not available, drug susceptibilities can be inferred by the drug susceptibility pattern of isolates from the adult source case. Data for guiding drug selection may not be available for foreign-born children or in circumstances of international travel. If this information is not available, a 4-drug initial regimen is recommended with close monitoring for clinical response.

Therapy for Drug-Resistant Tuberculosis Disease. Drug resistance is most common in the following: (1) people previously treated for tuberculosis disease; (2) people born in areas such as Russia and the former Soviet Union, Asia, Africa, and Latin America; and (3) contacts, especially children, with tuberculosis disease whose source case is a person from one of these groups (see also Box 143.5). Most cases of pulmonary tuberculosis in children that are caused by an isoniazid-resistant but rifampin- and pyrazinamide-susceptible strain of *M tuberculosis* complex can be treated with a 6-month regimen of rifampin, pyrazinamide, and ethambutol. For cases of MDR tuberculosis disease, the treatment regimen needed for cure should include at least 4 antituberculosis drugs to which the organism is susceptible administered for 12 to 24 months of therapy

from the time of culture conversion. Regimens in which drugs are administered 2 or 3 times per week are not recommended for drug-resistant disease; daily DOT is critical to prevent emergence of further resistance.

Extrapulmonary M tuberculosis Tuberculosis Disease. In general, extrapulmonary tuberculosis—with the exception of meningitis—can be treated with the same regimens as used for pulmonary tuberculosis. For suspected drug-susceptible tuberculous meningitis, daily treatment with isoniazid, rifampin, pyrazinamide, and ethambutol or ethionamide, if possible, or an aminoglycoside should be initiated. When susceptibility to all drugs is established, the ethambutol, ethionamide, or aminoglycoside can be discontinued. Pyrazinamide is given for a total of 2 months, and isoniazid and rifampin are given for a total of 9 to 12 months. Isoniazid and rifampin can be given daily or 2 or 3 times per week after the first 2 months of treatment.

Corticosteroids. The evidence supporting adjuvant treatment with corticosteroids for children with tuberculosis disease is incomplete. Corticosteroids are indicated for children with tuberculous meningitis, because corticosteroids decrease rates of mortality and long-term neurologic impairment. Corticosteroids can be considered for children with pleural and pericardial effusions (to hasten reabsorption of fluid), severe miliary disease (to mitigate alveolocapillary block), endobronchial disease (to relieve obstruction and atelectasis), and abdominal tuberculosis (to decrease the risk of strictures). Corticosteroids should be given only when accompanied by appropriate antituberculosis therapy. Most experts consider

2 mg/kg per day of prednisone (maximum, 60 mg/day) or its equivalent for 4 to 6 weeks followed by tapering to be adequate.

Tuberculosis Disease and HIV Infection.
Adults and children with HIV infection have an increased incidence of tuberculosis disease. Hence, *HIV testing is indicated for all patients with tuberculosis disease.* The clinical manifestations and radiographic appearance of tuberculosis disease in children with HIV infection tend to be similar to those in immunocompetent children, but manifestations in these children can be more severe and unusual and can include extrapulmonary involvement of multiple organs. In HIV-infected patients, a TST result of 5-mm induration or more is considered positive (see Box 143.1); however, a negative TST result attributable to HIV-related immunosuppression also can occur. Specimens for culture should be obtained from all HIV-infected children with suspected tuberculosis.

Most HIV-infected adults with drug-susceptible tuberculosis respond well to antituberculosis drugs when appropriate therapy is initiated early. However, optimal therapy for tuberculosis in children with HIV infection has not been established. Treating tuberculosis in an HIV-infected child is complicated by antiretroviral drug interactions with the rifamycins and overlapping toxicities caused by antiretroviral drugs and medications used to treat tuberculosis. Therapy always should include at least 4 drugs initially, should be administered daily, and should be continued for at least 6 months. Isoniazid, rifampin, and pyrazinamide, usually with ethambutol or an aminoglycoside, should be given for at least the first 2 months. Ethambutol can be discontinued once drug-resistant tuberculosis disease is excluded. Rifampin may be contraindicated in people who are receiving antiretroviral therapy. Rifabutin can be substituted for rifampin in some circumstances. Consultation with a specialist who has experience in managing HIV-infected patients with tuberculosis is strongly advised.

Evaluation and Monitoring of Therapy in Children and Adolescents. Careful monthly monitoring of clinical and bacteriologic responses to therapy is important. With DOT, clinical evaluation is an integral component of each visit for drug administration. For patients with pulmonary tuberculosis, chest radiographs should be obtained after 2 months of therapy to evaluate response. Even with successful 6-month regimens, hilar adenopathy can persist for 2 to 3 years; normal radiographic findings are not necessary to discontinue therapy. Follow-up chest radiography beyond termination of successful therapy usually is not necessary unless clinical deterioration occurs.

If therapy has been interrupted, the date of completion should be extended. Although guidelines cannot be provided for every situation, factors to consider when establishing the date of completion include the following: (1) length of interruption of therapy; (2) time during therapy (early or late) when interruption occurred; and (3) the patient's clinical, radiographic, and bacteriologic status before, during, and after interruption of therapy. The total doses administered by DOT should be calculated to guide the duration of therapy. Consultation with a specialist in tuberculosis is advised.

Untoward effects of isoniazid therapy, including severe hepatitis in otherwise healthy infants, children, and adolescents, are rare. Routine determination of serum transaminase concentrations is not recommended. However, for children with severe tuberculosis disease, especially children with meningitis or disseminated disease, transaminase concentrations should be monitored approximately monthly during the first several months of treatment. Other indications for testing include the following: (1) having concurrent or recent liver or biliary disease, (2) being pregnant or in the first 6 weeks postpartum, (3) having clinical evidence of hepatotoxic effects, or (4) concurrently using other hepatotoxic drugs (eg, anticonvulsant or HIV agents). In most other circumstances, monthly clinical evaluations to observe for signs or symptoms of hepatitis and other adverse effects of drug therapy without routine monitoring of transaminase concentrations is appropriate follow-up. In all cases, regular physician-patient contact to assess drug adherence, efficacy, and adverse effects is an important aspect of management. Patients should be given written instructions and advised to call a physician immediately if signs of adverse events, in particular hepatotoxicity (eg, vomiting, abdominal pain, jaundice), develop.

Immunizations. Patients who are receiving treatment for tuberculosis can be given measles and other age-appropriate attenuated live-virus vaccines unless they are receiving high-dose corticosteroids, are severely ill, or have other specific contraindications to immunization.

Tuberculosis During Pregnancy and Breast-feeding. Tuberculosis treatment during pregnancy varies because of the complexity of management decisions. During pregnancy, if tuberculosis disease is diagnosed, a regimen of isoniazid, rifampin, and ethambutol is recommended. Pyrazinamide commonly is used in a 3- or 4-drug regimen, but safety during pregnancy has not been established. At least 6 months of therapy is indicated for drug-susceptible tuberculosis disease if pyrazinamide is used; at least 9 months of therapy is indicated if pyrazinamide is not used. Prompt initiation of therapy is mandatory to protect mother and fetus.

Asymptomatic pregnant women with a positive TST or IGRA result, normal chest radiographic findings, and recent contact with a contagious person should be considered for isoniazid therapy. The recommended duration of therapy is 9 months. Therapy in these circumstances should begin after the first trimester. Pyridoxine supplementation is indicated for all pregnant and breastfeeding women receiving isoniazid.

Isoniazid, ethambutol, and rifampin are relatively safe for the fetus. The benefit of ethambutol and rifampin for therapy of tuberculosis disease in the mother outweighs the risk to the infant. Because streptomycin can cause ototoxic effects in the fetus, it should not be used unless administration is essential for effective treatment. The effects of other second-line drugs on the fetus are unknown, and ethionamide has been demonstrated to be teratogenic, so its use during pregnancy is contraindicated.

Although isoniazid is secreted in human milk, no adverse effects of isoniazid on nursing infants have been demonstrated. Breastfed infants do not require pyridoxine supplementation unless they are receiving isoniazid.

Congenital Tuberculosis. Women who have only pulmonary tuberculosis are not likely to infect the fetus but can infect their infant after delivery. Congenital tuberculosis is rare, but in utero infections can occur after maternal bacillemia.

If a newborn infant is suspected of having congenital tuberculosis, a TST, chest radiography, lumbar puncture, and appropriate cultures should be performed promptly. The TST result usually is negative in newborn infants with congenital or perinatally acquired infection. Hence, regardless of the TST or IGRA results, treatment of the infant should be initiated promptly with isoniazid, rifampin, pyrazinamide, and an aminoglycoside (eg, amikacin). The placenta should be examined histologically for granulomata and AFB, and a specimen should be cultured for *M tuberculosis* complex. The mother should be evaluated for presence of pulmonary or extrapulmonary disease, including uterine tuberculosis disease. If the physical examination and chest radiographic findings support the diagnosis of tuberculosis disease, the newborn infant should be treated with regimens recommended for tuberculosis disease. If meningitis is confirmed, corticosteroids should be added. Drug susceptibility testing of the organism recovered from the mother or household contact, infant, or both should be performed.

Management of the Newborn Infant Whose Mother (or Other Household Contact) Has LTBI or Tuberculosis Disease. Management of the newborn infant is based on categorization of the maternal (or household contact) infection. Although protection of the infant from exposure and infection is of paramount importance, contact between infant and mother should be allowed when possible. Differing circumstances and resulting recommendations are as follows:

- *Mother (or household contact) has a positive TST or IGRA result and normal chest radiographic findings.* If the mother (or household contact) is asymptomatic, no separation is required. The mother usually is a candidate for treatment of LTBI after the initial postpartum period. The newborn infant needs no special evaluation or therapy. Because the positive TST or IGRA result could be a marker of an unrecognized case of contagious tuberculosis within the household, other household members should have a TST or IGRA and further evaluation, but this should not delay the infant's discharge from the hospital. These mothers can breastfeed their infants.

- *Mother (or household contact) has clinical signs and symptoms or abnormal findings on chest radiograph consistent with tuberculosis disease.* Cases of suspected or proven tuberculosis disease in mothers (or household contacts) should be reported immediately to the local health department, and investigation of all household members should start within 7 days. If the mother has tuberculosis disease, the infant should be evaluated for congenital tuberculosis (see Congenital Tuberculosis), and the mother should be tested for HIV infection. The mother (or household contact) and the infant should be separated until the mother (or household contact) has been evaluated and, if tuberculosis disease is suspected, until the mother (or household contact) and infant are receiving appropriate antituberculosis therapy, the mother wears a mask, and the mother understands and is willing to adhere to infection control measures. Once the infant is receiving isoniazid, separation is not necessary unless the mother (or household contact) has possible MDR tuberculosis disease or has poor adherence to treatment and DOT is not possible. In this circumstance, the infant should be separated from the mother (or household contact), and BCG immunization should be considered for the infant if HIV infection is not present. If the mother is suspected of having MDR tuberculosis disease, an expert in tuberculosis disease treatment should be consulted. Women with tuberculosis disease

who have been treated appropriately for 2 or more weeks and who are not considered contagious can breastfeed.

- If congenital tuberculosis is excluded, isoniazid is given until the infant is 3 or 4 months of age, when a TST should be performed. If the TST result is positive, the infant should be reassessed for tuberculosis disease. If tuberculosis disease is excluded, isoniazid should be continued for a total of 9 months. The infant should be evaluated at monthly intervals during treatment. If the TST result is negative at 3 to 4 months of age and the mother (or household contact) has good adherence and response to treatment and no longer is contagious, isoniazid is discontinued.

- *Mother (or household contact) has abnormal findings on chest radiography but no evidence of tuberculosis disease.* If the chest radiograph of the mother (or household contact) appears abnormal but is not suggestive of tuberculosis disease and the history, physical examination, and sputum smear indicate no evidence of tuberculosis disease, the infant can be assumed to be at low risk of tuberculosis infection and need not be separated from the mother (or household contact). The mother and her infant should receive follow-up care and the mother should be treated for LTBI. Other household members should have a TST or IGRA and further evaluation.

Isolation of the Hospitalized Patient

Most children with tuberculosis disease, especially children younger than 10 years, are not contagious. Exceptions are the following: (1) children with cavitary pulmonary tuberculosis, (2) children with positive sputum AFB smears, (3) children with laryngeal involvement, (4) children with extensive pulmonary infection, or (5) children with congenital tuberculosis undergoing procedures that involve the oropharyngeal airway (eg, endotracheal intubation). In these instances, isolation for tuberculosis or AFB is indicated until effective therapy has been initiated, sputum smears demonstrate a diminishing number of organisms, and cough is abating. Children with no cough and negative sputum AFB smears can be hospitalized in an open ward. Infection control measures for hospital personnel exposed to contagious patients should include the use of personally "fitted" and "sealed" particulate respirators for all patient contacts. The contagious patient should be placed in an airborne infection isolation room in the hospital.

The major concern in infection control relates to adult household members and contacts who can be the source of infection. Visitation should be limited to people who have been evaluated medically. Household members and contacts should be managed with tuberculosis precautions when visiting until they are demonstrated not to have contagious tuberculosis. Nonadherent household contacts should be excluded from hospital visitation until evaluation is complete and tuberculosis disease is excluded or treatment has rendered source cases noncontagious.

Tuberculosis Caused by **M bovis.** Infections with *M bovis* account for approximately 1% to 2% of tuberculosis cases in the United States. Children who come from countries where *M bovis* is prevalent in cattle or whose parents come from those countries are more likely to be infected. Most infections in humans are transmitted from cattle by unpasteurized milk and its products, such as fresh cheese, although human-to-human transmission by the airborne route has been documented. In children, *M bovis* more commonly causes cervical lymphadenitis, intestinal tuberculosis disease, and meningitis. In adults, latent *M bovis* infection can progress to advanced pulmonary disease, with a risk of transmission to others.

An IGRA or TST typically is positive in a person infected with *M bovis*. However, the definitive diagnosis requires a culture isolate. The commonly used methods for identifying *M tuberculosis* complex do not distinguish *M bovis* from *M tuberculosis, M africanum,* and BCG; *M bovis* is identified in clinical laboratories routinely by its resistance to pyrazinamide. This approach can be unreliable, and species confirmation at a reference laboratory should be requested when *M bovis* is suspected. Molecular genotyping through the state health department may assist in identifying *M bovis*. Resistance to first-line drugs in addition to

pyrazinamide has been reported. BCG rarely is isolated from pediatric clinical specimens; however, it should be suspected from the characteristic lesions or localized BCG suppuration or draining lymphadenitis in children who have received BCG vaccine. Only a reference laboratory can distinguish an isolate of BCG from an isolate of *M bovis*.

Therapy for **M bovis** *Disease.* Controlled clinical trials for treatment of *M bovis* disease have not been conducted, and treatment recommendations for *M bovis* disease in adults and children are based on results from treatment trials for *M tuberculosis* disease. Although most strains of *M bovis* are pyrazinamide resistant and resistance to other first-line drugs has been reported, MDR strains are rare. Initial therapy should include 3 or 4 drugs besides pyrazinamide that would be used to treat disease from *M tuberculosis* infection. For isoniazid- and rifampin-susceptible strains, a total treatment course of at least 9 to 12 months is recommended.

Parents should be counseled about the many infectious diseases transmitted by unpasteurized milk and its products, and parents who might import traditional dairy products from countries where *M bovis* infection is prevalent in cattle should be advised against giving those products to their children. When people are exposed to an adult who has pulmonary disease caused by *M bovis* infection, they should be evaluated by the same methods as other contacts to contagious tuberculosis.

Control Measures

Control of tuberculosis disease in the United States requires collaboration between health care professionals and health department personnel, obtaining a thorough history of exposure(s) to people with infectious tuberculosis, timely and effective contact investigations, proper interpretation of TST or IGRA results, and appropriate antituberculosis therapy, including DOT services. A plan to control and prevent extensively drug-resistant tuberculosis has been published. Eliminating ingestion of unpasteurized dairy products will sprevent most *M bovis* infection.

Management of Contacts, Including Epidemiologic Investigation. Children with a positive TST or IGRA result or tuberculosis disease should be the starting point for epidemiologic investigation by the local health department. Close contacts of a TST- or IGRA-positive child should have a TST or IGRA, and people with a positive TST or IGRA result or symptoms consistent with tuberculosis disease should be investigated further. Because children with tuberculosis usually are not contagious unless they have an adult-type multibacillary form of pulmonary or laryngeal disease, their contacts are not likely to be infected unless they also have been in contact with an adult source case. After the presumptive adult source of the child's tuberculosis is identified, other contacts of that adult should be evaluated.

Therapy for Contacts. Children and adolescents exposed to a contagious case of tuberculosis disease should have a TST or IGRA and an evaluation for tuberculosis disease (chest radiography and physical examination). For exposed contacts with impaired immunity (eg, HIV infection) and all contacts younger than 4 years, isoniazid therapy should be initiated, even if the TST result is negative, once tuberculosis disease is excluded (see Therapy for LTBI, pages 577 and 580). Infected people can have a negative TST or IGRA result because a cellular immune response has not yet developed or because of cutaneous anergy. People with a negative TST or IGRA result should be retested 8 to 10 weeks after the last exposure to a source of infection. If the TST or IGRA result still is negative in an immunocompetent person, isoniazid is discontinued. If the contact is immunocompromised and LTBI cannot be excluded, treatment should be continued for 9 months. If a TST or IGRA result of a contact becomes positive, isoniazid should be continued for 9 months.

Child Care and Schools. Children with tuberculosis disease can attend school or child care if they are receiving therapy. They can return to regular activities as soon as effective therapy has been instituted, adherence to therapy has been documented, and clinical symptoms have diminished. Children with LTBI can participate in all activities whether they are receiving treatment or not.

BCG Vaccines. BCG vaccine is a live vaccine originally prepared from attenuated strains of *M bovis*. Use of BCG vaccine is recommended by the Expanded Programme on Immunization of the World Health Organization for administration at birth and is used in more than 100 countries. BCG vaccine is used to reduce the incidence of disseminated and other life-threatening manifestations of tuberculosis in infants and young children. Although BCG immunization appears to decrease the risk of serious complications of tuberculosis disease in children, the various BCG vaccines used throughout the world differ in composition and efficacy.

Two meta-analyses of published clinical trials and case-control studies concerning the efficacy of BCG vaccines concluded that BCG vaccine has relatively high protective efficacy (approximately 80%) against meningeal and miliary tuberculosis in children. The protective efficacy against pulmonary tuberculosis differed significantly among the studies, precluding a specific conclusion. Protection afforded by BCG vaccine in 1 meta-analysis was estimated to be 50%. Two BCG vaccines, one manufactured by Merck/Schering-Plough and the other by Sanofi Pasteur, are licensed in the United States. Comparative evaluations of these and other BCG vaccines have not been performed.

Indications. In the United States, administration of BCG vaccine should be considered only in limited and select circumstances, such as unavoidable risk of exposure to tuberculosis and failure or unfeasibility of other control methods. Recommendations for use of BCG vaccine for control of tuberculosis among children and health care personnel have been published by the Advisory Committee on Immunization Practices of the CDC and the Advisory Council for the Elimination of Tuberculosis. For infants and children, BCG immunization should be considered only for people with a negative TST result who are not infected with HIV in the following circumstances:

- The child is exposed continually to a person or people with contagious pulmonary tuberculosis resistant to isoniazid and rifampin, and the child cannot be removed from this exposure.

- The child is exposed continually to a person or people with untreated or ineffectively treated contagious pulmonary tuberculosis, and the child cannot be removed from such exposure or given antituberculosis therapy.

Careful assessment of the potential risks and benefits of BCG vaccine and consultation with personnel in local tuberculosis control programs are recommended strongly before use of BCG vaccine.

Healthy infants from birth to 2 months of age may be given BCG vaccine without a TST unless congenital infection is suspected; thereafter, BCG vaccine should be given only to children with a negative TST result.

Adverse Reactions. Uncommonly (1%–2% of immunizations), BCG vaccine can result in local adverse reactions, such as subcutaneous abscess and regional lymphadenopathy, which generally are not serious. One rare complication, osteitis affecting the epiphysis of long bones, can occur as long as several years after BCG immunization. Disseminated fatal infection occurs rarely (approximately 2 per 1 million people), primarily in people who are severely immunocompromised. Antituberculosis therapy is recommended to treat osteitis and disseminated disease caused by BCG vaccine. Pyrazinamide is not believed to be effective against BCG and should not be included in treatment regimens. Most experts do not recommend treatment of draining skin lesions or chronic suppurative lymphadenitis caused by BCG vaccine, because spontaneous resolution occurs in most cases.

Large-needle aspiration of suppurative lymph nodes can hasten resolution. People with complications caused by BCG vaccine should be referred for management, if possible, to a tuberculosis expert.

Contraindications. People with burns, skin infections, and primary or secondary immunodeficiencies, including HIV infection, should not receive BCG vaccine. Because an increasing number of cases of localized and disseminated BCG have been described in infants and children with HIV infection, the World Health Organization no longer recommends BCG in healthy, HIV-infected children. Use of BCG vaccine is contraindicated for people receiving immunosuppressive medications, including high-dose corticosteroids. Although no untoward effects of BCG vaccine on the fetus have been observed, immunization during pregnancy is not recommended.

Reporting of Cases. Reporting of suspected and confirmed cases of tuberculosis disease is mandated by law in all states. A diagnosis of LTBI or tuberculosis disease in a child is a sentinel event representing recent transmission of *M tuberculosis* in the community. Physicians should assist local health department personnel in the search for a source case and others infected by the source case. Members of the household, such as relatives, babysitters, au pairs, boarders, domestic workers, and frequent visitors or other adults, such as child care providers and teachers with whom the child has frequent contact, potentially are source cases.

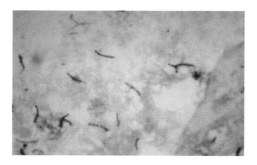

Image 143.1

This photomicrograph reveals *Mycobacterium tuberculosis* bacteria using acid-fast Ziehl-Neelsen stain (magnification x1,000). The acid-fast stains depend on the ability of mycobacteria to retain dye when treated with mineral acid or an acid-alcohol solution such as the Ziehl-Neelsen, or the Kinyoun stains that are carbolfuchsin methods specific for *M tuberculosis*. Courtesy of Centers for Disease Control and Prevention/Dr George P. Kubica.

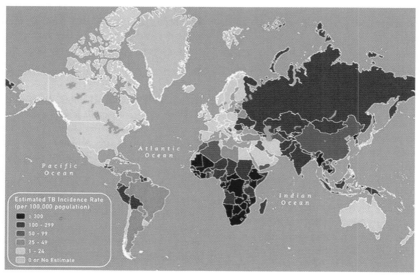

Image 143.2

Estimated tuberculosis incidence rates, 2009. Courtesy of Centers for Disease Control and Prevention.

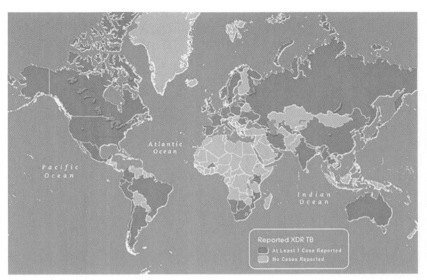

Image 143.3
Distribution of countries and territories reporting at least one case of extensively drug-resistant tuberculosis as of 2010. Courtesy of Centers for Disease Control and Prevention.

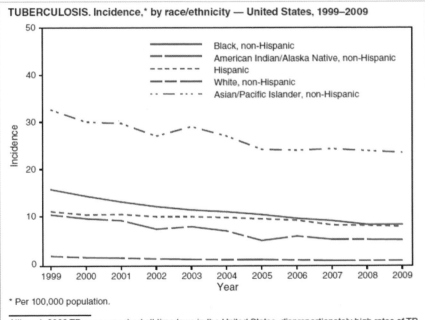

Image 143.4
Tuberculosis. Incidence per year by race/ethnicity—United States, 1999–2009. Courtesy of *Morbidity and Mortality Weekly Report.*

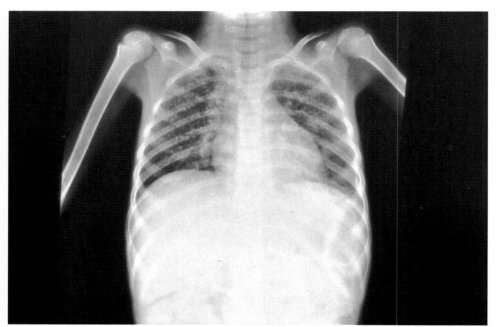

Image 143.5
Miliary tuberculosis. Courtesy of Gary Overturf, MD.

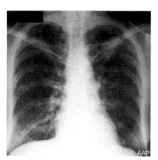

Image 143.6
Tuberculosis, miliary, in a 29-year-old woman 4 months after delivery. Tuberculosis may exacerbate during pregnancy.

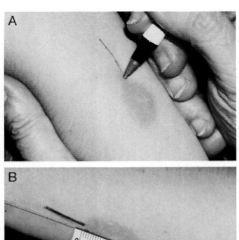

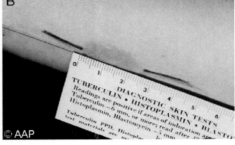

Image 143.7
(A) Interpreting the tuberculin skin test by the Sokol ballpoint pen method involves slowly approaching the site of induration using a ballpoint or felt tip pen in the direction perpendicular to the axis on which the test was placed until resistance is felt. The procedure is repeated on the opposite side. As shown in (B), the distance between the lines where resistance was noted is measured in millimeters. This measures the degree of induration found 48 to 72 hours after application of the test.

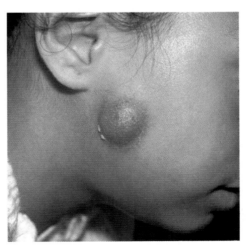

Image 143.8
Young woman with *Mycobacterium tuberculosis* scrofula.
Copyright Martin G. Myers, MD.

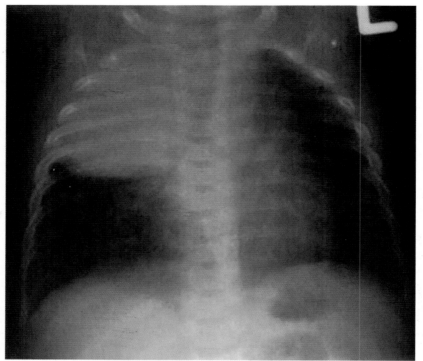

Image 143.9

A 3-month-old infant with tuberculosis. The child had a fever when first examined. Chest radiograph revealed right upper lobe consolidation. A purified protein derivative was placed and was positive. *Mycobacterium tuberculosis* grew from gastric aspirate culture. Copyright Barbara Jantausch, MD, FAAP.

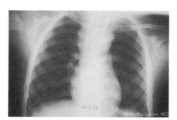

Image 143.10

Mycobacterium tuberculosis infection with paratracheal lymph nodes. Copyright Martha Lepow, MD.

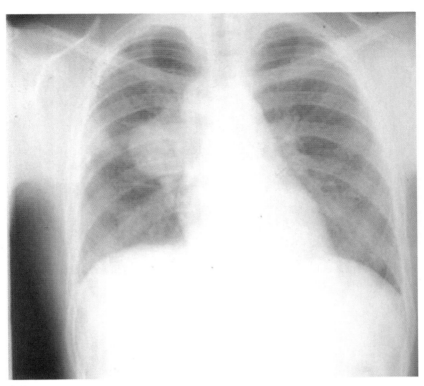

Image 143.11

A 13-year-old male with tuberculosis. The patient had a 1-week history of shortness of breath and sharp pain on his right side while riding his bicycle. A purified protein derivative revealed 20 by 25 mm of induration at 72 hours. The chest computed tomography scan revealed right hilar adenopathy and a primary complex in the right peripheral lung field. Copyright Barbara Jantausch, MD, FAAP.

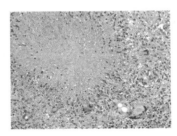

Image 143.12

Tuberculosis. Caseous necrosis and Langhans giant cells in a lymph node. Courtesy of Dimitris P. Agamanolis, MD.

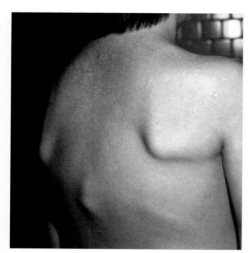

Image 143.13
Tuberculosis of the spine with paravertebral abscess (Pott disease).

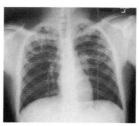

Image 143.14
Cavitary tuberculosis in a 15-year-old male. Copyright Benjamin Estrada, MD.

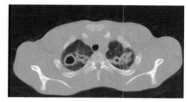

Image 143.15
Cavitary tuberculosis in a 15-year-old male delineated by computed tomography scan. Copyright Benjamin Estrada, MD.

144

Diseases Caused by Non-tuberculous Mycobacteria

(Atypical Mycobacteria, Mycobacteria Other Than *Mycobacterium tuberculosis*)

Clinical Manifestations

Several syndromes are caused by nontuberculous mycobacteria (NTM). In children, the most common of these syndromes is cervical lymphadenitis. Less common syndromes include soft tissue infection, osteomyelitis, otitis media, central line catheter–associated bloodstream infections, and pulmonary infection, especially in adolescents with cystic fibrosis. NTM, especially *Mycobacterium avium* complex (MAC [including *M avium* and *Mycobacterium avium-intracellulare*]) and *Mycobacterium abscessus,* can be recovered from sputum in 10% to 20% of adolescents and young adults with cystic fibrosis and can be associated with fever and declining clinical status. Disseminated infections almost always are associated with impaired cell-mediated immunity, as found in children with congenital immune defects (eg, interleukin-12 deficiency, NF-kappa-B essential modulator mutation and related disorders, and interferon-gamma receptor defects), hematopoietic stem cell transplants, or HIV infection. Disseminated MAC is rare in HIV-infected children during the first year of life. The frequency of disseminated MAC increases with increasing age and declining CD4+ T-lymphocyte counts, typically less than 50 cells/μL, in children older than 6 years. Manifestations of disseminated NTM infections depend on the species and route of infection but include fever, night sweats, weight loss, abdominal pain, fatigue, diarrhea, and anemia. In HIV-infected patients developing immune restoration with initiation of antiretroviral therapy (ART), local MAC symptoms can worsen. This immune reconstitution syndrome usually occurs 2 to 4 weeks after initiation of ART. Symptoms can include worsening fever, swollen lymph nodes, local pain, and laboratory abnormalities.

Etiology

Of the more than 130 species of NTM that have been identified, only a few account for most human infections. The species most commonly infecting children in the United States are MAC, *Mycobacterium fortuitum, M abscessus,* and *Mycobacterium marinum* (Table 144.1). Several new species that can be detected by nucleic acid amplification testing but cannot be grown by routine culture methods have been identified in lymph nodes of children with cervical adenitis. NTM disease in patients with HIV infection usually is caused by MAC.

Table 144.1
Diseases Caused by Nontuberculous *Mycobacterium* Species

Clinical Disease	Common Species	Less Common Species in the United States
Cutaneous infection	*M chelonae, M fortuitum, M abscessus, M marinum*	*M ulcerans*[a]
Lymphadenitis	MAC; *M haemophilum; M lenteflavum*	*M kansasii, M fortuitum, M malmoense*[b]
Otologic infection	*M abscessus*	*M fortuitum*
Pulmonary infection	MAC, *M kansasii, M abscessus*	*M xenopi, M malmoense,*[b] *M szulgai, M fortuitum, M simiae*
Catheter-associated infection	*M chelonae, M fortuitum*	*M abscessus*
Skeletal infection	MAC, *M kansasii, M fortuitum*	*M chelonae, M marinum, M abscessus, M ulcerans*[a]
Disseminated	MAC	*M kansasii, M genavense, M haemophilum, M chelonae*

Abbreviation: MAC, *Mycobacterium avium* complex.
[a]Not endemic in the United States.
[b]Found primarily in Northern Europe.

M fortuitum, Mycobacterium chelonae, and *M abscessus* commonly are referred to as "rapidly growing" mycobacteria, because sufficient growth and identification can be achieved in the laboratory within 3 to 7 days, whereas other NTM and *Mycobacterium tuberculosis* usually require several weeks before sufficient growth occurs for identification. Rapidly growing mycobacteria have been implicated in wound, soft tissue, bone, pulmonary, central venous catheter, and middle-ear infections. Other mycobacterial species that usually are not pathogenic have caused infections in immunocompromised hosts or have been associated with the presence of a foreign body.

Epidemiology

Many NTM species are ubiquitous in nature and are found in soil, food, water, and animals. Tap water is the major reservoir for *Mycobacterium kansasii, Mycobacterium lenteflavum, Mycobacterium xenopi, Mycobacterium simiae,* and health care–associated infections attributable to the rapidly growing mycobacteria *M abscessus* and *M fortuitum.* For *M marinum,* water in a fish tank or aquarium or an injury in saltwater are the major sources of infection. The environmental reservoir for *M abscessus* and MAC causing pulmonary infection is unknown. Although many people are exposed to NTM, it is unknown why some exposures result in acute or chronic infection. Usual portals of entry for NTM infection are believed to be abrasions in the skin (eg, cutaneous lesions caused by *M marinum*), penetrating trauma (needles and organic material most often associated with *M abscessus* and *M fortuitum*), surgical sites (especially for central vascular catheters), oropharyngeal mucosa (the presumed portal of entry for cervical lymphadenitis), gastrointestinal or respiratory tract for disseminated MAC, and respiratory tract (including tympanostomy tubes for otitis media). Pulmonary disease and rare cases of mediastinal adenitis and endobronchial disease do occur. NTM can be an important pathogen in patients with cystic fibrosis. Most infections remain localized at the portal of entry or in regional lymph nodes. Dissemination to distal sites primarily occurs in immunocompromised hosts. No definitive evidence of person-to-person transmission of NTM exists. Outbreaks of otitis media caused by *M abscessus* have been associated with polyethylene ear tubes and use of contaminated equipment or water. Buruli ulcer disease is a skin and bone infection caused by *Mycobacterium ulcerans,* an emerging disease causing significant morbidity and disability in tropical areas such as Africa, Asia, South America, Australia, and the western Pacific.

Incubation Period

Variable.

Diagnostic Tests

Definitive diagnosis of NTM disease requires isolation of the organism. Consultation with the laboratory should occur to ensure that culture specimens are handled correctly. Because these organisms commonly are found in the environment, contamination of cultures or transient colonization can occur. Caution must be exercised in interpretation of cultures obtained from nonsterile sites, such as gastric washing specimens, endoscopy material, a single expectorated sputum sample, or urine specimens and if the species cultured usually is nonpathogenic (eg, *Mycobacterium terrae* complex or *Mycobacterium gordonae*). An acid-fast bacilli smear-positive sample or repeated isolation of a single species on culture media is more likely to indicate disease than are culture contamination or transient colonization. Diagnostic criteria for NTM lung disease in adults include 2 or more separate sputum samples that grow NTM or 1 bronchial alveolar lavage specimen that grows NTM. These criteria have not been validated in children and apply best to MAC, *M kansasii,* and *M abscessus.* Unlike other bacteria, NTM isolates from draining sinus tracts or wounds almost always are significant clinically. Recovery of NTM from sites that usually are sterile, such as cerebrospinal fluid, pleural fluid, bone marrow, blood, lymph node aspirates, middle ear or mastoid aspirates, or surgically excised tissue, is the most reliable diagnostic test. With radiometric or nonradiometric broth techniques, blood cultures are highly sensitive in recovery of disseminated MAC and other bloodborne NTM species. Disseminated MAC disease should prompt a search for underlying immunodeficiency.

Patients with NTM infection, such as *M marinum* or MAC cervical lymphadenitis, can have a positive tuberculin skin test (TST) result because the purified protein derivative preparation derived from *M tuberculosis* shares a number of antigens with NTM species. These TST reactions usually measure less than 10 mm of induration but can measure more than 15 mm. The interferon-gamma release assays use 2 or 3 antigens to detect infection with *M tuberculosis*. Although these antigens are not found on *M avium-intracellulare*, cross-reactions can occur with infection caused by *M kansasii, M marinum,* and *Mycobacterium szulgai.*

Treatment

Many NTM relatively are resistant in vitro to antituberculosis drugs. In vitro resistance to these agents, however, does not necessarily correlate with clinical response, especially with MAC infections. Only limited controlled trials of antituberculous drugs have been performed in patients with NTM infections. The approach to therapy should be directed by the following: (1) the species causing the infection, (2) the results of drug-susceptibility testing, (3) the site(s) of infection, (4) the patient's immune status, and (5) the need to treat a patient presumptively for tuberculosis while awaiting culture reports that subsequently reveal NTM (Table 144.2).

For NTM lymphadenitis in otherwise healthy children, especially when the disease is caused by MAC, complete surgical excision is curative. Antimicrobial therapy has been shown in a randomized, controlled trial to provide no additional benefit. Therapy with clarithromycin or azithromycin combined with ethambutol or rifampin or rifabutin may be beneficial for children in whom surgical excision is incomplete or for children with recurrent disease.

Isolates of rapidly growing mycobacteria (*M fortuitum, M abscessus,* and *M chelonae*) should be tested in vitro against drugs to which they commonly are susceptible and that have been used with some therapeutic success (eg, amikacin, imipenem, sulfamethoxazole or trimethoprim-sulfamethoxazole, cefoxitin, ciprofloxacin, clarithromycin, linezolid, and doxycycline). Clarithromycin and at least one other agent is the treatment of choice for cutaneous (disseminated) infections attributable to *M chelonae* or *M abscessus.* Indwelling foreign bodies should be removed, and surgical debridement for serious localized disease is optimal. The choice of drugs, dosages, and duration should be reviewed with a consultant experienced in the management of NTM infections.

For patients with cystic fibrosis and isolation of MAC species, treatment is suggested only for those with clinical symptoms not attributable to other causes, worsening lung function, and chest radiographic progression. The decision to embark on therapy should take into consideration susceptibility testing results and involve consultation with an expert in cystic fibrosis care. *M abscessus* is difficult to treat, and the role of therapy in clinical benefit is unknown.

In patients with AIDS and in other immunocompromised people with disseminated MAC infection, multidrug therapy is recommended. Clinical isolates of MAC usually are resistant to many of the approved antituberculosis drugs, including isoniazid, but are susceptible to clarithromycin and azithromycin and often are susceptible to combinations of ethambutol, rifabutin or rifampin, and amikacin or streptomycin. Susceptibility testing to these agents has not been standardized and, thus, is not recommended routinely. The optimal regimen is yet to be determined. Treatment of disseminated MAC infection should be undertaken in consultation with an expert.

Table 144.2

Treatment of Nontuberculous Mycobacteria Infections in Children

Organism	Disease	Initial Treatment
Slowly Growing Species		
Mycobacterium avium complex (MAC); *Mycobacterium haemophilum*; *Mycobacterium lentiflavum*	Lymphadenitis	Complete excision of lymph nodes; if excision incomplete or disease recurs, clarithromycin or azithromycin plus ethambutol and/or rifampin (or rifabutin).
	Pulmonary infection	Clarithromycin or azithromycin plus ethambutol with rifampin or rifabutin (pulmonary resection in some patients who fail to respond to drug therapy). For severe disease, an initial course of amikacin or streptomycin often is included. Clinical data in adults support that 3-times-weekly therapy is as effective as daily therapy, with less toxicity for adult patients with mild to moderate disease. For patients with advanced or cavitary disease, drugs should be given daily.
	Disseminated	See page 597.
Mycobacterium kansasii	Pulmonary infection	Rifampin plus ethambutol with isoniazid daily. If rifampin resistance is detected, a 3-drug regimen based on drug susceptibility testing should be used.
	Osteomyelitis	Surgical debridement and prolonged antimicrobial therapy using rifampin plus ethambutol with isoniazid.
Mycobacterium marinum	Cutaneous infection	None, if minor; rifampin, trimethoprim-sulfamethoxazole, clarithromycin, or doxycycline[a] for moderate disease; extensive lesions may require surgical debridement. Susceptibility testing not routinely required.
Mycobacterium ulcerans	Cutaneous and bone infections	Daily intramuscular streptomycin and oral rifampin for 8 weeks; excision to remove necrotic tissue, if present; disability prevention.
Rapidly Growing Species		
Mycobacterium fortuitum group	Cutaneous infection	Initial therapy for serious disease is amikacin plus meropenem, IV, followed by clarithromycin, doxycycline,[a] or trimethoprim-sulfamethoxazole or ciprofloxacin, orally, on the basis of in vitro susceptibility testing; may require surgical excision. Up to 50% of isolates are resistant to cefoxitin.

Table 144.2

Treatment of Nontuberculous Mycobacteria Infections in Children, continued

Organism	Disease	Initial Treatment
Rapidly Growing Species, continued		
Mycobacterium abscessus	Catheter infection	Catheter removal and amikacin plus meropenem, IV; clarithromycin, trimethoprim-sulfamethoxazole, or ciprofloxacin, orally, on the basis of in vitro susceptibility testing.
	Otitis media; cutaneous infection	There is no reliable antimicrobial regimen because of variability in drug susceptibility. Clarithromycin plus initial course of amikacin plus cefoxitin or meropenem; may require surgical debridement on the basis of in vitro susceptibility testing (50% are amikacin resistant).
	Pulmonary infection (in cystic fibrosis)	Serious disease, clarithromycin, amikacin, and cefoxitin or meropenem on the basis of susceptibility testing; may require surgical resection.
Mycobacterium chelonae	Catheter infection	Catheter removal and tobramycin (initially) plus clarithromycin.
	Disseminated cutaneous infection	Tobramycin and meropenem or linezolid (initially) plus clarithromycin.

Abbreviation: IV, intravenously.

ªDoxycycline should not be given to children younger than 8 years unless no other therapeutic options are available. Only 50% of isolates of *M marinum* are susceptible to doxycycline.

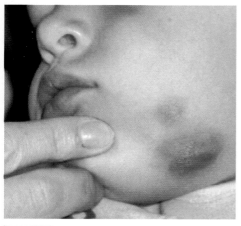

Image 144.1
Atypical mycobacterial tuberculosis (lymphadenitis) with ulceration.

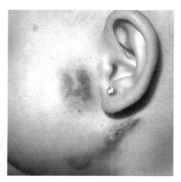

Image 144.2
Atypical mycobacterial lymphadenitis.

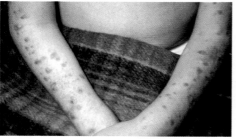

Image 144.3
Disseminated atypical mycobacterial tuberculosis with generalized cutaneous lesions in a boy with acute lymphoblastic leukemia in remission.

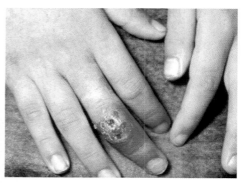

Image 144.4
The same patient as in Image 144.3 with atypical mycobacterial tuberculosis osteomyelitis of the right middle finger.

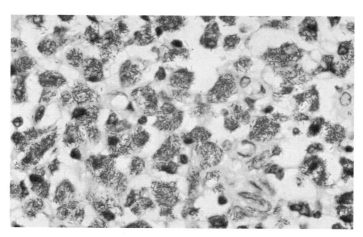

Image 144.5
Mycobacterium avium-intracellulare infection of the lymph node in a patient with AIDS (Ziehl-Neelsen stain). Histopathology of the lymph node shows tremendous numbers of acid-fast bacilli within plump histiocytes. Courtesy of Centers for Disease Control and Prevention/Dr Edwin P. Ewing, Jr.

145

Tularemia

Clinical Manifestations

Most patients with tularemia have abrupt onset of fever, chills, myalgia, and headache. Illness usually conforms to one of several tularemic syndromes. Most common is the **ulceroglandular syndrome,** characterized by a maculopapular lesion at the entry site, with subsequent ulceration and slow healing associated with painful, acutely inflamed regional lymph nodes, which can drain spontaneously. The **glandular syndrome** (regional lymphadenopathy with no ulcer) also is common. Less common disease syndromes are **oculoglandular** (severe conjunctivitis and preauricular lymphadenopathy), **oropharyngeal** (severe exudative stomatitis, pharyngitis, or tonsillitis and cervical lymphadenopathy), **vesicular** skin lesions that can be mistaken for herpes simplex virus or varicella zoster virus, typhoidal (high fever, hepatomegaly, and splenomegaly), **intestinal** (intestinal pain, vomiting, and diarrhea), and **pneumonic.** Pneumonic tularemia, characterized by fever, dry cough, chest pain, and hilar adenopathy, would be the typical syndrome after intentional aerosol release of organisms.

Etiology

Francisella tularensis is a small, weakly staining, gram-negative pleomorphic coccobacillus. Two subspecies cause human infection in North America: *F tularensis* subspecies *tularensis* (type A) and *F tularensis* subspecies *holartica* (type B).

Epidemiology

F tularensis can infect more than 100 animal species; vertebrates considered most important in enzootic cycles are rabbits, hares, and rodents, especially muskrats, voles, and beavers. In the United States, human infection usually is associated with direct contact with one of these species, the bite of an infected domestic cat, or the bite of arthropod vectors ticks and deer flies. Infection has been reported in commercially traded hamsters and in a child bitten by a pet hamster. Infection also can be acquired following ingestion of contaminated water or inadequately cooked meat, inhalation of contaminated aerosols generated during lawn mowing, brush cutting, or piling contaminated hay. At-risk people have occupational or recreational exposure to infected animals or their habitats, such as rabbit hunters and trappers, people exposed to certain ticks or biting insects, and laboratory technicians working with *F tularensis,* which is highly infectious and aerosolized easily when grown in culture. In the United States, most cases occur during June to October. Approximately two-thirds of cases occur in males, and one-quarter of cases occur in children 1 to 14 years of age. Since 2000, when tularemia was redesignated a nationally notifiable disease, there have been 90 to 154 cases reported per year. Organisms can be present in blood during the first 2 weeks of disease and in cutaneous lesions for as long as 1 month if untreated. Person-to-person transmission does not occur.

Incubation Period

Usually 3 to 5 days; range, 1 to 21 days.

Diagnostic Tests

Diagnosis is established most often by serologic testing. Most patients do not develop antibodies until the second week of illness. A single serum antibody titer of 1:128 or greater determined by microagglutination (MA) or of 1:160 or greater determined by tube agglutination (TA) is consistent with recent or past infection and constitutes a presumptive diagnosis. Confirmation by serologic testing requires a fourfold or greater titer change between serum samples obtained at least 2 weeks apart, with 1 of the specimens having a minimum titer of 1:128 or greater by MA or 1:160 or greater by TA. Nonspecific cross-reactions can occur with specimens containing heterophile antibodies or antibodies to *Brucella* species, *Legionella* species, or other gram-negative bacteria. However, cross-reactions rarely result in MA or TA titers that are diagnostic. Some clinical laboratories presumptively can identify *F tularensis* in ulcer exudate or aspirate material by PCR or direct fluorescent antibody (DFA) assays. Immunohistochemical staining is specific for detection of *F tularensis* in fixed tissues; however, this method is not available in most clinical laboratories. Isolation of *F tularensis* from specimens of blood, skin, ulcers, lymph node drainage, gastric washings, or respiratory tract secretions is best achieved by inoculation of cysteine-enriched media. Suspect growth on culture can be identified presumptively by PCR or DFA assays. Because of its propensity for causing laboratory-acquired infections, laboratory personnel should be alerted when *F tularensis* infection is suspected.

Treatment

Streptomycin or gentamicin is recommended for treatment of tularemia. Duration of therapy usually is 10 days. Ciprofloxacin is an alterna-tive for mild disease, but ciprofloxacin is not recommended in patients younger than 18 years. Doxycycline is another alternative agent. Treatment with doxycycline should be continued for at least 14 days because of a higher rate of relapses when compared with other therapies. Suppuration of lymph nodes can occur despite antimicrobial therapy. *F tularensis* is resistant to beta-lactam drugs and carbapenems.

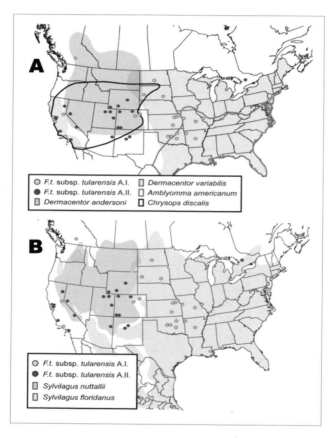

Image 145.1

Spatial distributions of isolates from the AI and AII subpopulations of *Francisella tularensis* subsp *tularensis* relative to (A) distribution of tularemia vectors *Dermacentor variabilis, Dermacentor andersoni, Amblyomma americanum,* and *Chrysops discalis* and (B) distribution of tularemia hosts *Sylvilagus nuttallii* and *Sylvilagus floridanus.* Courtesy of Farlow J, Wagner DM, Dukerich M, et al. *Francisella tularensis* in the United States. *Emerg Infect Dis.* 2005;11(12):1835–1841.

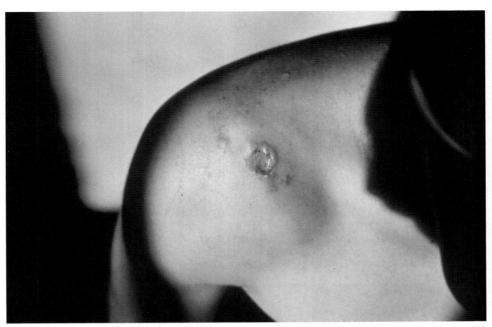

Image 145.2
Tularemia ulcer on the shoulder. Courtesy of Gary Overturf, MD.

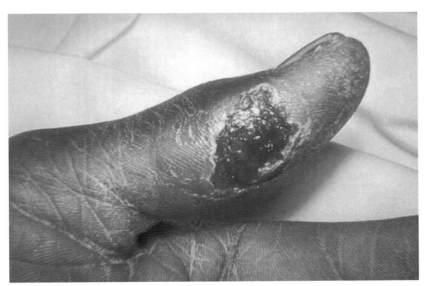

Image 145.3
Tularemia ulcer on the thumb. Irregular ulceration occurred at the site of entry of *Francisella tularensis.* Courtesy of Centers for Disease Control and Prevention/Dr Thomas F. Sellers, Emory University.

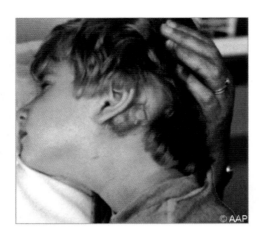

Image 145.4
Tularemia is a relatively rare infection that can manifest with painful cervical adenitis. This boy had a tick bite on his scalp that developed an ulcer followed by a large postauricular node. His tularemia titers were positive and he responded to treatment with gentamicin.

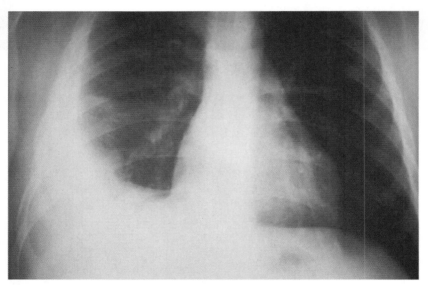

Image 145.5
Tularemia pneumonia. Posterior-anterior chest radiograph showing pneumonia and pleural effusion in the lower lobe of the right lung; the pneumonia was unresponsive to ceftriaxone, azithromycin, and nafcillin. The patient had a history of tick bite and a high fever for 8 days, and his tularemia agglutinin titer was 1:2,048. An outbreak of pneumonic tularemia should prompt consideration of bioterrorism.

146

Endemic Typhus
(Murine Typhus)

Clinical Manifestations

Endemic typhus resembles epidemic (louse-borne) typhus but usually has a less abrupt onset with less severe systemic symptoms. In young children, the disease can be mild. Fever, present in almost all patients, can be accompanied by a persistent, usually severe, headache and myalgia. Nausea and vomiting also develop in approximately half the patients. A rash typically appears on day 4 to 7 of illness, is macular or maculopapular, lasts 4 to 8 days, and tends to remain discrete, with sparse lesions and no hemorrhage. Rash is present in approximately 50% of patients. Illness seldom lasts longer than 2 weeks; visceral involvement is uncommon. Fatal outcome is rare except in untreated severe disease.

Etiology

Endemic typhus is caused by *Rickettsia typhi*.

Epidemiology

Rats, in which infection is unapparent, are the natural reservoirs for *R typhi*. The primary vector for transmission among rats and to humans is the rat flea, *Xenopsylla cheopis*, although other fleas and mites have been implicated. Cat fleas and opossums have been implicated as the source of some cases of endemic typhus caused by *Rickettsia felis*. Infected flea feces are rubbed into broken skin or mucous membranes or inhaled. The disease is worldwide in distribution and tends to occur most commonly in adults, in males, and during the months of April to October; in children, males and females are affected equally. Exposure to rats and their fleas is the major risk factor for infection, although a history of such exposure often is absent. Endemic typhus is rare in the United States, with most cases occurring in southern California, southern Texas, the southeastern Gulf Coast, and Hawaii.

Incubation Period

6 to 14 days.

Diagnostic Tests

Antibody titers determined with *R typhi* antigen by an indirect fluorescent antibody (IFA) assay, enzyme immunoassay, or latex agglutination test peak around 4 weeks after infection, but these test results often are negative up to 10 days after illness onset. A fourfold immunoglobulin (Ig) G titer change between acute and convalescent serum specimens taken 2 to 3 weeks apart is diagnostic. Although more prone to false-positive results, immunoassays demonstrating rises in specific IgM antibody can aid in distinguishing clinical illness from previous exposure if interpreted with a concurrent IgG test; use of IgM assays alone is not recommended. Serologic tests may not differentiate murine typhus from epidemic (louseborne) typhus, *R felis* infection, or infection with spotted fever rickettsiosis such as *R rickettsii* without antibody cross-absorption for IFA or western blotting analyses, which are not available routinely. Routine hospital blood cultures are not suitable for culture of *R typhi*. Molecular diagnostic assays on infected whole blood and skin biopsies can distinguish endemic and epidemic typhus and other rickettsioses and are performed at the Centers for Disease Control and Prevention.

Treatment

Doxycycline is the treatment of choice for endemic typhus, regardless of patient age. Treatment should be continued for at least 3 days after defervescence and evidence of clinical improvement is documented, usually for 7 to 14 days. Fluoroquinolones or chloramphenicol are alternative medications but may not be as effective.

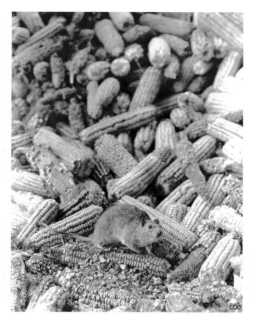

Image 146.1
A Norway rat, *Rattus norvegicus,* in a Kansas City, MO, corn storage bin. *R norvegicus* is known to be a reservoir of bubonic plague (transmitted to man by the bite of a flea or other insect), endemic typhus fever, rat-bite fever, and a few other dreaded diseases. Courtesy of Centers for Disease Control and Prevention.

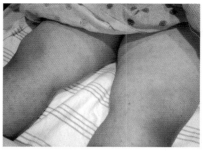

Image 146.2
A healthy 8-year-old boy had 5 days of fever, severe headache, and malaise before this rash began. He had been exposed to numerous cats with fleas before the onset of illness. Courtesy of Carol J. Baker, MD.

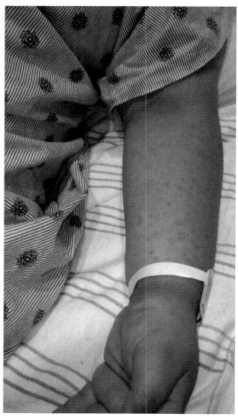

Image 146.3
The same boy who had rash involving palms and soles as well as pancytopenia. He recovered completely with doxycycline therapy. Courtesy of Carol J. Baker, MD.

147

Epidemic Typhus

(Louseborne or Sylvatic Typhus)

Clinical Manifestations

Epidemic louseborne typhus usually is characterized by the abrupt onset of high fever, chills, and myalgia accompanied by severe headache and malaise. A rash appears 4 to 7 days after illness onset, beginning on the trunk and spreading to the limbs. A concentrated eruption can be present in the axillae. The rash typically is maculopapular, becomes petechial or hemorrhagic, and then develops into brownish pigmented areas. The face, palms, and soles usually are not affected. There is no eschar, as often is present in many other rickettsial diseases. Changes in mental status are common, and delirium or coma can occur. Myocardial and renal failure can occur when the disease is severe. The fatality rate in untreated people is as high as 30%. Mortality is less common in children, and the rate increases with advancing age. Untreated patients who recover typically have an illness lasting 2 weeks. Brill-Zinsser disease is a relapse of epidemic louseborne typhus that can occur years after the initial episode. Factors that reactivate the rickettsiae are unknown, but relapse often is more mild and of shorter duration.

Etiology

Epidemic typhus is caused by *Rickettsia prowazekii.*

Epidemiology

Humans are the primary reservoir of the organism, which is transmitted from person to person by the human body louse, *Pediculus humanus corporis.* Infected louse feces are rubbed into broken skin or mucous membranes or inhaled. All ages are affected. Poverty, crowding, poor sanitary conditions, and poor personal hygiene contribute to the spread of body lice and, hence, the disease. Cases of epidemic louseborne typhus are rare in the United States but have occurred throughout the world, including Asia, Africa, some parts of Europe, and Central and South America. Epidemic typhus is most common during winter, when conditions favor person-to-person

transmission of the vector, the body louse. Rickettsiae are present in the blood and tissues of patients during the early febrile phase but are not found in secretions. Direct person-to-person spread of the disease does not occur in the absence of the louse vector. In the United States, sporadic human cases associated with close contact with infected flying squirrels, their nests, or their ectoparasites occasionally are reported in the eastern United States. Flying squirrel–associated disease, called sylvatic typhus, typically presents as a milder illness than body louse transmitted infection. *Amblyomma* ticks in the Americas and in Ethiopia have been shown to carry *R prowazekii,* but their vector potential is unknown.

Incubation Period

1 to 2 weeks.

Diagnostic Tests

R prowazekii can be isolated from acute blood specimens by animal passage or through tissue culture but can be hazardous. Definitive diagnosis requires immunohistochemical visualization of rickettsiae in tissues, isolation of the organism, detection of rickettsial DNA by PCR assay, or a fourfold change in antibody titer between acute and convalescent serum specimens obtained 2 to 3 weeks apart. The indirect fluorescent antibody test is the preferred serologic assay, but enzyme immunoassay and dot immunoassay tests also are available.

Treatment

Doxycycline is the drug of choice to treat epidemic typhus, regardless of patient age. Treatment should be continued for at least 3 days after defervescence and evidence of clinical improvement is documented, usually for 7 to 14 days. Ciprofloxacin is not recommended, because treatment failures have occurred. Chloramphenicol is an alternative drug. To halt the spread of disease to other people, louse-infested patients should be treated with cream or gel pediculicides containing pyrethrins or permethrin; malathion is prescribed most often when pyrethroids fail. In epidemic situations in which antimicrobial agents may be limited (eg, refugee camps), a single dose of doxycycline may provide effective treatment.

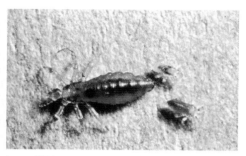

Image 147.1
This image depicts an adult female body louse, *Pediculus humanus,* and 2 larval young, which serve as the vector of epidemic typhus. Courtesy of World Health Organization.

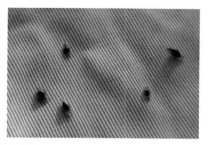

Image 147.2
Human body lice in clothes. Courtesy of Foucault C, Brouqui P, Raoult D. *Bartonella quintana* characteristics and clinical management. *Emerg Infect Dis.* 2006;12(2):217–223.

148

Varicella-Zoster Infections

Clinical Manifestations

Primary infection results in varicella (chickenpox), manifesting as a generalized, pruritic, vesicular rash typically consisting of 250 to 500 lesions in varying stages of development and resolution (crusting), low-grade fever, and other systemic symptoms. Complications include bacterial superinfection of skin lesions, pneumonia, central nervous system involvement (acute cerebellar ataxia, encephalitis), thrombocytopenia, and other rare complications, such as glomerulonephritis, arthritis, and hepatitis. Varicella tends to be more severe in infants, adolescents, and adults than in young children. Breakthrough chickenpox cases usually are mild and clinically modified and occur in immunized children. Reye syndrome can follow cases of chickenpox, although Reye syndrome currently is rare because of decreased use of salicylates during varicella. In immunocompromised children, progressive, severe varicella characterized by continuing eruption of lesions and high fever persisting into the second week of illness as well as encephalitis, hepatitis, and pneumonia can develop. Hemorrhagic varicella is much more common among immunocompromised patients than among immunocompetent hosts. Pneumonia is relatively less common among immunocompetent children but is the most common complication in adults. In children with HIV infection, recurrent varicella or disseminated herpes zoster can develop. Severe and even fatal varicella has been reported in otherwise healthy children receiving intermittent courses of high-dose corticosteroids for treatment of asthma and other illnesses. The risk especially is high when corticosteroids are given during the incubation period for chickenpox.

Varicella-zoster virus (VZV) establishes latency in the dorsal root ganglia during primary infection and/or breakthrough varicella that may develop despite immunization. Reactivation results in herpes zoster (shingles), characterized by grouped vesicular lesions in the distribution of 1 to 3 sensory dermatomes,

sometimes accompanied by pain or itching localized to the area. *Postherpetic neuralgia,* which may last for weeks to months, is defined as pain that persists after resolution of the zoster rash. Zoster occasionally can become disseminated in immunocompromised patients, with lesions appearing outside the primary dermatomes and with visceral complications. Childhood zoster tends to be milder than disease in adults and is less frequently associated with postherpetic neuralgia. The attenuated VZV in the varicella vaccine can also establish latent infection and reactivate as herpes zoster. However, data from immunocompromised children indicate that the risk of developing zoster is lower among vaccine recipients than among children who have experienced natural varicella. Postlicensure data also suggest a lower risk of herpes zoster among healthy vaccinees.

Fetal infection after maternal varicella during the first or early second trimester of pregnancy occasionally results in fetal death or varicella embryopathy, characterized by limb hypoplasia, cutaneous scarring, eye abnormalities, and damage to the central nervous system (congenital varicella syndrome). The incidence of congenital varicella syndrome among infants born to mothers with varicella is approximately 1% to 2% when infection occurs before 20 weeks of gestation. Two cases of congenital varicella syndrome have been reported in infants of women infected after 20 weeks of pregnancy, the latest occurring at 28 weeks. Children exposed to VZV in utero also can develop inapparent varicella and subsequent zoster early in life without having had extrauterine varicella. Varicella infection has a higher case fatality rate in infants when the mother develops varicella from 5 days before to 2 days after delivery, because there is little opportunity for development and transfer of antibody from mother to infant and the infant's cellular immune system is immature. When varicella develops in a mother more than 5 days before delivery and gestational age is 28 weeks or more, the severity of disease in the newborn infant is modified by transplacental transfer of VZV-specific maternal immunoglobulin (Ig) G antibody.

Etiology

VZV (also known as human herpesvirus 3) is a member of the herpesvirus family, the alphaherpes subfamily, and the *Varicellovirus* genus.

Epidemiology

Humans are the only source of infection for this highly contagious virus. Humans are infected when the virus comes in contact with the mucosa of the upper respiratory tract or the conjunctiva. Person-to-person transmission occurs by the airborne route from direct contact with patients with vesicular VZV lesions (varicella and herpes zoster); vesicles contain infectious virus that can be aerosolized. Transmission also can occur from infected respiratory tract secretions. There is no evidence of VZV spread from fomites, because the virus is extremely labile and is unable to survive long periods in the environment. In utero infection occurs as a result of transplacental passage of virus during maternal varicella infection. VZV infection in a household member usually results in infection of almost all susceptible people in that household. Children who acquire their infection at home (secondary family cases) often have more skin lesions than the index case. Health care–associated transmission is well documented in pediatric units, but transmission is rare in newborn nurseries.

In temperate climates in the prevaccine era, varicella was a childhood disease with a marked seasonal distribution, with peak incidence during late winter and early spring. In tropical climates, the epidemiology of varicella is different; acquisition of disease occurs at later ages, resulting in a higher proportion of adults being susceptible to varicella compared with adults in temperate climates. In the prevaccine era, most cases of varicella in the United States occurred in children younger than 10 years. Following implementation of universal immunization in the United States in 1995, varicella disease has declined in all age groups, with evidence of herd protection. The age of peak varicella incidence is shifting from children younger than 10 years of age to children 10 through 14 years, although the incidence in this and all age groups is lower than in the prevaccine era. Immunity generally is lifelong. Cellular immunity is more important than humoral immunity for limiting the extent of primary infection with VZV and for preventing reactivation of virus with herpes zoster. Symptomatic reinfection is uncommon in immunocompetent people; asymptomatic reinfection is more frequent.

Since 2007, coverage with 1 dose of varicella vaccine among 19- through 35-month-old children in the United States has been 90%. As vaccine coverage increases and the incidence of wild-type varicella decreases, a greater proportion of varicella cases are occurring in immunized people as breakthrough disease. This should not be confused as an increasing rate of breakthrough disease or as evidence of increasing vaccine failure. In the surveillance areas with high vaccine coverage, the rate of varicella disease decreased by approximately 90% from 1995 to 2005 with use of varicella vaccine. Since recommendation of a routine second dose of vaccine in 2006, the incidence of childhood varicella has declined further.

Immunocompromised people with primary (varicella) or recurrent (herpes zoster) infection are at increased risk of severe disease. Severe varicella and disseminated zoster are more likely to develop in children with congenital T-lymphocyte defects or AIDS than in people with B-lymphocyte abnormalities. Other groups of pediatric patients who may experience more severe or complicated disease include infants, adolescents, patients with chronic cutaneous or pulmonary disorders, and patients receiving systemic corticosteroids, other immunosuppressive therapy, or long-term salicylate therapy.

Patients are contagious from 1 to 2 days before onset of the rash until all lesions have crusted.

Incubation Period

14 to 16 days (range, 10–21 days) after exposure to rash; 9 to 15 days from onset of rash in a mother to illness in her neonate.

Diagnostic Tests

Diagnostic tests for VZV are summarized in Table 148.1. Vesicular fluid or a scab can be used to identify VZV using a PCR test. This testing also can be used to distinguish between wild-type and vaccine-strain VZV (genotyp-

Table 148.1
Diagnostic Tests for Varicella-Zoster Virus (VZV) Infection

Test	Specimen	Comments
Tissue culture	Vesicular fluid, CSF, biopsy tissue	Distinguishes VZV from HSV. Cost, limited availability, requires up to a week for result.
PCR	Vesicular swabs or scrapings, scabs from crusted lesions, biopsy tissue, CSF	Very sensitive method. Specific for VZV. Real-time methods (not widely available) have been designed that distinguish vaccine strain from wild-type (rapid, within 3 hours).
DFA	Vesicle scraping, swab of lesion base (must include cells)	Specific for VZV. More rapid and more sensitive than culture, less sensitive than PCR.
Tzanck smear	Vesicle scraping, swab of lesion base (must include cells)	Observe multinucleated giant cells with inclusions. Not specific for VZV. Less sensitive and accurate than DFA.
Serology (IgG)	Acute and convalescent serum specimens for IgG	Specific for VZV. Commercial assays generally have low sensitivity to reliably detect vaccine-induced immunity. gpELISA and FAMA are the only IgG methods that can readily detect vaccine seroconversion, but these tests are not commercially available.
Capture IgM	Acute serum specimens for IgM	Specific for VZV. IgM inconsistently detected. Not reliable method for routine confirmation but positive result indicates current/recent VZV activity. Requires special equipment.

Abbreviations: CSF, cerebrospinal fluid; DFA, direct fluorescent antibody; FAMA, fluorescent antibody to membrane antigen (assay); gpELISA, glycoprotein enzyme-linked immunoassay; HSV, herpes simplex virus; IgG, immunoglobulin G; IgM, immunoglobulin M; PCR, polymerase chain reaction.

ing), which may especially be desirable and informative in immunized children who develop herpes zoster. PCR assay currently is the diagnostic method of choice. During the acute phase of the illness, VZV also can be identified by PCR assay of saliva or buccal swabs, from both unimmunized and immunized patients. VZV also can be demonstrated by direct fluorescent antibody (DFA) assay or isolated in cell culture, using scrapings of a vesicle base during the first 3 to 4 days of the eruption. Viral culture and DFA assay both are less sensitive than PCR assay, and neither test has the capacity to distinguish vaccine strain from wild-type viruses. A significant increase in serum varicella IgG antibody between acute and convalescent samples by any standard serologic assay can confirm a diagnosis retrospectively. These antibody tests are reliable for diagnosing natural infection in healthy hosts but may not be reliable in immunocompromised people. Commercially available enzyme immunoassay tests are not sufficiently sensitive to demonstrate reliably a vaccine-induced anti-

body response. IgM tests are not reliable for routine confirmation or excluding acute infection, but positive results indicate current or recent VZV infection or reactivation.

Treatment

The decision to use antiviral therapy and the route and duration of therapy should be determined by specific host factors, extent of infection, and initial response to therapy. Antiviral drugs have a limited window of opportunity to affect the outcome of VZV infection. In immunocompetent hosts, most virus replication has stopped by 72 hours after onset of rash; the duration of replication may be extended in immunocompromised hosts. Oral acyclovir or valacyclovir are not recommended for routine use in otherwise healthy children with varicella. Administration within 24 hours of onset of rash results in only a modest decrease in symptoms. Oral acyclovir or valacyclovir should be considered for otherwise healthy people at increased risk of moderate to severe varicella, such as unvaccinated people older than 12 years, people with chronic cutaneous or pulmonary disorders, people receiving long-term salicylate therapy, and people receiving short, intermittent, or aerosolized courses of corticosteroids. Some experts also recommend use of oral acyclovir or valacyclovir for secondary household cases in which the disease usually is more severe than in the primary case.

Some experts recommend oral acyclovir or valacyclovir for pregnant women with varicella, especially during the second and third trimesters. Intravenous acyclovir is recommended for the pregnant patient with serious complications of varicella.

Intravenous acyclovir therapy is recommended for immunocompromised patients, including patients being treated with chronic corticosteroids. Therapy initiated early in the course of the illness, especially within 24 hours of rash onset, maximizes efficacy. Oral acyclovir should not be used to treat immunocompromised children with varicella because of poor oral bioavailability. Valacyclovir has improved bioavailability compared with oral acyclovir and can be used in selected immunocompromised patients perceived to be at lower risk of developing severe varicella, such as HIV-infected patients with relatively normal concentrations of CD4+ T-lymphocytes and children with leukemia in whom careful follow-up is ensured. Although the antiviral drug famciclovir is available for treatment of VZV infections in adults, its efficacy and safety have not been established for children. Infections caused by acyclovir-resistant VZV strains, which generally are limited to immunocompromised hosts, should be treated with parenteral foscarnet.

Children with varicella should not receive salicylates or salicylate-containing products, because administration of salicylates to such children increases the risk of Reye syndrome. Salicylate therapy should be stopped in a child who is exposed to varicella.

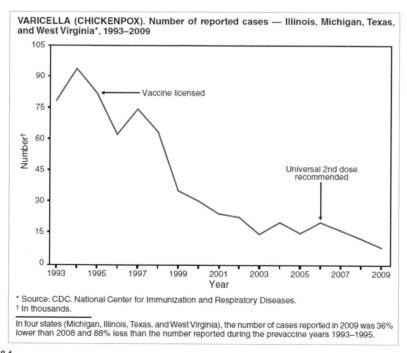

VARICELLA (CHICKENPOX). Number of reported cases — Illinois, Michigan, Texas, and West Virginia*, 1993–2009

* Source: CDC. National Center for Immunization and Respiratory Diseases.
† In thousands.

In four states (Michigan, Illinois, Texas, and West Virginia), the number of cases reported in 2009 was 36% lower than 2008 and 88% less than the number reported during the prevaccine years 1993–1995.

Image 148.1

Varicella (chickenpox). Number of reported cases—IL, MI, TX, WV, 1993–2009. Courtesy of *Morbidity and Mortality Weekly Report*.

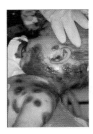

Image 148.2
This newborn has a secondary bacterial infection, which is a complication following infection with varicella (chickenpox). He contracted chickenpox from his infected mother.

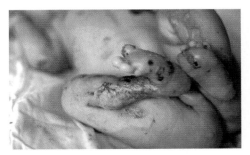

Image 148.3
Congenital varicella with short-limb syndrome and scarring of the skin. The mother had varicella during the first trimester of pregnancy. Copyright David Clark, MD.

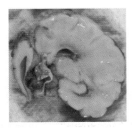

Image 148.4
Varicella embryopathy with involvement of the brain. Atrophy of the left cerebral hemisphere. Courtesy of Dimitris P. Agamanolis, MD.

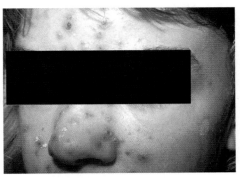

Image 148.5
Adolescent white female with varicella lesions in various stages.

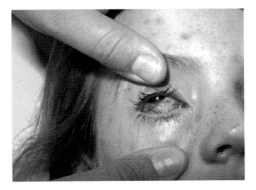

Image 148.6
Varicella with scleral lesions and bulbar conjunctivitis in the same patient as in Image 148.5.

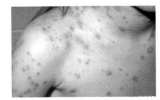

Image 148.7
An adolescent white female with varicella lesions in various stages. This is the same patient as in images 148.5 and 148.6.

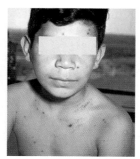

Image 148.8
Varicella with secondary thrombocytopenic purpura.

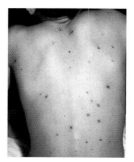

Image 148.9
Varicella with secondary thrombocytopenic purpura in the same Latin American child as in Image 148.8.

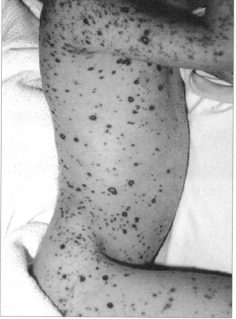

Image 148.10
Hemorrhagic varicella in a 6-year-old white male with eczema.

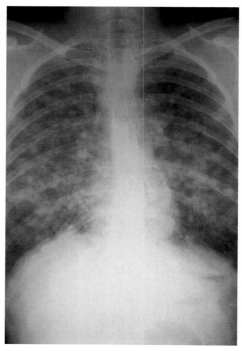

Image 148.11
Diffuse varicella pneumonia bilaterally shown in the chest radiograph of a patient with Hodgkin's disease. Courtesy of George Nankervis, MD.

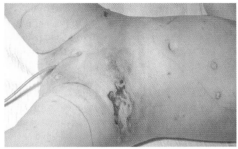

Image 148.12
Varicella complicated by necrotizing fasciitis. A blood culture was positive for group A streptococcus. The disease responded to antibiotics and surgical debridement followed by primary surgical closure.

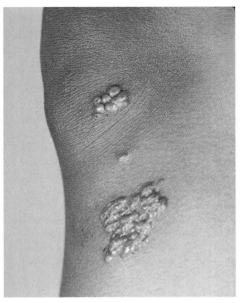

Image 148.13
Herpes zoster in an otherwise healthy child.

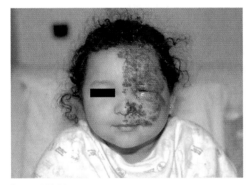

Image 148.14
Varicella zoster in a 7-year-old girl. The patient had an erythematous vesicular skin rash on the face on first examination. The dermatologic distribution suggested the diagnosis of herpes zoster. This image was taken 3 days after acyclovir therapy was initiated. The lesions were crusting. The child had no prior history of recurring infections and was growing well. Copyright Barbara Jantausch, MD, FAAP.

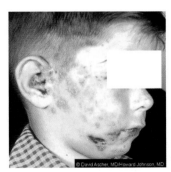

Image 148.15
Herpes zoster. Trigeminal nerve involvement. There may be significant pain associated with lesions in the trigeminal nerve distribution. Copyright David Ascher, MD/Howard Johnson, MD.

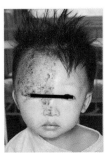

Image 148.16
Herpes zoster (shingles). Courtesy of C. W. Leung.

149

Vibrio cholerae Infections

Clinical Manifestations

Cholera is characterized by painless, voluminous watery diarrhea without abdominal cramps or fever. Severe dehydration, hypokalemia, metabolic acidosis and, occasionally, hypovolemic shock can occur within 4 to 12 hours if fluid losses are not replaced. Coma, seizures, hypoglycemia, and death also can occur, particularly in children. Stools are colorless, with small flecks of mucus ("rice-water") and contain high concentrations of sodium, potassium, chloride, and bicarbonate. Most infected people with toxigenic *Vibrio cholerae* O1 have no symptoms, and some have only mild to moderate diarrhea lasting 3 to 7 days.

Etiology

V cholerae is a gram-negative, curved or comma-shaped rod that is motile. There are more than 200 *V cholerae* serogroups, some of which carry the cholera toxin (CT) gene. Although those serogroups with the CT gene and others without the CT gene can cause acute watery diarrhea, only toxin-producing serogroups O1 and O139 cause epidemic clinical cholera, with O1 causing more than 98% of cases of cholera. There are 3 serotypes of *V cholerae* O1: Inaba, Ogawa, and Hikojima. The 2 biotypes of *V cholerae* are classical and El Tor. El Tor is present globally, and the classical biotype is limited to Bangladesh. Both El Tor and classical biotypes can be further classified into 2 serotypes: Ogawa and Inaba. Since 1992, toxigenic *V cholerae* serogroup O139 has been recognized as a cause of cholera in Asia. Nontoxigenic strains of *V cholerae* O1 and some toxigenic non-O1 serogroups (eg, O141) can cause sporadic diarrheal illness, but they have not caused epidemics.

Epidemiology

Since the early 1800s, there have been 7 cholera pandemics. During the last 5 decades, *V cholerae* O1 biotype El Tor has spread from India and Southeast Asia to Africa, the Middle East, Southern Europe, and the Western Pacific Islands (Oceania). In 1991, epidemic cholera caused by toxigenic *V cholerae* O1, serotype Inaba, biotype El Tor, appeared in Peru and spread to most countries in South, Central, and North America. After causing more than 1 million cases, the cholera epidemic in the Americas largely has subsided, with very few cases reported in the past decade. In the United States, cases resulting from travel to Latin America or Asia or ingestion of contaminated food transported from these regions have been reported. In addition, the Gulf Coast of Louisiana and Texas has an endemic focus of a unique strain of toxigenic *V cholerae* O1. Most cases of disease from this strain have resulted from consumption of raw or undercooked shellfish. In 2010, an outbreak of *V cholerae* serogroup O1, serotype Ogawa, biotype El Tor, began in Haiti.

Humans are the only documented natural host, but free-living *V cholerae* organisms can exist in the aquatic environment. The usual mode of infection is ingestion of large numbers of organisms from contaminated water or food (particularly raw or undercooked shellfish, raw or partially dried fish, or moist grains or vegetables held at ambient temperature). Direct person-to-person spread has not been documented. People with low gastric acidity and with blood group O are at increased risk of severe cholera infection.

Incubation Period

1 to 3 days; range, a few hours to 5 days.

Diagnostic Tests

V cholerae can be cultured from fecal specimens (preferred) or vomitus plated on thiosulfate citrate bile salts sucrose agar. Because most laboratories in the United States do not culture routinely for *V cholerae* or other *Vibrio* organisms, clinicians should request appropriate cultures for clinically suspected cases. Other tests, such as the vibriocidal assay and/or an anticholera toxin enzyme linked immunoassay, can be performed under certain circumstances. Both require the submission of acute and convalescent serum specimens. A fourfold increase in vibriocidal or anticholera toxin antibody titers between acute and convalescent serum can confirm the diagnosis.

Treatment

Oral or parenteral rehydration therapy to correct dehydration and electrolyte abnormalities is the most important therapeutic intervention and should be initiated as soon as the diagnosis is suspected. Oral rehydration is preferred unless the patient is in shock, is obtunded, or has intestinal ileus. The World Health Organization's reduced-osmolality oral rehydration solution (ORS) has been the standard, but data suggest that rice-based ORS or amylase-resistant starch ORS is more effective.

Antimicrobial therapy results in prompt eradication of vibrios, decreases the duration of diarrhea, and decreases fluid losses. Antimicrobial therapy should be considered for people who are moderately to severely ill. Oral doxycycline or azithromycin as a single dose or tetracycline for 3 days is recommended for cholera treatment. If strains are resistant to tetracyclines, then ciprofloxacin, ofloxacin, furazolidone, or trimethoprim-sulfamethoxazole can be used. Antimicrobial susceptibility testing of newly isolated organisms should be performed.

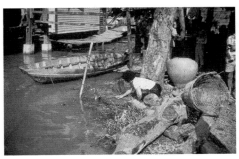

Image 149.1
Typical *Vibrio cholerae*-contaminated water supply. Ingestion of *V cholerae*-contaminated water is a typical mode of pathogen transmission. Courtesy of Centers for Disease Control and Prevention.

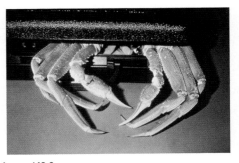

Image 149.2
In 1991, 17 persons in the United States were infected with *Vibrio cholerae* related to travel to Latin America. Of these, only 6 had actually traveled there (ie, 1 to Peru, 1 to Columbia, and 4 to Ecuador). The other 11 were family members in the United States who ate crab brought back from Latin America in the 4 travelers' suitcases. Courtesy of Centers for Disease Control and Prevention.

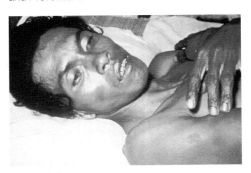

Image 149.3
An adult cholera patient with "washerwoman's hand" sign. Due to severe dehydration, cholera manifests itself in decreased skin turgor, which produces the so-called washerwoman's hand sign. Courtesy of Centers for Disease Control and Prevention.

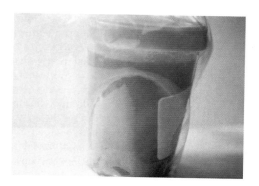

Image 149.4

Here, a cup of typical "rice-water" stool from a cholera patient shows flecks of mucus that have settled to the bottom. These stools are inoffensive, with a faint fishy odor. They are isotonic with plasma and contain high levels of sodium, potassium, and bicarbonate. They also contain extraordinary quantities of *Vibrio cholerae* bacterial organisms. Courtesy of Centers for Disease Control and Prevention.

150

Other Vibrio Infections

Clinical Manifestations

Several nontoxogenic *Vibrio* species (ie, those that do not cause cholera) can cause a variety of clinical syndromes, including gastroenteritis, wound infection, and bacteremia. Gastroenteritis is the most common syndrome and is characterized by acute onset of watery stools and crampy abdominal pain. Approximately half of those afflicted will have low-grade fever, headache, and chills; approximately 30% will have vomiting. Spontaneous recovery follows in 2 to 5 days. Primary septicemia is uncommon but can develop in immunocompromised people with preceding gastroenteritis or wound infection. Wound infections can be severe in people with liver disease or who are immunocompromised. Septicemia and hemorrhagic bullous or necrotic skin lesions can be seen in people with infections caused by *Vibrio vulnificus*, with associated high morbidity and mortality rates.

Etiology

Vibrio organisms are facultatively anaerobic, motile, gram-negative bacilli that are tolerant of salt. The most commonly reported nontoxigenic *Vibrio* species associated with diarrhea are *Vibrio parahaemolyticus* and *Vibrio cholerae* non-O1/non-O139. *V vulnificus* typically causes primary septicemia and severe wound infections; the other species can also cause these syndromes. *Vibrio alginolyticus* typically causes wound infections.

Epidemiology

Non-cholera *Vibrio* species are natural inhabitants of marine and estuarine environments. Most infections occur during summer and fall months when *Vibrio* populations in seawater are highest. Gastroenteritis usually follows ingestion of undercooked seafood, especially oysters, crabs, and shrimp. Wound infections can result from exposure of a preexisting wound to contaminated seawater or from punctures resulting from handling of contaminated shellfish. Exposure to contaminated water during natural disasters such as hurricanes has resulted in wound infections. Transmission of infection person to person has not been reported. People with liver disease, low gastric acidity, and immunodeficiency have increased susceptibility to infection with *Vibrio* species.

Incubation Period

For gastroenteritis, 23 hours; range, 5 to 92 hours; for septicemia, unknown.

Diagnostic Tests

Vibrio organisms can be isolated from stool of patients with gastroenteritis, from blood specimens, and from wound exudates. Because identification of the organism in stool requires special techniques, laboratory personnel should be notified when infection with *Vibrio* species is suspected.

Treatment

Most episodes of diarrhea are mild and self-limited and do not require treatment other than oral rehydration. Antimicrobial therapy can benefit people with severe diarrhea, wound infection, or septicemia. Septicemia with or without hemorrhagic bullae should be treated with a third-generation cephalosporin plus doxycycline. In children younger than 8 years, a combination of trimethoprim-sulfamethoxazole and an aminoglycoside is an alternative regimen. Wound infections require surgical debridement of necrotic tissue, if present.

151

West Nile Virus

Clinical Manifestations

Approximately 80% of human West Nile virus (WNV) infections are asymptomatic. Most symptomatic people experience an acute systemic febrile illness that often includes headache, myalgia, or arthralgia; gastrointestinal tract symptoms and a transient maculopapular rash also are common. Less than 1% of infected people develop neuroinvasive disease, which typically manifests as meningitis, encephalitis, or acute flaccid paralysis. WNV meningitis is indistinguishable clinically from aseptic meningitis caused by most other viruses. Patients with WNV encephalitis usually present with seizures, mental status changes, focal neurologic deficits, or movement disorders. WNV acute flaccid paralysis often is clinically and pathologically identical to poliovirus-associated poliomyelitis, with damage of anterior horn cells, and can progress to respiratory paralysis requiring mechanical ventilation. WNV-associated Guillain-Barré syndrome has also been reported and can be distinguished from WNV poliomyelitis by clinical manifestations and electrophysiologic testing. Cardiac dysrhythmias, myocarditis, rhabdomyolysis, optic neuritis, uveitis, chorioretinitis, orchitis, pancreatitis, and hepatitis have been described rarely after WNV infection.

Routine clinical laboratory results are generally nonspecific in WNV infections. In patients with neuroinvasive disease, cerebrospinal fluid (CSF) examination generally shows lymphocytic pleocytosis, but neutrophils may predominate early in the illness. Brain magnetic resonance imaging frequently is normal, but signal abnormalities may be seen in the basal ganglia, thalamus, and brain stem with WNV encephalitis and in the spinal cord with WNV poliomyelitis.

Most patients with WNV nonneuroinvasive disease or meningitis recover completely, but fatigue, malaise, and weakness can linger for weeks or months. Patients who recover from WNV encephalitis or poliomyelitis often have residual neurologic deficits. Among patients with neuroinvasive disease, the overall case fatality rate is approximately 10% but is significantly higher in WNV encephalitis and poliomyelitis than in WNV meningitis.

Most women known to have been infected with WNV during pregnancy have delivered infants without evidence of infection or clinical abnormalities. In the single known instance of confirmed congenital WNV infection, the mother developed WNV encephalitis during week 27 of gestation, and the infant was born with cystic destruction of cerebral tissue and chorioretinitis. If WNV disease is diagnosed during pregnancy, a detailed examination of the fetus and of the newborn infant should be performed.

Etiology

WNV is an RNA flavivirus which is related antigenically to St Louis encephalitis and Japanese encephalitis viruses.

Epidemiology

WNV is an arthropodborne virus (arbovirus) that is transmitted in an enzootic cycle between mosquitoes and amplifying vertebrate hosts, primarily birds. WNV is transmitted to humans primarily through bites of infected *Culex* mosquitoes. Humans usually do not develop a level or duration of viremia sufficient to infect mosquitoes. Therefore, humans are dead-end hosts. However, person-to-person WNV transmission can occur through blood transfusion and solid organ transplantation. Intrauterine and probable breastfeeding transmission has been described rarely.

WNV transmission has been documented on every continent except Antarctica. Since the 1990s, the largest outbreaks of WNV neuroinvasive disease have occurred in the Middle East, Europe, and North America. WNV first was detected in the Western Hemisphere in New York City in 1999 and subsequently spread across the continental United States and Canada. From 1999 through 2009, 12,208 cases of WNV neuroinvasive disease were reported in the United States, including 481 (4%) cases among children younger than 18 years. Neuroinvasive disease occurs more commonly in people older than 50 years.

In temperate and subtropical regions, most human WNV infections occur in summer or early fall. Although all age groups and both sexes are equally susceptible to WNV infection, the incidence of encephalitis and death are highest among older adults. History of solid organ transplantation, other immuno-compromising conditions, diabetes, and hypertension are other reported risk factors for WNV neuroinvasive disease.

Incubation Period

2 to 6 days; range, 2 to 14 days, and 21 days in immunocompromised people.

Diagnostic Tests

Anti-WNV immunoglobulin (Ig) M antibodies in serum or CSF are the preferred tests for diagnosis of WNV infection. The presence of anti-WNV IgM usually is good evidence of recent WNV infection but can indicate infection with another closely related flavivirus. Because anti-WNV IgM can persist in some patients for longer than 1 year, a positive test result occasionally can reflect past infection. Serum collected within 10 days of illness onset may lack detectable IgM, and the test should be repeated on a convalescent-phase sample. IgG antibody generally is detectable shortly after IgM and persists for years. Plaque-reduction neutralization tests can be performed to measure virus-specific neutralizing antibodies. A fourfold or greater increase in virus-specific neutralizing antibodies between acute- and convalescent-phase serum specimens collected 2 to 3 weeks apart may be used to confirm recent WNV infection and to discriminate between cross-reacting antibodies from closely related flaviviruses.

Viral culture and WNV nucleic acid amplification tests can be performed on acute-phase serum, CSF, or tissue specimens. However, by the time most immunocompetent patients present with clinical symptoms, WNV RNA no longer is detectable; the sensitivity of these tests is likely higher in immunocompromised patients.

WNV disease should be considered in the differential diagnosis of febrile or acute neurologic illnesses associated with recent exposure to mosquitoes, blood transfusion, or solid organ transplantation and of illnesses in neonates whose mothers were infected with WNV during pregnancy or while breastfeeding. In addition to other more common causes of aseptic meningitis and encephalitis (eg, herpes simplex virus and enteroviruses), other arboviruses should also be considered in the differential diagnosis.

Treatment

Management of WNV disease is supportive. Although various therapies have been evaluated or used for WNV disease, none has shown specific benefit thus far.

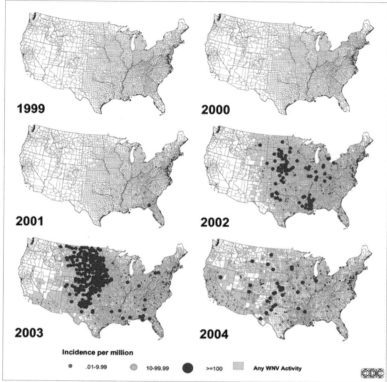

Image 151.1
Reported incidence of neuroinvasive West Nile virus disease by county in the United States, 1999–2004. Reported to Centers for Disease Control and Prevention by states through April 21, 2005. Courtesy of Hayes EB, Komar N, Nasci RS, Montgomery SP, O'Leary DR, Campbell GL. Epidemiology and transmission dynamics of West Nile virus disease. *Emerg Infect Dis.* 2005;11(8):1167–1173.

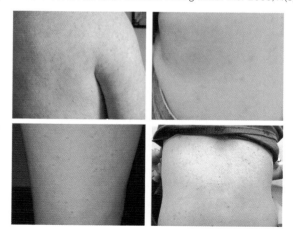

Image 151.2
Four patients with West Nile virus fever and erythematous, maculopapular rashes on the back (top left), flank (top right), posterior thigh (bottom left), and back (bottom right). Courtesy of Ferguson DD, Gershman K, LeBailly A, Petersen LR. Characteristics of the rash associated with West Nile virus fever. *Clin Infect Dis.* 2005;41(8):1204–1207. Reprinted with permission from Oxford University Press.

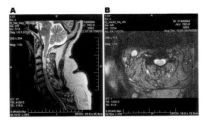

Image 151.3
West Nile virus–associated flaccid paralysis. Saggital (A) and axial (B) T2-weighted magnetic resonance images of the cervical spinal cord in a patient with acute asymmetric upper extremity weakness and subjective dyspnea. (A) Diffuse cervical cord signal abnormality. (B) Abnormal signal in the anterior horn region. Courtesy of Sejvar JJ, Bode AV, Marfin AA, et al. West Nile virus-associated flaccid paralysis. *Emerg Infect Dis.* 2005;11(7):1021–1027.

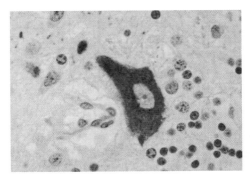

Image 151.4
Staining of West Nile virus antigen in the cytoplasm of a Purkinje cell in the cerebellum (immunohistochemistry, magnification x40). Courtesy of Centers for Disease Control and Prevention.

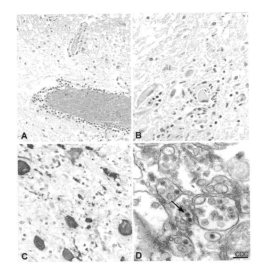

Image 151.5
Histopathologic features of West Nile virus (WNV) in human tissues. Panels A and B show inflammation, microglial nodules, and variable necrosis that occur during WNV encephalitis; panel C shows WNV antigen (red) in neurons and neuronal processes using an immunohistochemical stain; panel D is an electron micrograph of WNV in the endoplasmic reticulum of a nerve cell (arrow) (bar = 100 nm). These 4 images are from a fatal case of WNV infection in a 39-year-old African American female. Courtesy of Hayes EB, Sejvar JJ, Zaki SR, Lanciotti RS, Bode AV, Campbell GL. Virology, pathology, and clinical manifestations of West Nile virus disease. *Emerg Infect Dis.* 2005;11(8):1174–1179.

152

Yersinia enterocolitica and *Yersinia pseudotuberculosis* Infections
(Enteritis and Other Illnesses)

Clinical Manifestations

Yersinia enterocolitica causes several age-specific syndromes and a variety of other less common clinical illnesses. Infection with *Y enterocolitica* typically manifests as fever and diarrhea in young children; stool often contains leukocytes, blood, and mucus. Relapsing disease and, rarely, necrotizing enterocolitis also have been described. In older children and adults, a pseudoappendicitis syndrome (fever, abdominal pain, tenderness in the right lower quadrant of the abdomen, and leukocytosis) predominates. Bacteremia with *Y enterocolitica* most often occurs in children younger than 1 year and in older children with predisposing conditions, such as excessive iron storage (eg, desferrioxamine use, sickle cell disease, and beta-thalassemia) and immunosuppressive states. Focal manifestations of *Y enterocolitica* are uncommon and include pharyngitis, meningitis, osteomyelitis, pyomyositis, conjunctivitis, pneumonia, empyema, endocarditis, acute peritonitis, abscesses of the liver and spleen, and primary cutaneous infection. Postinfectious sequelae with *Y enterocolitica* infection include erythema nodosum, reactive arthritis, and proliferative glomerulonephritis. These sequelae occur most often in older children and adults, particularly people with HLA-B27 antigen.

Major manifestations of *Yersinia pseudotuberculosis* infection are fever, scarlatiniform rash, and abdominal symptoms. Acute pseudoappendiceal abdominal pain is common, resulting from ileocecal mesenteric adenitis, or terminal ileitis. Other findings include diarrhea, erythema nodosum, septicemia, and sterile pleural and joint effusions. Clinical features can mimic those of Kawasaki disease; in Hiroshima, Japan, nearly 10% of children with a diagnosis of Kawasaki disease have serologic or culture evidence of *Y pseudotuberculosis* infection.

Etiology

The genus *Yersinia* consists of 11 species of gram-negative bacilli. *Y enterocolitica*, *Y pseudotuberculosis*, and *Yersinia pestis* are the 3 recognized human pathogens. Fifteen pathogenic O groups of *Y enterocolitica* are recognized. Serotype O:3 now predominates as the most common *Y enterocolitica* type in the United States.

Epidemiology

Y enterocolitica infections are uncommon in the United States. According to the Foodborne Disease Active Surveillance Network, during the years 1996 through 2009, 3.5 laboratory-confirmed infections per 1 million people were reported to surveillance sites. The median age of reported people was 6 years; 30% were hospitalized, and 1% died. Most isolates were recovered from stool. In contrast, the average annual incidence of *Y pseudotuberculosis* was 0.04 cases per 1 million people; the median age was 47 years, 72% were hospitalized, and 11% died. Two-thirds of *Y pseudotuberculosis* isolates were recovered from blood.

The principal reservoir of *Y enterocolitica* is swine; feral *Y pseudotuberculosis* has been isolated from ungulates (deer, elk, goats, sheep, cattle), rodents (rats, squirrels, beaver), rabbits, and many bird species. Infection with *Y enterocolitica* is believed to be transmitted by ingestion of contaminated food (raw or incompletely cooked pork products, tofu, and unpasteurized or inadequately pasteurized milk), by contaminated surface or well water, by direct or indirect contact with animals, by transfusion with contaminated packed red blood cells and, rarely, by person-to-person transmission. Cross-contamination can lead to infection in infants if their caregivers handle raw pork intestines (chitterlings) and do not cleanse their hands adequately before handling the infant or the infant's toys, bottles, or pacifiers. *Y enterocolitica* and *Y pseudotuberculosis* are isolated most often during the cool months of temperate climates.

Incubation Period

4 to 6 days; range, 1 to 14 days.

Diagnostic Tests

Y enterocolitica and *Y pseudotuberculosis* can be recovered from stool, throat swabs, mesenteric lymph nodes, peritoneal fluid, and blood. *Y enterocolitica* also has been isolated from synovial fluid, bile, urine, cerebrospinal fluid, sputum, pleural fluid, and wounds. Stool cultures generally yield bacteria during the first 2 weeks of illness, regardless of the nature of gastrointestinal tract manifestations. Because of the relatively low incidence of *Yersinia* infection in the United States, *Yersinia* organisms are not sought routinely in stool specimens by most laboratories. Consequently, laboratory personnel should be notified when *Yersinia* infection is suspected so that stool can be cultured on suitable media (eg, CIN agar). Characteristic ultrasonographic features demonstrating edema of the wall of the terminal ileum and cecum help to distinguish pseudoappendicitis from appendicitis and can help avoid exploratory surgery.

Treatment

Patients with septicemia or sites of infection other than the gastrointestinal tract and immunocompromised hosts with enterocolitis should receive antimicrobial therapy. Other than decreasing the duration of fecal excretion of *Y enterocolitica* and *Y pseudotuberculosis,* a clinical benefit of antimicrobial therapy for immunocompetent patients with enterocolitis, pseudoappendicitis syndrome, or mesenteric adenitis has not been established. *Y enterocolitica* and *Y pseudotuberculosis* usually are susceptible to trimethoprim-sulfamethoxazole, aminoglycosides, cefotaxime, fluoroquinolones, doxycycline, and chloramphenicol. *Y enterocolitica* isolates usually are resistant to first-generation cephalosporins and most penicillin.

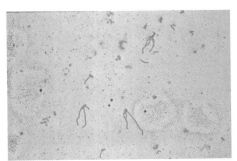

Image 152.1

A photomicrograph of *Yersinia enterocolitica* using flagella staining technique. Symptoms of yersiniosis are fever, abdominal pain, and diarrhea (often bloody), and *Y enterocolitica* is the cause of most *Yersinia*-related illnesses in the United States (mostly in children). Courtesy of Centers for Disease Control and Prevention.

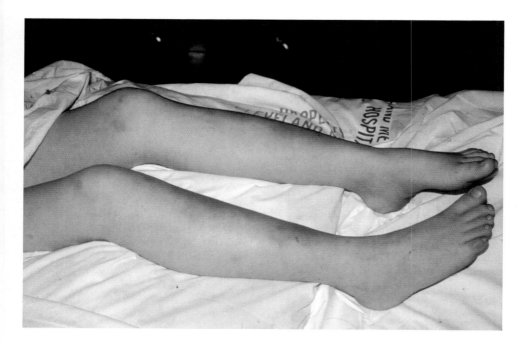

Image 152.2

Multiple erythema nodosum lesions over both lower extremities of a 10-year-old female following a *Yersinia enterocolitica* infection. This immunoreactive complication may also occur in association with *Campylobacter jejuni* infections, tuberculosis, leprosy, coccidioidomycosis, histoplasmosis, and other infectious diseases. Courtesy of George Nankervis, MD.

Index

Page numbers followed by *f* indicate a figure.
Page numbers followed by *i* indicate an image.
Page numbers followed by *t* indicate a table.

A

Abdominal abscess
  from *Bacteroides* infection, 47
  from *Prevotella* infection, 47
Abdominal actinomycosis, 1
Abdominal cramps
  from *Bacillus cereus,* 43
  from *Clostridium difficile,* 99
  from cryptosporidiosis, 116
  from cyclosporiasis, 122
  from human calicivirus infections, 65
  from microsporidia infections, 312
  from *Salmonella* infections, 426
  from *Shigella* infections, 440
Abdominal discomfort
  from *Balantidium coli* infection, 49
  from *Clostridium difficile,* 99
  from trichinellosis, 553
  from *Yersinia pseudotuberculosis* infection, 624
Abdominal distention
  from *Escherichia coli,* 151
  from *Giardia intestinalis* infections, 163
Abdominal pain
  from anthrax, 17
  from astrovirus infections, 38
  from babesiosis, 40
  from *Blastocystis hominis* infections, 54
  from brucellosis, 60
  from *Campylobacter* infections, 67
  from cystoisosporiasis, 253
  from dengue, 130
  from enterovirus infections, 142
  from *Escherichia coli* diarrhea, 155
  from *Giardia intestinalis* infections, 163
  from hemorrhagic fever, 186
  from hemorrhagic fever with renal syndrome, 188
  from hepatitis E, 204
  from hookworm infections, 220
  from influenza, 246
  from isosporiasis, 253
  from malaria, 294
  from nontuberculous mycobacteria, 595
  from Q fever, 399
  from Rocky Mountain spotted fever, 415
  from schistosomiasis, 436
  from smallpox, 443
  from *Strongyloides,* 498
  from tapeworm infections, 521
  from *Trichomonas vaginalis* infections, 557
  from trichuriasis, 560
  from tuberculosis, 567
Abortion
  lymphocytic choriomeningitis and, 292
  mumps and, 316
  syphilis and, 502

Abscesses
  abdominal
    from actinomycosis, 1
    from *Bacteroides* infection, 47
    from *Prevotella* infection, 47
  actinomycotic, 2i
  from *Bacteroides* infection, 47
  from blastomycosis, 56
  brain
    from *Arcanobacterium haemolyticum* infections, 29
    from *Bacillus cereus,* 43
    from *Bacteroides* infection, 47
    from *Escherichia coli,* 151
    from Lemierre disease, 160
    from melioidosis from *Burkholderia pseudomallei,* 62
    from *Prevotella* infection, 47
  hepatic, from *Pasteurella* infections, 357
  intra-abdominal, from non–group A or B streptococcal and enterococcal infections, 493
  liver, 10i
    from amebiasis, 7
    from *Yersinia enterocolitica,* 624
  lung
    from *Bacteroides* infection, 47
    from *Burkholderia* infections, 62
    from nocardiosis, 326
    from *Prevotella* infection, 47
  orbital, 462i
  from paracoccidioidomycosis, 336
  paravertebral, 594i
  peritonsillar
    from *Arcanobacterium haemolyticum* infections, 29
    from *Bacteroides* infection, 47
    from group A streptococcal infections, 473
    from *Prevotella* infection, 47
  from *Prevotella* infection, 47
  prostatic, from melioidosis from *Burkholderia pseudomallei,* 62
  pulmonary, from *Pasteurella* infections, 357
  from rat-bite fever, 406
  retropharyngeal, from group A streptococcal infections, 473
  scalp
    from staphylococcal infections, 450
    from tinea capitis, 530
  spleen, from *Yersinia enterocolitica,* 624
Acalculous cholecystitis from Q fever, 399
Acanthamoeba species, 12
Acid-fast bacillus (AFB), 570
  smear for nontuberculous mycobacteria, 596
Acid-fast staining for cyclosporiasis, 122
Acidosis from rotavirus infections, 418
Acid-Schiff stain for microsporidia infections, 312
Acquired immunodeficiency syndrome (AIDS) from *Cryptococcus neoformans* infections, 113
Acquired syphilis, 501
  follow-up and management of, 506
  primary stage, 501
  secondary stage, 501
Actinobacillus actinomycetemcomitans, 2i
Actinomyces israelii, 1, 2i, 326

Vibrio cholerae infections (cholera), continued
tetracycline for, 617
treatment of, 617
trimethoprim-sulfamethoxazole for, 617
Vibriocidal antibody titers for *Vibrio cholerae* infections, 616
Vibrio infections, 619
aminoglycosides for, 619
antimicrobial therapy for, 619
cephalosporins for, 619
clinical manifestations of, 619
diagnostic tests for, 619
doxycycline for, 619
epidemiology of, 619
etiology of, 619
incubation period of, 619
treatment of, 619
trimethoprim-sulfamethoxazole for, 619
Vibrio parahaemolyticus, 619
Vibrio vulnificus, 619
Vincent stomatitis, 162*i*
Viral antigen
in nasopharyngeal specimens for respiratory syncytial virus, 410
for parainfluenza virus infections, 342
Viral cultures for West Nile virus, 621
Viral gastroenteritis from *Campylobacter* infections, 67
Viral meningitis from poliovirus infections, 392
Viral nucleic acid
for hemorrhagic fever, 187
for human papillomaviruses, 332
Viral shedding
from influenza, 247
in respiratory syncytial virus, 410
Viridans streptococci from non–group A or B streptococcal and enterococcal infections, 493
Visceral leishmaniasis, 265, 266
Visual impairment from tapeworm diseases, 516
Vitamin A supplementation for measles, 301
Vitamin B_{12} deficiency from tapeworm infections, 521
Vitiligo, pityriasis versicolor and, 373
Vittaforma, 312
Vomiting. *See also* Nausea
from anthrax, 17
from astrovirus infections, 38
from babesiosis, 40
from *Bacillus cereus,* 43
from *Balantidium coli* infection, 49
from *Clostridium perfringens* food poisoning, 101
from cryptosporidiosis, 116
from cyclosporiasis, 122
from cystoisosporiasis, 253
from dengue, 130
from *Ehrlichia* and *Anaplasma* infections, 137
from enterovirus infections, 142
from *Escherichia coli,* 151
from hantavirus pulmonary syndrome, 179
from *Helicobacter pylori* infections, 184
from hookworm infections, 220
from influenza, 246
from isosporiasis, 253
from leptospirosis, 273
from malaria, 294
from pertussis, 365
from Q fever, 399
from rat-bite fever, 406
from rickettsialpox, 413
from Rocky Mountain spotted fever, 415
from rotavirus infections, 418
from smallpox, 443
from *Strongyloides,* 498
from trichinellosis, 553
Vulvitis from bacterial vaginosis, 45
Vulvovaginal burning from *Trichomonas vaginalis* infections, 557
Vulvovaginal candidiasis, treatment for, 71
Vulvovaginal infections
from *Bacteroides* infection, 47
from *Prevotella* infection, 47
Vulvovaginal itching from *Trichomonas vaginalis* infections, 557

W

Warts, 331
anogenital, 331
cutaneous, 331
cutaneous nongenital, 331
filiform, 331
flat, 331
nongenital, 332
plantar, 331, 332
skin, 331
thread-like, 331
tretinoin for, 333
Washer woman's hand, 617*i*
Water contamination as cause of *Escherichia coli* diarrhea, 155–156
Wayson stain for plague, 376
Weakness
from brucellosis, 60
from Q fever, 399
from West Nile virus, 620
Weight loss
from African trypanosomiasis, 561
from babesiosis, 40
from brucellosis, 60
from cryptosporidiosis, 116
from cyclosporiasis, 122
from cystoisosporiasis, 253
from histoplasmosis, 216
from isosporiasis, 253
from leishmaniasis, 265
from nontuberculous mycobacteria, 595
from paracoccidioidomycosis, 336
from tuberculosis, 567
Weil syndrome from leptospirosis, 273
West African infection, 561
Western blot assays
for hantavirus pulmonary syndrome, 180
for human herpesvirus 8, 229
Western blot serologic antibody test for paragonimiasis, 339
Western equine encephalitis virus, disease caused by arboviruses in Western hemisphere, 24*t*
West Nile encephalitis virus, 24*t*